CRITICAL CARE INFECTIOUS DISEASES TEXTBOOK

CRITICAL CARE INFECTIOUS DISEASES TEXTBOOK

Edited by

Jordi Rello, M.D., Ph.D.

HOSPITAL UNIVERSITARI JOAN XXIII.
AND
UNIVERSITY ROVIRA & VIRGILI
TARRAGONA, SPAIN

Jordi Valles, M.D., Ph.D.

CORPORACIO SANITARIA PARC TAULI,
SABADELL, BARCELONA, SPAIN

Marin H. Kollef, M.D.

WASHINGTON UNIVERSITY SCHOOL OF MEDICINE
AND
BARNES-JEWISH HOSPITAL
ST LOUIS, MISSOURI, USA

Springer-Science+Business Media, B.V.

Library of Congress Cataloging-in-Publication Data
Critical care infectious diseases textbook / edited by Jordi Rello, Jordi Valles, Marin H. Kollef.
p. ; cm.
Includes bibliographical references and index.
ISBN 978-1-4613-5674-5 ISBN 978-1-4615-1679-8 (eBook)
DOI 10.1007/978-1-4615-1679-8
1. Communicable diseases. 2. Critical care medicine. 3. Intensive care units. 4. Nosocomial infections. 5. Opportunistic infections. I. Rello, Jordi. II. Valles, Jordi, 1953– III. Kollef, Marin H.
[DNLM: 1. Cross Infection – therapy. 2. Anti-Infective Agents – therapeutic use. 3. Community-Acquired Infections – therapy. 4. Critical Care – methods. 5. Infection Control – methods. 6. Intensive Care Units. WX 167 C934 2001]
RC112 .C75 2001
616.9 – dc21

00-066407

Originally published by Kluwer Academic Publisher in 2001
Softcover reprint of the hardcover 1st edition 2001

Printed on acid-free paper.

CONTENTS

PREFACE

Infections and their complications are a very important clinical area in the intensive care unit setting. Community-acquired infections and nosocomial infections both contribute to the high level of disease acquity common among critically ill patients. The importance of accurately diagnosing nosocomial infections and providing appropriate therapies, to include antimicrobial therapy effective against the identified agents of infection, have been shown to be important determinants of patient outcome. Critical care practitioners are in a unique position in dealing with infectious diseases. They are often the initial providers of care to seriously ill patients with infections. Additionally, they have a responsibility to ensure that nosocomial infections are prevented and that antimicrobial resistance is minimized by prudently employing antibiotic agents. It is our hope that this textbook will provide clinicians practicing in the intensive care unit a reference to help guide their care of infected patients. To that end we have brought together a group of international authors to address important topics related to infectious diseases for the critical care practitioner.

Jordi Rello, M.D., Ph.D.
Jordi Valles, M.D., Ph.D.
Marin H. Kollef, M.D.

SECTION 5: BLOODSTREAM INFECTIONS

J. Valles

31. NOSOCOMIAL BLOODSTREAM INFECTION IN THE ICU

Jordi Vallés

Introduction

Nosocomial infections occur in 5%–10% of patients admitted to hospitals in the Unites States [1]. The endemic rates of nosocomial infections vary markedly between hospitals and between areas of the same hospital. Patients in intensive care units (ICUs), representing 8% to 15% of hospital admissions, suffer a disproportionately high percentage of nosocomial infections compared with patients in non-critical care areas [2–7]. Wenzel *et al.* [3] reported that patients admitted to ICUs account for 45% of all nosocomial pneumonias and bloodstream infections, although the critical-care units comprise only 5% to 10% of all hospital beds. Severity of underlying disease, invasive diagnostic and therapeutic procedures, contaminated life-support equipment, and the prevalence of resistant microorganisms are critical factors in the high rate of infection in the ICUs [8].

Donowitz *et al.* [5] reported a three-fold increase in the risk of nosocomial infection for ICU patients when compared with ward patients (18% *versus* 6%; $p < 0.001$); and bloodstream infections were 7.4 times as likely to occur in ICU patients as in ward patients, with an infection rate in the ICU of 5.2 episodes per 100 admissions compared with 0.7 episodes per 100 admissions in a general ward ($p < 0.001$). Trilla *et al.* [9], in a study of the risk factors for nosocomial bloodstream infection in a large Spanish university hospital found that among other variables, the admission to an ICU was linked with a marked increase in the risk of nosocomial bloodstream infection (OR = 2.37; CI 95%: 1.67 to 3.38; $p = 0.02$).

The aim of this chapter is to discuss the clinical importance of bloodstream infection in the ICU, and the current epidemiology, microbiology, systemic response, risk factors and prognosis of ICU-acquired nosocomial bloodstream infections.

Pathophysiology of Bloodstream Infection

Invasion of the blood by microorganisms usually occurs via one of two mechanisms: drainage from the primary focus of infection via the lymphatic system to the vascular system, or direct entry from needles (e.g., in intravenous drug users) or other contaminated intravascular devices such as catheters or graft material. The presence of bloodstream infection represents either the failure of an individual's host defenses to localize an infection at its primary site or the failure of a physician to remove, drain, or otherwise sterilize that focus. Ordinarily, host defenses respond promptly to a sudden influx of microorganisms, particularly by efficient phagocytosis by macrophages or the mononuclear phagocytic system that help clear the blood within minutes to hours. Clearance may be less efficient when microorganisms are encapsulated, or it may be enhanced if the host has antibodies specific for the infecting organism. Clearance of the bloodstream is not always successful. Examples of this problem are bloodstream infections associated with intravascular foci and endovascular infections and episodes that occur in individuals whose host defense mechanisms either are too impaired to respond efficiently or are simply overwhelmed [10].

For that reason, the presence of living microorganisms in blood is of substantial clinical importance; it is an indicator of disseminated infection and, as such, generally indicates a poorer prognosis than that associated with localized disease.

Definitions

Nosocomial bloodstream infection in the ICU is defined in a patient with a clinically significant blood culture positive for a bacterium or fungus that is obtained more than 72 hours after admission in the ICU or previously, if it is directly related to a invasive manipulation on admission in the ICU (e.g., urinary catheterization or insertion of intravenous line). When a culture is unexpectedly positive (in the absence of signs or symptoms) or when only one of several cultures is positive for a microorganism, it can often be dismissed as a contaminant. Every positive blood culture, however, should be carefully evaluated before being dismissed as insignificant [11].

Nosocomial bloodstream infections may be classified as primary or secondary according to the source of the infection [12]. Primary bloodstream infection occurs without any recognizable focus of infection with the same organism at another site at the time of positive blood culture, and secondary bloodstream infections are infections that developed subsequent to a documented infection with the same microorganism at another site. Episodes secondary to intravenous or arterial lines have traditionally been classified as primary bloodstream infections; however, if local infection (defined as redness, tenderness, and pus) is present at the site of an intravascular line, and if the semiquantitative (yielding > 15 colonies) or quantitative culture of a segment catheter is positive to the same strain as in the blood cultures, they may be classified as secondary bloodstream infections. According to this definition, in the absence of an identified source, primary bloodstream infections should be designated bloodstream infections of unknown origin [13–15].

According to clinical patterns of bloodstream infection, it may also be useful to categorize bloodstream infection as transient, intermittent, or continuous [10]. Transient bloodstream infection, lasting minutes to hours, is the most common and occurs after manipulation of infected tissues (e.g., abscesses); during certain surgical procedures; when procedures are undertaken that involve contaminated or colonized mucosal surfaces (e.g., gastrointestinal endoscopy); and, predictably, at the onset of acute bacterial infections such as pneumonia, meningitis, and complicated urinary infections. Intermittent bloodstream infection is that which occurs, clears, and then recurs in the same patient due to the same microorganism. Classically, this type of bloodstream infection is associated with undrained closed space infections, such as intrabdominal abscesses. Continuous bloodstream infection is characteristic of infective endocarditis as well as other endovascular infections such as arterial graft infections, and suppurative thrombophlebitis associated with intravenous line infections commonly seen in critically ill patients.

Bloodstream infections may also be categorized as unimicrobial or polymicrobial depending of the number of microoganisms isolated during a single bacteremic episode.

Blood cultures which are found to be positive in the laboratory but which do not truly reflect bloodstream infection in the patient have been termed contaminant bloodstream infections or, more recently, pseudobloodstream infections [11]. Several techniques are available to assist the clinician and microbiologist in interpreting the clinical importance of a positive blood culture. The categorical decision to consider the bloodstream infection as true-infection or a contaminant should take into account, at least: the patient's clinical history, physical findings, body temperature at the time of the blood culture, leukocyte count and differential cell counts, the identity of microorganism isolated and the result of cultures of specimens from other sites. Indeed, the type of microorganism isolated may have some predictive value: common blood isolates that always or nearly always (>90%) represent true infection include *S. aureus*, *E. coli* and other members of the *Enterobacteriaceae*, *Pseudomonas aeruginosa*, *Streptococcus pneumoniae*, and *Candida albicans*. Other microoganisms such as *Corynebacterium* spp., *Bacillus* spp., and *Propionibacterium acnes* rarely (<5%) represent true bloodstream infection. More problematic are the viridans group streptococci that represent true bloodstream infection in 38% of cases, enterococci in 78%, and coagulase-negative staphylococci (CNS) in 15% [16, 17].

The number of positive blood cultures out of the total number performed is frequently used to determine the clinical significance of the isolate, but recent data suggest that this technique is flawed. Mirret *et al.* [18] examined the significance of CNS in blood cultures. For conventional two-bottle culture sets, 49% of those classified as significant infections and 68% classified as contaminants grew in one bottle, whereas 51% of pathogens and 68% of contaminants grew in both bottles. The degree of overlap is so great that it is difficult to predict the clinical significance based on the number of positive bottles. It is important to note that although CNS have frequently been considered as contaminants in the past, recent studies have shown that even a single blood-culture positive for these microorganisms is frequently associated with clinically relevant episodes of bloodstream infections [19–21].

Epidemiology

Nosocomial infection in ICU patients is a frequent event with potentially lethal consequences. Because patients in ICUs are severely ill and undergo invasive procedures, they suffer a disproportionate percentage of nosocomial infections [5, 7, 22–24]. Compared with patients in general medical/surgical wards, who have been found to have an overall risk of 6% of acquiring an infection during their hospital stay, the risk in critically ill patients in the ICU is around 18% [5]. The nosocomial infection rates among ICU patients are as much as 5–10 times higher than those recorded for patients admitted to other wards, meaning that nearly 25% of all hospital-acquired infections occur in ICU patients [25]. Nosocomial infections are more common in ICUs because of the severity of the underlying disease, the duration of hospital stay, the use of invasive procedures, contaminated life-support equipment, and the prevalence of multiply resistant microorganisms. Data from the European Prevalence of Infection in Intensive Care study (EPIC) collected in 1992 shows that on the day of study a total of 21% of patients admitted to the ICU had an infection acquired in the ICU [26].

Patients in the ICU not only have a higher endemic rates of nosocomial infection than patients in general wards, but the distribution of their nosocomial infections also differs. The two most important nosocomial infections in general wards are urinary tract infections and surgical wound infections, whereas in the ICU lower respiratory tract and bloodstream infections are the most frequent [25] (Figure 1). This distribution is related to the widespread use of mechanical ventilation and intravenous catheters. Recent data compiled through the National Nosocomial Infections Surveillance System (NNIS) of the Centers for Disease Control and Prevention between 1992–1997 in the USA revealed that bloodstream infections accounted for almost 20% of nosocomial infections in ICU patients, 87% of which were associated with a central line [27].

Despite the higher incidence of nosocomial bloodstream infection in ICUs, few studies have adequately analyzed this infection in this selected population. The studies conducted in critically ill patients in recent years show that the incidence rate of nosocomial bloodstream infection in the ICU ranges from 27 to 67

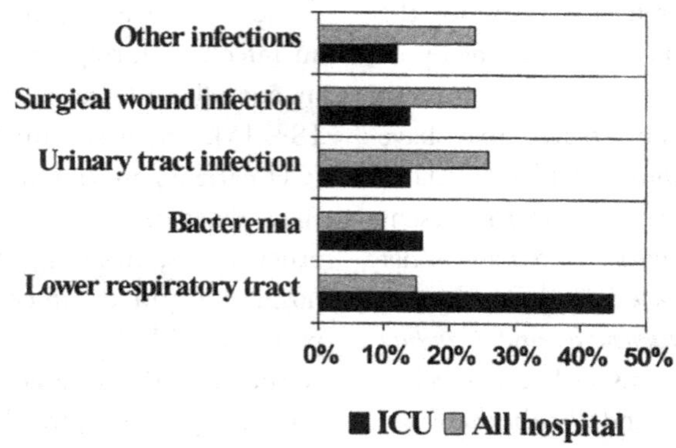

FIGURE 1. Distribution of nosocomial infections in the ICU versus the whole hospital (NNIS). (From [25], with permission.)

episodes per 1000 admissions [14, 15, 28, 29] (Table 1), depending on the type of ICU (surgical or medical or coronary care unit), the severity of patients, the use of invasive devices and the length of ICU stay. These infection rates among ICU patients are as much as 5–10 times higher than those recorded for patients admitted to general wards.

Microbiology

The spectrum of microorganisms that invade the bloodstream in patients with nosocomial infections during their stay in the ICU has been evaluated in several recent studies. Although almost any microorganism can produce bloodstream infection, staphylococci and Gram-negative bacilli account for the vast majority of cases. However, among the staphylococci, CNS has recently become a clinically significant agent of bloodstream infection in the ICU [14–17]. The ascendance of this group of staphylococci has increased the interpretative difficulties for clinicians, since a high number of CNS isolations represent contamination rather than true bloodstream infection. The increased importance of CNS bloodstream infection seems to be related to the high incidence of utilization of multiple invasive devices in critically ill patients and to the multiple antimicrobial therapy used for Gram-negative infections in ICU patients, which results in selection of Gram-positive microorganisms. The change in the spectrum of organisms causing nosocomial bloodstream infection in an adult ICU is confirmed in the recent study by Edgeworth *et al.* [30], which

TABLE 1. Rates of nosocomial bloodstream infection in the ICU

Year	Type of ICU	Episodes of nosocomial bloodstream infection per 1000 admissions	Reference
1993	Medical-surgical ICU	67.2	Rello
1994	Surgical ICU	26.7	Pittet
1996	Adult ICUs Multicenter study	41	Brun-Buisson
1997	Adult ICUs Multicenter study	36	Vallés

analyzed the evolution of nosocomial bloodstream infection over 25 years in the same ICU. Between 1971 and 1990, the frequency of isolation of individual organisms changed little, with *S. aureus*, *P. aeruginosa*, *E. coli* and *K. pneumoniae* species predominating. However, between 1991 and 1995, the number of bloodstream infections doubled, largely due to the increased isolation of CNS, *Enterococus* spp., and intrinsically antibiotic-resistant Gram-negative organisms, particularly *P. aeruginosa* and *Candida* spp.

Currently, the leading pathogens among cases of monomicrobial nosocomial bloodstream infection in the ICU are Gram-positive microorganisms, representing nearly half of the organisms isolated [14, 15, 28, 31] (Table 2). CNS, *S. aureus* and enterococci are the most frequent Gram-positive bacteria in all studies, and CNS is isolated in 20–30% of all episodes of bloodstream infection. Gram-negative bacilli are responsible for 30–40% of bloodstream infection episodes, and the remaining cases are mostly due to *Candida* spp. Polymicrobial episodes are relatively common, representing about 10%. Anaerobic bacteria are isolated in fewer than 5% of cases.

Among Gram-positive bloodstream infections, the incidence of the pathogens is similar in the different ICUs, CNS being the most frequently isolated organism, and *S. aureus* the second most common pathogen in all studies. Only the incidence of strains with antibiotic resistance such as methicillin-resistant *Staphylococcus aureus* (MRSA) or vancomycin-resistant enterococci (VRE) differs substantially according to the characteristics of individual institutions, and depending on whether they become established as endemic nosocomial pathogens in the ICU. On the other hand, the Gram-negative species isolated from nosocomial bloodstream infections in the ICUs of different institutions show marked variability. The relative contribution of each Gram-negative species to the total number of isolates from blood varies from hospital to hospital and over time. The antibiotic policy of the institution may induce the appearance of highly resistant microorganisms and the emergence of endemic nosocomial pathogens, in particular *Pseudomonas* spp., *Acinetobacter* spp., and *Enterobacteriaceae* with extended-spectrum beta-lactamase (ESBL).

The incidence of polymicrobial and anaerobic bloodstream infections depends on the incidence of surgical patients in each ICU, because in 2/3 of these bacteremic episodes the origin is an intrabdominal infection.

TABLE 2. Microorganisms causing nosocomial bloodstream infection in adult ICUs

Reference	Gram-positive microorganisms	Gram-negative microorganisms	Fungi	Polymicrobial episodes
Rello (1993)	44.1% CNS *S. aureus* Enterococci	40 5% *P. aeruginosa* *E. coli* *Enterobacter* spp.	5.4% *Candida* spp.	9.9%
Pittet (1994)	51.0% CNS *S. aureus* Enterococci	39.0% *Enterobacter* spp. *Klebsiella* spp. *S. marcescens*	4.8% *Candida* spp.	21%
Vallés (1997)	49.8% CNS *S. aureus* Enterococci	32.6% *P. aeruginosa* *A. baumannii* *K. pneumoniae*	4.4% *Candida* spp.	12.7%
Jamal (1999)	46.8% CNS *S. aureus* Enterococci	36.6% *Enterobacter* spp. *S. marcescens* *K. pneumoniae*	17.6% *Candida* spp.	9.8%

CNS: Coagulase-negative staphylococci.

TABLE 3. Major sources of nosocomial bloodstream infection in the ICUs

Type of infection causing bloodstream infection	Rello (%)	Pittet (%)	Vallés (%)	Edgeworth (%)
Intravenous catheter	35	18	37.1	62
Respiratory tract	10	28	17.5	3
Intrabdominal infection	9	NA	6.1	6.9
Genitourinary tract	3.6	5.4	5.9	2.4
Surgical wound or soft tissue	8	8	2.4	3
Other	7	14.5	2.9	–
Unknown origin	27	20	28.1	22.4

Sources

According to a more recent analysis, the vast majority (70%) of nosocomial bloodstream infections in the ICU are secondary bloodstream infections, including the bloodstream infections related to an intravascular catheter-infection, and nearly 30% are bloodstream infections of unknown origin. Table 3 summarizes the sources of nosocomial bloodstream infections in the ICU in several recent series [14, 15, 28, 30]. As shown, intravascular catheter-related infections and respiratory tract infections are the leading sources of secondary bloodstream infections.

The source of bloodstream infections varies according to microorganism. CNS and *Staphylococcus aureus* secondary bloodstream infections commonly complicate intravenous-related infections, whereas Gram-negative bacilli are the main etiology for secondary bloodstream infections following respiratory tract, intrabdominal and urinary tract infections. Among bloodstream infections of unknown origin, most are caused by Gram-positive microorganisms, mainly CNS, and they may originate in device-related infections not diagnosed at the time of the development of the bloodstream infection.

Systemic Response to Bloodstream Infection

The host reaction to invading microbes involves a rapidly amplifying polyphony of signals and responses that may spread beyond the invaded tissue. Fever or hypothermia, chills, tachypnea and tachycardia often herald the onset of the systemic inflammatory response to microbial invasion, also called sepsis. However, the interchangeable use of terms as "bloodstream infection", "sepsis", and "septicemia" has led to confusion.

A recent definition of bloodstream infection classifies patients with severe infection and its sequelae [32]. Bloodstream infection and fungemia have been simply defined as the presence of bacteria or fungi in blood cultures, and four stages of systemic response increasing severity have been described: the systemic inflammatory response syndrome (SIRS), which is identified by a combination of simple and readily available clinical signs and symptoms (i.e., fever or hypothermia, tachycardia, tachypnea, and changes in blood leukocyte count); sepsis, in patients in whom the SIRS is caused by documented infection; severe sepsis when patients have a dysfunction of the major organs; and septic shock, which describes patients with hypotension and organ dysfunction in addition to sepsis. As sepsis progresses to septic shock, the risk of death increases substantially. Early sepsis is usually reversible, whereas many patients with septic shock succumb despite aggressive therapy.

The presence of organisms in the blood is one of the most reliable criteria for characterizing a patient presenting with SIRS as having sepsis or one of its more severe presentations, such as severe sepsis or septic shock.

In a recent multicenter study, Brun-Buisson *et al.* [29] analyzed the relationship between bloodstream infection and severe sepsis in adults ICUs and general wards in 24 hospitals in France. In this study, of the 842 episodes of clinically significant bloodstream infection recorded, 162 (19%) occurred in patients hospitalized in ICUs. Three hundred and seventy seven episodes (45%) of bloodstream infection were nosocomial, and their incidence was 12 times greater in ICUs than in wards. The frequency of severe sepsis during bloodstream infection differed markedly between wards and ICUs (17% *versus* 65%, $p < 0.001$). The nosocomial episodes acquired in the ICU represented an incidence rate of 41 episodes per 1000 admissions and the incidence rate of severe sepsis among patients with nosocomial bloodstream infection in the ICU was 24 episodes per 1000 admissions.

Another recent multicenter study reported by our group [15] analyzed exclusively nosocomial bloodstream infections acquired in adult ICUs of 30 hospitals in Spain, and classified their systemic response according to new definitions as sepsis, severe sepsis and septic shock. Among 590 episodes of nosocomial bloodstream, the host reaction was classified as sepsis in 371 episodes (62.8%), severe sepsis in 109 episodes (18.5%), and septic shock in the remaining 110 (18.6%). The systemic response differed markedly according to source of bloodstream infection (Table 4). The episodes of bloodstream infection associated with intravascular catheters showed the lowest rate of septic shock (12.8%), whereas the episodes of bloodstream infection secondary to lower respiratory tract, intrabdominal or genitourinary tract infections showed the highest incidence of severe sepsis and septic shock. In the study by Brun-Buisson *et al.* [29], in patients hospitalized in ICUs, intravascular catheter-related bloodstream infection was also associated with a lower risk of severe sepsis (OR = 0.2; 95% CI: 0.1 to 0.5; $p < 0.01$).

The systemic response may differ according to the microorganism causing the episode of bloodstream infection. Gram-negative and *Candida* spp. have been associated with a higher incidence of severe sepsis and septic shock in our multicenter study [15], whereas CNS was the microorganism causing the lowest incidence of septic shock. The multicenter study of Brun-Buisson *et al.* [29] analyzed ICU bloodstream infections separately and found the episodes caused by CNS also to be associated with a reduced risk of severe sepsis (OR = 0.2; $p = 0.02$) relative to other organisms.

These results suggest that the source of infection and probably the type of microorganism causing the episode of bloodstream infection, especially if a species other than CNS is involved, may be important in the development of severe sepsis and septic shock.

TABLE 4. Distribution of systemic response according to source of 590 episodes of ICU nosocomial bloodstream infection

	Number (%) of episodes			
Source	Sepsis	Severe sepsis	Septic shock	Total
Intravenous catheter	158 (68.5)	41 (18.7)	28 (12.8)	219 (37.1)
Lower respiratory tract	53 (51.5)	27 (26.2)	23 (22.3)	103 (17.5)
Intrabdominal infection	12 (33.3)	9 (25)	15 (41.7)	36 (6.1)
Urinary tract	23 (65.7)	5 (14.3)	7 (20)	35 (5.9)
Surgical wound and soft tissue	7 (50)	2 (14.3)	5 (35.7)	14 (2.4)
Other	11 (64.7)	4 (23.5)	2 (11.8)	17 (2.9)
Unknown	115 (69.3)	21 (12.6)	30 (18.1)	166 (28.1)
Total	371 (62.8)	109 (18.5)	110 (18.6)	590 (100)

Risk Factors for Nosocomial Bloodstream Infection

The conditions that predispose an individual to bloodstream infection include not only host underlying conditions but therapeutic, microbial and environmental factors as well. The illnesses that have been associated with an increased risk of bloodstream infection include hematologic and nonhematologic malignancies, diabetes mellitus, renal failure requiring dialysis, chronic hepatic failure, immune deficiency syndromes, and conditions associated with the loss of normal skin barriers such as serious burns and decubitus ulcers. In the ICU, therapeutic maneuvers associated with an increased risk of nosocomial bloodstream infection include procedures such as placement of intravascular and urinary catheters, endoscopic procedures, and drainage of intrabdominal infections.

Several risk factors have been associated with the acquisition of bloodstream infection by specific pathogens. CNS are mainly associated with central venous line infection and with the use of intravenous lipid emulsions. *Candida* spp. infections are related to the exposure to multiple antibiotics, hemodialysis, isolation of candida species from sites other than the blood, azotemia, and the use of indwelling catheters [33]. In a recent analysis of risk factors for nosocomial candidemia in ICU patients with nosocomial bloodstream infections we found that exposure to more than four antibiotics during the ICU stay (OR: 4.10), parenteral nutrition (OR: 3.37), previous surgery (OR: 2.60) and the presence of solid malignancy (OR: 1.57) were the variables that were independently associated with the development of *Candida* spp. infection [34].

Prognosis

The crude mortality associated with bacteremic sepsis averages 35% (range 20 to 50%) [13, 35, 36]. The mortality directly attributable to the nosocomial bloodstream infection averaged 27% (range 14 to 38%) [37]. Although one-third of the deaths occur within the first 48 hours after the onset of symptoms, mortality can occur 14 or more days later. Late deaths are often due to poorly controlled infection, complications during the stay in the ICU, or failure of multiple organs [38]. Nosocomial bloodstream infection is associated with higher crude mortality rates than community-acquired infection [11, 36]. In a recent study, Bueno-Cavanillas *et al.* [39] analyzed the impact of nosocomial infection on the mortality rate in an ICU. In that study, overall crude relative risk of mortality was 2.48 (95% CI = 1.47 to 4.16) in patients with a nosocomial infection compared with noninfected patients. When the type of infection was evaluated, the risk of mortality for patients with bloodstream infection was 4.13 (95% IC = 2.11 to 8.11).

The risk of dying is influenced by the prior clinical condition of the patient and the rate at which complications develop. Analysis using prognostic stratification systems (such as APACHE scoring system) indicate that factoring in the patient's age and certain physiologic variables results in more accurate estimates of the risk of dying. Variables associated with the high care-fatality rates include acute respiratory distress syndrome (ARDS), disseminated intravascular coagulation (DIC), renal insufficiency, and multiple organ dysfunction (MOD). Microbial variables are less important, although high care-fatality rates have been observed for patients with bloodstream infection due to *Pseudomonas aeruginosa*, *Candida* spp. and for patients with polymicrobial bloodstream infection.

In a recent study of bloodstream infection in an adult ICU of a teaching hospital in UK over a 12-year period, Crowe *et al.* [40] analyzed 315 episodes of bloodstream infection, of which 82% were hospital-acquired, and found an overall mortality related to bloodstream infection of 44.4%. They also observed that ICU stay was longer in bacteremic patients (12 days) than non-bacteremic patients (three days).

The crude mortality from bloodstream infection is often 35% to 60%, ranging from 12% to

80%. The attributable mortality defines the mortality directly associated with the episode of bloodstream infection, and excludes the mortality attributable to underlying conditions. It averages 26%, but varies according to the specific microorganisms involved: CNS averaged 13.6%; enterococci, 31%; and Candida spp., 38% [19, 41, 42].

Pittet *et al.* in 1994 [28] analyzed the attributable mortality, excess of length and extra costs to nosocomial bloodstream infection in a surgical ICU. In this case-control study, the crude mortality rate was 50%, differing significantly from the matched controls (15%, $p < 0.01$). In consequence, the attributable mortality associated with nosocomial bloodstream infection was 35%. Those authors also observed that median length of hospital stay for cases was 14 days longer than for controls. Furthermore, nosocomial bloodstream infection was associated with a doubling of time of SICU stays, and consequently with a significant economic burden.

This study demonstrates that nosocomial bloodstream infections cause excess mortality and significantly prolong ICU and hospital stay among critically ill patients.

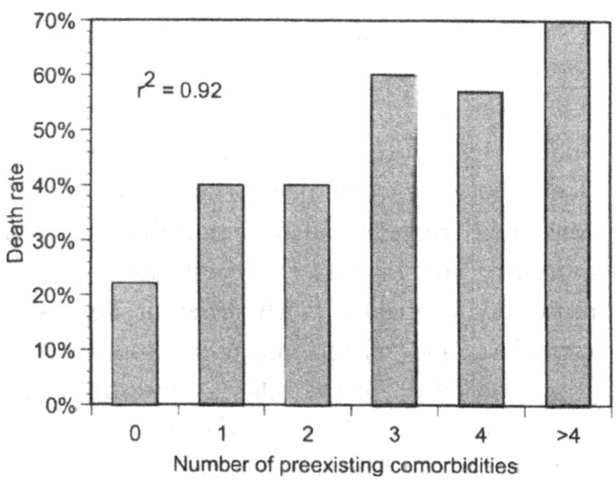

FIGURE 2. Importance of pre-existing co-morbidities for prognosis of septicemia in critically ill patients. (From [43], with permission.)

In another study of nosocomial bloodstream infection in a medical-surgical ICU reported by Rello *et al.* [14], the overall mortality was 31.5%, and 65.7% of all deaths were directly attributable to infection. Bloodstream infection from intrabdominal, lower respiratory tract or unknown origin were associated with a poor prognosis. A logistic regression analysis defined intrabdominal origin ($p = 0.01$, OR: 15.7), and presence of shock ($p < 0.004$, OR: 3.3) as independently influencing the risk of death.

In a more recent study, Pittet *et al.* [43] analyzed the importance of pre-existing co-morbidities for the prognosis of bloodstream infection in critically ill patients. The study was performed in a surgical ICU, and the authors analyzed 176 patients with bloodstream infection, of which 125 (71%) were nosocomially acquired. The mean total length of ICU stay of bacteremic patients was also four times longer than that of non-bacteremic patients (17.6 days *versus* 4.3 days). The overall mortality rate of non-bacteremic was 8.8%, whereas that of bacteremic patients was 44.3%. Thus, bacteremic patients had a five-fold increased risk of dying when compared with non-bacteremic patients (RR = 5.03, CI 95% 4.17 to 6.07, $p < 0.0001$). In this study they found a close correlation between the number of co-morbidities and fatality rates (Figure 2). In addition, APACHE II $\geq$ 20 was also identified as an independent predictor of mortality.

A number of factors have been suspected as being associated with mortality in bloodstream infection. The most widely recognized prognostic factors are age, severity of the patient's underlying disease, and the appropriateness of antimicrobial therapy. Among other factors potentially related to the outcome of bloodstream infection, a multiple source of infection, secondary infection, bloodstream infection caused by some difficult-to-treat organisms such as *Pseudomonas* or *Serratia* spp., polymicrobial bloodstream infection, and factors related to host response such as the occurrence of hypotension, shock, or organ failure have all been described as

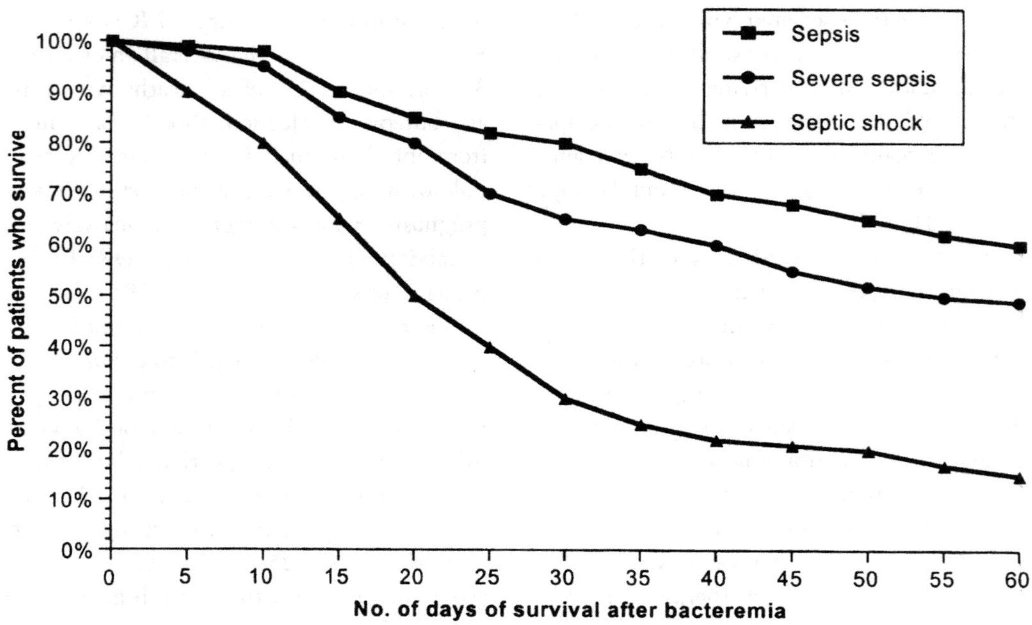

FIGURE 3. Survival after bloodstream infection according to systemic response.

prognostically important. In a French multicenter study of bloodstream infection and severe sepsis in ICUs and wards of 24 hospitals, Brun-Buisson *et al.* [29] reported that bloodstream infection due to *E. coli* or CNS was associated with a lower risk of severe sepsis and death, whereas *S. aureus* and Gram-positive organisms other than CNS were associated with an increased risk of death. The results of that study emphasize the impact of end-organ dysfunction (i.e., severe sepsis and septic shock) on prognosis in bloodstream infection.

In the multicenter study on nosocomial bloodstream infection carried out by our group [15] in 30 Spanish ICUs, crude mortality was 41.6%, and 56% of all deaths were directly attributable to the bloodstream infection. The crude mortality was correlated to the severity of systemic response; it was as high as 80% among patients with septic shock, compared with 26% among patients whose bacteremic episodes were manifested exclusively as sepsis. The cumulative probability of survival stratified according to the grade of systemic response is showed in Figure 3. In addition, bloodstream infections originating in the abdomen or respiratory tract were associated with the highest mortality ($p = 0.04$).

Because crude mortality cannot differentiate between mortality directly related to bloodstream infection and mortality attributable to underlying conditions, we were aware that different factors may influence the prognosis if we considered directly related mortality or crude mortality. For this reason we performed a double multivariate analysis with different dependent variables: one, related mortality, and another, crude mortality. In the related mortality analysis, in addition to the level of systemic response and associated complications, we found that the type of microorganisms involved and the source of bloodstream infection played an important role in the prognosis. In the crude mortality analysis, we found that in addition to the systemic response and associated complications, mechanical ventilation at the time of development of bloodstream infection, chronic hepatic failure, and APACHE II > 15 at the time of diagnosis of bloodstream infection were chosen as factors by the statistical model; this seems to indicate that underlying diseases and the severity of patient's conditions markedly influence crude mortality among ICU patients with nosocomial bloodstream infection. On the other hand, the immediate prognosis after an episode of nosocomial bloodstream infection (related mortality) correlated with level of systemic response, type of microorganism involved and the different sources of bloodstream infection.

Pittet *et al.* [44] recently conducted a large cohort study to determine prognostic factors of mortality in ICU patients with positive blood cultures. They analyzed 173 patients with bacteremia, of which 53.1% were nosocomially acquired. Among patients with bacteremic sepsis, 75 died (43%); in 81% of them, the cause of death was considered to be directly or indirectly related to the infection. In this study, the best two independent prognostic factors were the APACHE II score at the onset of sepsis (OR, 1.13; CI 95%, 1.08 to 1.17; $p < 0.001$) and the number of organ dysfunctions developing thereafter (OR, 2.39; CI 95%, 2.02 to 2.82; $p < 0.001$). This study suggests that in ICU patients with positive blood cultures, outcome can be predicted by the severity of illness at onset of sepsis and the number of vital organ dysfunctions developing subsequently.

Conclusions

1. Nosocomial bloodstream infections occur two to seven times more often in ICU patients than in ward patients. Recent studies have shown that the incidence rate range between 26 and 67 episodes per 1000 ICU admissions, depending on the type of ICU.
2. Patients with nosocomial ICU bloodstream infection have a higher prevalence of intravenous lines and respiratory sources of infection than ward patients in whom urinary tract infection is the most prevalent source of bloodstream infection.
3. Gram-positive microorganisms are the most prevalent cause of nosocomial bloodstream infection in ICU patients. This high incidence is related to the high prevalence of bloodstream infection associated with intravascular catheters in critically ill patients, and to the multiple antibiotic therapy used for Gram-negative infections in ICU patients, which result in the selection of Gram-positive microorganisms.
4. Currently, Gram-negative microorganisms cause between 30% and 40% of ICU-acquired bloodstream infections, and multiresistant organisms, such as *P. aeruginosa*, *Serratia* spp., or *A. baumannii*, are the most frequently isolated pathogens.
5. Approximately 40% of ICU patients with nosocomial bloodstream infection show a severe systemic response, such as severe sepsis or septic shock, associated with high mortality.
6. The attributable mortality from nosocomial bloodstream infections is high in critically ill patients, and the infection is associated with excessively long ICU and hospital stays, and a significant economic burden.

References

1. Wenzel RP. Organization for infection control. In Mandell GL, Douglas RG Jr, Bennett JE (eds). Principles and practice of infectious diseases. 3rd edn, New York: Churchill Livingstone, 1990:2176.
2. Weinstein RA. Epidemiology and control of nosocomial infections in adult intensive care units. Am J Med 91(suppl 3B):179S, 1991.
3. Wenzel RP, Thompson RL, Landry SM, *et al.* Hospital-acquired infection in intensive care unit patients: an overview with emphasis on epidemics. Infect Control 4:371, 1983.
4. Maki DG. Risk factors for nosocomial infection in intensive care: "devices vs nature" and goals for the next decade. Arch Intern Med 149:30, 1989.
5. Donowitz LG, Wenzel RP, Hoyt JW. High risk of hospital-acquired infection in the ICU patient. Crit Care Med 10:355, 1982.

6. Brown RB, Hosmer D, Chen HC, *et al.* A comparison of infections in the different ICUs within the same hospital. Crit Care Med 13:472, 1985.
7. Daschner F. Nosocomial infections in intensive care units. Intensive Care Med 11:284, 1985.
8. Massanari RM, Hierholzer WJ Jr. The intensive care unit. In Bennett JV, Brachman PS (eds). Hospital infections. 2nd edn, Boston: Little, Brown and Company, 1986:285.
9. Trilla A, Gatell JM, Mensa J, *et al.* Risk factors for nosocomial bacteremia in a large Spanish teaching hospital: A case-control study. Infect Control Hosp Epidemiol 12:150, 1991.
10. Reimer LG, Wilson ML, Weinstein MP. Update on detection of bacteremia and fungemia. Clin Microbiol Rev 10:444, 1997.
11. Pittet D. Nosocomial bloodstream infections. In Wenzel RP (ed). Prevention and control of nosocomial infections. 2nd edn, Baltimore: Williams & Wilkins; 1993:512.
12. Garner JS, Jarvis WR, Emori TG, *et al.* CDC definitions for nosocomial infections. Am J Infect Control 16:128, 1988.
13. Gatell JM, Trilla A, Latorre X, *et al.* Nosocomial bacteremia in a large Spanish teaching hospital: analysis of factors influencing prognosis. Rev Infect Dis 10:203, 1988.
14. Rello J, Ricart M, Mirelis B, *et al.* Nosocomial bacteremia in a medical-surgical intensive care unit: epidemiologic characteristics and factors influencing mortality in 111 episodes. Intensive Care Med 20:94, 1994.
15. Vallés J, León C, Alvarez-Lerma F, *et al.* Nosocomial bacteremia in critically ill patients: a multicenter study evaluating epidemiology and prognosis. Clin Infect Dis 24:387, 1997.
16. Towns ML, Quartey SM, Weinstein MP, *et al.* The clinical significance of positive blood cultures: a prospective, multicenter evaluation. In Abstracts of the 93rd General Meeting of the American Society for Microbiology. Washington, D.C.: American Society for Microbiology, 1993: Abstr. C-232.
17. Weinstein MP, Towns ML, Quartey SM, *et al.* The clinical significance of positive blood cultures in the 1990s: a prospective comprehensive evaluation of the microbiology, epidemiology, and outcome of bacteremia and fungemia in adults. Clin Infect Dis 24:584, 1997.
18. Mirret S, Weinstein MP, Reimer LG, *et al.* Interpretation of coagulase-negative staphylococci in blood cultures: does the number of positive bottles help? In Abstracts of the 93rd General meeting of the American Society for Microbiology. Washington, D.C.: American Society for Microbiology, 1994: Abstr. C-69.
19. Martin MA, Pfaller MA, Wenzel RP. Coagulase-negative staphylococci bacteremia. Mortality and hospital stay. Ann Intern Med 110:9, 1989.
20. Ponce de León S, Wenzel RP. Hospital-acquired bloodstream infections with Staphylococcus epidermidis. Am J Med 77:639, 1984.
21. Domínguez-de Villota E, Algora-Weber A, Millan I, *et al.* Early evaluation of coagulase-negative staphylococci in blood samples of intensive care unit patients. A clinically uncertain judgement. Intensive Care Med 13:390, 1987.
22. Craven DE, Kunches LM, Lichtenberg DA, *et al.* Nosocomial infections and fatality in medical and surgical intensive care unit patients. Arch Intern Med 148:1161, 1988.
23. Constantini M, Donisi PM, Turrin MG, *et al.* Hospital-acquired infections surveillance and control in intensive care services. Results of an incidence study. Eur J Epidemiol 3:347, 1987.
24. Daschner FD, Frey P, Wolff G, *et al.* Nosocomial infections in intensive care wards: A multicenter prospective study. Intensive Care Med 8:5, 1982.
25. Trilla A. Epidemiology of nosocomial infections in adult intensive care units. Intensive Care Med 20:S1, 1994.
26. Vincent JL, Bihari DJ, Suter PM, *et al.* The prevalence of nosocomial infection in intensive care units in Europe. JAMA 274:634, 1995.
27. Richards MJ, Edwards JR, Culver DH, *et al.* Nosocomial infections in medical intensive care units in the United States. Crit Care Med 27:887, 1999.
28. Pittet D, Tarara D, Wenzel RP. Nosocomial bloodstream infection in critically ill patients. Excess length of stay, extra costs, and attributable mortality. JAMA 271:1598, 1994.
29. Brun-Buisson C, Doyon F, Carlet J, *et al.* Bacteremia and severe sepsis in adults: A multicenter prospective survey in ICUs and wards of 24 hospitals. Am J Respir Crit Care Med 154:617, 1996.
30. Edgeworth JD, Treacher DF, Eykyn SJ. A 25-year study of nosocomial bacteremia in an adult intensive care unit. Crit Care Med 27:1421, 1999.
31. Jamal WY, El-Din K, Rotimi VO, *et al.* An analysis of hospital-acquired bacteraemia in intensive care unit patients in a university hospital in Kuwait. J Hosp Infect 43:49, 1999.
32. Bone RC, Balk RA, Cerra FB, *et al.* Definitions for sepsis and organ failure and guidelines for the

use of innovative therapies in sepsis. Chest 101:1644, 1992.
33. Wenzel RP. Isolation of Candida species from sites other than the blood. Clin Infect Dis 20:1531, 1995.
34. Díaz E, Villagrá A, Martínez M, *et al.* Nosocomial candidemia risk factors. Intensive Care Med 24(Suppl 1):S143, 1998.
35. Leibovici L, Konisberger H, Pitlik SD. Bacteremia and fungemia of unknown origin in adults. Clin Infect Dis 14:436, 1992.
36. Weinstein MP, Reller LB, Murphy JR, *et al.* The clinical significance of positive blood cultures: a comprehensive analysis of 500 episodes of bloodstream infection and fungemia in adults. I. Laboratory and epidemiologic observations. Rev Infect Dis 5:35, 1983.
37. Wenzel RP. The mortality of hospital-acquired bloodstream infections: need for a new vital statistic? Int J Epidemiol 17:225, 1988.
38. Munford RS. Sepsis and septic shock. In Isselbacher KJ, Braunwald E, Wilson JD, Martin JB, Fauci AS, Kasper DL (eds). Harrison's Principles of Internal Medicine. 13th edn, New York: McGraw-Hill Inc., 1994:511.
39. Bueno-Cavanillas A, Delgado-Rodríguez M, López-Luque A, *et al.* Influence of nosocomial infection on mortality rate in an intensive care unit. Crit Care Med 22:55, 1994.
40. Crowe M, Ispahani P, Humphreys H, *et al.* Bacteraemia in the adult intensive care unit of a teaching hospital in Nottingham, UK, 1985–1996. Eur J Clin Microbiol Dis 17:377, 1998.
41. Landry SL, Kaiser DL, Wenzel RP. Hospital stay and mortality attributed to nosocomial enterococcal bacteremia: a controlled study. Am J Infect Control 17:323, 1989.
42. Wey SB, Motomi M, Pfaller MA, *et al.* Hospital-acquired candidemia: the attributable mortality and excess length of stay. Arch Intern Med 148:2642, 1988.
43. Pittet D, Thiévent B, Wenzel RP, *et al.* Importance of pre-existing co-morbidities for prognosis of septicemia in critically ill patients. Intensive Care Med 19:265, 1993.
44. Pittet D, Thiévent B, Wenzel RP, *et al.* Bedside prediction of mortality from bacteremic sepsis. A dynamic analysis of ICU patients. Am J Respir Crit Care Med 153:684, 1996.

32. HEMODIALYSIS CATHETER-RELATED INFECTIONS

Raúl Lombardi

Introduction

Infection is one of the most serious and frequent complications associated with the use of central venous catheter for hemodialysis. Bacteremia, which is 80–90% of the times related to vascular access, is responsible for three-quarters of deaths caused by infection in end stage-renal disease (ESRD) patients [1].

ESRD patients are more susceptible to infection due to defects in the immune system, particularly at the skin barrier and the cellular immunity [2]. On the other hand, dialysis procedure itself that requires repeated access to the bloodstream and exposed blood to the extracorporeal circuit, acts as a relevant associated risk factor [3]. Malnutrition and old age are supplementary risk factors.

Currently, it is estimated that 15% of hemodialysis patients use central venous catheters, whether as a temporary access until placement or maturation of an arteriovenous fistula or graft, or as a permanent access due to the exhaustion of the native vascular bed [1].

Definitions

Catheter colonization: Growth of ≥15 colony-forming units by semiquantitative culture of the extraluminal segment of the catheter tip [4] or $>10^3$ by quantitative culture of the intraluminal surface [5, 6], in the absence of clinical symptoms. It could be considered as a localized infection. A lower count corresponds to contamination of the catheter. Some studies have suggested that combination of different catheter-segments cultures increases sensitivity and specificity for the diagnosis of colonization. Rello *et al.* [7] found that combination of the semiquantitative culture of the external surface of the tip with the quantitative culture of the intraluminal surface of the subcutaneous segment has the best performance to detect catheter colonization.

Exit site infection: Erythema, tenderness, edema and suppuration within 2 cm from the exit site.

Tunnel infection: Inflammation or suppuration along the catheter subcutaneous tunnel, more than 2 cm from the exit site.

Catheter-related bloodstream infection (CR-BSI): Isolation of the same microorganism from the catheter and from blood drawn through a peripheral vein, in absence of another evident source of infection. An equivalent of the CR-BSI occurs when there is a blood culture negative and defervescence of the clinical picture after the catheter removal.

Catheter-related sepsis: It is defined by the association of one or more organ dysfunctions with colonization of the catheter. It corresponds with so-called severe sepsis, in accordance with the definitions of the Consensus Conference of the American College of Chest Physicians/Society of Critical Care Medicine [8].

Epidemiology

The number of ESRD patients is increasing all over the world. In addition to that, survival in dialysis has increased, which leads to more frequent problems with the definitive vascular access, and therefore, to an increase in the use of catheters for temporary or prolonged vascular access.

The available information about the incidence of hemodialysis catheter-related infections is diverse, and there are few controlled trials. In general, publications show a frequency of infections that exceeds that reported for other indications [9, 10]. Variations on the type of catheters used (tunneled, non-tunneled, cuffed or non-cuffed), the material of which catheters are made (polyethylene, polyurethane, silicone), the time of permanence (temporary, prolonged), as well as the insertion site could explain, among other reasons, the differences found in the bibliography (Table 1).

On the other hand, the way to express the frequency with which these complications occur also varies and this rends the comparison between series difficult. The frequency is often expressed through the ratio of infection episodes per patient-year or patient-month. Relative frequency is also used, that is, the number of events in relation to the number of patients exposed. Density of incidence is the most appropriate way to express the frequency with which an event occurs, since it normalizes the incidence to the duration of exposure to the risk. Density of incidence is the quotient of the number of episodes (CR-BSI, catheter colonization, exit-site infection, etc.) and the total duration of exposure to the risk (sum of days each catheter remained) referred to 1000 days:

number of episodes/days of exposure × 1000

Bacteremia is one of the most serious complications in dialysis patients and it is mainly related to vascular access, being caused more often by temporary or permanent catheters than by the arteriovenous fistula or the graft [11, 12]. On the other hand, vascular access related infection represents the most common cause of bacteremia in the patient undergoing dialysis [11–15]. A comprehensive study carried out in Denmark showed that out of 14,387 cases of *S. aureus* bacteremia, 5.5% occurred in hemodialysis patients and 80% were catheter-related [16].

Incidence of bacteremia ranges between 1.6 and 13.5 episodes per 1000 catheter-days, using non-tunneled, non-cuffed devices. Other investigators have found that tunneled, cuffed catheters are associated with lower risk of infection that ranges between 0.2 and 0.8 episodes per 1000 catheter-days [17]. In a non-published series of the author of 123 non-cuffed, non-tunneled catheters CR-BSI occurred with a density of incidence of 1.9 episodes per 1000 catheter-days [18].

Catheter colonization is seen more frequently than CR-BSI, especially if the catheter tip is cultivated routinely when removed. Figures range between 10.3 [19] and 30 colonization episodes per 1000 catheter-days [10]. In the personal series mentioned above, the colonization incidence was 11.9 per 1000 catheter-days.

Exit-site infection is another frequent and potentially severe complication. The density of incidence ranges between 0.4 and 4.5 episodes

TABLE 1. Epidemiology of catheter related-bloodstream infection (references in text)

Author	Date	Number of catheter	Type of catheter	Incidence (CR-BSI/1000 catheter-days)
Vanherweghem	1986	200	Non-tunneled	6/1000 catheter-days
Almirall	1989	53	Non-tunneled	10/1000 catheter-days
Capello	1989	107	Hickman	0.8/1000 catheter-days
Kinnaert	1990	19	Hickman	07/1000 catheter-days
Marr	1997	102	Cuffed-tunneled	3.9/1000 catheter-days
Lombardi	1998	123	Non-tunneled	1.9/1000 catheter-days

per 1000 catheter-days [20]. The frequency of episodes per patient-year has been estimated between 0.36 [21] and 0.57 [22]. Exit site infection represents a potential risk for the colonization of the intravascular segment of the catheter and bacteremia. Likewise, it may determine the loss of access, unless controlled by treatment.

Pathogenesis

The development of catheter-related infection depends on the occurrence of three conditions: microorganism invasion at the catheter, its adherence to synthetic material and its multiplication. Infective organisms can migrate into the endovascular segment of the catheter through the insertion site (*periluminal*); through the catheter hub during its manipulation (*endoluminal*) or by a distant focus of infection that leads to bacteremia and subsequent colonization of the tip (*hematogenous*). The type of catheter and the setting in which it is inserted could determine the mechanism of colonization. In short-term catheters (less than one month) periluminal way is the more likely mechanism of colonization [23]. In long-term catheter and, particularly, when it is used for parenteral nutrition, colonization is more frequent through the catheter hub [24].

Staphylococcus aureus and *negative-coagulase Staphylococcus* are the prevailing microrganism, so it is reasonable to think in the muco-cutaneous origin of catheter-related infections. Hemodialysis patients are *S. aureus* nasal carriers more frequently than the general population. The frequency has been estimated to be 50 to 60% [25, 26], and therefore, periluminal colonization is likely to take place. Likewise, the high frequency of *S. aureus* carriage in these patients endures the risk of auto-contamination at the time of connection, unless appropriate preventive measures are applied (use of surgical mask by the patients). In a study [27], the same strain of *S. aureus* was identified simultaneously in the nares and in blood of patients in 50% of cases. This study demonstrated the predictive value of colonization of the insertion site by *S. aureus* for the development of bacteremia. Finally, staff member hands might be a vehicle for transmission during catheter connection and disconnection, especially *negative-coagulase Staphylococcus*.

There is little and contradictory information available about the colonization mechanism of hemodialysis catheters [9, 10, 28, 29]. According to Almirall *et al.* [10], the prevailing mechanism would seem to be periluminal, from migration of skin flora to the tip (correspondence skin/tip: 58.6%; hub/tip: 17.2%). Cheesbrough *et al.* [9] found a greater relationship between the hub cultures (57%) and the tip than the skin (36%). Studying a group of patients with weekly quantitative cultures taken through the catheter, Dittmer *et al.* [28] found a high incidence of endoluminal catheter colonization (68%) and bacteremia (35%). Other investigators assume that skin colonization plays a very important role, since they found a relation between the condition of the skin at the exit site and the frequency of catheter colonization and bacteremia [29]. Typing organisms by phage, Nielson *et al.* [27] also found evidence favoring the periluminal via.

End-stage renal disease patients are prone to infection, due to defense mechanism dysfunction cause by uremia, as well as for specific risk associated to renal replacement therapies.

Uremia affects the barrier function of skin and mucosa, as well as the humoral immunity, even though the typical disorder is the cellular immunity impairment. Lymphopenia, decrease of delayed hypersensitivity, lymphoid system and thymus atrophy are the characteristic disorders in ESRD, and experimental data suggests the existence of immune inhibitor factors in the serum of uremic patients [2, 30]. It has not been possible to establish which are the substances responsible for such disorders, but they are very likely not to be related to the well known markers of uremia (urea, creatinine), but to other factors such as phosphate, potassium, indoles, phenols, PTH and others [2]. Deficiencies in vitamins E and C and folic acid, as well as the increase in seric levels of trace elements (copper, cadmium) and zinc depletion, have been related to immune disorders in uremic patients [31]. Malnutrition, which also develops in end-state renal disease patients, has been proven to be a risk factor for infection [32].

Iron overload, caused by excessive iron replacement or repeated blood transfusions, leads to granulocyte malfunction and infection [12, 14, 33], making the risk of bacteremia increase by up to three times [34].

Nasal carriage of *S. aureus* is another risk factor for infection in this group of patients, as was already mentioned. Approximately 15% of healthy individuals are nasal carriers of *S. aureus* but this percentage could rise to more than 60% in dialysis patient [25].

The contact of blood with the material of the dialysis circuit triggers an inflammatory-antiinflammatory response mediated by citokines, complement and other mediators of the inflammatory cascade which leads to a decrease in the granulocyte function and the release of oxygen-free radicals. These disturbances have been associated with a higher risk of bacterial infection, as well as catabolic stress and β-2 microglobuline amyloidosis, particularly if cellulosic membranes are used [3, 35] and that is why some authors have suggested the use of more biocompatible membranes in order to decrease the risk. The results of these studies are exciting, but the efficacy of this practice has not been yet definitively proven [12].

Microbiology

Hemodialysis catheter-related infections are caused mainly by Gram-positive cocci, especially *Staphylococcus spp. Negative-coagulase Staphylococcus* is a prevalent organism as in other settings, but the incidence of *S. aureus* is comparatively higher due to the frequent skin and nasal colonization with this agent among dialysis patients. Both represent approximately 70% of total catheter colonization. Bacteremia is caused by *negative-coagulase Staphyloccocus* in 14% to 76% of cases, while *S. aureus* has been isolated in 12% to 44%, according to different authors [10, 13, 19, 36–38]. However, in a large series of 63 CR-BSI, *S. aureus* was prevailing (43%) compared to *S. epidermidis* (14%) [13].

Enterococcus is the second most frequent Grampositive cocci after *Staphyloccus* (5% to 13%) and finally, Gram-negative aerobic bacilli (11% to 24%), among which *Pseudomonas* species prevail since it frequently contaminates dialysis water. Other bacteremia-causing agents less frequently isolated, are fungi and diphteroids. In our unit we have had eight catheter-related bacteremia episodes due to *Bacillus spp.*, which has also been reported by other authors [38, 39].

In our series already mentioned, the prevailing organisms in the catheter tip were *negative-coagulase Staphyloccocus* (43%) and *S. aureus* (25%). In bacteremia, *S. aureus* prevailed.

Table 2 shows microbiological data of different authors.

TABLE 2. Organisms isolated in blood cultures (references in text)

Author	Date	Number of bacteremias	S. aureus (%)	Coagulase-negative Staphyloccocus (%)	Enteroccocus (%)	Gram-negative bacilli (%)
Marr	1997	63	43	14	5	24
Robinson	1998	23	35	22	13	13
Capdevilla	1993	13	16	3		38
Almirall	1989	9	44	33	11	11
Schaffer	1995	8	12	62	12	12
Lombardi	1998	7	57	14		14

Diagnosis

The diagnosis criteria for the different forms of catheter-related infections are mentioned elsewhere in this section. Diagnosis of catheter-related infection by semiquantitative or quantitative methods requires removal of the device. However, if catheter removal is undesirable, quantitative blood culture is an alternative diagnostic method. Blood is drawn through the device and from a peripheral vein simultaneously. Capdevilla and colleagus [40] demonstrated that a count four-fold greater or more in the catheter blood culture than in the peripheral blood has a sensitivity of 94% and a specificity of 100% for the diagnosis of catheter-related infection. Likewise, a count of >100 cfu/ml in the catheter blood with the same organism in peripheral blood also has a high predictive value. Other authors suggest cutoff seven-fold greater [41]. The quantitative culture methods are safer, but less practical so they are not recommended for clinical practice.

Complications of Catheter-Related Infections

Catheter-related infections may get complicated with metastatic localization, especially when there is persistent bacteremia or associated thrombophlebitis. The most frequent complications are infective endocarditis, osteomyelitis, suppurative arthritis, spinal epidural abscess, and pulmonary septic emboli, among others.

Osteomyelitis and osteoarthritis are frequent localizations. They are observed in 5% to 15% of all hemodialysis catheter-related bacteremias [13, 16, 27, 33, 42]. Vertebral, clavicular, and pelvic involvement are the most common ones. Pain is the most frequent symptom, while fever is only seen in 30% of cases [42]. The most reliable methods for the diagnosis are bone scintigraphy and computarized tomography. Recently, the use of labeled human polyclonal IgG has been suggested and preliminary studies have shown promising results [43].

Infective endocarditis is a serious complication that is associated with high rates of morbimortality. The real incidence of endocarditis is not yet known with certitude, because there are not well designed epidemiological studies and the criteria for diagnosis have been modified since the introduction of the Duke's diagnosis criteria [44]. According to the scarce bibliography available, the incidence ranges between 3 and 4.4% [16, 45]. Diagnosis may be difficult due to the low frequency of classical symptoms of endocarditis, and the high frequency of pre-existing cardiac murmur in these patients. Infective endocarditis should be suspected in all dialysis patients who have fever or bacteremia of unexplained origin. The most sensitive and specific diagnosis method is the transesophageal echocardiography. The largest series published is that of Robinson *et al.* [45], consisting of 20 cases in which catheter infection was the cause in 55% of patients. Fever and cardiac murmur were the most frequent manifestations, and the most affected valve was the mitral valve. The germ most frequently isolated was *S. aureus*, followed by *S. epidermidis*. Only five patients underwent valve replacement and the mortality rate was 30%. The above data is very similar to that from an unpublished series studied by the author in 1993, the results of which are shown in Table 3 [46].

Spinal epidural abscess is a rare and serious infection. However, its frequency has been increasing due to the more extensive use of hemodialysis catheters, especially when catheter salvage has been used [47]. The main symptom is persistent and intense back pain [47, 48]. Fever and leukocytosis are not constant. In some cases, neurological manifestations due to medullar compression (paresis, hypoestesia or paresthesia) could be observed. The prevailing organism is *S. aureus*, which is isolated in 60% of the cases. The diagnostic test of choice is magnetic resonance imaging. Treatment consists of a prolonged course of antibiotics for four to six weeks, the antibiotic being selected according to the susceptibility of the causative organism and

TABLE 3. Infective endocarditis in a serie of ESRD patients (non published)

Number of cases	20
Age	53.8 ± 12.4yr.
Source of infection	
Catheter	8
Fistula	3
Other	6
Unknown	3
Microbiology	
S. aureus	6
Enteroccocus	5
Gram-negative bacilli	5
Enteroccocus + GN bacilli	1
Negative	3
Valve affected	
Aortic	9
Mitral	5
Aortic + mitral	5
Tricuspid	1
Surgery	2 (10%)
Mortality rate	7 (35%)

its tissue penetration. Surgery for drainage of the epidural space is indicated when symptoms of medullar compression are observed. Diagnosis and treatment must be done without delay to minimize the risk of neurological sequelae, which are in fact frequent.

Prevention

Strategies for the prevention of catheter-related infections in hemodialysis have been less studied than those related to other settings.

Due to the high prevalence of *S. aureus* carriers among dialysis patients, skin antisepsis at the time of catheter insertion is very important. Maximal barrier precaution during placement of catheter minimizes the risk of subsequent infection. Catheter site dressing regimens are controversial and a very active topic of research. There is general agreement about not using transparent adhesive dressing at the insertion site because of the risk of increase microbial colonization [49]. Levin *et al.* [50] have demonstrated that the use of povidone-iodine ointment and sterile gauze on the catheter exit site has significantly decreased the frequency of catheter-related infection. Exite site infection fall from 5 to 1.23 episodes/1000 catheter-days, tip colonization from 11.26 to 5.33/1000 catheter-days, and bacteremia from 4.59 to 0.41 episodes/1000 catheter-days. Decrease of the relative risk was 72%, 52% and 93% respectively. On the other hand, they proved the reduction to be more evident in *S. aureus* nasal carriers. Other authors have studied the effect of mupirocin, an active antistaphylococcal topical antibiotic, in the form of an ointment at the exit site level, for the prevention of infections caused by *S. aureus*. Sesso *et al.* [51] randomized 136 ESRD patients to disinfect their skin with povidone-iodine versus 2% mupirocin ointment after catheter placement and in every hemodialysis. They found significantly less catheter-colonization (1.76 vs. 14.27 episodes/1000 catheter-days) and bacteremia (0.71 vs. 8.92 episodes/1000 catheter-days) with the use of mupirocin.

There is general agreement that tunneled, cuffed catheters are associated with less risk of infection. However, the available data are scarce and methodologically questionable. In a non-controlled study [52] using Hickman catheters, the authors found a lower rate of CR-BSI (0.8 episodes/1000 catheter-days) than that previously reported by the same group. In another paper [53], eighty tunneled, cuffed catheters were compared prospectively to standard double-lumen catheters. Incidence of bacteremia was significantly lower in the tunneled device group (1.3% vs. 3.6%), but exit site infection was higher (29% vs. 9%). Recently has been introduced a two separated single lumen catheter by Canaud *et al.* [54] in an attempt to provide a higher blood flow and prolonge its duration; infection rates are similar to other types of tunneled devices.

Likewise, there is not enough information to sustain the use of antiseptic or antimicrobial-impregnated catheters(silver, clorhexidine, cefa-

TABLE 4. Guidelines for the treatment of CR-BSI

Type of catheter	Management of Catheter	Antibiotics
Temporary catheter	Remove	Systemic antibiotic for 2 weeks
Prolonged catheter	1. Remove	Systemic antibiotic for 2 weeks
	2. Non-remove (salvage)	Systemic antibiotic for 2–3 weeks plus antibiotic-lock
	3. Change over guidewire 3.1. same tunnel (non-infected) 3.2. new tunnel (if infected)	Systemic antibiotic for 2–3 weeks

zoline, etc.). Even though there are studies that show beneficial effects in other kind of patients [55], there is no evidence to prove the results are similar in hemodialysis setting. A randomized study carried out in 100 patients using silver-impregnated catheters could not demonstrate any preventive effect of this type of catheter on colonization rate, which, on the other hand, are more expensive [56]. Finally, a small series of four patients with silver-impregnated cuffed catheters was compared to another four patients with regular catheters. The latter had less infectious complications that the study group [57].

Replacement of the catheter over a guidewire, which is common practice and is safe in critically ill patients [58], has not been studied enough in hemodialysis patients. Uldall [59] compared the weekly replacement over a guidewire with the clinically indicated replacement, and did not find differences in the infection rates between the two groups.

There are no data about the effect of prophylactic antibiotics in hemodialysis catheters, but if we take into account the results in others settings [17], such practice is not recommended.

Several studies have shown that infection rate is less frequent when the subclavian vein is used as the placement site [17], and that is the reason why it has been the insertion site of choice until recently. The frequency with which subclavian vein stenosis and thrombosis occurs [60–62] has determined the preference for the internal jugular vein. There is controversy about the femoral vein, traditionally considered to be more risk and used for just a few days. However, some studies shown that it can be used as a prolonged access without major infection risk. Montagnac *et al.* [63] found a colonization rate of 21.8% in a group of 55 patients with silicone-rubber femoral catheters that in average stayed for 41 days. In another study [64] carried out with polyurethane double-lumen catheters in hospitalized patients, the rate of infection found was not higher than usual, even though the time of permanence was seven days.

In 1995, the National Kidney Foundation established a Task Force to define guidelines for improving the dialysis patient quality of life and life expectancy. The NKF-DOQI (National Kidney Foundation – Dialysis Outcomes Quality Initiative) review all literature pertinent available and developed these evidence-based clinical practice guidelines [65]. Recommendations formulated regarding the prevention of infection related to catheters are:

a) Trained dialysis staff should only perform hemodialysis-catheter dressing changes and catheter manipulations (evidence/opinion).
b) Catheter exit site should be examined at each hemodialysis treatment for signs of infection (opinion).
c) Catheter exit site dressings should be changed at each hemodialysis session (opinion).
d) Use of sterile gauze and povidone-iodine ointment at the catheter exit site is recommended (evidence/opinion).

e) During catheter connection and disconnection procedures, nurses and patients should wear a surgical mask. Nurses should also wear sterile gloves (opinion).
f) Manipulating a catheter and accessing the patient's bloodstream should be performed in a manner that minimizes contamination. Hubs should be disinfected with povidone-iodine during three to five minutes. Hubs should be covered in order to prevent exposure.

Treatment

Standard treatment of catheter-related infections consists of removing the catheter and the use of systemic antibiotics, followed by the placement of another catheter in a new site. However, this modality of treatment implies the loss of venous access, which is critical in ESRD, because of the need to preserve the vascular bed.

The therapeutic approach of CRI implies making decisions in two different issues: 1) selection of the appropriate antibiotic and via of administration; 2) management of the infected catheter, which includes three alternatives: removal, permanence, or replacement over a guidewire [66].

1) **Antibiotic therapy.** When a catheter-related infection is suspected, systemic empiric antibiotic therapy must be started, based upon the prevailing organisms and its sensitivity pattern. As was previously mentioned, in 70–80% of the cases, the causative organisms are *Staphylococci*, which are frequently resistant to methicillin, and *Entherococcus*. For that reason, the antibiotic of choice is vancomycin, which has the supplementary advantage of low dosage requirement (1 g weekly), because of the impairment of renal function and no extraction by standard dialysis membranes [67]. An aminoglycoside must be added in order to cover Gram-negative aerobic bacilli; dosage must also be adapted to renal function and body mass (amikacin: 7 mg/kg body-weight, post-dialysis). Seric levels of vancomycin and aminoglycoside must be monitored to avoid toxicity. Once the agent has been identified and susceptibility data are available, therapy should be adjusted accordingly. The widespread use of vancomycin must be discouraged because their relatively less antimicrobial activity, with regard to anti-staphyloccocal beta-lactamines and the risk of vancomycin-resistant enterococcus selection [68, 69], which is emerging as a frequent pathogen in this population. Cefazolin, in a schedule of 20 mg/kg post-dialysis, has shown satisfactory results in the case of methicillin-sensitive *S. aureus* [70, 71].

Some authors have suggested the use of antibiotics in the lumen of the catheter (antibiotic-lock) [36, 72], in an attempt to salvage the catheter in patients with limited sites for placement of future accesses, but the results have not been satisfactory.

2) **Catheter management.** This is a controversial issue in the treatment of catheter-associated infections. The common practice in CR-BSI is the immediate removal of the colonized device, which implies the elimination of the infectious focus and enhances the chances of cure. However, this practice reduces the vascular bed of the patient and limits the possibilities of future accesses. Alternative modalities of treatment have been proposed with the aim to preserve the venous site access. The type of catheter to be used is of uttermost importance in the decision making process.

Non-tunneled catheter. There is a general agreement in that single-lumen or double-lumen, non-tunneled, non-cuffed catheters must be removed [58], placing a new catheter in another venous access.

Tunneled catheter. On the contrary, when prolonged, tunneled, cuffed, double-lumen or twin catheters are used, salvage of catheter or the venous access where it is placed could be attempted. Two alternatives have been suggested: 1) maintenance of catheter in place, 2) replacement over guidewire using the same venous access. Some authors [36, 72, 73] have obtained satisfactory results using the catheter salvage technique (catheter maintenance and systemic antibiotics), but the reports are brief and do not include many cases. Other researchers did not get satisfactory results. Marr *et al.* [74], successfully achieved cure without removing the catheter in only 32% of 62 episodes of CR-BSI. Swartz *et al.* [75] were able to keep the catheter in place in 31% of his patients and Moss *et al.* [21] in 25%. Based on these results, catheter replacement over a guidewire keeping the same venous access has been suggested. This procedure may be rehearsed if the access is not severely infected (sepsis, endocarditis or other metastatic colonizations) and if the tunnel or the exit site is not infected. In these cases, the catheter may be placed in the same vein through a new tunnel [76]. In a series of 21 catheters, the replacement over a guidewire failed in the four cases in which the exit site was infected [77]. Robinson *et al.* [37] achieved a resolution rate of 92% in a series of 23 cases of CR-BSI without infection on the exit site, treated with replacement over a guidewire and three weeks of systemic antibiotics. In a short series of 13 episodes of persistent bacteremia in spite of the systemic antibiotic and in which the tunnel was not infected, Schaffer [38] achieved cure of infection in all the cases by combining the replacement over a guidewire with a new tunnel and a short systemic antibiotic course (one to two weeks), even in those cases of mycotic infection. In a recent work, Beathard [76] prospectively studied a series of CR-BSI in hemodialysis patients that he divided into three categories: 1) minimal symptoms without skin infection, in which he replaced the catheter over a guidewire after a 48-hour-treatment with systemic antibiotics; 2) minimal symptoms with tunnel or exit site infection, in which he replaced the catheter over a guidewire and created a new tunnel; 3) severe clinical symptoms, which were treated by removing and delayed replacement. In all cases systemic antibiotics were used for three weeks. According to these practices, cure rates were 87.8%, 75%, and 86.5% respectively.

Infection of the exit site without systemic infection is treated topically. If it persists, systemic antibiotics are prescribed. Tunnel suppuration is treated with systemic antibiotics.

To summarize:

1. *CR-BSI in non-tunneled catheters:* catheter removal, with replacement in other venous site, associated with systemic antibiotics.
2. *CR-BSI in tunneled catheters: 2.1. Catheter removal*; with replacement of a new non-tunneled catheter and systemic antibiotics. Criteria for the removal are severe infection (sepsis, endocarditis, osteoarthritis, spinal epidural abscess); persistent bacteremia beyond 48–72 hours of antibiotic therapy or worsening of clinical status; blood cultures positives to fungi; tunnel suppuration.

   2.2. Non-removal of catheter; 2.2.1. Salvage of catheter with systemic antibiotics and antibioticlock (not recommended) 2.2.2. Replacement over a guidewire and insertion of a new tunneled catheter in the same venous site. If there is tunnel suppuration it can be tried to maintain the venous site and do the replacement through a new tunnel.

   In all cases, systemic antibiotic therapy selected according to susceptibility of the offending organism must be associated during 2–3 weeks.
3. *Exit site infection.* Antiseptic or local antibiotic treatment (mupirocin, yodo-povidone, chlorhexidine).
4. *Tunnel infection.* It is recommended to remove the catheter and administrate systemic antibiotics, but replacement over a guidewire with a new tunnel could be attempted.

References

1. U.S. Renal Data System. USRDS 1997 Annual Data Report. National Institutes of Health, NIDDK, Bethesda, April, 1997.
2. Vanholder R, Van Loo A, Dhondt AM, De Smet R, Ringoir S. Influence of uremia and haemodialysis on host defense and infection. Nephrol Dial Transplant 11:593, 1996.
3. Hakim RM. Clinical implications of hemodialysis membrane bioincompatibility. Kidney Int 44:484, 1993.
4. Maki DG, Weise CE, Sarafin HW. Semiquantitative culture method for identifying intravenous

catheter-related infections. N Engl J Med 196:1305, 1977.

5. Cleri DJ, Corrado ML, Seligrnan SJ. Quantitative culture of intravenous catheters and other intravascular inserts. J Infect Dis 141:781, 1980.
6. Brun-Bussion C, Abroug F, Legrand P, Huet Y, Larabe S, Rapin M, Diagnosis of central venous catheter-related sepsis. Critical level of quantitative tips cultures. Arch Intern Med 47:873, 1987.
7. Rello J, Gatell JM, Almirall J, Campistol JM, González J, Puig de la Bellacasa J. Evaluation of cultures techniques for identification of catheter-related infection in hemodialysis patients. Eur J Clin Microbiol Infect Dis 8:620, 1989.
8. American College of Chest Physicians, Society of Critical Care Medicine Consensus Conference. Definitions for sepsis and organ failure and guidelines for the use of innovative therapies in sepsis. Crit Care Med 20:864, 1992.
9. Cheesbrough JS, Finch RG, Burden RP. A prospective study of the mechanisms of infection associated with hemodialysis catheters. J Infect Dis 154:579, 1986.
10. Almirall J, Conzalez J, Rello J, Campistol JM, Montoliu J, Puig de la Bellacasa J, Revert L, Gatell JM. Infection of hemodialysis catheters: incidence and mechanisms. Am J Nephrol 9:454, 1989.
11. Power NR, Jaar B, Furth SL, Hermann J, Briggs W. Septicemia in dialysis patients: incidence, risk factors, and prognosis. Kidney Int 55:1081, 1999.
12. Hoen B, Paul-Dauphin A, Hestin D, Kessler M. EPIBACDIAL: A multicenter prospective study of risk factors for bacteremia in chronic hemodialysis patients. J Am Soc Nephrol 9:869, 1998.
13. Marr KA, Kong LK, Fowler VG, Gopal A, Sexton DJ, Conlon PJ, Corey GR. Incidence and outcome of Staphylococcus aureus bacteremia in hemodialysis patients. Kidney Int 54:1684, 1998.
14. Hoen B, Kessler M, Hestin D, Mayeux D. Risk factors for bacterial infections in chronic hemodialysis adult patients: a multicenter prospective survey. Nephrol Dial Transplant 10:377, 1995.
15. Taylor GD, McKenzie M, Buchanan-Chell M, Caballo L, Chui L, Kowalewska-Grochowska K. Central venous catheter as a source of hemodialysis-related bacteremia. Infect Control Hosp Epidemiol 19:643, 1998.
16. Nielsen J, Kolmos HJJ, Espersen F. Staphylococcus aureus bacteraemia among patients undergoing dialysis – focus on dialysis catheter-related cases. Nephrol Dial Transplant 13:139, 1998.
17. Pearson ML and the Hospital Infection Control Practices Advisory Committee. Guideline for prevention of intravascular device-related infections. Am J Infect Control 24:262, 1996.
18. Lombardi R. Unpoblished.
19. Vanherweghem JL, Dhaene M, Goldman M, Stolear JC, Sabot JP, Waterlot Y, Serruys E, Thayse C. Infections associated with subclavian dialysis catheters: the key role of nurse training. Nephron 42:116, 1986.
20. Dryden MS, Samson A, Ludlam HA, Wing AJ, Phillips I. Infective complications associated with the use of Quínton Permcath for long-term central vascular access for hemodialysis patients. J Hosp Infect 19:257, 1991.
21. Moss AH, Vasilakis C, Holley JL, Foulks CJ, Pillai K, McDowell DE. Use of a silicone dual-lumen catheter with a Dacron cuff as a long-term vascular access for hemodialysis patients. Am J Kidney Dis 16:211, 1990.
22. Prabhu PN, Kems SR, Sabatelli FW, Hawkins IF, Ross EA. Long-term performance and complications of the Tease twin catheter system for hemodialysis access. Am J Kidney Dis 30:213, 1997.
23. Raad I, Costerton W, Sabharwal U, Sacilowski M, Anaissie E, Bodey GP. Ultraestructural analysis of indwelling vascular catheters: a quantitative relationship between luminal colonization and duration of placement. J Infect Dis 168:400, 1993.
24. Sitges-Serra A, Puig P, Liñares J, Pérez JL, Farreró N, Jaurrieta E, Garau J. Hub colonization as the initial step in an outbreak of catheter-related sepsis due to coagulase negative Staphylococci during parenteral nutrition. J Parent Enter Nutrit 8:668, 1984.
25. Bargman JM. Nasal carriage of Staphylococcus aureus in dialysis patients. Seminars in Dialysis 8:220, 1995.
26. Wanten GJA, Schneeberger PM, Bevers A, van Ginneken E, Koolen MI. Optimizing screening procedures for Staphylococcus aureus nasal carriage in patients on hemodialysis. Nephrol Dial Transplant 13:1256, 1998.
27. Nielsen J, Daustrand Ladefoged S, Kolmos HJJ. Dialysis catheter-related septicaemia – focus on Staphylococcus aureus septicaemia. Nephrol Dial Transplant 13:2847, 1998.
28. Dittmer ID, Sharp D, McNulty CAM, Williams

AJ, Banks RA. A prospective study of central venous hemodialysis catheter colonization and peripheral bacteremia. Clin Nephrol 51:34, 1999.

29. Hung KY, Tsai TJ, Yen CJ, Yen TS. Infection associated with double lumen catheterization for temporary haemodialysis: experience of 168 cases. Nephrol Dial Transplant 10:247, 1995.
30. Goldblum SE, Reed WP. Host defenses and immunologic alterations associated with chronic hemodialysis. Ann Intern Med 93:597, 1980.
31. Briggs WA, Pedersen MM, Mahajan SK, Sillix DH, Prasad AS, McDonald FD. Lymphocyte and granulocyte function in zinc-treated and zinc-deficient hemodialysis patients. Kidney Int 21:827, 1982.
32. Churchill DN, Taylor W, Cook RJ, LaPlante P, Barre P, Cartier P, Fay WP, Goldstein MB, Jindal K, Mandin H, McKenzie JK, Muirhead N, Parfrey PS, Posen GA, Slaughter D, Ulan RA, Werb R. Canadian hemodialysis morbidity study. Am J Kidney Dis 19:214, 1992.
33. Kessler M, Hoen B, Mayeux D, Hestin D, Fontenaille C. Bacteremia in patients on chronic hemodialysis. Nephron 64:95, 1993.
34. Boelaert JR, Daneels RF, Schugers ML, Matthys EG, Goedts BZ, Van Landuyt HW. Iron overload in hemodialysis patients increase the risk of bacteremia: a prospective study. Nephrol Dial Transplant 5:130, 1990.
35. Bonomini V, Coli Ren, Scolari MP, Stefoni S. Structure of dialysis membranes and long-term clinical outcome. Am J Nephrol 15:455, 1995.
36. Capdevila JA, Segarra A, Planes AM, Ramirez-Arellano M, Pahissa A, Piera L, Martínez-Vázquez JM. Successful treatment of hemodialysis catheter-related sepsis without catheter removal. Nephrol Dial Transplant 8:231, 1993.
37. Robinson D, Suhocki P, Schwab SJ. Treatment of infected tunneled venous access hemodialysis catheters with guidewire exchange. Kidney Int 53:1792, 1998.
38. Shaffer D. Catheter-related sepsis complicating long-term, tunneled central venous dialysis catheters: management by guidewire exchange. Am J Kidney Dis 25:593, 1995.
39. Curtis JR, Wing AJ, Coleman JC. Bacillus cereus bacteraemia. A complication of intermittent haemodialysis. Lancet i:136, 1967.
40. Capdevila JA, Planes AM, Palomar M, Gasser I, Almirante B, Pahissa A, Crespo E, Martínez-Vázquez JM. Value of differential quantitative blood culture in the diagnosis of catheter-related sepsis. Eur J Clin Microbiol Infect Dis 11:403, 1992.
41. Fan ST, Teoh-Chan CH, Lau KF. Evaluation of central venous catheter sepsis by differencial quantitative blood culture. Eur J Clin Microbiol Infect Dis 8:142, 1989.
42. Torda AJ, Gottlieb T, Bradbury R. Pyogenic vertebral osteomyelitis: analysis of 20 cases and review. Clin Infect Dis 20:320, 1995.
43. Palermo F, Boccaletto, Paolin A, Carniato A, Zoli P, Giusto F, Turra S. Comparison of Technetium-99m-MDP, technetium-99m-WBC and technetium-99m-HIG in musculoeskeletal inflammation. J Nuclear Med 39:516, 1998.
44. Durack, DT, Lukes AS, Bright DK. New criteria for diagnosis of infective endocarditis: utilization of specific echocardiographic findings. Duke Endocarditis Service. Am J Med 96:200, 1994.
45. Robinson DL, Fowler VG, Sexton DJ, Corey RG, Conlon PJ. Bacterial endocarditis in hemodialysis patients. Am J Kidney Dis 30:521, 1997.
46. Lombardi R, Mautone M, Rodríguez O, Alvarez A, Kuster F, Zinno E. 2° Congreso Uruguayo de Nefrología. Montevideo, 1993.
47. Kovalik EC, Raymond JR, Albers FJ, Berkoben M, Butterly DW, Montella B, Conlon PJ. A clustering of epidural abscesses in chronic hemodialysis patients: risk of salvaging access catheters in cases of infection. J Am Soc Nephrol 7:2264, 1996.
48. Obrador GT, Levenson DJ. Spinal epidural abscess in hemodialysis patients: report of three cases and review of the literature. Am J Kidney Dis 27:75, 1996.
49. Conly JM, Grieves K, Peters B. A prospective, randomized study comparing transparent and dry gauze dressings for central venous catheters. J Infect Dis 159:310, 1989.
50. Levin A, Mason AJ, Jindal KK, Fong IW, Goldstein MB. Prevention of hemodialysis subclavian vein catheter infections by topical povidone-iodine. Kidney Int 40:934, 1991.
51. Sesso R, Barbosa D, Leme IL, Sader H, Canzani ME, Manfredi S, Draibe S, Pignatari AC. Staphylococcus aureus prophylaxis in hemodialysis patients using central venous catheter: effect of mupirocin ointment. J Am Soc Nephrol 9:1085, 1998.
52. Capello M, De Pauw L, Bastin G, Prospert F, Delcour C, Thaysse C, Dhaene M, Vanherweghem JL, Kinnaert P. Central venous access for hemodialysis using the Hickman catheter. Nephrol Dial Transplant 4:988, 1989.

53. Schwab SJ, Buller GL, McCann RL, Bollinger PR, Stickel DL. Prospective evaluation of a dacron cuffed hemodialysis catheter for prolonged use. Am J Kidney Dis 11:166, 1988.
54. Canaud B, Beraud JJ, Joyeux H, Mion C. Internal jugular vein cannulation with two silicone rubber catheters: A new and safe temporary vascular access for hemodialysis. Thirty month's experience. Artif Organs 10:397, 1986.
55. Maki DG, Stolz SM, Wheeler S, Mermel LA. Prevention of central venous catheter-related bloodstream infection by use of an antiseptic-impregnated catheter. Ann Int Med 127:257, 1997.
56. Trerotola SO, Kraus M, Johnson MS, Harris VJ, Snidow JJ, Shah H, McKusky M. Randomized study of silver coating (Silvergard) for prevention of infection in tunneled hemodialysis catheters. J Am Soc Nephrol 7:1422, 1996.
57. Diskin CJ, Stokes TJ. Efficacy of an attachable silver impregnated subcutaneous cuff for the prevention of catheter-associated infections in patients on chronic maintenance hemodialysis. Nephron 69:357, 1995.
58. Hagley MT, Martin B, Gast P, Traeger SM. Infectious and mechanical complications of central venous catheters placed by percutaneous venipuncture and over guidewires. Crit Care Med 20:1426, 1992.
59. Uldall PR. Subclavian cannulation for hemodialysis. Int Artif Org 4:213, 1981.
60. Clark DD, Albina JE, Chazan JA. Subclavian vein stenosis and thrombosis: a potential serious complication in chronic hemodialysis patients. Am J Kidney Dis 15:265, 1990.
61. Cimochowski GE, Worley E, Rutherford WE, Sartain JA, Blondin J, Harter H. Superiority of the internal jugular over the subclavian access for temporary dialysis. Nephron 54:154, 1990.
62. Hernandez, D, Díaz F, Suria S, Machado M, Lorenzo V, Losada M, González-Posada JM, De Bonis E, Domínguez ML, Rodríguez AP, Torres A. Subclavian catheter-related infection is a major risk factor for the late development of subclavian vein stenosis. Nephrol Dial Transplant 8:227, 1993.
63. Montagnac R, Bernard C, Gullaumie J, Hanhart P, Clavel P, Yazji J, Martínez LM, Schillinger F. Indwelling silicone femoral catheters: experience of three hemodialysis centers. Nephrol Dial Transplant 12:772, 1997.
64. Kirkpatrick WG, Culpepper RM, Sirmon MD. Frequency of complications with prolonged femoral vein catheterization for hemodialysis access. Nephron 73:58, 1996.
65. NKF-DOQI Clinical Practice Guidelines for Vascular access. Am J Kidney Dis 30(supp 3):S167, 1997.
66. Schwab SJ, Beathard G. The hemodialysis catheter conundrum: hate living with them, but can't live without them. Kidney Int 56:1, 1999.
67. DeSoi CA, Sahm DF, Umans JG. Vancomycin elimination during high-flux hemodialysis: kinetic model and comparison of four membranes. Am J Kidney Dis 20:354, 1992.
68. Brady JP, Snyder JW, Hasbargen JA. Vancomycin-resistant enterococcus in end-stage renal disease. Am J Kidney Dis 32:415, 1998.
69. Tokars JI. Vancomycin use and antimicrobial resistance in hemodialysis centers. Am J Kidney Dis 32:521, 1998.
70. Marx MA, Frye RF, Matzke GR, Golper TA. Cefazolin as empiric therapy in hemodialysis-related infections: efficacy and blood concentrations. Am J Kidney Dis 32:410, 1998.
71. Fogel MA, Nussbaum PB, Feintzeig ID, Hunt WA, Gavin JP, Kim RC. Cefazolin in chronic hemodialysis patients: a safe, effective alternative to vancomycin. Am J Kidney Dis 32:401, 1998.
72. Domoto DT, Kennedy DJ. Antibiotic treatment of chronic central venous hemodialysis catheter infection without catheter removal. Int J Artif Org 10:239, 1987.
73. Donnelly PK, Hoenich NA, Lennard TWJ, Proud G, Taylos RMR. Surgical management of long-term central venous access in uraemic patients. Nephrol Dial Transplant 3:57, 1988.
74. Marr KA, Sexton DJ, Conlon PJ, Corey GR, Schwab SJ, Kirkland KB. Catheter-related bactereima and outcome of attempted catheter salvage in patients undergoing hemodialysis. Ann Intern Med 127:275, 1997.
75. Swartz RD, Messana JM, Boyer CJ, Lunde NM, Weitzel WF. Successful use of cuffed central venous hemodialysis catheters inserted percutaneously. J Am Soc Nephrol 4:1719, 1994.
76. Beathard GA. Management of bacteremia associated with tunneled-cuffed hemodialysis catheters. J Am Soc Nephrol 10:1045, 1999.
77. Carlisle EJ, Blake P, McCarthy F, Vas S, Uldall R. Septicemia in long-term jugular hemodialysis catheters; eradicating infection by changing the catheter over a guidewire. Int J Artif Organs 14:150, 1991.

33. INFECTION OF PULMONARY ARTERIAL CATHETER AND PERIPHERAL ARTERIAL CATHETER

Alejandro Rodríguez, Sandra Arcieri and Jordi Rello

Background

The pulmonary arterial catheter (PAC) and peripheral arterial catheter (AC) are used frequently in the management of critically ill patients, but not without risk. The use of the catheter has been associated with complications such as infection of the catheter insertion site and catheter-related infection with and without subsequent catheter-related bacteremia (CRB) [1].

Current information about infections associated with the central venous catheter is extensive. However, less information is available about arterial catheters used temporarily in specific hospital areas like the intensive care unit (ICU). Insertion complications may occur during central venous catheterization, while infectious complications have occurred with catheter maintenance. Recently, Raad [2] estimated that in the USA at least 400,000 episodes of vascular catheter-related bloodstream infection occur every year. The estimated cost of treating one episode for a patient in ICU increased from US$8000 in 1988 to more than US$28,000 in 1994.

In 1979, Band and Maki [3] reported a 4% incidence of catheter-related bacteremia (CRB) associated with an arterial catheter that had remained in place for over 96h. Myres *et al.* [4] reported a catheter-related infection (CRI) rate of 5.8% when the mean duration of catheterization was 4.2 days, while Hudson-Civetta *et al.* [1] reported a 10% rate of positive catheter segment cultures at three days in a large group of patients with sepsis. At the same time, Pinilla *et al.* [5] reported that the rate of infectious complications associated with the internal jugular site (29%) and the antecubital site (20%), was higher than with the subclavian approach (7%). The rates of PAC related-infection and CRB reportedly range from 1.7% to 35% [1–7], which may reflect differences in the patient population and the methods used to recognize infection.

While the most frequently selected arteries for peripheral arterial catheterization are the radial and femoral arteries, there are currently no specific guidelines on the type of catheter (venous/arterial) to use to prevent a catheter-associated infection. Few studies have evaluated the incidence and pathogenesis of colonization and bloodstream infection secondary to the placement of AC.

In this chapter, we summarize current knowledge of infectious complications associated with these catheters and focus on laboratory diagnosis and clinical approach.

Pulmonary Arterial Catheter (PAC)

The benefits of arterial catheterization in critically ill patients must be balanced by the potential technical and septic risks. The risk of CRI from PAC has been difficult to assess due to the reported variable incidence of catheter colonization (ranging from 5.8 [4] to 40% [8]) and bloodstream infection (ranging from 0% [4, 9–11] to 10% [13]). Characteristics of pulmonary arterial catheter colonization or bloodstream infection are shown in Table 1. As Rello *et al.* [14] state, these results are heterogeneous and cannot be compared since they have used different methods of diagnosis, incomplete data or too few cases. Also, they have different populations and risk factors.

The cumulative incidence of bloodstream infection associated with PAC is generally low, i.e. <5% in most reports (Table 1). In contrast, the cumulative incidence of colonization is generally high, ranging from 5.8% to 40%. Given that in most series the period of catheterization is short, the incidence of colonization 1.3 to 15.5 per 100 days of catheterization [4, 8]. Local inflammation at the insertion site (erythema, cellulitis, etc) occurs in 0.9 to 16% of patients [14, 19] and is usually resolved by withdrawing the catheter.

In CRI, bacteria may gain access to the bloodstream in two ways: they may migrate from the catheter-skin interface over the external surface or down the internal surface of the catheter to the catheter tip. Widmer [27] thinks that the physician should adhere strictly to the recommendation that PAC should be replaced after five days, because the risk of CRI or CRB after five days is substantial, i.e. up to 80% after 14 days of catheterization.

There are several potential sources of microorganism contamination for catheter colonization and bloodstream infection. Maki *et al.* [28] believe that the external surface is the most important source of infection because [27]:

1. The colonization of the catheter is mainly detected by microorganisms on the external surface.
2. Bacteria have been shown to move along the outer surface, possibly by capillary action.
3. There is a strong link between the semi-quantitative culture (SQC) of the external surface and CRB.
4. Colonization of the skin is a strong predictor of CRI and CRB.
5. Topical disinfectants reduce the rate of infection.
6. Maximal barrier precautions taken at the time of catheter insertion prevent infection.

The catheter may be colonized internally secondary to contamination of the hub or infusate derivate from skin or infusate. Nevertheless, cutaneous colonization of the device at the insertion site is the main source of microorganism contamination. Hubs are frequently colonized, and their contribution as a primary source of infection is well established [25, 26]. Recently, Liñares *et al.* [29] have highlighted the importance of hubs as a source of microorganism contamination in parenteral nutrition catheters. Similarly, PAC hubs are frequently manipulated by caregivers, usually without optimal aseptic technique. Moreover, repeatedly injecting a frozen saline solution to monitor cardiac output, drawing multiple blood samples for biochemical tests, measuring oxygen pressure in mixed venous blood and repeatedly manipulating the catheter to administer drugs to critically ill patients increase the risk of bloodstream infection from hubs [14]. Bacteria can migrate from the hub to the tip of the catheter while protected from any host-defense mechanism. This hypothesis is also supported by findings in animal models [30] and clinical studies [31]. Furthermore, higher rates of CRI have been reported with triple-lumen catheters (three hubs) than with single-lumen catheters (one hub) [32].

Finally, as Widmer [27] states, contamination of the skin at the insertion site may be the most important variable in short-term catheterization, whereas the hub becomes more important as a source of infection as the duration of catheterization increases.

The microbes involved in both catheter colonization and bloodstream infection include: coagulase-negative staphylococci, *Staphylococcus aureus*, *Streptococcus* sp, Gram-negative bacilli (such as *Pseudomonas* sp., *Proteus* sp., *Escherichia coli*, or *Klebsiella* sp.) and *Candida albicans*. [8, 18]. In a prospective study, Rello *et al.* [7]

TABLE 1. Characteristics of pulmonary arterial colonization or bloodstream infection. Adapted from [14]

Ref.	ICU[a]	Design[b]	Culture[c]	Nr. cases	Days[d]	Bacteremia (%)	Colonization (%)	Colonization (×100 d)
15	Q	P	Qual.	57	3.2	0	25	7.81
16	C	R	Qual.	152	2.5	0	30	12.00
17	G	P	–	71	2.8	2.8	–	–
18	M	P	Qual.	153	–	0	19	–
19	G	P	Semi.	37	3.5	–	8.1	2.31
20	G	P	Semi.	133	2.6	2	10	3.84
21	G	P	Semi.	31	2.9	–	6.4	2.2
5	Q	P	Semi.	37	–	2.7	16	–
13	G	P	Quan.	10	–	10	20	–
22	G	P	Semi.	12	6.0	0	33.3	5.55
4	Q	P	Semi.	170	4.4	0	5.8	1.31
23	Q	P	Semi.	63	3.0	0	6.1	2.03
8	G	P	Quan.	20	2.6	–	40	15.83
1	Q	P	Semi.	49	3.0	0	10.2	3.4
24	G	P	Semi.	272	–	5	12	–
9	Q	P	Semi	102	3.5	0	5.9	1.68
11	Q	P	Semi	50	2.5	0	6	2.4
25	Q	P	Semi	297	3.0	0.7	21.9	–
7	G	P	Semi	69	4.5	2.9	21.7	4.98
26	Q	P	Semi.	442	3.1	1.1	21.7	6.8
12	G	P	Semi.	66	5.0	0	28.7	5.6

[a] Intensive Care Unit: Q: Surgical, C: Coronary, G: General, M: Medical.
[b] Design: P: prospective; R: Retrospective.
[c] Culture: Qual.: qualitative; Semi.: Semiquantitative; Quan.: Quantitative.
[d] Mean days of catheterization.

analyzed 69 PAC that remained *in situ* over 24 h in a general ICU. Eighteen strains of microorganisms were isolated from 15 catheters. In 13 (72.2%) cases, the pathogens identified were coagulase-negative staphylococci, which were simultaneously recovered from the skin around the insertion site in 10 cases. The remaining five pathogens isolated were Gram-negative bacilli, which were isolated from the hubs but not from the insertion site. These findings suggest the need to culture hubs when pulmonary arterial catheter-related bloodstream infection is suspected.

Henderson [33] grouped risk factors for CRI and CRB into patient-related factors and hospital-related factors. Age, altered host defense mechanism, the severity of the underlying disease, remote infections and sepsis are all considered patient-related risk factors and cannot usually be altered but should be considered when developing catheter maintenance protocols [34].

Hospital-related factors include catheter type and material, insertion sites, type of placement (percutaneous vs cutdown), duration of site use, emergency vs selective placement, the skill of the individual who places the catheter and alteration in skin microflora [34].

In particular, several risk factors have been considered regarding PAC infection, but the most frequently analyzed variable is probably the length of catheterization. This may be a co-factor in the severity of the underlying illness; septic patients are at a much higher risk than nonseptic patients. The length of hospitalization prior to catheter insertion may also be a risk factor, but this is difficult to distinguish from the severity of illness [34].

A decade ago the Center of Disease Control recommended in its guidelines for preventing intravascular infections "the proper and frequent changing of central venous cannulas that are used for pressure monitoring" [35]. Several studies have demostrated a significant increase in the rate of positive PAC aspirate cultures [15], catheter-related infection [36] and intra-arterial catheter-related infection [3] after 72h *in situ*. In their study, Hudson-Civetta *et al.* [1] evaluated the risk of PAC infection in septic surgical patients but found no cases of bloodstream infection after 72h of catheterization and no relationship between the percentage of positive catheter-aspirate cultures and the duration of catheterization. However, all subjects received antibodies to treat their primary infection. On the other hand, Sise *et al.* [37], using a qualitative culture method, found that local and other septic complications are infrequent within the first 72h but rise significantly thereafter. Another study [38] used a protocol to determine whether PAC sites (and those of other types of catheters) could be used for longer periods to avoid the risk of repeating central venopunctures. The rate of CRI increased in nonseptic patients when catheter use was extended from four days to six (33% vs 12%, $p < 0.05$). There was also a strong relationship between number of days of catheter placement in ICU and the likelihood of subsequent CRI, e.g. catheters placed at ≤ six days versus those placed after seven days ($p < 0.05$).

Infections are probably more frequent when catheters are exposed to bloodstream infections from other sites [1, 15], or where there are local signs of inflammation at the insertion site [15]. Senagore *et al.* [23] prospectively studied the infection rate by evaluating two different vascular accesses (subclavian vein vs jugular vein) and whether they were replaced by new puncture or through a wide guide; they found no significant differences. An earlier randomized trial [39] to evaluate scheduled replacement was carried out on 112 patients and 460 catheters. It compared the changes performed every seven days either with guide-assistance or new puncture sites with the changes performed with new puncture sites when indicated clinically. There were no significant differences in the complication rates between the three groups, but infections and mechanical complications were slightly more frequent in patients in the scheduled-change group than in the group whose catheters were changed when indicated clinically. Recently, in another randomized trial, Cobb *et al.* [40] compared four methods of catheter exchange. These were: replacement every three days either by insertion at a new site (group 1), exchange over a guide wire (group 2), replacement when clinically indicated by insertion at a new site (group 3) or exchange over a guide wire (group 4). The incidence rates (per 100 days of catheter use) of bloodstream infection were: 3 in group 1, 6 in group 2, 2 in group 3 and 3 in group 4. The incidence rates of mechanical complications were 14%, 4%, 8% and 3% for groups 1, 2, 3, and 4 respectively, and the patients randomly assigned to guide-wire-assisted exchange were more likely to have bloodstream infection after the first three days of catheterization (6% vs 0%, $p < 0.05$). The authors concluded that routinely replacing central vascular catheters every three days does not prevent infection, but exchanging catheters with a guide-wire increased the risk of bloodstream infection.

Since most of the clinical and epidemiologic variables often cited affect the risk of CRI and CRB, a multivariate statistical analysis such as multiple logistic regression is the only way to identify which variables independently influence the risk after adjustment has been made for all others. Table 2 summarizes the results of three reports [7, 9, 41] that evaluated potential risk factors by multivariate analysis. In the study by Rello *et al.* [7] twenty potential risk factors were analyzed. Only seven variables had an odds ratio (OR) >2. These were: 1) the duration of catheterization over 5 days 2) jugular access 3) insertion technique 4) complications 5) diurnal insertion

6) absence of microbial use, and 7) cardiorespiratory arrest. However, when these variables were included in the logistic regression analysis only the duration of catheterization (>5 days) was statistically linked to a greater risk of PAC colonization. In contrast, antimicrobial use was associated with negative cultures.

It is difficult to diagnose CRI and CRB. Clinical criteria alone, such as fever or inflammation at the catheter insert site, are nonspecific and usually of little help [42, 43]. When CRI is suspected it is common practice to remove the catheter and replace it at a new site. However, 80 to 90% of new febrile episodes in patients in intensive care are not caused by catheter infection. It has therefore been estimated that 75 to 85% of catheters are removed unnecessarily during new fever episode [40, 42, 44]. So the increased risks of infection or traumatic complications secondary to unnecessary catheter replacement should also be considered.

TABLE 2. Risk factors for colonization of pulmonary-artery catheter. Adapted from [14]

Risk Factors for Colonization for Multivariate Analyses		
Ref.	Risk Factor	Odds Ratio
9	Children	–
	Long catheterization	–
	Inotropic use	–
40	Skin colonization	5.5
	Jugular access	4.3
	>3 days	3.1
	Antisepsis violation	2.1
7	>5 days	2.1
	Antibiotic use	0.2

"Catheter-related infection" is an imprecise term. Erroneous delineation of contamination, colonization and true catheter-related infection can lead to confusion and an incorrect interpretation of this paper. Table 3 shows, therefore, which definitions of catheter infection are now generally accepted [27, 34]. Clinical markers show a poor correlation with infection associated with PAC or central-venous lines. Laboratory tests are therefore needed to confirm a clinically suspected diagnosis of CRI. Interpretation of the laboratory results depends on the culture method and the gold standard used. Diagnostic methods can be classified as:

a) *Qualitative broth culture*, when colonies are not counted. This method is highly sensitive but not very specific and does not help to distinguish contamination from infection.
b) *Semi-quantitative culture*, when the specimen is cultured directly and the colonies are counted on agar plates to allow an enumeration just within a limited range. This technique has several important limitations: only the external surface of the catheter is

TABLE 3. Definitions on catheter infection

Term	Definition
Catheter-related infection (CRI)	Catheter segment culture with presence of = or > 15 colonies on a blood-agar by semiquantitative culture*
Catheter-related bacteremia (CRB)	Isolated of the same organism from a catheter segment quantitative or semiquantitative culture and from a peripheral blood culture in a patient with sepsis syndrome
Catheter Contamination	Presence in a specimen taken for culture, of organisms introduced by the person collecting the specimen during the course of obtaining the sample
Catheter Colonization	Catheter segment culture with presence of <15 colonies on blood agar by semiquantitative culture

(* For the Centers of Disease Control and Prevention (CDC) definition include necessary sings of infection, fever or elevated white blood cells count, and local signs of inflammation such as erythema).

explored, so endoluminal infections may be undetected. Sensitivity is optimal (almost 100%) but specificity is low (20 to 50%) [43].

c) *Quantitative culture*, when the serial dilutions of original specimen are used for culture. This technique only explores the internal part of the catheter. The quantitative culture technique has been simplified with catheter vortexing in sterile water by Brun-Buisson *et al.* [45]. Both specificity (88%) and sensitivity (97%) are high.

In 1979, Wing *et al.* [46] had the idea of performing cultures of blood withdrawn from the catheter and a peripheral vein. More recently, Hudson-Civetta *et al.* [1] evaluated multiple samples from 49 patients with PAC to confirm the hypothesis that bloodstream infection could be diagnosed on the basis of qualitative catheter-drawn cultures. However, neither blood cultures from peripheral veins, arterial blood, or catheter-drawn blood were found to be useful. This study concluded that pulmonary arterial catheter-related bloodstream infection should only be evaluated with segment-catheter cultures and blood samples drawn by direct venipuncture. Several authors [2, 43, 47], however, state that paired quantitative blood cultures should be used to diagnose CRI. These techniques are based on the premise that, when a bacteremia is linked to a CRI, the number of microorganisms retrieved by the blood culture drawn from the catheter is higher than in the blood peripheral culture. A diagnosis is preposed when the number of colonies isolated from the cultures of blood taken through the vascular catheter is at least five times the number in the culture of a concurrent peripheral blood sample. The predictive value of this method has been studied using threshold for positive between 15 to 10^3 UFC/ml with a specificity of 99% but a sensitivity of just 20% for diagnosing CRI in cancer patients [48]. Fan *et al.* [49] found that differential blood cultures correctly identified seven out of nine infected catheters. In this study, sensitivity was 77.8% and specificity was 100%, with no false-positive results. Similarly, Douard *et al.* [50] found that differential blood cultures had a specificity and positive predictive value of 100%, while their sensitivity (38%) and negative predictive value (78%) were slightly lower. Despite their accuracy, paired cultures are not routinely used in clinical practice, mainly because of their relative complexity and cost.

Passerini *et al.* [8] used electron microscopy and the quantitative culture method in the CRI. They showed that the extent of catheter colonization in internal and external surfaces is different. Even more important is the fact that colonization is not uniform along the length of the catheter surface. This method has no clinical interest, but it questions the real value of using a single segment of the catheter to diagnose colonization. Rello *et al.* [51] evaluated the usefulness of semiquantitative cultures of distal, intradermal and atrial segments (3 cm around the proximal orifice) for diagnosing PAC colonization. In this study, the semiquantitative culture of the tip detected 66% of colonized catheters. Results were similar when the other segment was considered independently. Rello *et al.* therefore concluded that a combination of both intradermal and distal segment cultures is the most practical and reliable method for identifying colonized PAC. In another study, the same authors [52] showed the need to culture both the catheter tip and the introducer segment to obtain an accurate diagnosis of PAC colonization when an indwelling introducer is present. A recent meta-analysis [44] confirmed the superiority of quantitative techniques for catheter segment culture. This method had a higher pooled sensitivity and specificity (above 90%), than semiquantitative or qualitative cultures.

In summary, the optimal way to diagnose CRI and replace PAC is unknown. If temperature inexplicably increases more than 48 h after catheter insertion and there is evidence of local signs of infection with or without positive blood culture, the catheter and introducer can be exchanged and treated according to the results of semiquantitative culture. However, because of

TABLE 4. Preventive Strategies for catheter-related infections

* Maximum sterile barriers
* Cutaneous antimicrobials and antiseptic
* Tunneling
* Ionic silver cuffs
* Infusion therapy team
* Intraluminal antibiotic locks
* Antiseptic hubs
* Antimicrobial coating of catheter

the particularly high colonization rate of the PAC and the introducers, it is recommended that Swan-Ganz catheters be removed before the fifth day of placement.

Infection of short-term catheters is mainly prevented by avoiding contamination of the catheter by the skin flora at the catheter insertion site. As Rello [53] indicated in a recent editorial the best strategy for protecting against colonization from the hub or the skin depends on the conservative affinities (skin hypothesis) or otherwise (hub hypothesis) of the physician. However, the pathogenesis of colonization is probably different in each type of catheter and the results cannot be extrapolated. The full barrier precautions during central-venous catheter insertion significantly reduce the risk of intravenous CRI and CRB [25, 27, 41]. These precautions have been linked to a four-fold decrease in the rate of CRB to PAC [41] and a more than six-fold decrease in the rate of sepsis related to central-venous catheters [54]. Table 4 shows preventive strategies for catheter-related infections. All these preventive strategies should be evaluated at the time of selection. They should never be considered as a substitute for the traditional practice of adhering to an aseptic and careful technique during insertion and maintenance of the catheters [53].

Peripheral Arterial Catheter (AC)

Peripheral arterial catheters (AC) for measuring intra-arterial pressure and monitoring arterial gases are some of the most common devices in an ICU setting. However, few studies have evaluated the true incidence and pathogenesis of colonization and bloodstream infection secondary to the placement of AC.

ACs have a low rate of catheter colonization and bloodstream infection. The incidence of colonization is reported to range from 0% to 22.5% and from 1.1 to 8.8 episodes per 100 days of catheterization (Table 5) [3, 60]. Bloodstream infection associated with AC is uncommon and its incidence ranges from 0 to 0.95 episodes per

TABLE 5. Summary of studies on peripheral catheter. Adapted from [14]

Ref.	ICU[a]	Design[b]	Culture[c]	No. Cases	Days[d]	Bacteremia (%)	Colonization (%)	Colonization (×100 d)
3	G	P	Semi.	130	4.4	3.8	18.0	4.4
19	–	P	Semi.	52	3.3	–	11.1	2.6
5	Q	P	Semi.	172	3.0	0	4.0	1.2
55	P	P	Qual/Semi.	70	2.9	0	0	0
56	Q	P	Semi.	75	4.0	0	9.5	1.19
57	G	P	Semi.	164	6.4	0	22.5	3.49
58	C	P	Semi.	340	2.7	0	2.3	8.8
59	O	P	Semi.	71	–	5.6	16.0	–
60	G	P	Semi.	71	10.6	7.0	36.0	3.4

[a] Intensive care unit: G, polyvalent; Q, surgical; P, pediatric; C, coronary; O, oncologic.
[b] Design: P, prospective.
[c] Culture: Semi., semiquantitative; Qual., qualitative.
[d] Mean period of catheterization.

100 days of catheterization [5, 59]. In the study by Pinilla *et al.* [5], ACs showed a very low rate of catheter infection and were not associated with bacteremia. This infection rate is low possibly because: a) most of the catheters were removed within 4 days b) the vessel is deeply situated c) the catheter shaft is short d) the catheter is secured and inserted more easily (especially in the radial site) e) the staff are more familiar with maintenance, or f) high flow-pressure conditions in the artery may be effective in flushing out potential pathogens and a fast arterial flow may help to prevent bacterial adherence [27].

The skin is probably the most common source of the microorganisms that cause peripheral arterial bloodstream infection [55, 58]. Many clinical and microbiologic data indicate that most catheter-related bacteremias are caused by microorganisms that invade the intracutaneous area surrounding the catheter. Several studies [55, 56, 58] have shown a strong correlation between organisms present on the skin surrounding the catheter wound and microorganisms recovered from a catheter that has been linked to bacteremia.

The organisms responsible are usually coagulase-negative staphylococci and *Staphylococcus aureus* [42]. When rare organisms such as *Candida parapsilosis*, *Serratia marcescens*, *Klebsiella oxytoca*, *Pseudomonas cepacia*, *Acinetobacter baumannii*, or *Flavobacterium* spp. are isolated, contamination of the fluid should be considered, especially inside the transducer assembly [57]. The risk of developing bloodstream infection from infusate contamination is reported to be low and generally occurs in epidemics, especially during summer time [27, 57]. Using normal saline solution in intraarterial infusion, which does not support the growth of most microbial pathogens, probably provides protection against contamination in hemodynamic monitoring [14]. The official recommendations by the CDC [35] that the flush solution be replaced every 24 h and that the tubing and continuous flow device be changed every 48 h are questionable as they are not based on evidence. For instance, Shinozaki *et al.* [61] reported no instance of bacterial fluid contamination irrespective of the duration of catheterization. Ducharme *et al.* [55] reported that manipulating the system as little as possible probably reduces the risk of contamination of both the infusate and insertion site significantly. Good aseptic technique during insertion is therefore much more important than any systematic change.

As with PAC, few studies have attempted to identify the risk factors associated with AC colonization and bloodstream infection. Several studies [3, 55, 57, 59] agreed that systemic antimicrobial therapy does not protect against arterial catheter-related infection. In fact, most episodes of bloodstream infection in these studies occurred in patients receiving antibiotics. In 1979 Band and Maki [3] studied catheter-related infection from AC and determined that three factors were associated with a significant increase in both local and bloodstream catheter-related infections: 1) insertion of the catheter by surgical cutdown (ninefold increase in catheter-related bacteremia) 2) cannulation that exceeded 4 days, and 3) inflammation of the insertion site. The incidence of catheter-related infection was 18%, while 70% of infections occurred in catheters that had been used for more than 96 h. All catheter-related bacteremias in this study occurred in patients whose catheter sites were used for over 96 h. These observations led the Center of Disease Control and Prevention to recommend that AC used for hemodynamic monitoring should not be left in place for longer than four days [62], although bloodstream infection associated with long-term radial artery is extremely uncommon [57].

Most ICU policies recommend the radial artery as first choice, but there are no guidelines that relate site selection to the prevention of catheter-related infection. The femoral artery access is frequently selected in patients with multiple underlying diseases or shock. Some of the advantages of this artery are; the catheters are easy to place, blood specimens can be taken and the incidence of thromboembolism is low.

However, this site is frequently avoided because of the increased possibility of bacterial contamination from the perineal area [19, 63]. Thomas *et al.* [63] conducted a study to evaluate the risk of infection related to radial versus femoral sites for arterial catheterization. They found that the incidence of local infection was similar for both insertion sites. Recently, Frezza and Mezghebe [64] compared the complications rate of AC in an ICU medical to those in an ICU surgical. They found that the rate of infection was similar in both ICUs and between radial and femoral sites (43% in ICU medical and 50% in ICU surgical).

Several researchers have studied the duration of cannulation. Some found that long periods of catheterization increased the cumulative incidence of colonization (%) but did not increase the incidence rate when the days of catheterization were considered [19, 57, 63]. Band and Maki [3] reported that the duration of the arterial catheterization was a major determinant but Thomas *et al.* [63] found no correlation between the incidence of catheter infection and duration of catheterization and questioned whether it was necessary to remove the arterial catheter systematically every four days. In the opinion of Ducahrme *et al.* [55], the risk of catheter infection in children is very low and does not demand systemic replacement. Consequently, the efficacy of periodically changing the arterial catheters as a measure of prevention is still unconfirmed. Leroy *et al.* [57] and Thomas *et al.* [63] have suggested that each hospital should determine its own rate of AC infection and the time of placement that is followed by a significant increase in the infection rate.

The issue of whether the catheter should be replaced remains controversial. However, peripheral arterial catheters and the entire infusion apparatus must be changed if there is: a) ischemia of the distal extremity b) evidence of microembolization c) sign of inflammation at the insertion site d) unsafe location e) unexplained fever, or f) positive blood cultures without an obvious source [14, 34].

As with PAC, the semiquantitative culture technique reported by Maki *et al.* [36] seems to be the best method for diagnosing AC colonization. Bloodstream infection is found almost exclusively among patients with positive semiquantitative AC culture. Fever with no obvious other source is how AC bloodstream infection is most frequently presented.

Acknowledgement

We are indebted to Sandra Trefler B.D. for her active participation in this paper.

References

1. Hudson-Civetta J, Civetta JM, Martines OV, Hoffman TA. Risk and detection of pulmonary artery catheter-related infection in septic surgical patients. Crit Care Med 15:29, 1987.
2. Raad I. Intravascular-catheter-related infections. Lancet 351:893, 1998.
3. Band JD, Maki DG. Infection caused by arterial catheters used for hemodynamic monitoring. Am J Med 67:735, 1979.
4. Myres ML, Austin TW, Sibbald WJ. Pulmonary artery catheter infections. Ann Surg 201:237, 1985.
5. Pinilla JC, Ross DF, Martin T, Crump H. Study of the incidence of intravascular catheter infection and associated septicemia in critically ill patients. Crit Care Med 11:21, 1983.
6. Elliott CG, Zimmerman GA, Clemmer TP. Complications of pulmonary artery catheterization in the care of critically ill patients. Chest 76:647, 1979.
7. Rello, J, Coll P, Net A, Prats G. Infection of pulmonary artery catheters. Chest 103:132, 1993.
8. Passerini L, Phang PT, Jackson Fl, *et al.* Biofilms on right heart flow-directed catheters. Chest 92:440, 1987.
9. Damen J. The microbiologic risk of invasive haemodynamic monitoring in open-heart patients requiring prolongated ICU treatment. Intensive Care Med 14:156, 1988.
10. Jarvis WR, Edwaros JR, Culuer DH, *et al.* Nosocomial infection rates in aduit and pediatsic ICVs in the united states. NNIS system. Am J Med 91:1855–1915, 1991.

11. Levy JH, Nagle DM, Curling PE, *et al.* Contamination reduction during central venous catheterization. Crit Care Med 16:165, 1988.
12. Vallés J, Rello J, Matas L, *et al.* Pulmonary artery catheter colonization: influence of using an indwelling introducer. Eur J Clin Microbiol Infect Dis 15:71, 1996.
13. Miller JJ, Venus B, Mathru M. Comparison of the sterility of long-term central venous catheterization using single lumen, triple lumen and pulmonary artery catheters. Crit Care Med 12:634, 1984.
14. Rello J, Jubert P, Esandi M, Vallés J. Specific problems of arterial, Swan-Ganz, and hemodialysis catheters. Nutrition 13(suppl):36S, 1997.
15. Applefeld JJ, Caruters RE, Reno DJ, Civetta JM. Assessment of the sterility of long-term cardiac catheterization using the thermodilution Swan-Ganz catheter. Chest 74:377, 1978.
16. Prachar H, Dittel M, Jobst CH, *et al.* Bacterial contamination of central venous catheter. Intensive Care Med 4:79, 1978.
17. Puri V, Carlson R, Bamder J, Weil MH. Complications of vascular catheterization in critically ill. Crit Care Med 8:495, 1980.
18. Michel L, Marsh M, McMichan JC, Southorn P, Brewer N. Infection of pulmonary artery catheters in critically ill patients. JAMA 245:1032, 1982.
19. Singh S, Nelson N, Acosta I, Check E, Puri V. Catheter colonization and bacteriemia with pulmonary and arterial catheters. Crit Care Med 10:736, 1982.
20. Kaye W, Wheateon M, Potter-Bynoe G. Radial and pulmonary artery catheter-related sepsis (abstract). Crit Care Med 11:249, 1983.
21. Nelson N, Singh S, Check F, Puri V. Colonization and catheter-related sepsis with pulmonary and arterial sepsis (abstract). Crit Care Med 11:144, 1981.
22. Samsoondar W, Freeman J, Coultish I, Oxley C. Colonization of intravascular catheter in the intensive care unit. Am J Surg 145:730, 1985.
23. Senagore A, Waller J, Bonnel B, Bursch L, Scholten D. Pulmonary artery catheterization: a prospective study of internal jugular and subclavian approach. Crit Care Med 15:35, 1987.
24. Hilton E, Haslett T, Borenstein M, *et al.* Central catheter infections: single versus triple-lumen catheters. Am J Med 84:662, 1988.
25. Mermel LA, Maki DG. Infectious complications of Swan-Ganz pulmonary artery catheters. Pathogenesis, epidemiology, prevention and management. Am J Respir Crit Care Med 149:1020, 1994.
26. Maki DG, Stolz SS, Wheeler S, Mermel LA. A prospective randomized trial of gauze and two polyurethane dressings for site care of pulmonary artery catheters: implications for catheter management. Crit Care Med 15:1729, 1994.
27. Widmer AF. Intravenous-related infections. In Wenzel RP (ed). Prevention and Control of Nosocomial Infections. Williams and Wilkins 1997:771.
28. Maki DG, Goldmann DA, Rhame FS. Infection control in intravenous therapy. Ann Intern Med 79:867, 1973.
29. Liñares J, Sitges-Serra A, Garau J, Pérez JL, Martín R. Pathogenesis of catheter sepsis: a prospective study with quantitative and semiquantitative cultures of catheter hub and segment. J Clin Microbiol 21:357, 1985.
30. Segura M, Alia C, Valverde J, *et al.* Assessment of a new hub design and the semiquantitative catheter culture method using an in vivo experimental model of catheter sepsis. J Clin Microbiol 28:2551, 1990.
31. Segura M, Alvarez-Lerma F, Tellado JM, *et al.* Clinical trail of the effect of a new catheter hub on the prevention of central venous catheter-related sepsis. Interscrience Conference on Antimicrobial Agents and Chemotherapy. San Francisco 1995:258 (Abstract).
32. Yeung C, May J, Hughes R. Infection rate for single lumen versus triple lumen subclavian catheter. Infect Control Hosp Epidemiol 9:154, 1988.
33. Hendreson DK. Intravascular device-associated infection: current concepts and controversies. Infect Surg 7:365, 1988.
34. Norwood S, Ruby A, Civetta J, Cortes V. Catheter-related infections and associated septicemia. Chest 99:968, 1991.
35. Simmons BP, Hooton TM, Wong ES, Allen JR. Guidelines for prevention of intravascular infections. 1982. Springfield, Va: National Technical information service.
36. Maki DG, Weise CE, Sarafin HW. A semiquantitative method for identifying intravenous-catheter-related infection. N Engl J Med 296:1305, 1977.
37. Sise MJ, Hollinhsworth P, Brimm JE. Complications of the flow-directed pulmonary artery catheter: a prospective analysis in 219 patients. Crit Care Med 9:315, 1981.
38. Civetta JM, Hudson-Civetta JA, Dion L. Duration of illness effects catheter-related infection and bacteriemia (abstract). In Program and abstracts of the 27th interscience conference on

antimicrobial agents and chemotherapy. Atlanta, October 11–12 1998.
39. Eyer S, Brummitt C, Crossley K, Siegel R, Cerra F. Catheter related-sepsis: prospective, randomized study of three methods of long-term catheter maintenance. Crit Care Med 18:1073, 1990.
40. Cobb D, High K, Sawyer RG, Sable CA, Adams RB, Lindley DA, *et al.* A controlled trial of scheduled replacement of central venous and pulmonary-artery catheters. NEJM 327:1062, 1992.
41. Mermel L, Stolz S, Maki DG. Epidemiology of infection with PA/Swan-Ganz catheter: a prospective study using molecular epidemiology. Am J Med 91(31B):197S, 1991.
42. Raad II, Bodey GP. Infectious complications of indwelling vascular catheters. Clin Infect Dis 15:197, 1992.
43. Blot F, Brun-Buisson C. Current approaches to the diagnosis and prevention of catheter-related infections. Curr Opin Crit Care 5:341, 1999.
44. Siegman-Igra Y, Anglim AM, Shapiro DE, Adal KA, Strain BA, Farr BM. Diagnosis of vascular catheter-related bloodstream infection: a meta-analysis. J Clin Microbiol 35:928, 1997.
45. Burn-Buisson C, Abroug F, Legrand P, Huet Y, Larabi S, Rapin M. Diagnosis of central venous catheter-related sepsis: critical level of quantitative tip cultures. Arch Inten Med 147:873, 1987.
46. Wing EJ, Norden CW, Shadduck RK, Winkelstein A. Use of quantitative bacteriologic techniques to diagnose catheter-related sepsis. Arch Intern Med 139:482, 1979.
47. Moyer MA, Edwards LD, Farley L. Comparative culture methods on 101 intravenous catheters: routine, semi-quantitative and blood cultures. Arch Intern Med 143:66, 1983.
48. Andremont A, Paulet R, Nitenberg G, Hill C. Value of semi-quantitative cultures of blood drawn through catheter hubs for estimating the risk of catheter tip colonization in cancer patients. J Clin Microbiol 26:2297, 1988.
49. Fan ST, Teoh-Chan CH, Lau KF. Evaluation of central venous catheter sepsis by differential quantitative blood culture. Eur J Clin Microbiol Infec Dis 8:142, 1989.
50. Douard MC, Arlet G, Leverger G, Paulien R, Waintrop C, Eurin E, *et al.* Quantitative blood culture for diagnosis and management of catheter-related sepsis in pediatric hematology and oncology patients. Intensive Care Med 17:30, 1991.
51. Rello J, Coll P, Net A, Prats G. Evaluation of different catheter parts for identification of pulmonary artery catheter colonization. Scand J Infect Dis 23:655, 1991.
52. Vallés J, Rello J, Matas L, *et al.* Pulmonary artery catheter colonization: influence of using an indwelling introducer. Eur J Clin Microbiol Infect Dis 15:71, 1996.
53. Rello J. Prevención de las infecciones por catéter: ha llegado la hora del cambio? Enferm Infecc Microbil Clin 16:53, 1998.
54. Raad II, Honh DC, Gilbreath BJ, *et al.* Prevention of central venous catheter-related infections by using maximal sterile barrier precautions during insertion. Infect Control Hosp Epidemiol 15:231, 1994.
55. Ducharme F, Gauthier M, Lacroix J, Lafleur L. Incidence of infection related to arterial catheterization in children: a prospective study. Crit Care Med 16:272, 1988.
56. Norwood S, Cormier B, McMahon N, Moss A, Moore V. Prospective study of catheter-related infection during prolonged arterial catheterization. Crit Care Med 16:836, 1988.
57. Leroy O, Billiau V, Beuscart C, *et al.* Nosocomial infections associated with long-term radial artery cannulation. Intnsive Care Med 15:241, 1989.
58. Furfaro S, Gauthier M, Lacroix J, *et al.* Arterial catheter-related infections in children. Am J Dis Child 145:1037, 1991.
59. Raad I, Umphrey J, Khan A, Truett LJ, Bodey G. The duration of placement as a predictor of peripheral and pulmonary arterial catheter infection. J Hosp Infect 23:17, 1993.
60. León MA, León C, Mateu A, Olaechea P, Insausti JM, Martínez Pellús A, *et al.* Infecciones relacionadas con catéteres intravasculares en el paciente crítico. Estudio multicéntrico. Med Intensiva 17:531, 1993.
61. Shinozaki T, Deane RS, Mazuzan JE, *et al.* Bacterial contamination of arterial lines. JAMA 249:223, 1983.
62. Centers for Disease Control Working Group. Guidelines for prevention of intravenous therapy-related infection. Infect Control 3:62, 1981.
63. Thomas F, Burke JP, Parker J, Orme JE, Gardner RM, Clemmer TP, *et al.* The risk of infection related to radial vs femoral sites for arterial catheterization. Crit Care Med 11:807, 1983.
64. Frezza EE, Mezghebe H. Indications and complications of arterial catheter use in surgical or medical intensive care units: analysis of 4932 patients. Am Surg 64:127, 1998.

34. CATHETER-RELATED BLOODSTREAM INFECTIONS IN TOTAL PARENTERAL NUTRITION

Meritxell Girvent and Antonio Sitges-Serra

Historical Aspects

Early after the introduction of intravenous feeding (TPN) it became clear that one of the most serious complications of this new modality treatment was bacteremia arising from the central venous catheter or the infusion devices or mixtures administered. Initial papers on this topic properly reflect the efforts by pioneers of TPN to make it a safe treatment for prolonged periods of time [1, 2]. Strategies to prevent catheter-related bloodstream infections (CRBI) in patients on TPN met, however, with different success due to the fact that at that time the pathogenesis of these infections was incompletely understood. Endemics of CRBI due to coagulase negative staphylococci were reported during the late 1970s and early 1980s from several parts of the world [3–6]. Uniform belief in the extraluminal origin of CRBI led to inefficient prevention measures such as long subcutaneous tunnelization or routine catheter exchange. Work done in the 1980s revealed that most infections associated with the administration of TPN originate at the catheter hub level and, consequently, in recent years the junction(s) between the catheter and the giving set(s) has become the main target for developing new prevention strategies. In addition, new devices have appeared in the market incorporating antiseptic or antibiotic barriers to prevent attachment of microorganisms to the internal catheter surface.

TPN has become a safe therapy from the metabolic point of view. Metabolic complications can now effectively be prevented by avoiding hyperalimentation, administering the appropriate doses of vitamins and trace elements, avoiding salt and carbohydrate overload and using all-in-one mixtures [7]. CRBI, however, remains the most common and disturbing complication of TPN administration both in hospital and at home and efforts should be pursued to make it totally preventable [8].

While in the home setting single lumen catheters are used and there are no major difficulties in diagnosing and treating CRBI, in the hospital setting, and particularly in the ICU setting, TPN-related CRBI is a more complex issue. The current use of multilumen catheters makes it more and more difficult to differentiate infections due to conventional catheters from those arising in "TPN catheters" and, consequently, most of the concepts developed on studies on multipurpose central venous catheters can be applied to currently used "TPN catheters".

In the paragraphs that follow, the main concepts relating to CRBI due to central venous lines will be discussed underlining, when required, the specific issues that apply to TPN administration.

General Pathophysiological Concepts

EXTRALUMINAL VERSUS ENDOLUMINAL CONTAMINATION ROUTE

Intravascular catheters are contaminated through intraluminal or extraluminal routes [9]. In extraluminal contamination, microorganisms migrate along the external surface of the catheter from an infected cutaneous exit site or, more rarely, they seed the catheter after reaching the bloodstream from a distant septic focus. Microorganisms reach the lumen of the catheter if the infusate is contaminated or during non-aseptic manipulation of the junction between the catheter and the giving set. The intraluminal route of catheter contamination is by far the most common origin of CRBI associated with the administration of TPN.

Extraluminal Contamination

HEMATOGENOUS SEEDING. This has traditionally been considered as the least common pathway of contamination of the external surface of the catheter. It occurs because bacteria are present in the blood coming from distant septic focus such as intrabdominal collections, urinary sepsis and adhere to the intravascular segment of the catheter. In critically ill patients, however, the hematogenous seeding of an intravascular catheter may be more common than initially thought. In a recent Spanish prospective study [10], about 25% of CRBI observed in the ICU setting were considered to have origin in a catheter contaminated by the hematogenous route.

SKIN CONTAMINATION AND EXIT SITE INFECTION. Skin contamination with site infection, the best known route of catheter contamination, was described more than 40 years ago [11]. Since then data have accumulated in favor of this route of contamination, which is the most relevant for catheters inserted for less than a week or infected within that period [12]. Due to poor skin preparation, defective surgical technique, or inappropriate dressing of the fresh skin puncture, the wound gets contaminated at catheter insertion or shortly afterwards. This contamination develops into a subdermal infection, which spreads along the subcutaneous tract surrounding the catheter and reaches the catheter tip. If the catheter has been tunneled to the anterior chest wall, insertion-site infection may give rise to a clinically evident soft-tissue infection, also called tunnelitis. The organisms most often involved are skin commensals such coagulase-negative staphylococci and *S. aureus*, but in hospitalized patients the skin flora may also include other pathogens, such as *Enterococcus* spp., Enterobacteriaceae, or *Pseudomonas* spp., all of which are also found in skin-originated CRBI.

Extraluminal contamination due to site infection is uncommon during intravenous feeding since TPN catheters are, more and more, inserted in an operating room or in the ICU using maximal aseptic barriers. Maximizing aseptic care at catheter insertion results in complete prevention or in very low rates of extraluminally originated CRBI in patients on TPN [13].

Endoluminal Contamination

CONTAMINATED INFUSATE. Intrinsic infusate contamination occurring at the time of industrial manufacturing of intravenous solutions is rare but may cause outbreaks of catheter related sepsis [14]. More often, extrinsic contamination of the infusate happens in hospital during the addition of pharmaceuticals or during mixing parenteral nutrition solutions. Although coagulase negative staphylococci may be responsible, contamination is more often caused by Gram-negative bacilli (see below). Isolation of *Enterobacter* spp., *Klebsiella* spp. and *Pseudomonas* spp. in patients with suspected CRBI should remind the physician to consider infusate contamination as a potential cause [9]. A contaminated infusate may give rise to severe septic shock, if the innoculum is massive, or it may lead to contamination of the inner catheter surface, resulting in CRBI some time after its administration.

HUB CONTAMINATION. Since the early 1980s, hub contamination has been progressively recognized as a very common precursor of CRBI and as the main contamination route for long dwelling intravascular catheters such as TPN central venous lines [15–18]. Hub-related CRBI tends to appear after the first or second week of catheter insertion. The microorganisms most commonly causing hub contamination are the coagulase-negative staphylococci which account for over two thirds of the CRBI associated with TPN. Other microorganisms have been cultured from hubs, however, such as *Proteus* spp., *Pseudomonas* spp., *S. aureus*, *Serratia marcescens* and *Candida albicans* [18–21]. This variety reflects the hospital flora potentially colonizing the hands of health care personnel manipulating catheter junctions. Initial epidemiological studies suggest that hub contamination is caused by handling of catheter junctions during connections and disconnections. In one study [18], some of the microorganisms found to contaminate the hubs were also isolated from the hands of the nurses who manipulated the catheters.

BACTERIAL ADHERENCE TO INTRAVASCULAR CATHETERS

In recent years much information has accumulated on the intimate mechanisms whereby microorganisms attach to the inner and outer catheter surfaces [22]. The host rapidly produces a coating or biofilm over the intravascular external catheter surface consisting of plasma proteins mostly fibrin and fibronectin to which microorganisms become eaisly attached. The latter seem particularly relevant in promoting the adherence of Gram-positive cocci [23]. In addition to this host component, the coagulase negative staphylococci and other bacteria are able to secrete a glycocalix matrix or slime which enables them to attach and grow on catheter surfaces and become rather inaccesible to the host natural defenses or to antibiotics. Attachment of microorganisms to catheter surfaces is followed by replication and eventually blood seeding.

BACTERIAL PROLIFERATION IN TPN MIXTURES

Compounding of TPN mixtures is a very sensitive step in the overall TPN administration scheme. Aseptic mixing of different TPN components is essential to avoid infusate-related infections that can be fatal. Many environmental (mesophilic) microorganisms such as *Candida* spp., coagulase negative staphylococci, *Bacillus* spp., *E. cloacae* or *E. coli* can grow luxuriously in TPN bags at room temperature. Bacterial growth in TPN solutions, however, is very sensitive to temperature [24]. At 4°C all bacterial growth ceases and, for this reaseon, storage of up to a week of TPN mixtures is allowed at this temperature [25]. Some psycrophilic bacteria, however, such as *Pseudomonas cepacia*, *Pseudomonas fluorescens* or *Stenotrophomonas maltophilia* grow at rather low temperatures (8°C) and their isolation from blood in patients receiving TPN should alert the physician to look for potential infusate contamination.

Risk Factors for CRBI in TPN

Indwelling time has been repeatedly shown to be one of the most important risk factors for CRBI [26, 27]. For this simple reason, TPN catheters have been incriminated as causing more infections that conventional central lines. In addition to indwelling time, epidemiological and experimental studies [28–30] have demonstrated other relevant risk factors for CRBI due to venous central lines such as: 1) access site (internal jugular > femoral > subclavian vein); 2) setting (emergency > elective); 3) number of hubs (multilumen > single lumen); 4) transparent semi-permeable dressings; 5) material (in experimental studies silicone > others) and 6) venous cutdown > direct puncture.

Multiple lumen catheters have been associated with an increased infection rate in some studies [30–32] but not in others [33–35]. Since increased CRBI rates for multiple lumen catheters can be ascribed basically to the increased likelihood of endoluminal contamination through the double or triple ports, studies such as that of Gil *et al.* [33] with a mean indwelling time of less than a week may not appropriately reflect the higher potential for CRBI of these devices. With increased dwelling time, however, the number of hubs can make a difference, particularly if hub handling is less than adequate. Unfortunately, there are no studies comparing single vs multilumen conventional or TPN catheters in which hub cultures have been implemented.

TPN has not been identified as an independent risk variable for CRBI in multivariate analysis [26]. Increased sepsis rates attributable to lipid administration was suggested in one epidemiological study in which *S. epidermidis* bacteremia was detected more often in infants neonates receiving lipids [36]. However, the most probable culprit of these higher CRBI rates was the lipid administration system and not fat *per se* [37]. Thus, the higher risk of CRBI occasionally found in patients on TPN can be attributed to confounding factors such as the catheterization time, which is uniformly superior for TPN catheters than for other kinds of intravascular devices, and frequent manipulation of hubs.

Clinical Presentation

INFUSION-RELATED SYMPTOMS

The clinical symptoms associated with CRBI during TPN often present shortly (one or two hours) after starting the infusion. This is due to the fact that during infusion the microorganisms lying in the inner surface of the catheter are shed off to the circulation by the infusate flow. This causes spiking fever, rigors, tachycardia, sweating, malaise and in some cases septic shock. All these symptoms tend to clear after stopping the infusion, a maneuver that we find very helpful in the diagnosis of TPN-related CRBI, particulalry when TPN is administered through a separate line [21].

PERSISTENT FEVER OF UNKNOWN ORIGIN

In a few cases fever may persist after removing the central line and giving the appropriate antibiotics. In this case a systematic investigation should be made to make sure that:

1. The patient has no other source of infection
2. The microorganism isolated from blood and catheter was sensitive to the antibiotics given
3. The patient does not have a fungal infection
4. There is no metastatic infection such as endocarditis, phlebitis, arthritis or osteomyelitis.

TUNNELITIS

Tunnelitis refers to a soft tissue infection originated from an exit site infection tracing down the subcutaneous tunnel. It can also be associated with a subcutaneous abscess and, in immunocompromised hosts, it can have devastating consequences. In this case – often due to *S. aureus* – removal of the central line is mandatory and systemic antibiotics should be given according to a Gram stain of the prulent exudate. Surgical debridement of the anterior chest wall should always be considered in the presence of loculated pus or spreading soft tissue infection.

Complications of CRBI

CRBI is the leading cause of hospital-acquired bacteremias and accounts for more than 40% of all bacteremias in ICUs [38].

One-third of patients may experience severe complications secondary to CRBI such as septic shock, sustained bacteriemia, suppurative thrombophebitis, metastatic infection, endocarditis and arteritis. The risk of major complications is highest in episodes of CRBI caused by *Candida* spp., *P. aeruginosa*, *S. aureus* or multiple pathogens, and the most severe complications are usually due to *S. aureus* [39]. The approach to these severe complications of CRBI requires immediate removal of the central line, even if the patient is on home parenteral nutrition, and starting intravenous antibiotics and eventually antithrombotic agents to treat suppurative thrombophlebitis.

THROMBOPHLEBITIS

Deep venous thrombosis is not a rare complicacion associated to parenteral nutrition. Its real prevalence is difficult to ascertain because it is often asymptomatic. Routine venography has shown that venous thrombosis complicate 45–65% of long-term catheters and 2.5–6% of patients have symptoms and clinical signs of deep vein thrombosis [40–42].

Subclavian vein thrombosis is heralded by arm edema, collateral circulation and pain around the shoulder. It is more prevalent in the left than in the right side [42]. A confirmative diagnosis can be obtained by doppler ultrasound or an upper limb venogram. In the context of a CRBI, the presence of signs suggesting venous obstruction often translates the presence of thrombophlebitis. Treatment of subclavian vein thrombosis in a febrile patient requires withdrawal of the line, systemic antibiotics and heparin.

SEPTIC METASTASES-ENDOCARDITIS

Septic metastases are usually observed in patients with a relatively long history of fever and untreated bacteremia. The Gram-positive cocci, and particularly *S. aureus*, are the organisms most commonly found. Septic metastases have been described almost everywhere, but the most common ones sit in lungs, joints (septic arthritis) and bones. They should be looked for in patients with persistent bacteremia and fever despite line removal and appropriate antibiotic coverage.

TABLE 1. Indication for catheter removal in the ICU patient

Severe sepsis with no other likely focus
Bacteremia due to Gram-positive cocci
Fungemia
Fever of unknow origin
Sudden unexplained clinical deterioration:
Septic shock
Unexplained tachycardia
Metabolic acidosis
Clinical signs of skin infection:
Purulence
Tunnelitis
Phlebitis (particularly for PICCs)
Limb edema/colateral circulation
Isolation of psycrophilic organisms from blood culture

Infective endocarditis on native valves associated with CRBI has a mortality close to 50% [44]. Endocarditis is diagnosed on the basis of persistent positive blood cultures, positive ultrasound findings and a murmur. Transesophageal echocardiography is becoming the current standard for the diagnosis of endocardial abnormalities in patients with *S. aureus* bacteremia and should be considered in all patients with this type of CRBI [43]. Signs of cardiac failure tanslate advanced valve destruction and may be the presenting symptomatology. Prompt line removal is the best preventive strategy against endocarditis. Surgery and systemic antibiotics are the best therapy for established endocarditis [44].

Diagnosis

The cornerstone for the diagnosis of CRBI continues to be the identification of the same microorganism (species and antibiotype) in the tip of the intravscular catheter and in the blood using conventional microbiological techinques. This requires catheter withdrawal which particularly applies to the ICU patient (Table 1) in whom conservative diagnosis of CRBI leaving the catheter *in situ* is not recommended. The minimum set of cultures that should be done in the microbiology laboratory to ascertain the occurrence of CRBI are: two peripheral blood cultures, culture of the catheter tip and culture of the inner surface of the catheter hub(s). We prefer peripheral blood cultures to cultures of blood taken from the catheter because they reflect more accurately the presence of bacteremia. Blood cultures drawn through the catheter use blood as a "washing" culture medium for microorganisms present on the inner catheter surface. Instead of taking blood cultures drawn through the catheter, we culture the catheter hub with a cotton swab without running the risk of catheter blockade or increase catheter manipulation. Although there are no comparative studies between these two techniques, we suspect that their results are fairly similar. In addition, in the ICU patient, many blood cultures through different catheters would have to be taken since these patients usually require several vascular accesses.

Although controversy exists as to which is the most appropriate culture method for catheter tips, there is increasing consensus that a quantitative technique culturing the inner and the outer catheter surfaces is to be preferred [45–48]. Despite the difficulty of standardization, sonication of catheter tips seems to be the most promising method in order to obtain a thorough bacteriological assessment of the catheter tip. Tips of catheters responsible for CRBI will almost invariably yield more than 1000 colony forming units [45, 46].

There is no universally accepted method for culturing the catheter hub. We perform semiquantitative cultures by swabing its inner surface with a cotton swab which is then streaked onto an agar plate. A periorificial small-surface (2 sq cm) semiquantitative skin culture of the catheter entry site is very valuable to define the origin of the bacteremia (skin vs hub vs mixed). It is compulsory if the skin site shows inflammation or purulence. A too wide skin sampling, however, may give false postive results. If the patient is receiving TPN, a high volume (at least 10 ml) culture of the mixture should be added to rule out mixture contamination [49]. All-in-one compounding in suboptimal conditions may result in bacterial contamination of the nutrient solutions; however, only high volume culture may detect low grade contamination of the infusate [50].

Recently, the time to positivity of blood cultures has been proposed as a useful tool to diagnose CRBI. Blot and colleagues [51] evaluated prospectively the differential time to positivity of paired blood cultures drawn simultaneously via the catheter hub and from a peripheral venous site. A diagnosis of CRBI was made in 16 of the 17 patients in whom a positive hub-blood culture was detected at least two hours earlier than peripheral-blood culture. CRBI was excluded in ten of the 11 patients with a differential time to positivity lower than 2 h.

There seems to be no role for sophisticated microbiological genetic identification techniques – such as pulsed field electrophoresis – for the diagnosis of CRBI in the clinical setting [50]. Current evidence suggests that device-related infections – particularly those caused by the coagulase negative staphylococci – are polyclonal. This means that although standard bacteriological cultures and antibiotype from a clinical isolate may suggest the presence of a single strain of *S. epidermidis*, genetic studies may uncover different strains based on genetic differences. A recent report [52], investigated the clonality of coagulase negative staphylococci obtained from surveillance cultures of central venous catheters. In over 80% of the hub isolates, there was proof of polyclonality indicating that genetic analysis, if not exhaustive, may lead to erroneous conclusions based on the isolation of "different" microorganisms at the skin, hub, tip or blood.

Conservative Diagnosis

Withdrawal of catheters suspected of being infected results in the loss of many "innocent" sterile devices that could have been preserved. This has prompted the development of *in situ* bacteriological tests aiming at the diagnosis of CRBI without removing the line. These techniques are particularly useful in patients in good condition, with a single line inserted, and in patients equipped with tunneled implanted catheters for long-term administration of TPN. These circumstances rarely apply to an ICU patient but occasionally a patient (i.e., single line in a blood marrow transplant patient, TPN line) may be a candidate suitable for a try of conservative diagnosis.

In a prospective study we investigated fifty-nine patients with suspected CRBI while receiving TPN via a single-lumen line [21]. Forty-one (Group I) were managed conservatively: swab cultures were taken from the catheter hub lumen, exit site and peripheral blood, and the catheter was heparinized and locked. The catheter was withdrawn only if cultures were positive, if not TPN was resumed. In 18 patients the catheter was immediately withdrawn (Group II). Thirteen patients of Group I had positive hub or skin cultures, their catheters were subsequently removed and 12 had blood cultures matching for the same microorganism. CRBI was diagnosed in 11 patients out of the 18 in whom catheters were immediately withdrawn (Group II). Thus, one out of 41 catheters and 7 out of 18 catheters were unnecessarily removed in Groups I and II respectively ($p = 0.001$). Negative skin and hub cultures, in patients with suspected CRBI, had a negative predictive value for CRBI of 96%. This has been confirmed in other studies [50, 52]. A positive hub culture in a symptomatic patient had a 100% positive predictive value for CRBI.

Other diagnostic strategies rely on quantitation of bacterial growth or time to positivity from blood cultures drawn through the suspected line or drawn from a peripheral vein [51, 53].

Treatment

Indications for immediate catheter withdrawal are shown in Table 1 and particularly apply to critically ill patients in whom leaving the catheter(s) *in situ* may lead to complications of persistent bacteremia such as septic shock or endocarditis. After catheter removal empiric antibiotic treatment is advisable until the responsible microorganism has been isolated. Antimicrobials should be selected on the basis of the microorganisms more often found in each unit and on the basis of the prevalence of methicillin-resistant *S. aureus*. Cloxacillin, eventually associated with an aminoglycoside, may be a good initial choice if resistance is not anticipated. Because methicillin-resistant *S. aureus* is increasing in many hospitals, vancomycin is also an appropiate antibiotic to start with. In cases of septic shock, coverage against Gram-negative bacteria and fungi should be considered until definitive culture data are available. Antibiotic treatment should be given for at least 5 to 7 days after catheter removal if microorganisms other than *S. aureus* or *Candida* have been isolated [54].

The is no consensus on the length of antibiotic treatment for CRBI due to *S. aureus*. For early-diagnosed, uncomplicated *S. aureus* bacteremia, treatment for at least 10–14 days to prevent endocarditis and metastatic infection seems appropriate [55, 56]. After this period, close follow-up is required to detect relapse. If fever persists for more than 72 h after starting the appropriate antibiotics metastatic infection is likely. If septic or thrombotic complications are diagnosed treatment should continue for at least four weeks [56, 57].

Prevention of Extraluminal Contamination

Reduction of CRBI must be one of the main goals of infection control practitioners. A sound understanding of the pathogenesis of CRBI is essential for a successful approach to this nosocomial infection. Effective prevention of CRBI can only be achieved if effective barriers are established to prevent bacteria from reaching the infusion system by either extraluminal or intraluminal routes [9, 58].

INSERTION TECHNIQUE

The most important single step in preventing CRBI is aseptic catheter insertion [13]. Most cases of skin-related CRBI, as happens with any clean surgical wound infection, appear within the first week of the procedure as a consequence of poor aseptic technique. To avoid this, the skin and the insertion field must be prepared as for a surgical intervention. The individual doing the procedure must perform a thorough hand scrub and use sterile gloves. The value of wearing gown, cap, and mask was recently addressed in a randomized study carried out at M.D. Anderson Cancer Center. Raad and coworkers [13] showed that maximal sterile barrier precautions, including a full-body sterile drape, during catheter insertion reduce the risk of CRBI, particularly during the first two months after catheter insertion. The absence of appropriate hub cultures, however, obscures the results of this study. Late episodes of CRBI were attributed to skin contamination without properly ruling out endoluminal contamination.

The technical expertise of the nurse or physician inserting the catheter also influences the incidence of CRBI. As with any clean surgical procedure, the amount of tissue trauma and the duration of the operation are directly related to the rate of wound infection.

SITE MAINTENANCE

Probably the only other single measure useful for the prevention of skin-related CRBI is the use of an antiseptic to keep the puncture site sterile while the catheter is in place. An antiseptic should be applied to the entry site. Chlorhexidine, alcohol and povidone-iodine are the best choice [59]. Povidone-iodine ointment achieves a low incidence of skin colonization by the coagulase negative staphylococci [60], with one report noting a significantly decreased rate of bacteremia [61].

Transparent dressings have not yet been demonstrated to provide an advantage over sterile gauze and tape in terms of reducing bacteremia, catheter-tip contamination, or skin colonization rates [26, 62].

Dressings of the catheter and replacement of the tubing should be done whenever required, but twice-weekly routine changes appear to be safe even for total parenteral nutrition administration [38, 60] with the added advantage of decreasing the risk of hub contamination.

Prevention of Endoluminal Contamination

ASEPTIC HUB HANDLING

Hubs of the luer Lock-type currently used were designed to improve tightness of the catheter-tubing junction but not to prevent endoluminal bacterial contamination. Therefore, they must be handled with extreme care to prevent bacteria from gaining access to the lumen. Prevention of hub-related CRBI depends on avoidance of bacterial contamination during connection and disconnection and on protection of the hub while the catheter is in place. Hub handling should be kept to a minimun and should be done by nurses wearing sterile gloves and mask. Catheter hubs should be protected against external contamination. Wherever implemented, proper junctional care has resulted in a significant decrease of CRBI [17, 38, 60, 63, 64].

Three-way stopcocks have become a popular means of intravascular access for administering drugs because they eliminate the use of rubber side ports and reduce the risk of needle puncture associated with these ports. Repeat connections and disconnections of three-way stopcocks for administration of drugs or withdrawal of blood may be a major mechanism of hub contamination. As with any type of conventional hub, three-way stopcocks should be handled asseptically and must remain protected when not connected to a giving set. Three-way stopcocks should only be used when absolutely required however, because they increase the number of open points and thus potentially facilitate endoluminal contaminations [65, 66].

ANTISEPTIC HUBS

Although effective preventive measures taken at the hub level were reported more than a decade ago [17, 60, 64], the current CDC guidelines do not consider this to be a relevant issue since no advice is offered to specifically prevent endoluminal contamination [67]. In addition, there has been very little response of the industry to this issue. The scenario, however, is changing and in the future this will be an area of both conceptual and technological progress.

Inoue *et al.* [68] reported on the use of a new connector incorporating the piggyback concept. They were able to reduce CRBI rates from 12% to 2%. Our group designed a new hub incorporating a chamber with a biocompatible antiseptic (3% iodinated alcohol) which is now available in Spain. Experimental studies and a first clinical trial are encouraging. CRBI of endoluminal origin was reduced from 9% to 1% [69] in newly inserted subclavian lines with a mean dwelling time of 15 days, the longest catheterization time for in-hospital trials published to date.

Antibiotic and Antiseptic-Coated Catheters

In the evolving scenario of prevention of CRBI, new technologies have appeared aiming at confering the intravascular devices more resistance against contamination. In 1991, Kamal *et al.* [70] published a first trial comparing a catheter impregnated with cephazolin with a conventional one. There were no differences in CRBI rates. The prevalence of colonization, however, was significantly reduced (2 vs 14%). This method did not popularize due to the cumbersome bonding maneuvers and the short duration of the protective effect. A second generation of coated catheters was manufactured already incorporating an external coating of chlorhexidine and silver sulfadiazine. These have been tested in several randomized trials with controversial and often negative results [71–77] attributed either to the sterilization process [76] or to the loss of the antiseptic coating [72]. A recent meta-analysis [77] of twelve randomized studies (11 of which failed to show a statistical difference) suggests, however, that CHX may be effective in reducing the CRBI rates (Odds ratio 0.56; $p = 0.005$). In the base-case analysis, use of antiseptic impregnated catheters resulted in a decrease in the incidence of CRBI of 2.2% (5.2% for standard vs 3.0% for CHX). A cost-effectiveness analysis of CHX has been published recently [78] suggesting savings ranging from $68 to $391 per catheter used. Caution should be taken, however, because CHX is approved as an antiseptic for external use; anaphylactic reactions have been reported in patients equipped with chlorhexidine-coated catheters [79].

Raad *et al.* [80] published a first randomized double-blind trial of catheters coated with minocycline and rifampin with a mean indwelling time of six days. CRBI was significantly reduced from 5 to 0% and colonization from 26% to 8%. Later on, the same group [81] compared CHX with RM catheters with a mean indwelling time of eight days. The rate of CRBI was significantly lower for RM (0.3 vs 3.4%; $p < 0.002$). It was claimed that the superiority of RM over CHX was mostly due to the fact that RM are coated on both surfaces while CHX are coated only externally.

Some issues in the Darouiche *et al.* [81] paper, however, deserve comment. Despite the better protection offered by the RM catheters, the number of devices that were withdrawn on the basis of suspicion of CRBI was similar in both groups. Quite a number of catheters (15%) were withdrawn for unknown reasons. Finally, despite the mean catheterization time in both groups being eight days, the actuarial curves of catheters free of CRBI diverge only from day 10. This suggests that the advantage of RM over CHX is restricted to catheters with an indwelling times over 10 days, when the endoluminal contamination route becomes predominant.

Antiseptic and antibiotic-coated catheters are currently under continuous evaluation. Initial results suggest that they may prevent CRBI mostly of the skin type, originating during the first 10–14 days of catheter placement. Studies on long dwelling TPN catheters are either not available or have reported disappointing results [71].

References

1. Holm I, Wretlind A. Prophylaxis against the infection and septicemia in parenteral nutrition via central intravenous catheter. Acta Chir Scand 141:173, 1975.
2. Sanderson I, Deitel M. Intravenous hyperalimentation without sepsis. Surg Gynecol Obstet 136:577, 1973.
3. Forse RA, Dixon C, Bernard K, Martínez L, McLean APH, Meakins JL. *Staphylococcus epidermidis*: An important pathogen. Surgery 86:507, 1979.
4. Sitges-Serra A, Puig P, Jaurrieta E, Garau J, Alastrue A, Sitges-Creus A. Catheter sepsis due to *Staphylococcus epidermidis* during parenteral nutrition. Surg Gynecol Obstet 151:481, 1980.
5. Deitel M, Krajden S, Saldanha CF, Gregory WD, Fuksa M, Cantwell E. An outbreak of *Staphylococcus epidermidis* septicemia. JPEN 7:569, 1983.
6. Garden OJ, Sim AJW. A comparison of tunnelled and non-tunnelled catheters: A prospective study of complications during parenteral feeding. Clin Nutr 2:51, 1983.
7. Sitges-Serra A. Parenteral mutrition and the surgical patient. Presses Agronomiques. Brussels, 1999.
8. Mughal MM. Complications of intravenous feeding catheters. Br J Surg 76:15, 1989.
9. Sitges-Serra A, Pi-Suñer T, Garcés JM, Segura M. Pathogenesis and prevention of catheter-related septicemia. Am J Infect Control 23:310, 1995.
10. León Regidor MA, León C, Mateu A, Olaechea P, Insausti JM, Martínez Pellús A, González V, lópez V, Alvarez B y GEIRCI. Infecciones relacionadas con catéteres intravasculares en el paciente crítico. Estudio Multicéntrico. Medicina Intensiva 17:531, 1993.
11. Crane Ch. Venous interruption for septic thrombophlebitis. N Engl J Med 262:947, 1960.
12. Maki DG. Pathogenesis, prevention and management of infections due to intravascular devices used for infusion therapy. In Bisno AL, Waldvogel FA (eds). Infections associated with indwelling medical devices. Washington DC: American Society for Microbiology, 1989: 171
13. Raad II, Hohn DC, Gilbreath J, Suleiman N, Hill LA, Bruso PA, Marts K, Mansfiel P, Bodey GP. Prevention of central venous catheter-related infections by using maximal sterile barrier precaustions during insertion. Inf Control Hosp Epidemiol 15:231, 1994.
14. Maki DG. Infections due to infusion therapy. In Benett JV, Brachman PS (eds). Hospital infections. Boston: Little, Brown, 1992: 849.
15. Sitges-Serra A, Liñares J, Garau J. Catheter sepsis: The clue is the hub. Surgery 97:355, 1985.
16. Liñares J, Sitges-Serra A, Garau J, Pérez JL, Martín R. Pathogenesis of catheter sepsis: a prospective study using quantitative and semiquantitaive cultures of catheter hub and segments. J Clin Microbiol 21:357, 1985.
17. Stotter AT, Ward H, Waterfield AH, Hilton J, Sim AJ. Junctional care: the key to prevention of cahteter sepsis in intravenous feeding. JPEN J Parenter Nutr 11:159, 1987.
18. Cicco M, Panarello G, Chiaradia V, Fracasso A, Veronesi A, Testa V, Santini G, Tesio F. Source and routed of microbial colonisation of parenteral nutrition catheters. Lancet 2:1258, 1989.
19. Salzman MK, Isenberg HD, Shapiro JF, Lipsitz PJ, Rubin LG. A prospective study of the catheter-related sepsis in neonates. J Infect Dis 167:487, 1993.
20. Tan TQ, Musser JM, Shulman RJ, Mason EO Jr, Mahoney DH Jr, Kaplan SL. Molecular epidemiology of coagulase-negative *Staphylococcus* blood isolates from neonates with persistent bacteremia and children with central venou catheter infections. J Infect Dis 169:1393, 1994.
21. Segura M, Lladó L, Guirao X, Piracés M, Herms R, Alía C, Sitges-Serra A. A prospective study of a new protocol for in situ diagnosis of central venous catheter related bacteriemia. Clin Nutr 12:103, 1993.
22. Lewis WJ, Sherertz RJ. Microbial interactions with catheter material. Nutrition 13(Suppl.):5S, 1997.
23. Vaudaux P, Pittet D, Haeberli A, Lerch PG, Morgenthaler JJ, Proctor RA, Waldvogel FA, Lew DP. Fibronectin is more active than fibrin or fibrinogen in promoting *Staphylococcus aureus* adherence to inserted intravascular catheters. J Infect Dis 167:633, 1993.
24. Jeppson R, Johansson M, Tengborn J. Bacterial growth properties in refrigerated all-in-one TPN mixtures. Clin Nutr 6:25, 1987.
25. Weil DC, Arnow PM. Safety of refrigerated storage of admixed parenteral fluids. J Clin Microbiol 26:1787, 1988.
26. Moro ML, Franco E, Cozzi A. The central venous catheter-related infections study group. Risk

factors for central venous catheter-related infections in surgical and intensive care patients. Inf Control Hosp Epidemiol 15:253, 1994.

27. Richet H, Hubert B, Nitemberg G, Andremont A, Buu-Hoi A, Ourbak P, Galicier C, Veron M, Boisivon A, Bouvier AM, Ricome JC, Wolff MA, Pean Y, Berardi L, Bourdain JL, Hautefort B, Laaban JP, Tillant D. Prospective multicenter study of vascular-catheter-related complications and risk factors for positive central-catheter cultures in intensive care unit patients. J Clin Microbiol 28:2520, 1990.
28. Hilton E, Haslett TM, Borenstein MT, Tucci V, Isenberg HD, Singer C. Central catheter infections: Single versus triple-lumen catheters. Influence of guide wires on infection rates when used for replacement catheters. Am J Med 84:667, 1988.
29. Hoffmann KK, Weber DJ, Samsa GP, Rutala W. Transparent polyurethane film as an intravenous catheter dressing. A meta-analysis of the infection risks. JAMA 267:2072, 1992.
30. Clark-Christoff N, Watters VA, Sparks W, Snyder P, Grant JP. Use of triple-lumen catheters for administration of total parenteral nutrition. JPEN 16:403, 1992.
31. McCarthy MC, Shives JK, Robison RJ, Broadie TA. Prospective evaluation of single and triple lumen catheters in total parenteral nutrition. JPEN 11:259, 1987.
32. Pemberton LB, Lyman B, Lander V, Covinsky J. Sepsis from triple- vs single-lumen catheters during total parenteral nutrition in surgical or critically ill patients. Arch Surg 121:591, 1986.
33. Gil RT, Kruse JA, Thill-Baharozian MC, Carlson RW. Triple- vs single-lumen central venous catheters. A prospective study in a critically ill population. Arch Intern Med 149:1139, 1989.
34. Savage AP, Picard M, Hopkins CC, Malt RA. Complications and survival of multilumen central venous catheters used for total parenteral nutrition. Br J Surg 80:1287, 1993.
35. Farkas JC, Liu N, Bleriot JP, Chevret S, Goldsterin FW, Carlet J. Single- versus triple-lumen central catheter-related sepsis: a prospective randomized study in a critically ill population. Am J Med 93:277, 1992.
36. Freeman J, Goldmann DA, Smith NE, Sidebottom DG, Epstein MF, Platt R. Association of intravenous lipid emulsion and coagulase-negative staphylococcal bacteremia in neonatal intensive care units. N Engl J Med 323:301, 1991.
37. Pérez JL, Liñares J, Pallarés R, Sitges-Serra A, Martín R. Lipid emulsions and bacteremia in the neonatal intensive care unit (letter). N Engl J Med 324:267, 1991.
38. Widmer AF. IV-related infections. In Wenzel RP (ed). Prevention and control of nosocomial infections. Baltimore: Williams and Wilkins 1993:556.
39. Arnow PM, Quimosing EM, Beach M. Consequences of intravascular catheter sepsis. Clin Infect Dis 16:778, 1993.
40. Ladefoged K, Efsen F, Krogh Christoffersen J, Jarnum S. Long-term parenteral nutrition II. Catheter-related complications. Scand J Gastroenterol 16:913, 1981.
41. Freund HR. Chemical phlebothrombosis of large veins. A not uncommon complication of total parenteral nutrition. Arch Surg 116:1220, 1981.
42. De Cicco M, Matovic M, Balestreri L, Fanarello G, Fanmtin D, Morassut S, Testa V. Central venous thrombosis: an early and frequent complication in cancer patients bearing long-term silastic catheters. A prospective study. Thromb Res 86:101, 1997.
43. Fowler VG Jr, Li J, Corey GR, Boley J, Marr KA, Gopal AK, Kong LK, Gottlieb G, Donovan CL, Sexton DJ, Ryan T. Role of echocardiography in evaluation of patients with *Staphylococcus aureus* bacteremia: experience in 103 patients. J Am Coll Cardiol 30:1072, 1997.
44. Lamas CC, Eykyn SJ. Hospital acquired native valve endocarditis: analysis of 22 cases presenting over 11 years. Heart 79:442, 1998.
45. Sherertz RJ, Heard SO, Raad II. Diagnosis of triple-lumen catheter infection: comparison of roll plate, sonication, and flushing methodologies. J Clin Microbiol 35:641, 1997.
46. Brun-Buisson CH, Abrouk F, Legrand P, Huet Y, Larabi S, Rapin M. Diagnosis of central venous catheter-related sepsis. Critical level of quantitative tip cultures. Arch Int Med 147:873, 1987.
47. Kelly M, Wciorka LR, McConico S, Peterson LR. Sonicated vascular catheter tip cultures. Quantitative association with catheter related sepsis and the non-utility of an adjuvant cytocentrifuge Gram stain. Am J Clin Pathol 105:210, 1996.
48. Siegman-Igra Y, Anglim AM, Shapiro DE, Adal KA, Strain BA, Farr BM. Diagnosis of vascular catheter-related bloodstream infection: a meta-analysis. J Clin Microbiol 35:928, 1997.
49. Maki DG, Alvarado CJ. The role of the clinical microbiology laboratory in diagnosis of infusion-related sepsis. Clin Microbiol Newsletter 4:89, 1982.

50. Liñares J, Domínguez MA, Martín R. Current laboratory techniques in the diagnosis of catheter-related infections. Nutrition 13(Suppl.):10S, 1997.
51. Blot F, Nitenberg G, Chachaty E, Raynard B, Germann N, Antoun S, Laplanche A, Brun-Buisson C, Tancrede C. Diagnosis of catheter-related bacteraemia: a prospective comparison of the time to positivity of hub-blood versus peripheral-blood cultures. Lancet 354:1071, 1999.
52. Atela I, Coll P, Rello J, Quintana E, Barrio J, March F, Sánchez F, Barraquer P, Ballús J, Cotura A, Prats G. Serial surveillance cultures of skin and catheter hub specimens from critically ill patients with central venous catheters: Molecular epidemiology of infection and implications for clinical management and research. J Clin Microbiol 35:1784, 1997.
53. Capdevila JA. Catheter-related infecion: An update on diagnosis, treatment and prevention. Int J Infect Dis 2:230, 1998.
54. Sitges-Serra A, Girvent M. Catheter-related bloodstream infections. World J. Surg 23:589, 1999.
55. Ehni WF, Reller LB. Short-course therapy for catheter-associated *Staphylococcus aureus* bacteremia. Arch Intern Med 149:533, 1989.
56. Malanoski GJ, Samore MH, Pefanis A, Karchmer AW. *Staphylococcus aureus* catheter-associated bacteremia. Minimal effective therapy and unusual infectious complications associated with arterial sheath catheters. Arch Intern Med 155:1161, 1995.
57. Raad I, Narro J, Khan A, Tarrand J, Vartivarian S, Bodey GP. Serious complications of vascular catheter-related *Staphylococcus aureus* bacteremia in cancer patients. Eur J Clin Microbiol Infect Dis 11:675, 1992.
58. Sitges-Serra A, Hernández R, Maestro S, Pi-Suñer T, Garcés JM, Segura M. Prevention of catheter sepsis: the hub. Nutrition 13(Suppl.):30S, 1997.
59. Maki DG, Ringer M, Alvarado CJ. Prospective randomised trial of povidone-iodine, alcohol, and clorhexidine for prevention of infection associated with central venous and arterial catheters. Lancet 338:339, 1991.
60. Sitges-Serra A, Liñares J, Pérez JL, Jaurrieta E, Lorente L. A randomised trial on the effect of tubing changes on hub contamination and catheter sepsis during parenteral nutrition. J Parent Enter Nutr 9:322, 1985.
61. Levin A, Mason AJ, Jindal KK, Fong IW, Goldstein MB. Prevention of hemodialysis subclavian vein catheter infections with topical povidone-iodine. Kidney Int 40:934, 1991.
62. Hoffmann KK, Weber DJ, Samsa GP, Rutala W. Transparent polyuretane film as an intravenous catheter dressing. JAMA 267:2072, 1992.
63. Hanrahan TO, Irving MH. The role of home parenteral nutrition in the management of intestinal failure – report of 400 cases. Clin Nutr 11:331, 1992.
64. Halpin DP, O'Byrne P, MaEntee G, Hennessy ThPJ, Stephens RB. Effect of a betadine connection shield on central venous catheter sepsis. Nutrition 7:33, 1991.
65. Brismar B, Jordahl L, Nystrom B, Petterson N. Bacterial contamination of intravenous line side ports of different designs. Clin Nutr 6:31, 1987.
66. Snydman DR, Murray SA, Kornfeld EJ, Majka JA, Ellis CA. Total parenteral nutrition-related infections. Am J Med 73:695, 1982.
67. Pearson ML, the Hospital Infection Control Practices Advisory Committee. Guideline for prevention of intravascular-device-related infections. Infect Control Hosp Epidemiol 17:438, 1996.
68. Inoue Y, Nezu R, Matsuda H, Fujii M, Nakai S, Wasa M, Takagi Y, Okada A. Prevention of catheter-related sepsis during parenteral nutrition: effect of a new connection device. JPEN 16:581, 1992.
69. Segura M, Alvarez F, Tellado JM, Jiménez-Farreres J, Oms L, Rello J, Baró T, Sánchez R, Morera A, Mariscal D, Marrugat J, Sitges-Serra A. A clinical trial on the prevention of catheter-related sepsis using a new hub model. Ann Surg 223:363, 1996.
70. Kamal GD, Pfaller MA, Rempe LE, Jebson PJ. Reduced intravascular catheter infection by antibiotic bonding. A prospective, randomized, controlled trial. JAMA 265:2364, 1991.
71. Pemberton LB, Ross V, Cuddy P, Kremer H, Fessler T, McGurk E. No differences in catheter sepsis between standard and antiseptic central venous catheters. A prospective randomized trial. Arch Surg 131:986, 1996.
72. Heard SO, Wagle M, Vijayakumar E, McLean S, Brueggemann A, Napolitano LM, Edwards LP, O'Connell FM, Puyana JC, Doern G. Influence of triple-lumen central venous catheter coated with chlorhexidine and silver sulfadiazine on the incidence of catheter-related bacteremia. Arch Int Med 158:81, 1998.
73. Tenneberg S, Lieser M, McCurdy B, Boomer G, Howington E, Newman C, Wolf I. A prospec-

tive randomized trial of an antibiotic and antiseptic-coated central venous catheter in the prevention of catheter related infections. Arch Surg 132:1348, 1997.

74. Ciresi DL, Albrecht RM, Volkers PA, Scholten DJ. Failure of antiseptic bonding to prevent central venous catheter-related infection and sepsis. Am Surg 62:641, 1996.
75. Maki DG, Stolz SM, Wheeler S, Mermel LA. Prevention of central venous catheter-related bloodstream infection by use of an antiseptic-impregnated catheter. Ann Int Med 127:257, 1997.
76. Sherertz RJ, Heard SO, Raad II, Gentry L, Bowton D, Scuderi P, Hu, J, Carruth W, Satishchandra B, Pepe J, Mosenthal A, Burke T, Dupuis J. Gamma radiation-sterilized, triple lumen catheters coated with a low concentration of clorhexidine were not efficacious at preventing catheter infections in intensive care unit patients. Antimicrob Agents Chemother 40:1995, 1996.
77. Veenstra DL, Saint S, Lumley T, Sullivan SD. Efficacy of antiseptic-impregnated central venous catheters in preventing catheter-related bloodstream infection: a meta-analysis. JAMA 281:261, 1999.
78. Veentra DL, Saint S, Sullivan SD. Cost-effectiveness of antiseptic impregnated central venous catheters for the prevention of catheter-related bloodstream infections. JAMA 282:554, 1999.
79. Terazawa E, Nagase K, Masue T, Niwa Y, Fukao I, Shimonaka H, Yokoi T, Kondoh N, Dohi S. Anaphylactic shock associated with a central venous catheter impregnated with chlorhexidine and silver sulfadiazine. Masui 47:556, 1998.
80. Raad I, Darouiche R, Dupuis J, Abi-Said D, Gabrielli A, Hachem R, Wall M, Harris R, Jones J, Buzaid A, Robertson C, Shenaq S, Curling P, Burke T, Ericsson C. Central venous catheters coated with minocycline and rifampin for the prevention of catheter-related colonization and bloodstream infections. A randomized, double-blind trial. Ann Int Med 127:267, 1997.
81. Darouiche RO, Raad II, Heard SO, Thornby JI, Wenker OC, Gabrielli A, Berg J, Khardori N, Hanna H, Hachem R, Harris RL, Mayhall G, for the Catheter Study Group. A comparison of two antimicrobial-impregnated central venous catheters. N Engl J Med 340:1, 1999.

35. PREVENTION OF CATHETER-RELATED INFECTIONS

Hend A. Hanna and Issam I. Raad

During the pre-intravascular catheter era, administration of drugs for critically ill patients used to take place through a small peripheral venous line. This practice was often complicated by extravasation of vesicants and toxic agents which eventually led to thrombosis of peripheral veins; and with the necrosis and scarring of the veins, they were rendered useless for further intravenous therapy. Since the introduction of the Broviac catheter in the early 1970s [1], followed by various forms of tunneled silicone catheters, physicians and patients alike have become dependent on the use of central venous catheters (CVCs) especially for the management of critically ill and cancer patients. CVCs are used frequently for the administration of blood products, fluids, parenteral nutrition, antibiotics, chemotherapeutic drugs, as well as for monitoring the hemodynamic status of critically ill patients.

However, the enthusiasm and benefits associated with these useful and essential tools are often clouded by the morbidity and mortality attributed to catheter-related infections, particularly catheter-related bloodstream infections.

Rates of Catheter-Related Bloodstream Infections (CRBSI)

It is estimated that more than five million CVCs are inserted annually in the United States [2]. About half a million of these are cuffed silastic catheters [3]. It is difficult to evaluate with accuracy the rate of CRBSI [3]. It ranges from 4% to 14% for noncuffed CVCs [4–7], yet reporting catheter infections in percentages of infected catheters ignores the duration of catheterization. Therefore, it is preferable to report CRBSI in terms of numbers of CRBSI per 1000 days of catheter use. Decker and Edwards reviewed 21 studies, including pediatric patients [8]. These studies collectively report 260,578 catheter days with 455 septic episodes, representing an overall rate of 1.7 CRBSI per 1000 days of catheter use. Clarke and Raffin combined data from multiple studies and calculated a rate of 1.37 infections per 1000 days of long-term CVC use [9].

Peripheral intravenous catheters are associated with higher infection rates than long-term CVCs. In one study, a rate of 27.7 infections for peripheral intravenous catheters per 1000 catheter days was observed [10]. Also, the use of short-term CVCs was associated with 5.35 infections per 1000 catheter days as reported in a review of three studies [11–13].

Given the above figures, at least 400,000 episodes of CRBSI are expected to occur annually [14]. Therefore, it becomes obvious that CRBSI cause morbidity and mortality which can clearly prolong hospitalization, leading to an added financial burden. A study published in 1994 estimated the cost of treating a single episode of CRBSI in critically ill patients to be $28,690 (1994 dollars) with an additional 6.5 days in the intensive care unit (ICU) [15].

In spite of the magnitude of the problem, CRBSI are preventable in most cases. It is essential to comprehend the possible risk factors that

TABLE 1. Risk factors for catheter-related bloodstream infection

- Prolonged catheterization
- Catheter dressings
- Catheter material
- Number of catheter lumens
- Location of catheter
- Improper aseptic techniques

TABLE 2. Preventive measures proven to decrease CRBSI

Aseptic measures
- Expert infusion therapy team
- Use of maximal sterile barrier precautions
- Use of topical disinfectants

New technologies
- Flush solutions: anticoagulant/antimicrobial
- Silver impregnated cuffs
- Aseptic hub mode
- Coated catheters: antiseptics and antimicrobials

attribute to the occurrence of CRBSI. Also, a thorough and comprehensive understanding of the different preventive techniques is essential to its application and, hence, to harvesting the coveted lower catheter-related infection rates. We will discuss the risk factors (Table 1) and preventive measures (Table 2) that have been shown to protect against CRBSI.

Risk Factors Associated with CRBSI

Prolonged catheterization has been shown to be a risk factor for infection. Catheters remaining in place for longer than 72 hours were shown to be at a significantly higher risk for infection [16, 17].

It has been suggested that catheter material may play a role in the process of thrombogenesis and adherence of organisms to the catheter surface and, hence, has a role in the pathogenesis of CRBSI. In a study by Linder *et al.*, polyvinylchloride catheters were shown to be more thrombogenic than soft silicone and polyurethane catheters [18]. Staphylococci and fungi were shown to adhere better to polyvinylchloride surfaces than to Teflon surfaces [19, 20]. Several studies have also examined the issue of comparing different CVC dressings and the role they play in CRBSI. Conly *et al.* compared transparent and dry gauze dressings in a prospective randomized trial. The authors showed that transparent dressings were associated with significantly increased rates of insertion site colonization ($P = 0.009$), local catheter-related infection ($P = 0.002$) and systemic catheter-related bacteremia ($P = 0.015$) than dry gauze dressings [21]. These findings were supported by a study that presented the outcome of meta-analysis of many randomized controlled trials comparing transparent polyurethane film and gauze dressings for hospitalized patients with central and peripheral venous catheters [22]. It was shown that the risk for catheter-related infections was increased with the use of occlusive transparent polyurethane film compared with gauze dressings. This could be due to the fact that occlusive transparent polyurethane films encourage a warm, moist environment at the catheter insertion site which is optimal for increasing the microbial burden and, hence, the increased risk of catheter colonization and septicemia. This finding may not be valid for the nonocclusive transparent dressings.

Some controversial issues that have been suggested to have a role in the risk of CRBSI include the number of catheter lumens and the site of catheter insertion. Retrospective studies have found that triple lumen CVCs were associated with higher risk of CRBSI than were single lumen CVCs [23–26]. On the other hand, some prospective randomized trials did not find significant differences in the infection rates between them [27–29]. While CVCs placed in internal jugular vein were found in one study more likely to become infected than those placed in subclavian veins [30], other researchers have presented contradictory data [31]. Frequent manipulation of the catheter, either for drawing blood, flushing the catheter, or administration of medication may also increase the risk of contamination [32].

Preventive Measures

ASEPTIC MEASURES

Skilled Infusion Therapy Team. Insertion and maintenance of CVCs by a skilled and trained infusion therapy team have become a desired approach in several medical centers. This practice has been shown to decrease infection rates associated with CVCs five- to eight-fold [33, 34]. Skilled infusion therapy teams are usually trained to insert and maintain catheters aseptically. They are also experienced in recognizing early signs of catheter-related infections which, when identified early, many times can be treated without having to remove the catheter. This approach can be cost-effective in hospitals with high rates of CRBSI or with immunocompromised patient populations. At M. D. Anderson Cancer Center (Houston, Texas), the use of nontunneled CVCs was associated with an infection rate of 1.3 per 1000 catheter days [35]. It is of interest to note that this low infection rate is similar to that associated with the tunneled Hickman CVC [36]. Achieving that low infection rate with the use of nontunneled CVCs was in part attributed to the availability of an expert and skilled infusion therapy team.

Maximal Sterile Barrier Precautions. During the insertion of nontunneled CVCs, including subclavian catheters and peripherally inserted central catheters, in most hospitals, minimal precautions are practiced which include wearing sterile gloves and using small sterile drapes. However, Raad *et al.*, in a prospective randomized study showed that the use of maximal sterile barriers during catheter insertion was associated with more than a six-fold decrease in the incidence of CRBSI and with a four-fold decrease in that of catheter-related pulmonary artery bacteremia [37]. Most (67%) CRBSI in the control arm occurred during the first week after insertion, while all infections in the sterile barrier arm occurred more than two months following insertion ($P < 0.01$). The maximal sterile barrier measures used were sterile gloves, gowns, masks, caps and large sterile drapes and as precautionary measures they proved to be cost-effective. Thus, one may conclude that the utilization of a skilled specialized infusion therapy team in the process of insertion of nontunneled silicone catheters under maximal sterile barrier precautions, results in a low infection rate associated with CVCs.

Topical Disinfectants and Antimicrobials. Skin is the most common source for short-term catheter colonization and infection [38]. Organisms migrate from the skin at the catheter insertion site along the catheter surface, colonizing the tip of the catheter and eventually causing CRBSI [39]. Therefore, techniques that are successful in lowering the microbial burden at the catheter insertion site may reduce CRBSI. Data concerning the efficacy of topical antimicrobial preparations are controversial. Povidone-iodine ointment applied at the insertion site failed to significantly decrease the rate of CRBSI [40]. Maki and Band, on the other hand, in a prospective trial, randomized patients to three arms of catheter care: 1) polymixin-neomycin-bacitracin ointment was applied at catheter insertion site at insertion and every 48 hours, 2) iodophor ointment applied at insertion and every 48 hours, or 3) no ointment applied. The authors found no difference in either catheter-related sepsis or local inflammation. However, in the topical polyantibiotic arm, there was a decrease in catheter tip colonization by semiquantitative cultures [41]. The difference was greatest for the catheters left in place for more than four days. This protection against bacterial infection took place at the expense of an increased risk of fungal colonization and infection, mostly with *Candida* [40, 41]. In another study, Maki and colleagues compared the efficacy of 2% chlorhexidine gluconate, 70% alcohol, and 10% povidone iodine in a prospective, randomized study [42]. The 2% chlorhexidine gluconate succeeded in lowering CRBSI about four-fold more than the 70% alcohol or the 10% povidone iodine.

NOVEL TECHNOLOGIES

Flush Solutions (Intraluminal Antibiotic Locks). This technique involves flushing the lumen of the CVC with a combination of antimicrobial and thrombolytic agents. The process of pathogenesis of catheter colonization involves a thrombin sheath formation on the catheter tip which acts as the adhesive medium that facilitates bacterial and fungal growth [43]. Therefore, regular heparin flushes have been shown to reduce bacterial growth on catheter tips [44]. In another study, Schwartz *et al.* have used a daily solution containing heparin and vancomycin to flush long-term tunneled CVCs [45]. The combination decreased the frequency of catheter-related bacteremia caused by luminal colonization with vancomycin-susceptible Gram-positive organisms more than flushing with heparin alone. However, it is prudent to avoid using vancomycin prophylactically due to the increase in the emergence of vancomycin-resistant organisms. It is also interesting to note that another study failed to show that flushing catheters with heparin/vancomycin flush solutions reduced the risk of bacteremia due to luminal colonization with organisms susceptible to vancomycin [46]. Raad *et al.* used a solution of 3 mg minocycline (M) and 30 mg ethylenediaminetetraacetate (EDTA) per milliliter of water (M-EDTA) as prophylaxis for three patients with recurrent CVC bacteremia [47]. The mixture was used as a flush solution and was also used to coat polyurethane catheters. The authors showed that *in vitro* and *in vivo* experiments proved that M-EDTA has broad-spectrum antimicrobial activity against methicillin-resistant staphylococci, Gram-negative bacilli and *Candida*. M-EDTA also has synergistic activity against *Enterobacter aerogenes* and *Candida albicans* as well as high bactericidal activity against *Staphylococcus epidermidis*. EDTA has an anticoagulant activity that was not diminished by the addition of minocycline. The study also showed that serum samples collected soon after administering the M-EDTA flush solution failed to show detectable levels of minocycline or EDTA and, hence, the emergence of resistant organisms is of no practical concern. Therefore, the use of novel flush solutions such as M-EDTA may be useful in preventing catheter infections as well as in maintaining the patency of the CVC.

Silver Impregnated Cuffs. A collagen cuff impregnated with silver ions and attached to the CVC can provide protection against catheter colonization and infection. The cuff is situated in the subcutaneous tunnel and creates both antimicrobial and physical barrier to microorganisms. Studies have shown that the incidence of catheter-related colonization and infections among critically ill patients was reduced by using the attachable silver impregnated cuff [48, 49]. In these studies, this was proven to be true for short-term CVCs where the mean duration of catheterization was 5.6 to 9.1 days. However, silver cuffs did not show protection against infections for long-term CVCs where mean duration of catheterization was 20 days [50] or for long-term tunneled Hickman catheters [51]. The collagen to which the silver ions are chelated is biodegradable in nature and, hence, catheters with silver impregnated cuffs failed to provide protection against infection when used for long-term catheterization. When Groeger *et al.* compared silver cuffed catheters to other cuffed catheters in a prospective randomized trial of more than 200 oncology patients, they failed to show an added protection associated with the silver cuffed catheters against infection [51]. This finding may suggest that the beneficial effect of silver cuffed catheters is due to the presence of the cuff itself rather than to the presence of silver ions, which are short-lived. In a rabbit model, silver iontophoretic catheters showed broad-spectrum antimicrobial inhibitory activity with long durability thus protecting against catheter colonization [52, 53]. In these catheters silver ions are generated by connecting silver wires to an electric power source along the intercutaneous segment of the catheter, preventing the migration of organisms from the skin to the catheter [52]. Silver ions are released over a period of several months. This catheter also provided *in vitro* broad-spectrum inhibitory activity against bacteria and *Candida*. However, this model needs to be tested for safety and efficacy through prospective randomized clinical trials.

Aseptic Hub Model. Since organisms migrate through the hub along the internal surface of the catheter to colonize the tip, a new antiseptic hub model was designed to provide protection to the hub and lumen against colonization and infection [54]. The hub model consists of two parts: a female component made out of a plastic cylinder closed at both ends with latex rubber. This cylinder contains 0.2 ml of 3% iodinated alcohol with 6 mg iodine. The male component is a 20 gauge needle that connects to the female port on one end and to the infusion tube on the other. The needle passes the antiseptic chamber and, thus, becomes sterilized by the antiseptic solution. In a study, catheter-related sepsis was shown to decrease four-fold with the use of this hub model in patient populations at high risk for hub-related sepsis [55]. This model, however, does not provide protection against the migration of skin organisms along the external intercutaneous segment of the catheter, hence, its limited contribution.

Catheters Coated with Antimicrobial Agents. Microbial organisms such as *S. epidermidis* and *C. parapsilosis* have the ability to adhere to the catheter surface by producing what is known as extracellular slime or glycocalyx through which the microorganisms become tightly embedded [56–58]. The microorganisms remain there protected from macrophages, phagocytic neutrophils, antibodies, and glycopeptide antibiotics [59–61] and, hence, the catheter becomes colonized and ultimately this process leads to CRBSI. Understanding this aspect of the pathogenesis of CRBSI, researchers tried to interfere with this process through coating catheters. In the early 1980s, Greco and Harvey successfully bonded a negatively charged antibiotic oxacillin to polytetrafluroethylene grafts (PTFE) by using benzalkonium chloride, a surfactant [62, 63]. Bonded PTFE grafts were then compared to control grafts by challenging both with *S. aureus* after being placed in the infrarenal aorta of dogs. Bonded grafts proved to be superior to the control ones in negative cultures, patency and survival. Pretreatment of catheter segments with tridodecylmethylammonium chloride (TDMAC) increased the bonding of another antibiotic, penicillin, to both polyethylene and silicone elastomer catheter segments. When tested against control catheters, the TDMAC-antibiotic-bonded catheters proved to be significantly superior in resisting colonization ($P < 0.005$) [64].

Darouiche and Raad impregnated the internal and external surfaces of vascular catheters using organic solvents as penetrating agents [65]. Scherertz *et al.* found that dicloxacillin, clindamycin, fusidic acid and chlorhexidine, when used to coat catheters in a rabbit model, led to a decrease in the risk of infection compared to uncoated control catheters ($P < 0.05$) [66]. In another study, Kamal *et al.* coated catheters that had been pre-treated with TDMAC by dipping them just prior to insertion into a cefazolin solution. The rate of catheter colonization was about seven-fold less in the cefazolin-coated catheter arm than in the control uncoated arm [67]. Nonetheless, the efficacy of this technique could not be validated since there were no cases of CRBSI in either of the study arms. Also, the technique is quite impractical for use in critically ill patients since the catheters need to be coated just prior to insertion. Maki and colleagues used catheters that had been coated only externally with antiseptics, chlorhexidine gluconate and silver sulfadiazine (CG/SS). The catheters were compared in a clinical trial to uncoated catheters and were less likely to be colonized (P = 0.005) and nearly five-fold less likely to cause CRBSI (P = 0.03) [68].

Maki and colleagues reported slightly more erythema around the catheter insertion site in the study arm due to a possible chemical irritation, but the difference between the two arms was small. Further prospective randomized studies failed to confirm the findings of Maki's study [69–71]. A recent meta-analysis of twelve studies found that these catheters were efficacious in preventing CRBSI [72]. However, in most of the studies analyzed in the meta-analysis, only the external surfaces coated with antiseptics were cultured. Therefore, the organisms from the internal uncoated catheter surfaces were not retrieved for culture. This may bias the results and represents one of the disadvantages of the CG/SS catheters in that they are coated only on the external surface while their lumens remain uncoated. The antimicrobial durability of these catheters is also less than one week which could be problematic if used in critically ill patients who may require longer use of CVCs [73]. There have also been reports of anaphylaxis and possible related death associated with the use of CG/SS catheters which resulted in these catheters being banned in Japan [74, 75].

However, a novel CG/SS catheters, whereby the internal and external surfaces are coated, have been developed and approved. This may represent an improved version of antiseptic catheters.

The synergistic combination of minocycline and rifampin (M/R) was tested by Raad *et al.* and was found to prevent bacterial colonization of slime-producing strains of *S. epidermidis* and *S. aureus* on catheter surfaces [76]. Raad *et al.* also found that the *in vitro* inhibitory activities of catheters coated with minocycline and rifampin against *S. epidermidis*, *S. aureus* and *Enterococcus faecalis* strains were significantly superior to those of catheters coated with vancomycin (P < 0.05). The inhibitory activities of catheters coated with minocycline and rifampin against Gram-negative bacilli and *C. albicans* were compared to those of catheters coated with ceftazidime and amphotericin B, respectively [76]. Catheters coated with minocycline/rifampin combination proved *in vitro* to have broad spectrum activity against Gram-positive, Gram-negative bacteria and *C. albicans* which were significantly superior to those coated with CG/Ss (P < 0.01) [73]. Because of these results, a recent multicenter prospective randomized clinical trial was conducted comparing the efficacy and safety of catheters impregnated with minocycline/rifampin with catheters coated with CG/SS [77].

Darouiche *et al.* found that catheters impregnated with minocycline/rifampin were at least three times less likely to be colonized than catheters impregnated with CG/SS (7.9% versus 22.8%, P < 0.001). Catheters coated with minocycline/rifampin were also 12-fold less likely to be associated with CRBSI than those coated with CG/SS (0.3% versus 3.4%, P < 0.002). No evidence of emergence of antibiotic resistance was found among bacteria recovered from patients who had received the catheters coated with minocycline/rifampin. These catheters have an antimicrobial durability that extends up to four weeks, which is an important advantage when used in critically ill patients [73, 78]. It is important to note that both the internal and external surfaces of the catheters were coated with the minocycline/rifampin combination which provides for protection of both surfaces of the catheter against colonization. So far, there are no reports of adverse events or anaphylaxis associated with the minocycline/rifampin-impregnated catheters.

After having reviewed the evolution of the technology aiming at the protection against CRBSI through preventing catheter colonization, the importance of novel techniques and approaches becomes evident. In the search of the optimal technique, new ideas should be tested for safety and efficacy through well designed clinical trials that are able to effectively challenge the validity of novel approaches.

References

1. Broviac JW, Cole JJ, Scribner BH. A silicone rubber atrial catheter for prolonged parenteral alimentation. Surg Gynecol Obstet 136:602, 1973.
2. Maki DG. Infection caused by intravascular devices: pathogenesis, strategies for prevention. London: Royal Society of Medicine Services, 1991.
3. Groeger JS, Lucas AB, Coit D. Venous access in the cancer patient. In DeVita VT Jr, Hellman S, Rosenbert SA (eds). Cancer: Principles and Practice of Oncology. 3rd edn, Philadelphia, PA: JB Lippincott. 1991:1.
4. Maki DG, Cobb L, Garman JK, Shapiro JM, Ringer M, Helgerson RB. An attachable silver-impregnated cuff for prevention of infection with central venous catheters: a prospective randomized multicenter trial. AM J Med 85:307, 1988.
5. Gill RT, Kruse JA, Thill-Baharozian MC, Carlson RW. Triple vs single-lumen central venous catheters. Arch Intern Med 149:1139, 1989.
6. Powell C, Kudsk KA, Kulich PA. Mandelbaum JA, Fabri PJ. Effect of frequent guidewire changes on triple-lumen catheter sepsis. JPEN J Parenter Enteral Nutr 112:464, 1988.
7. Raad II, Bodey GP. Infectious complications of indwelling vascular catheters. Clin Infect Dis 15:197, 1992.
8. Decker MD, Edwards KM. Central venous catheter infections. Ped Clin North Am 35:579, 1988.
9. Clarke DE, Raffin TA. Infections complications of indwelling long-term central venous catheters. Chest 4:966, 1990.
10. Band JD, Maki DG. Steel needles used for intravenous therapy: morbidity in patients with hematologic malignancy. Arch Intern Med 140:31, 1980.
11. Ryan JA, Abel RM, Abbot WM, Hoplins CC, Chesney TMcC, Colley R, *et al*. Catheter complications in TPN: a prospective study of 200 consecutive patients. N Engl J Med 290:757, 1974.
12. Kovacevich DS, Faubion WC, Bender JM, Schaberg DR, Wesley JR. Association of parenteral nutrition catheter sepsis with urinary tract infections. J JPEN 10:639, 1986.
13. Faubion WC, Wesley JR, Khaldi N, Silva J. Total parenteral nutrition catheter sepsis: impact of the term approach. J Paerenter Enteral Nutr 10:642, 1986.
14. Raad II, Darouiche R. Prevention of infections associated with intravascular devices. Curr Opin Crit Care 2:361, 1996.
15. Heiselman D. Nosocomial bloodstream infections in the critically ill [letter]. JAMA 272:1819, 1994.
16. Rhame FS, Maki DG, Bennett JV. Intravenous cannula-related infections. In Bennett JV, Brachman PS (eds). Hospital Infections. Boston: Little Brown, 1979:433.
17. Maki DG, Goldmann DA, Rhame FS. Infection control in intravenous therapy. Ann Intern Med 79:867, 1973.
18. Linder LE, Curelaru I, Gustavsson B, Hansson HA, Stenqvist O, Wojciechowski J. Material thrombogenicity in central venous catheterization: a comparison between soft, antebrachial catheters of silicone elastomer and polyurethane. J Parenter Enter Nutr 8:399, 1984.
19. Sheth NK, Franson TR, Rose HD, Buckmire FL, Cooper JA, Sohnle PG. Colonization of bacteria on polyvinyl chloride and Teflon intravascular catheter in hospitalized patients. J Clin Microbiol 18:1061, 1983.
20. Rotrosen D, Calderone RA, Edwards JE Jr. Adherence of *Candida* species to hose tissues and plastic surfaces. Rev Infect Dis 8:73, 1986.
21. Conly JM, Grieves K, Peters B. A prospective, randomized study comparing transparent and dry gauze dressings for central venous catheters. J Infect Dis 159:310, 1989.
22. Hoffmann KK, Weber DJ, Samsa GP, Rutala WA. Transparent polyurethane film as an intravenous catheter dressing. A meta-analysis of the infections rates. JAMA 167:2072, 1992.
23. Pemberton LB, Lyman B, Lander V, Covinsky J. Sepsis from triple vs. single-lumen catheters during total parenteral nutrition in surgical or critically ill patients. Arch Surg 121:591, 1986.
24. Hilton E, Haslett TM, Borenstein MT, Tucci V, Isenberg HD, Singer C. Central catheter infections: single vs. triple-lumen catheters-influence of guidelines on infection rates when used for replacement of catheters. Am J Med 84:667, 1988.
25. Yeung C, May J, Hughes R. Infection rate for single-lumen vs. triple-lumen subclavian catheters. Infect Control Hosp Epidemiol 9:154, 1988.
26. Mantese VA, German DS, Kruminski DL, *et al.* Colonization and sepsis from triple-lumen catheters in critically ill patients. Am J Surg 154:597, 1987.

27. Powell C, Fabri PJ, Kudsk KA. Risk of infection accompanying the use of single-lumen vs. double-lumen subclavian catheters: a prospective randomized study. J Parenter Enter Nutr 12:127, 1988.
28. MacCarthy MC, Shives JK, Robison RJ, Broadie TA. Prospective evaluation of single and triple lumen catheters in total parenteral nutrition. J Parenter Enter Nutr 11:259, 1987.
29. Farkas JC, Liu N, Bleriot JP, Chevret S, Goldstein FW, Carlet J. Single-versus triple-lumen central catheter-related sepsis: a prospective randomized study in a critically ill population. Am J Med 93:277, 1992.
30. Mermel LA, McCormick RD, Springman SR, Maki DG. The pathogenesis and epidemiology of catheter-related infection with pulmonary artery Swan-Ganz catheters: a prospective study utilizing molecular subtyping. Am J Med 91(Suppl 3B):197S, 1991.
31. Senagore A, Waller JD, Bonell BW, Bursch LR, Scholten DJ. Pulmonary artery catheterization: a prospective study of internal jugular and subclavian approaches. Crit Care Med 15:35, 1987.
32. Hampton AA, Sherertz RJ. Vascular-access infection in hospitalized patients. Surg Clin North Am 68:57, 1988.
33. Faubion WC, Wesley JR, Khalidi N, *et al.* Total parenteral nutrition catheter sepsis: impact of the team approach. J Parenter Enter Nutr 10:642, 1986.
34. Nelson DB, Kien CL, Mohr B, *et al.* Dressing changes by specialized personnel reduce infection rates in patients receiving central venous parenteral nutrition. J Parenter Enter Nutr 10:220, 1986.
35. Raad I, Davis S, Becker M, Hohn D, Houston D, Umphrey J, Bodey GP. Low infection rate and long durability of nontunneled silastic catheters: a safe and cost-effective alternative for long-term venous access. Arch Intern Med 15:1791, 1991.
36. Press OW, Ramsey RG, Larson EB, Fefer A, Hickman RO. Hickman catheter infections in patients with malignancies. Medicine 63:189, 1984.
37. Raad II, Hohn DC, Gilbreath BJ, *et al.* Prevention of central venous catheter-related infections using maximal sterile barrier precautions during insertion. Infect Control Hosp Epidemiol 15:1, 1994.
38. Maki DG. Sources of infection with central venous catheters in an ICU: a prospective study. In Program and Abstracts of the 28th Interscience Conference on Antimicrobial Agents and Chemotherapy, Los Angeles, October 23–26, 1988: Abstract 269, p. 157.
39. Maki DG. Infection caused by intravascular devices: Pathogenesis, strategies for prevention. Royal Society of Medicine Services Limited, London, England, 1991.
40. Maki DG, Band JD. A comparative study of polyantibiotic and iodophor ointments in prevention of vascular catheter-related infection. Am J Med 70:739, 1981.
41. Levy RS, Goldstein J. Value of a topical antibiotic ointment in reducing bacterial colonization of percutaneous venous catheters. J Alb Enst Med Center 18:67, 1979.
42. Maki DG, Ringer M, Alvarado CJ. Prospective randomized trial of povidone-iodine, alcohol, and chlorhexidine for prevention of infection associated with central venous and arterial catheters. Lancet 338:339, 1991.
43. Stillman RM, Soliman F, Garcia L, *et al.* Etiology of catheter-associated sepsis: correlation with thrombogenicity. Arch Surg 112:1497, 1977.
44. Bailey MJ. Reduction of catheter-associated sepsis in parenteral nutrition using low-dose intravenous heparin. Br Med J 1:1671, 1979.
45. Schwartz C, Henrickson KJ, Roghmann K, Powell K. Prevention of bacteremia attributed to luminal colonization of tunneled central venous catheters with vancomycin-susceptible organisms. J Clin Oncol 8:591, 1990.
46. Rackoff WR, Weiman M, Jakobowski D, *et al.* A randomized, controlled trial of the efficacy of a heparin and vancomycin solution in preventing central venous catheter infections in children. J Pediatr 127:147, 1995.
47. Raad I, Buzaid A, Rhyne J, Hachem R, Darouiche R, Safar H, Albitar M, Sherertz R. Minocycline and ethylenediaminetetraacetate for the prevention of recurrent vascular catheter infections. Clin Infect Dis 25:149, 1997.
48. Maki DG, Cobb L, Garman JK, *et al.* An attachable silver-impregnated cuff for prevention of infection with central venous catheters: a prospective randomized multicenter trial. Am J Med 85:307, 1988.
49. Flowers RH III, Schwenzer KJ, Kopel RF, *et al.* Efficacy of an attachable subcutaneous cuff for the prevention of intravascular catheter-related infection. JAMA 261:878, 1989.
50. Clementi E, Marie O, Arlet G, *et al.* Usefulness of an attachable silver-impregnated cuff for prevention of catheter-related sepsis (CRS). In Program and Abstracts of the 31st Interscience

Conference on Antimicrobial Agents and Chemotherapy, Chicago, III. 1991: Abstract 460, p. 175.

51. Groeger JS, Lucas AB, Coit D, *et al.* A prospective randomized evaluation of silver-impregnated subcutaneous cuffs for preventing tunneled chronic venous access catheter infections in cancer patients. Ann Surg 218:206, 1993.
52. Raad I, Hachem R, Zermeno A, Dumo M, Bodey GP. *In vitro* antimicrobial efficacy of silver iontophoretic cathere. Biomaterials. 17:1055, 1996.
53. Raad I, Hachem R, Zermeno A, Stephens LC, Bodey GP. Silver iontrophoretic catheter: a prototype of a long-term antiinfective vascular access device. J Infect Dis 173:495, 1996.
54. Segura M, Alia C, Oms L, Sancho JJ, Torres-Rodriguez JM, Sitges-Serra A. *In vitro* bacteriological study of a new hub model for intravascular catheters and infusion equipment. J Clin Microbiol 27:2656, 1989.
55. Segura M, Alvarez-Lerma F, Tellaco JM, Ferreres JJ, Oms L, Rello J, Baro T, Sanchez R, Morerea A, Mariscal D, *et al.* Advances in surgical technique. A clinical trial on the prevention of catheter-related sepsis using a new hub model. Ann Surg 223:363, 1996.
56. Christensen GD, Simpson WA, Bisno AL, Beachey EH. Adherence of slime-producing strains of *Staphylococcus epidermidis* to smooth surfaces. Infect Immunol 37:318, 1992.
57. Christensen GD, Simpson WA, Younger JJ, Baddour LM, Barrett FF, Melton DM, Beachey EH. Adherence of coagulase-negative staphylococci to plastic tissue culture plates: a quantitative model for the adherence of staphylococci to medical devices. J Clin Microbiol 22:996, 1985.
58. Pfaller MA, Messer SA, Hollis RJ. Variations in DNA subtype, antifungal susceptibility, and slime production among clinical isolates of *Candida parapsilosis*. Diag Microbiol Infect Dis 21:9, 1995.
59. Sheth NK, Franson TR, Sohnle PG. Influence of bacterial adherence to intravascular catheters on in vitro antibiotic susceptibility. Lancet 2:1266, 1985.
60. Farber BF, Kaplan MH, Clogstron AG. *Staphylococcus epidermidis* extracted slime inhibits the antimicrobial action of glycopeptide antibiotics. J Infect Dis 161:37, 1990.
61. Costerton JW, Lappin-Scott HM. Behavior of bacteria in biofilms. Am Society Microbiol News 55:650, 1989.
62. Greco RS, Harvey RA. The role of antibiotics bonding in the prevention of vascular prosthetic infections. Ann Surg 195:168, 1982.
63. Harvey RA, Greco RS. The noncovalent bond-ing of antibiotics to a polytetrafluoroethylene-benzalkonium graft. Ann Surg 194:642, 1981.
64. Trooskin SZ, Donetz AP, Harvey RA, Greco RS. Prevention of catheter sepsis by antibiotic bonding. Ann Surg 97:547, 1984.
65. Darouiche RO, Raad I. Antimicrobial impregnated catheters and other medical implants and methods for impregnating catheters and other medical implants with an antimicrobial agent. United States Patent #5,624,704, 1997.
66. Sherertz RJ, Carruth WA, Hampton AA, Byron MP, Solomon DJ. Efficacy of antibiotic coated catheters in preventing subcutaneous Staphylococcus aureus infection in rabbits. J Infect Dis 167:98, 1993.
67. Kamal GD, Pfaller MA, Rempe LE, Jebson PJR. Reduced intravascular catheter infection by antibiotic bonding. JAMA 265:2364, 1991.
68. Maki DG, Stolz SM, Wheeler S, Mermel LA. Prevention of central venous catheter-related bloodstream infection by use of antiseptic-impregnated catheter: a randomized, controlled study. Ann Intern Med 127:257, 1997.
69. Ciresi D, Albrecht RM, Volkers PA, Scholten DJ. Failure of an antiseptic bonding to prevent central venous catheter-related infection and sepsis. Am Surg 62:641, 1996.
70. Pemberton LB, Ross V, Cuddy P, Kremer H, Fessler T, McGurk E. No difference in catheter sepsis between standard and antiseptic central venous catheters: a prospective randomized trial. Arch Surg 131:986, 1996.
71. Heard SO, Wagle M, Vijayakumar E, *et al.* The influence of triple-lumen central venous catheters coated with chlorhexidine/silver sulfadiazine on the incidence of catheter-related bacteremia: a randomized, controlled clinical trial. Arch Intern Med 158:81, 1998.
72. Veenstra DL, Saint S, Saha S, Lumley T, Sullivan SD. Efficacy of antiseptic-impregnated central venous catheters in preventing catheter-related bloodstream infection. A meta-analysis. JAMA 281:261, 1999.
73. Raad I, Darouiche R, Hachem R, Mansour M, Bodey GP. The broad spectrum activity and efficacy of catheters coated with minocycline and rifampin. J Infect Dis 173:418, 1996.
74. Oda T, Junichiro H, Noami K, Mikami K. Anaphylactic shock induced by an antiseptic-coated

central venous catheter. Anesthesiology 87:1242, 1997.

75. World Heath Organization. Central venous catheters (Arrowguard) recalled: Anaphylactic shock. Geneva, Switzerland: World Health Organization; Alert 62, 1997.
76. Raad I, Darouiche R, Hachem R, Sacilowski M, Bodey GP. Antibiotics and prevention of microbial colonization of catheters. Antimicrob Agents Chemother 39:2397, 1995.
77. Darouiche RO, Raad II, Heard SO, Thornby JI, Wenker OC, Gabrielli A, Berg J, Khardori N, Hanna H, Hachem R, Harris RL, Mayhall G. For the catheter study group. A comparison of two antimicrobial-impregnated central venous catheters N Engl J Med 340:1, 1999.
78. Raad II, Darouiche RO, Hachem R, Abi-Said D, Safar H, Darnule T, Mansouri M, Morck D. Antimicrobial durability and rare ultrastructural colonization of indwelling central catheters coated with minocycline and rifampin. Crit Care Med 26:219, 1998.

SECTION 6: RESPIRATORY INFECTIONS

J. Rello

36. TRACHEOBRONCHITIS IN THE ICU

Dan Schuller and Subramanian Paranjothi

Introduction

Tracheobronchitis can be broadly defined as an inflammatory process of the airways between the larynx and the bronchioles. Clinically, this is a syndrome recognized by an increase in the volume and purulence of the lower respiratory tract secretions frequently associated with signs of variable airflow obstruction. In the intensive care unit (ICU), tracheobronchitis is a relatively common problem related to multiple potential insults to the airway of a critically ill host. For instance, the presence of an endotracheal tube, the frequent suctioning needed to maintain airway clearance, the process of bacterial colonization and the aspiration of contaminated secretions are only a few of the multiple triggers of an inflammatory response in the airway.

In contrast to ventilator-associated pneumonia (VAP), nosocomial tracheobronchitis is not associated with parenchymal involvement and thus, no radiographic pulmonary infiltrates. However, high quality portable chest radiographs may be difficult to obtain in the ICU, where poor patient cooperation, inconsistent technique and other obstacles may lead to inadequate studies [1]. Furthermore, common processes such as atelectasis, pulmonary edema, pleural effusions or pulmonary embolism can cause infiltrates that mimic pneumonia making this clinical distinction difficult [2].

The pathogenesis, diagnosis, preventive strategies and management of nosocomial or ventilator-associated pneumonia (VAP) are addressed extensively in various chapters of this textbook. For bacterial tracheobronchitis, the risk factors, routes and mechanisms of bacterial airway colonization are the same and will not be repeated in this section.

Bacterial Tracheobronchitis

Bacteria are among the most common causes of infectious tracheobronchitis in the ICU. Infectious tracheobronchitis is diagnosed when a patient develops fever, purulent respiratory secretions, and leukocytosis but the chest radiograph shows no new infiltrate [3]. However, when a patient lacks fever or leukocytosis the differentiation between colonization and active infection can be difficult and controversial. Furthermore the specific role that tracheobronchial colonization plays in predisposing a patient to develop a subsequent lower respiratory tract infection is unclear.

Colonization of the oropharynx has been associated with several factors including age, severity of acute and chronic illness, and hospitalization [4–6]. One study of outpatients with chronic tracheostomy concluded that patients could be managed with a low risk for developing severe respiratory tract infections, despite massive airway colonization with potentially pathogenic bacteria [7]. However, hospitalized patients with a tracheostomy or a translaryngeal endotracheal tube have both a higher frequency of tracheobronchial colonization, especially with Gram-negative enteric bacteria and *P. aeruginosa*, and also a higher risk of developing a severe lower respiratory tract infection [4, 8–11]. The upper airways and tracheobronchial tree serve a mechanical barrier function and also provide a mucociliary mechanism for removing particulate matter and microbes that have been deposited within the respiratory tract. Mucociliary clearance depends on the composition of airway secretions, an effective mucociliary escalator apparatus, and the presence of an effective cough reflex [12]. Artificial airways create a setting that is optimal for both colonization and the subsequent development of tracheobronchitis or pneumonia. Artificial airways provide direct access for bacteria to the lower respiratory tract, reduce effective cough reflex, and compromise the mucociliary escalator [13, 14]. Furthermore, endotracheal tube insertion and suctioning may cause tracheal epithelial cell damage allowing bacterial adherence and increased mucus secretion and stagnation [15, 16]. Respiratory therapy devices including medication nebulizers, ventilator spirometer, and ventilatory circuit and condensate may play a role in harboring and transmitting bacteria [17, 18].

While colonization with Gram-positive organisms occurs, Gram-negative bacilli are much more common in ICU patients with many studies showing *Pseudomonas* species as the most commonly isolated organism [19–21]. While there are no useful parameters to objectively predict which of those patients who have tracheobronchial colonization will go on to develop infectious tracheobronchitis, it is clear that tracheobronchitis often develops in those patients who are colonized. In one study seven of 15 patients with a chronic tracheostomy had colonization with *Pseudomonas* species and all of them developed an episode of purulent tracheobronchitis [22]. George *et al.*, found that tracheal colonization preceded ventilator-associated pneumonia in 93.5% and was a significant independent risk factor for ventilator-associated pneumonia [23].

While as a group, aerobic enteric Gram-negative bacilli account for most of the respiratory infections in ventilated patients, *Staphylococcus aureus* remains a very important nosocomial pathogen accounting for 20% of nosocomial respiratory infections. *S. aureus* is found in the nasopharynx in 20–40% of adults at any time with the carrier rate as high as 70% in hospitalized patients. Furthermore, patients with underlying lung disease, such as cystic fibrosis or chronic obstructive pulmonary disease, are frequently observed to have tracheobronchial colonization with *S. aureus*. The emergence of methicillin-resistant strains of *Staphylococcus aureus* (MRSA) has posed a special therapeutic problem. Manifestations are not limited to nosocomial pneumonia but also have been reported to cause a fulminant tracheobronchitis [24].

Acinetobacter baumannii (formerly *A. calcoaceticus* var. *anitratus*) has emerged as an important nosocomial pathogen that is most commonly seen in the ICU setting in those patients with impaired host defenses requiring mechanical ventilation. In addition to tracheobronchitis and pneumonia, other resulting illnesses include endocarditis, peritonitis, skin and soft tissue infection, urinary tract infection, and bloodstream infection. *A. baumannii* infections have been linked to contaminated respiratory therapy equipment, intravascular access devices, and transmission via hands of hospital personnel [25]. Seifert *et al.* observed that tracheobronchitis was the presumed portal of entry for nosocomial *A. baumannii* bacteremia in 19 of 87 (22%) episodes. This study also confirmed the results of other studies suggesting that the major determinants for developing *A. baumannii* bacteremia included treatment in an ICU, major surgery, mechanical ventilation, hyperalimentation, broad-spectrum antimicrobial therapy, and intravascular catheters [26]. Multi-drug resistance is common among these organisms limiting therapeutic options and resulting in mortality as high as 46% [27, 28].

Although *Mycoplasma pneumoniae* infection is best known for its ability to produce atypical pneumonia in young adults it may result in bronchitis about 30 times more often than it causes pneumonia [29]. *M. pneumoniae* is associated with both acute bronchiolitis and bronchiolitis obliterans in the infant and child as well as in the adult population. In children it is a relatively infrequent but significant cause of bronchiolitis accounting for 11% of cases of bronchiolitis due to a known agent [30]. *M. pneumoniae* outbreaks occur sporadically but have a predilection for the late fall and early winter [31]. Isolated bronchiolitis or bronchiolitis obliterans with organizing pneumonia (BOOP) without a patchy or lobar alveolar pneumonia is uncommon. Furthermore acute infectious bronchiolitis requiring hospitalization is relatively unusual in adults. Nonetheless *M. pneumoniae* should be considered as a cause for acute bronchitis or bronchiolitis in hospitalized patients.

The typical case of *Mycoplasma* infection begins insidiously with fever, nonproductive cough, headache, malaise and occasional chills. Upper respiratory symptoms of rhinitis and sore throat are present in 50% of cases. Myalgias, arthralgias, skin rash or gastrointestinal symptoms are rare; bullous myringitis and ARDS develop occasionally [32]. Rare cases of profound hypoxemia with airflow obstruction and hypercapnia have been reported presumably as a result of widespread bronchiolitis [33].

Fungal Tracheobronchitis

Fungal infections limited to the tracheobronchial tree are relatively uncommon. Clark *et al.*, [34] reported that of a total of 207 patients, only 15 (7%) had infection solely or predominantly within the airways [34–38]. The incidence of *Candida* infection localized to the tracheobronchial tree must be much lower as reported cases are very rare. Furthermore, some cases are poorly documented pathologically and the diagnosis of bronchial candidiasis was made solely on the basis of repeatedly positive sputum cultures and clinical improvement after treatment with antifungal agents [39, 40]. To our knowledge, there are no reported cases of *Mucor* spp. causing tracheobronchitis. In a case series of nine patients with fungal tracheobronchitis, the observations of Clark *et al.* confirmed other literature that *Aspergillus* was the predominant pathogen occurring alone in six of the cases and in combination with Candida spp. in one case. *Candida* spp. and *Rhizopus* spp. were each the sole responsible pathogen in one case [34].

Fungal tracheobronchitis can have two different morphological manifestations. The first consists of intraluminal growth involving more or less the entire circumference of the airway wall with only superficial mucosal invasion. Pathologically, such infection can appear as a peudomembrane in which a fibrinous exudate related to airway ulceration is prominent, or as tenacious mucus/fungus plugs more or less completely occluding the tracheobronchial tree. This is perhaps the most likely form of serious fungal infection to be missed clinically, as patients may only complain of increasing dyspnea with or without hemoptysis. Because the parenchyma is unaffected the chest roentgenograms may be normal. Thus it is important to send bronchial casts and airway debris for culture and histological analysis, especially in immunocompromised patients [34].

The second morphological form consists of one or several discrete plaques localized to a relatively small portion of the tracheobronchial tree. Although in the early stages of infection, invasion is limited to the airway mucosa, with progression of disease fungi penetrate beyond the bronchial wall into the adjacent lung parenchyma where they may result in focal pneumonia or abscess formation. Vascular invasion is not uncommon and may lead to parenchymal or pleural hemorrhage [34].

The explanation for why fungi colonize and invade the tracheobronchial tree in certain patients is unclear. However, given the underlying disorders that patients with fungal tracheobronchitis commonly have, it is clear that a deficiency in the host immune system is a common denominator among these patients. Fungal tracheobronchitis has been seen in patients with lung and bone marrow transplantation, AIDS and hematological malignancies

[41]. Prolonged neutropenia occurring either secondary to the malignancy or chemotherapy has been shown to be a risk factor for developing invasive pulmonary aspergillosis [42]. Even in the absence of neutropenia, impaired leukocyte mobilization and function may contribute to the predisposition to fungal infection in cancer patients [43]. Corticosteroids predispose to the development of fungal invasion by inhibiting macrophage killing of spores, inhibiting phagocyte migration to the site of infection, and by suppressing antibody production, delayed hypersensitivity reaction, and wound healing [34, 44]. Broad-spectrum antibiotics change the normal flora and predispose to the development of fungal colonization. Cellular and humoral immune deficiency are additional risk factors [45].

Viral Tracheobronchitis

Many respiratory infections caused by viruses begin in the upper respiratory tract usually without producing lower respiratory symptoms. A variety of clinical syndromes including rhinitis, pharyngitis, laryngotracheitis (croup), bronchitis or tracheobronchitis, bronchiolitis and pneumonia can occur depending on the specific virus involved, the viral load, virulence, host resistance and extent of respiratory mucosal involvement [46].

The patient's age is also an important factor in the form and severity of infection; for example, rhinovirus typically causes only coryza in immunocompetent adults, whereas it is a cause of croup, bronchitis, bronchiolitis and pneumonia in children. The attack rates for respiratory sincitial virus (RSV), parainfuenza virus types 1 and 3 and adenovirus is also several folds higher in the first two years of life [46].

In the ICU, viral tracheobronchitis is usually seen in one of two situations: (a) primary viral infection usually acquired in the community, such as influenza, parainfluenza, adenovirus or RSV that is either severe or complicates underlying pulmonary disease or, (b) reactivation of a latent virus in the nosocomial setting, such as herpes simplex virus (HSV) or cytomegalovirus (CMV). Either situation can further be complicated by bacterial co-infection or superinfection [47].

INFLUENZA VIRUS

Influenza virus infection usually involves only the upper respiratory tract, including trachea and major bronchi; however in a small percentage of patients, particularly the chronically ill or the elderly, it may be responsible for severe pneumonia. It can occur in pandemics, epidemics or sporadically. Almost all severe epidemics and all pandemics are caused by type A influenza. Typical winter outbreaks occur every year in temperate climates with a less predictable seasonal variation in tropical areas. Transmission occurs from person to person with an incubation period of 24–48 hours and is highly contagious. Viral shedding and infectivity can persist for as long as two weeks in children, but probably less in adults [48]. Antibody formation to specific strains by either immunization or infection confers immunity for 1–2 years. Serologic studies have found a higher incidence of antibodies to influenza A and B in health care workers than controls [49]. The risk of developing a complicated course is increased in older individuals, those with a significant history of tobacco smoking, comorbidities and pregnancy [50–52].

The clinical manifestations are variable and depend on the virulence of the influenza virus strain, the underlying condition and response of the host. The flu-like syndrome with rapid onset of dry cough, myalgias, headache, chills and fever without major pulmonary complaints affects predominantly young adults. Another syndrome seen in influenza is the bronchitis/tracheobronchitis with no radiographic abnormality but with more respiratory distress and sometimes associated with hemoptysis, exacerbation of underlying asthma or COPD. In more severe cases, spread of the virus to the pulmonary parenchyma causes clinical worsening within

12–36 hours with worsening dyspnea, tachypnea, cyanosis and hypoxemia [53, 54]. Finally, it is well recognized that superinfection with *Staphylococcus aureus*, *Streptococcus pneumoniae*, *Hemophilus influenzae* or other bacterias can occur after influenza [55].

The diagnosis can be confirmed by culturing the virus from respiratory secretions. More rapid diagnostic methods available consist of direct immunofluorescence assay (DFA), polymerase chain reaction (PCR) or the new rapid assays that detect activity of influenza neuraminidase or viral nucleoproteins [56].

Influenza vaccination is the mainstay of protection against the disease. The older drugs available for the prevention and treatment of influenza are amantadine and rimantadine. However, their use is limited by by lack of activity against Influenza B, rapid emergence of resistance and, especially with amantidine, central nervous sytem toxicity. New agents available for the treatment of influenza A and B include the neuraminidase inhibitors zanamivir that is delivered by inhalation and oseltamivir phosphate available orally [57].

PARAINFLUENZA VIRUS

In adults, parainfluenza is responsible for pharyngitis and coryza; in infants and children it is the predominant cause of severe croup. Immunocompromised individuals are at increased risk for more severe presentations. Parainfluenza type 1 and 2 occur predominantly in the autumn and early winter. Parainfluenza type 3 occurs in the spring and is an important cause of bronchiolitis or pneumonia in infants and children. Lower respiratory tract involvement in adults is uncommon.

The clinical manifestations in adults are acute pharyngitis and tonsillitis. When complicated by pneumonia it is indistinguishable from other viral or *Mycoplasma* infection. The radiographic findings are nonspecific. The organism can be isolated by culture of sputum or nasopharyngeal secretions. Immunofluorescent antibody is useful for rapid identification.

There are currently no available antiviral agents with proven effectiveness against parainfluenza virus. Ribavirin is active against the virus *in vitro*, but there have been no randomized controlled trials in humans.

RHINOVIRUS

Rhinovirus causes approximately 40–50% of common cold cases. Clinically significant lower respiratory tract infection in adults is uncommon but includes acute bronchitis, bronchiolitis and pneumonia. Perhaps more important is the indirect effect that such an infection may have in patients with asthma, COPD or other medically debilitating states. Rhinovirus infection has been associated with exacerbation of COPD and respiratory failure [58].

ADENOVIRUS

Adenovirus can cause pharyngitis, pharyngoconjuntivitis, laryngotracheo-bronchitis, bronchiolitis, pneumonia or a non-specific acute respiratory syndrome; there is also some evidence that it may cause some cases of bronchiectasis, bronchiolitis obliterans and hyperlucent lung syndrome [59]. Infections can occur sporadically or in epidemics. Localized nosocomial outbreaks have also been reported.

The adenoviruses are the most common cause of the ARDS, a poorly defined condition consisting of fever, pharyngitis, cough, hoarseness, chest pain, and conjunctivitis. Chills and myalgias may be present. In some cases, tracheobronchitis is prominent and may be indistinguishable from the classic whooping cough caused by *Bordetella pertussis*. When pneumonia occurs it is typically mild and associated with upper respiratory symptoms. However, a few fatal cases have been seen with autopsy studies revealing extensive areas of hemorrhagic consolidation with alternating areas of atelectasis and hyperinflation. The airways frequently show marked airway congestion with mucopurulent or hemorrhagic material. In most cases the infection is self-limited and the treatment is supportive.

RESPIRATORY SYNCYTIAL VIRUS

Respiratory syncytial virus (RSV) is particularly important as a cause of bronchiolitis in infants and small children. Infection occurs predominantly during the winter months and early spring. Transmission occurs by airborne droplets or hand-to-hand contact. The disease is highly contagious and there is evidence that health care workers are at increased risk for infection [49].

In adults, the disease is usually mild and limited to the upper respiratory tract. However, in the elderly, chronically ill, immunocompromised or hospitalized patient, lower tract involvement can occur [60]. Rarely, RSV can cause acute pneumonia with rapid progression to ARDS [61].

The clinical manifestations reflect the extent of airway involvement. Nasal congestion and discharge usually precede the cough and wheezing by 2–3 days, but may occur simultaneously. In contrast to Influenza infection, RSV is associated with relatively little risk of bacterial superinfection. The radiological findings usually reflect a disparity between the severity of respiratory symptoms and a paucity of abnormalities. However, bronchial wall thickening, peribronchial infiltrates or lobular consolidation may occur.

RSV can be cultured from nasopharyngeal or lower respiratory secretions. In adults and transplant patients, bronchoalveolar lavage is more sensitive than throat swabs [62]. The shell-vial culture has been shown to be a rapid and sensitive method. PCR and immune based assays including antigen detection by immunofluorescence or enzyme-linked immunosorbent assay (ELISA) are available for rapid diagnosis.

In addition to supportive care, severe cases of RSV infection have been treated with aerosolized ribavirin (6 g reconstituted in 300 ml of sterile water to a final concentration of 20 mg/ml and administered 12 to 18 hours per day for 3–7 days); although no clinical trials have been conducted in this patient population. There is no data regarding the use of oral ribavirin.

HERPES SIMPLEX VIRUS

Herpes simplex virus (HSV) was first recognized as a pulmonary pathogen by Morgan and Finland almost a half century ago [63]. Stern *et al.* [64] first focused attention on the possibility of herpetic involvement of the trachea and its transmission via contaminated secretions from an infected patient to a health care worker, causing herpetic whitlow. Later reports of herpetic respiratory infections have included patients with underlying diseases [65, 66], extensive burns [67], underlying malignancy, chemotherapy and radiation therapy [68], and critically ill patients with ARDS [69–72].

Herpetic tracheobronchitis has also been reported in immunocompetent patients without history of chronic lung disease [73–75], in patients after extracorporeal circulation for cardiac surgery [76], and following general surgery [77–79].

Despite the apparent increasing prevalence of pulmonary HSV, the relationship between respiratory HSV isolation, pulmonary function, and clinical outcome is not well documented. HSV type 1 in lower respiratory secretions has been associated with unresolved acute bronchospasm [73], prolonged requirement for mechanical ventilation [73–79], tracheal stenosis, and increased mortality [79, 80]. However, asymptomatic viral shedding of HSV also occurs in approximately one per cent to five per cent of asymptomatic normal individuals [81].

The concept of airway injury leading to viral reactivation has been reported previously in autopsy series [67, 82, 83] and in patients who have undergone surgery [73, 79]. One reason for this susceptibility of "traumatized" epithelium to viral colonization and potential subsequent inflammation may be that HSV typically infects squamous epithelium [84]. Thus, factors that promote squamous metaplasia, such as trauma, smoking, radiation therapy, or chemotherapy, may predispose the patient to lower respiratory tract infection with HSV [84].

At the present time, to our knowledge, there are no defined criteria for the diagnosis or treatment of herpetic tracheobronchitis. Simple isolation of HSV from respiratory secretions is clearly insufficient to make this diagnosis, since HSV can be asymptomatically shed in up to five per cent of asymptomatic adults, and the incidence of reactivation or shedding is increased in patients with airway injury. Thus, one usually makes the diagnosis based on a combination of the viral cultures, direct bronchoscopic examination of the endobronchial tree, cytological examination of tracheal or bronchial washings, and the clinical status of the patient.

The most frequent clinical manifestations exhibited by the patients are fever, productive cough and dyspnea. Frequency of these symptoms does not differ between the immunocompromised and immunocompetent patients. However, immunocompetent patients have significantly more bronchospasm. These data imply that the pathogenicity of HSV in the respiratory tract may vary depending on underlying immune status and the host response [85].

In addition, the role of primary infection versus reactivation in the spectrum of clinical manifestations of tracheobronchitis is unclear. One could speculate that respiratory HSV isolation in the immunocompromised patients most often represents "asymptomatic" shedding, perhaps due to reactivation, with less airway inflammation and, consequently, less bronchial hyperactivity. For unclear reasons, the clinical manifestations of HSV infection are more severe in the immunocompetent population; this may represent a more exuberant local immune response.

Whether to treat critically ill patients with lower respiratory tract HSV isolation with acyclovir is uncertain and controversial at this time. At the present time, it seems reasonable to treat with intravenous acyclovir (8 mg/Kg every 8 hours for 10 days) those patients with HSV isolation from lower respiratory secretions if, in addition, they have a clinical syndrome or bronchoscopic findings consistent with tracheobronchitis. However, future prospective, randomized trials that assess the impact of treatment on the outcome of both the apparently asymptomatic HSV "carrier" and those patients with clinical HSV tracheobronchitis are needed to clarify this issue. In addition, given the risk of horizontal transmission of HSV-1 to health care workers, full compliance with infection control measures, including use of gloves and goggles when there is any potential for contact with secretions, is recommended [86].

CYTOMEGALOVIRUS

Cytomegalovirus (CMV) has been cultured with increasing frequency from patients on prolonged mechanical ventilatory support [87]. Similarly to the case of HSV, the clinical spectrum of CMV can range from asymptomatic viral shedding to a severe disease with profound immunosupression, pneumonitis and multi-organ dysfunction syndrome. In contrast to HSV where the predominant involvement occurs in the airways, CMV typically involves the pulmonary parenchyma, leading to interstitial pneumonitis or diffuse alveolar damage. CMV infection has been shown to potentiate effects of bacterial infections, possibly through impairment of neutrophil migration or macrophage activation, and has been implicated in promoting bacterial translocation [79]. Cardiac surgery patients with CMV infection complicating mediastinitis have been shown to have persistence of local infection, prolonged hospitalization and increased mortality [88]. Trauma patients with HSV or CMV reactivation have also been shown to have increased ventilator dependence and increased superimposed bacterial pneumonias [89].

As with other organisms, several techniques are available to detect CMV. The virus can be isolated from various body fluids (e.g. blood, urine, respiratory secretions) and buffy coat culture may be useful. Use of shell-vial technique yields results within 24–36 hours. Additional, even more sensitive techniques include immunoglobulin-labeled immunomagnetic beads, fluorescent antibody staining, *in situ* hybridization, and PCR have also been utilized to identify CMV antigens. However, a major limitation of these tests is that it does not differentiate infection from disease. Thus, it is sometimes necessary to obtain tissue in order to assess the cytopathic effects.

The drugs effective against CMV are ganciclovir and foscarnet. However, the decision to treat an individual patient has to balance the risk of the patient, the evidence of disease and the potential toxicity associated with treatment.

Summary

Tracheobronchitis is increasingly recognized as a common syndrome in the ICU. The most common etiology is infection caused by bacterial, fungal, or viral pathogens. The clinical manifestations are variable and not specific for individual pathogens. The clinical distinction between incidental airway colonization and significant infection is difficult but carries important therapeutic and prognostic implications. A high index of suspicion with the appropriate diagnostic and treatment intervention can lead to an improved outcome.

Acknowledgment

We are indebted to Margie Galkowski for preparing the manuscript.

References

1. Siegal MD, Tocino I. Chest radiology in the intensive care unit. Clin Pulmonary Med 6:347, 1999.
2. Santos E, Talusan A, Brandestetter RD. Radiographic mimics of pneumonia in the critical care unit. Crit Care Clin 14:91, 1998.
3. Niederman MS, Craven DE, Fein AM, *et al.* Respiratory infection complication long-term tracheostomy: the implication of persistent Gram-negative tracheobronchial colonization. Chest 85:39, 1984.
4. Johanson WG, Pierce AK, Sanford JP, *et al.* Nosocomial respiratory infections with gram-negative bacilli. Ann Intern Med 77:701, 1972.
5. Örtqvest Å, Hammers-Berggren S, Kalin M. Respiratory tract colonization and incidence of secondary infection during hospital treatment of community-acquired pneumonia. Eur J Clin Microbiol Infect Dis 9:725, 1990.
6. Salata RA, Ellner JJ. Bacterial colonizaton of the tracheobronchial tree. Clin Chest Med 91:623, 1988.
7. Harlid R, Andersson G, Frostell CG, *et al.* Respiratory tract colonization and infection in patients with chronic tracheostomy: a one-year study in patients living at home. Am J Respir Crit Care Med 154:124, 1996.
8. Rogers RM, Weiler C, Ruppenthal B. Impact of the respiratory intensive care unit on survival of patients with acute respiratory failure. Chest 62:94, 1972.
9. Cross AS, Roup B. Role of respiratory assistance devices in endemic nosocomial pneumonia. Am J Med 70:681, 1981.
10. Niederman MS, Ferranti RD, Zeigler A, *et al.* Respiratory infection complicating long-term tracheostomy. Chest 85:39, 1984.
11. Bartlett JT, Faling LJ, Willey S. Quantitative tracheal bacteriological and cytologic studies in patients with long-term tracheostomies. Chest 74:635, 1978.
12. Levine SA, Niederman MS. The impact of tracheal intubation on host defenses and risks for nosocomial pneumonia. Clin Chest Med 12:523, 1991.
13. Gal TJ. How does tracheal intubation alter respiratory mechanics? Probl Anesth 2:191, 1988.
14. Klainer AS, Turndorf H, Wu WH, *et al.* Surface alterations due to endotracheal intubation. Am J Med 58:674, 1975.
15. Ramphal R, Guay P. *Pseudomonas aeruginosa* adhesions for tracheobronchial mucin. Infect Immun 55:600, 1987.
16. Ramphal R, Pyle M. Adherence of mucoid and nonmucoid *Pseudomonas aeruginosa* to acid-injured tracheal epithelium. Infect Immun 41:345, 1983.
17. Craven DE, Goularte TA, Make BJ. Contaminated condensate in mechanical ventilator circuits: a risk factor for nosocomial pneumonia. Am Rev Respir Dis 129:625, 1984.
18. Craven DE, Lichtenberg DA, Goularte TA, *et al.* Contaminated medication nebulizers in mechanical ventilator circuits: source of bacterial aerosols. Am J Med 77:834, 1984.
19. Schwartz SN, Dowling JN, Benkovic C, *et al.* Sources of gram-negative bacilli colonizing the trachea of intubated patients. J Infect Dis 138: 227, 1978.

20. Niederman MS, Mantovani R, Schoch P, *et al.* Patterns and routes of tracheobronchial colonization in mechanically ventilated patients: the role of nutritional status in colonization of the lower airway by *Pseudomonas* species. Chest 95:155, 1989.
21. Johanson WG Jr, Pierce AK, Sanford JP, *et al.* Nosocomial respiratory infections with gram-negative bacilli: the significance of colonization of the respiratory tract. Ann Intern Med 77:701, 1972.
22. Niederman MS, Ferranti RD, Ziegler A, *et al.* Respiratory infection complicating long-term tracheostomy: The implication of persistent gram-negative tracheobronchial colonization. Chest 85:39, 1984.
23. George DL, Falk PS, Wunderink RG, *et al.* Epidemiology of ventilator-acquired pneumonia based on protected bronchoscopic sampling. Am J Respir Crit Care Med 158:1839, 1998.
24. Namba Y, Mihara N, Tanaka M. Fulminant tracheobronchitis caused by methicillin-resistant *Staphylococcus aureus* (MRSA) (Japanese). Nihon Kyobu Shikkan Gakkai Zasshi. Jap J Thoracic Dis 35:969, 1997.
25. Cefai C, Richads J, Gould FK, *et al.* An outbreak of *Acinetobacter* respiratory tract infection resulting from incomplete disinfection of ventilatory equipment. J Hosp Infect 15:177, 1990.
26. Seifert H, Strate A, Pulverer G. Nosocomial bacteremia due to *Acinetobacter baumannii*: Clinical features, epidemiology, and predictors of mortality. Medicine 74:340, 1995.
27. Seifert H, Baginski R, Schulze A, *et al.* Antimicrobial susceptibility of *Acinetobacter* species. Antimicrob Agents Chemother 37:750, 1993.
28. Chen YC, Chang SC, Hsieh WC, *et al. Acinetobacter calcoaceticus* bacteremia: analysis of 48 cases. J Formosan Med Assoc 90:958, 1991.
29. Leigh MW, Clyde WA. Chlamydial and mycoplasmal pneumonias. Semin Respir Infect 2:152, 1987.
30. Glezen WP, Loda FA, Clyde WA, *et al.* Epidemiologic patterns of acute lower respiratory disease of children in a pediatric practice. J Pediatr 78:397, 1971.
31. Rose RM, Pinkston P, O'Donnell C, *et al.* Viral infection of the lower respiratory tract. Clin Chest Med 8:405, 1987.
32. Fischman RA, Marschall KE, Kislak JW, *et al.* Adult respiratory distress syndrome caused by *Mycoplasma* pneumonia. Chest 74:471, 1978.
33. Zack MB, Kazemi H. Carbon dioxide retention in *Mycoplasma* pneumonia. Am Rev Respir Dis 107:1052, 1973.
34. Clarke A, Skelton J, Fraser RS. Fungal tracheobronchitis: report of 9 cases and review of the literature. Medicine 70:1, 1991.
35. Meyer RD, Young LS, Armstrong D *et al.* Aspergillosis complicating neoplastic disease. Am J Med 54:6, 1973.
36. Orr DP, Myerowitz RL, Dubois PJ Pathoradiologic correlation of invasive pulmonary aspergillosis in the compromised host. Cancer 41:2028, 1978.
37. Young RC, Bennett JE, Vogel CL, *et al.* Aspergillosis. The spectrum of the disease of 98 patients. Medicine 49:149, 1970.
38. Dubois PJ, Myerowitz RL, Allen CM. Pathoradiologic correlation of pulmonary candidiasis in immunosuppressed patients. Cancer 40:1026, 1977.
39. Chakravarty SC. Bronchopulmonary candidiasis: Clinical aspects. Dis Chest 51:608, 1967.
40. Wengrower D, Or R, Segal E, Kleinman Y. Bronchopulmonary candidiasis exacerbating asthma. Case report and a review of the literature. Respiration 42:209, 1985.
41. Kramer MR, Denning DW, Marshall SE, *et al.* Ulcerative tracheobronchitis after lung transplantation: a new form of invasive aspergillosis. Am Rev Respir Dis 144:552, 1991.
42. Gerson SL, Talbot GH, Hurwitz S, *et al.* Prolonged granulocytopenia: the major risk factor for invasive pulmonary aspergillosis in patients with acute leukemia. Ann Intern Med 100:345, 1984.
43. Lehrer RI, Cline MJ. Leukocyte candidacidal activity and resistance to systemic candidiasis in patients with cancer. Cancer 27:1211, 1971.
44. Dale DC, Petersdorf RG. Corticosteroids and infectious diseases. Med Clin North Am 57:1277, 1973.
45. Bodey GP. Candidiasis in cancer patients. Am J Med 77(Suppl 4D):13, 1984.
46. Denny FW Jr. The clinical impact of human respiratory virus infections. Am J Respir Crit Care Med 152:S4, 1995.
47. Ellenbogen C, Graybill JL, Silva J, *et al.* Bacterial pneumonia complicating viral pneumonia. Am J Med 56:169, 1974.
48. Frank AL, Taber LH, Wells CR, *et al.* Patterns of shedding of myxoviruses and paramyxoviruses in children. J Infect Dis 144:433, 1981.
49. Davies KJ, Herbert AM, Westmoreland D, *et al.* Seroepidemiological study of respiratory virus

infections among dental surgeons. Br Dent J 176:262, 1994.
50. Kark JD, Lebiush M, Rannon L. Cigarette smoking as a risk factor for epidemic $A(H_1N_1)$ influenza in young men. N Engl J Med 307: 1042, 1982.
51. Mullooly JP, Barker WH, Nolan TF Jr. Risk of acute respiratory disease among pregnant women during influenza A epidemics. Public Health Rep 101:205, 1986.
52. Conway SP, Simmonds EJ, Littlewood JM. Acute severe deterioration in cystic fibrosis associated with influenza A virus infection. Thorax 47:112, 1992.
53. O'Brien TG, Sweeney DF. Interstitial viral pneumonitis complicated by severe respiratory failure: successful management using intensive dehydration and steroids. Chest 63:314, 1973.
54. Roberts GBS. Fulminating influenza. Lancet 2:944, 1957.
55. Winther B, Brofeldt S, Gronborg H, *et al.* Study of bacteria in the nasal cavity and nasopharynx during naturally acquired common cold. Acta Otolaryngol 98:315, 1984.
56. The Medical Letter, Inc. Rapid diagnostic tests for influenza 41:121, 1999.
57. Calfee DP, Hayden FG. New approaches to influenza chemotherapy. Neuraminidase inhibitors. Drugs 56:537, 1998.
58. Smith CB, Kanner RE, Golden CA, *et al.* Effect of viral infection on pulmonary function in patients with chronic obstructive pulmonary diseases. J Infect Dis 141:271, 1980.
59. Bateman ED, Hayashi S, Kuwano K, *et al.* Latent adenoviral infection in follicular bronchiectasis. Am J Respir Crit Care Med 151:170, 1995.
60. Morales F, Calder MA, Inglis JM, *et al.* A study of respiratory infections in the elderly to assess the role of respiratory syncytial virus. J Infect 7:236, 1983.
61. Zaroukian MH, Kashyap GH, Wentworth BB. Case report: respiratory syncytial virus infection: a case of respiratory distress syndrome and pneumonia in adults. Am J Med Sci 295:218, 1988.
62. Englund JA, Piedra PA, Jewell A, Patel K, Baxter BB, Whimbey E. Rapid diagnosis of respiratory syncytial virus infection in immunocompromised adults. J Clin Microbiol 34:1649, 1996.
63. Morgan HR, Finland M. Isolation of herpes virus from a case of atypical pneumonia and erythema multiforme exudativum: with studies of four additional cases. Am J Med Sci 217:92, 1949.
64. Stern H, Elek SD, Millar DM, Anderson HF. Herpetic whitlow: a form of cross-infection in hospitals. Lancet 2:871, 1959.
65. Lheureux P, Verhest A, Vincent JL, Liénard C, Levivier M, Kahn RJ. Herpes virus infection, an unusual source of adult respiratory distress syndrome. Aur J Respir Dis 67:72, 1985.
66. Benjamin DR. Herpes simplex tracheobronchitis and pneumonitis. Pediatr Pathol 9:773, 1989.
67. Nash G, Foley FD. Herpetic infection of the middle and lower respiratory tract. Am J Clin Pathol 54:857, 1970.
68. Ramsey PG, Fife KH, Hackman RC, Mayers JD, Corey L. Herpes simplex virus pneumonia: clinical, virologic, and pathologic features in 20 patients. Ann Intern Med 97:813, 1982.
69. Frable WJ, Frable MA, Seney FD Jr. Virus infections of the respiratory tract: cytopathologic and clinical analysis. Acta Cytol 21:32, 1977.
70. Tuxen DV, Wilson JW, Cade JF. Prevention of lower respiratory herpes simplex virus infection with acyclovir in patients with the adult respiratory distress syndrome. Am Rev Respir Dis 136:402, 1987.
71. Tuxen DV, Cade JF, McDonald MI, Buchanan MR, Clark RJ, Pain MC. Herpes simplex virus from the lower respiratory tract in adult respiratory distress syndrome. Am Rev Respir Dis 126:416, 1982.
72. Prellner T, Flamholc L, Haidl S, Lindholm K, Widell A. Herpes simplex virus – the most frequently isolated pathogen in the lungs of patients with severe respiratory distress. Scand J Infect Dis 24:283, 1992.
73. Sherry MK, Klainer AS, Wolff M, Gerhard H. Herpetic tracheobronchitis. Ann Intern Med 109:229, 1988.
74. Legge RH, Thompson AB, Linder J, Woods GL, Robbins RA, Moulton AL, *et al.* Acyclovir-responsive herpetic tracheobronchitis. Am J Med 85:516, 1988.
75. Chakraborty A, Forker A, Reese H, Casey J. Tracheobronchitis and pneumonia due to herpes simplex virus (HSV) infection. Nebr Med J 73:347, 1988.
76. Vaxelaire JF, Brunet F, Armaganidis A, Pochard F, Giraud T, Lanore JJ, *et al.* The role of herpes simplex virus in respiratory complications after cardiac surgery (abstract). Am Rev Respir Dis 143:A474, 1991.
77. Porteous C, Bradley JA, Hamilton DN, Ledingham IM, Clements GB, Robinson CG. Herpes simplex virus reactivation in surgical patients. Crit Care Med 12:626, 1984.

78. Avery RK, Longworth DL. Viral pulmonary infections in thoracic and cardiovascular surgery. Sem Thoracic Cardiovasc Surg 7:88, 1995.
79. Cook CH, Yenchar JK, Kraner TO, Davis EA, Ferguson RM. Occult herpes family viruses may increase mortality in critically ill surgical patients. Am J Surg 176:357, 1988.
80. St. John RC, Pacht ER. Tracheal stenosis and failure to wean from mechanical ventilation due to herpetic tracheitis. Chest 98:1520, 1990.
81. Corey L, Spear PG. Infections with herpes simplex viruses. N Engl J Med 314:749, 1986.
82. Nash G. Necrotizing tracheobronchitis and bronchopneumonia consistent with herpetic infection. Hum Pathol 3:283, 1972.
83. Graham BS, Snell JD Jr. Herpes simplex virus infection of the adult lower respiratory tract. Medicine 62:384, 1983.
84. Herout V, Vortel V, Vondrackova A. Herpes simplex involvement of the lower respiratory tract. Am J Clin Pathol 46:411, 1966.
85. Schuller D, Spessert C, Fraser JV, Goodenberger DM. Herpes simplex virus from respiratory tract secretions: epidemiology, clinical characteristics, and outcome in immunocompromised and non-immunocompromised hosts. Am J Med 94:29, 1993.
86. Perl TM, Haugen TH, Pfaller MA, Hollis R, Lakeman AD, Whitley RJ, *et al.* Transmission of herpes simplex virus type 1 infection in an intensive care unit. Ann Intern Med 117:584, 1992.
87. Papazian L, Fraisse L, *et al.* Cytomegalovirus. An unexpected cause of ventilator-associated pneumonia. Anesthesiology 84:280, 1996.
88. Domart Y, Trouillet JL, Fagan JY, Chastre J, Brun-Vezinet F, Gilbert C. Incidence and morbidity of cytomegaloviral infection in patients with mediastinitis following cardiac surgery. Chest 97:18, 1990.
89. Cushing D, *et al.* Herpes simplex virus and cytomegalovirus excretion associated with increased ventilator days in trauma patients. J Trauma 35:161, 1993.

37. SEVERE COMMUNITY-ACQUIRED PNEUMONIA

Miguel Gallego and Jordi Rello

Introduction

Pneumonia remains a common illness and a major cause of morbidity and mortality in the United States. In 1995, 82,900 deaths were caused by pneumonia [1]. The incidence of community-acquired pneumonia (CAP) is about 2 to 4/1000 persons/year, about 20% of whom require hospitalization [2].

The steady increase in the number of senior citizens and immunocompromised patients (those receiving corticosteroids, organ transplant recipients, HIV infection) and the better survival rates of patients affected by chronic illness are reasons that justify research in this field. Current investigations focus on improving diagnosis, defining risk factors that influence outcome and assessing new therapies.

In the last decade, a number of medical societies have sought to broaden our understanding of pneumonia by producing and publishing sets of guidelines. The first set of guidelines that avoided the traditional classification into "typical and atypical" pneumonia was published in 1993 by the American Thoracic Society (ATS) [3]. These guidelines classify patients into four categories on the basis of the most probable etiology: a) community-acquired pneumonia in patients younger than 60, without chronic associated illness; b) community-acquired pneumonia in patients older than 60 or patients with chronic associated conditions; c) pneumonia that requires hospitalization and d) pneumonia that requires ICU admission. In Europe similar guidelines have been produced, seeking to identify patients at risk of death or complications [4]. This chapter focuses on the subgroup of CAP patients that are admitted to the ICU – approximately 10% of patients hospitalized for CAP [5] – and reviews the most important factors regarding etiology, prognosis, diagnostic tools and treatments.

Definition

No consensus has been reached among researchers as regards the definition of severe pneumonia. Obviously, the condition of patients admitted to the ICU for control of vital constants, shock correction or mechanical ventilation can be considered severe, but criteria for ICU admission may differ from hospital to hospital. Therefore percentages of hospitalized patients requiring admission to the ICU obtained in different studies fluctuate between 5% and 35% [6], and may well reflect differences not only in clinical criteria, but in infrastructure as well. Some authors have tried to define criteria of severe pneumonia. In 1987 the British Thoracic Association [7] published the first guidelines based on a survey of 453 patients admitted to hospital for CAP. Using multivariate analysis the study concluded that three variables were associated with an increased risk of mortality: respiratory rate ≥30 breaths/min, blood urea >7 mmol/l and diastolic blood pressure ≤60 mmHg. The association of at least two of these variables increased the mortality risk 21 times. Subsequent studies have identified other factors that are related to mortality. The ATS guidelines, only recently validated, suggested 10 items for definition of severity (shown in Table 1); patients presenting any of them were diagnosed as cases of severe pneumonia. In a study conducted in Barcelona, Ewig *et al.* [8] studied 331 hospitalized CAP and 64 severe CAP admitted to the ICU. The presence of at least one of 10 criteria was 98% sensitive but only 32% specific, and the positive predictive value was as low as 24%. Moreover, both factors reflecting respiratory failure (respiratory rate >30 and PaO_2/FiO_2 <250 mm Hg) were found to be poorly sensitive and specific regarding to pneumonia severity. The authors suggested that definition of severity would need a "major" criterion (requirement of vasopressors >4 hours or requirement of mechanical ventilation) or at least two minor criteria (systolic blood pressure <90 mm Hg, PaO_2/FiO_2 <250 mm Hg, involvement of >two lobes in chest radiograph). These criteria had a sensitivity of 78% and specificity of 94%. Positive predictive value was 75% and negative predictive value 95%.

TABLE 1. Criteria of severity in CAP

Respiratory rate >30/minutes
Severe respiratory failure (PaO_2/FiO_2 < 250)
Requirement for mechanical ventilation
Bilateral involvement in chest radiograph
Increase in the size of the opacity by 50% or greater within 48 hours
Systolic blood pressure <90 mmHg
Diastolic blood pressure <60 mmHg
Requirement of vasopresors >4 hours
Urine output lower than 20 ml/h, or total urine output lower than 80 ml in 4 hours
Acute renal failure requiring dialysis

Aside from the need to validate these rules, there is no doubt that considering pneumonia as a dynamic process (which in the first 24–48 hours may worsen and require ICU admittance) can improve our approach to, and management of, this clinical entity. In a study of the influence of adherence to British guidelines on mortality, Hirani and Macfarlane [9] reported that 7% of CAP admitted in ICU were in cardiac arrest. In a previous study, cardiac arrest was present in 25% of cases [10]. In our own experience [11], pneumonia was documented in 24% of patients admitted to the ICU by cardiac arrest. This emphasizes the need for careful follow-up and respiratory monitoring of patients hospitalized by CAP.

Etiology and Risk Factors

The spectrum of causative agents of severe CAP is similar to that found in hospitalized patients or outpatients with CAP. The main difference is the relative importance of each microorganism. Table 2 [9, 12–17] shows that *S. pneumoniae* and *Legionella spp* account for 50% of cases with etiologic diagnosis. Likewise, Gram-negative microorganisms are the third most frequent cause in most series in the ICU. Interestingly, in some countries, ICU admission for tuberculosis may reach 10% of total cases [14].

The most important risk factors for *S. pneumoniae* infection are chronic hepatic disease, alcoholism, influenza, cigarette smoking and COPD [18]. In patients with HIV infection, the risk of pneumococcal infection correlates with the CD4 count. CD4 count below 200 or AIDS diagnosis significantly increases the risk of pneumococcal pneumonia. As many as 25% of these infections can produce bacteremia; the diagnosis of pneumococcal bacteremia should alert us to the possibility of HIV infection.

Pneumonia caused by *Legionella spp* is the second most frequent etiology, though there are significant regional variations. It is more common in Mediterranean countries and the US than in the north of Europe or South America.

The most important risk factors are smoking and corticotherapy. El-Ebiary *et al.* [19] reported COPD to be a more frequent risk factor in nosocomial pneumonia than in CAP caused by *Legionella pneumophila* (64% versus 41%). Infection in previously healthy patients has also

TABLE 2. Causative agents of severe CAP

Author	Pachón	Torres	Rello	Moine	Leroy	Rello	Hirani
Year	1990	1991	1993	1994	1995	1996	1997
Episodes	(n = 67)	(n = 92)	(n = 58)	(n = 132)	(n = 229)	(n = 95)	(n = 57)
Ref.	12	13	14	15	16	17	9
Intubation	–	61	87.5	61	50	87.3	96.4
Etiological diagnosis	48	52	60.3	72	66	39	67
S. pneumoniae	37.5	15	37	45	30.8	29.4	18
Legionella spp.	22	14	22.8	4.2	–	3.1	16
Enterobacteriaceae	25	4	11.4	14.7	18.1	6.3	–
H. influenzae	6	–	–	14.7	10	–	–
P. aeruginosa	–	5	–	–	3	–	1.7
Staphylococci	3	–	–	5.2	22**	1	12
Atypical pathogens*	–	6	–	7.3	3	3.1	5.2
P. carinii	–	–	8.5	–	–	1	5.2
M. tuberculosis	–	–	11.4	–	–	–	1.7
Virus	3	–	2.8	7.3	–	1	7
Others	–	5	5.6	10.5	12.7	–	1.7

* *M. pneumoniae, C. psitacci, C. pneumoniae, Rickettsia conorii, Coxiella burnetti.*
** Coagulase-negative staphylococci obtained from endotracheal aspirates that suggest contamination.
Values are presented as percentages.

been reported, even in cases of nosocomial acquisition.

H. influenzae accounts for between 6% and 15% [9, 12–17] of pneumonia that require ICU admission. COPD, elderly and HIV patients are mainly affected. Pneumonia caused by *S. aureus* is usually a severe infection, requiring ventilatory support in up to 90% of cases. The infection can occur after epidemic influenza or via bloodstream spread. Enterobacteriaceae are usually involved in nosocomial pneumonia and in some studies of CAP, are the third most important cause (25%) [12]. The microorganism most frequently involved is *Klebsiella pneumoniae*, which mainly affects COPD patients, alcoholics and in general patients suffering from consuming diseases. Blood isolation is reported in up to 38% of cases, especially in alcoholic patients.

Among Gram-negative bacteria, *P. aeruginosa* stand out on account of their extreme virulence. Fortunately the incidence in the community setting is low. In our opinion, this etiology should be considered only in patients with structural lung disease (bronchiectasis and cystic fibrosis), patients with neutropenia due to chemotherapy and HIV patients.

Finally, in a high percentage of patients the causative agent is impossible to determine even after extensive research. New microorganisms such as *C. pneumoniae* do not seem to play a role in severe pneumonia. A recent study [20] using PCR techniques confirmed that in the subgroup of patients with unknown etiology *S. pneumoniae* was the most probable cause.

Diagnosis

Empiricism is the usual approach in patients suffering from CAP. Indeed, some guidelines strongly recommend it [3]. However, a knowledge of causative agent is useful, given the possibility of adjusting antibiotic treatment on the basis of the antibiogram. Despite intensive etiologic research, the causative agent is not isolated in as many as 40% of cases. However, no study has concluded that outcome may be influenced by microorganism isolation.

From our point of view, the knowledge of etiology is useful, either for epidemiological purposes or to improve management in cases with poor clinical evolution. In severe CAP we recommend obtaining (at least) blood cultures and respiratory samples for cultures and Gram stain. However, it is extremely difficult to obtain a good sputum sample for the Gram stain from these patients (more than 25 neutrophils and ≤10 epithelial cells per microscopic field (×100)). In severe CAP a respiratory sample is available in only 40% of patients and in only 50% of these is it considered good enough for analysis [21].

Sputum induced by hypertonic saline serum has proved to be a good tool for *Pneumocystics carinii* and tuberculosis research, especially in AIDS patients. The success of this approach depends on the skill of the nurse and patient cooperation; an accuracy between 40–80% has been reported [22]. The usefulness of this method in the detection of other pulmonary pathogens has not been established.

The proper interpretation of Gram stain can be affected by staff training and by previous use of antibiotics; that is to say, previous antibiotic use may sterilize cultures, particularly in cases due to *H. influenzae* and *S. pneumoniae*. Furthermore, the interpretation of results in populations with high levels of bacterial colonization, such as COPD patients, can be difficult.

Blood cultures are positive in around 10–30% of patients with SCAP [2]. In spite of low sensitivity, the convincing nature of the isolation of a respiratory pathogen from blood, the opportunity to test the antimicrobial sensitivity of the isolate and the relative simplicity of drawing blood for cultures are all arguments in favor of the practice of obtaining blood cultures in patients requiring hospital admission. At least two cultures should be drawn by direct venopunction at separate sites. The main drawback is the time required, which means that the results are of no use in guiding initial treatment.

Other noninvasive techniques are based on antigen detection of some microorganisms in urine, plasma or sputum. The most useful is antigen detection of *Legionella spp* in urine. Sensitivity is around 50% and specificity is near to 100%. Likewise, this test is not influenced by previous use of the right antibiotic and can still remain positive for a long time after pulmonary infection has occurred (usually several weeks). The main drawback is that only serogroup 1 can be detected, though this serogroup accounts for >70% of *Legionella* infection [23]. More recently a colorimetric technique has been validated, allowing antigen detection at the bedside [24].

Other useful diagnostic tools that can be applied in etiologic investigation are based on invasive tests. Among these, fiberoptic bronchoscopy and transthoracic needle aspiration (TNA) are the most frequently used. Bronchoscopy is easy to perform when a patient is intubated, but it tends to be little used, because of the absence of laboratory equipment and well-trained bronchoscopic staff. Furthermore, in non-intubated patients, respiratory failure constitutes a relative contraindication, given the possibility of speeding up urgent intubation. In order to avoid this complication, a method that makes bronchoscopy safer in patients treated with CAP has recently been described [25]. This approach avoids the decline of positive end expiratory pressure and maintains correct levels of PaO_2.

The few studies undertaken in severe CAP have reported that the reliability of bronchoscopic tests is high. In one study, the authors reported isolation of causative agents in up to 70% of cases [26]. Likewise, correlation between bronchoalveolar lavage (BAL) and protected specimen brush (PSB) was good. In that study, none of the patients was receiving antibiotic treatment. In another study [27] performed in 193 patients affected by CAP of different degrees of severity, diagnosis was achieved in 71% of cases; the most reliable test was PSB. Other authors have tried to define the role of bronchoscopy as a rescue tool for pneumonia with poor clinical evolution. Örtqvist *et al.* [28]

evaluated the role of bronchoscopic techniques in patients with therapeutic failure. The authors considered failure to be early if it occurred before 72 hours, and late if it occurred after 72 hours. 277 patients were included in the study. Early failure was identified in 6% of cases and late failure in 7%. In 41% of these patients the performance of bronchoscopy gave useful information.

In the context of immunocompromise (HIV infection, stepidal therapy, transplantation) or high suspicion of atypical microorganism, performance of bronchoscopy with bronchoalveolar lavage (BAL) is the first step in the diagnostic approach. The accuracy of this test to detect *Pneumocystis carinii* is close to 90% [22].

Another invasive technique is TNA. Although few studies have evaluated its role in CAP, good results have been reported in nosocomial pneumonia and immunocompromised patients. In patients requiring ICU admission, the need for ventilatory support may preclude the performance of this technique, due to the high risk of barotrauma. Respiratory failure and severe bleeding diathesis are contraindications for this test. In general, sensitivity is around 40–50% and specificity is near to 100%. The prior use of antibiotic treatment and the size of pulmonary infiltrate are the main factors that can affect the diagnostic yield of this technique [29]. Pneumothorax and hemoptysis are the main complications; utilization of G25 needles reduces the number of adverse events.

Currently, it is possible to increase sensitivity of this procedure by means of techniques based on polymerase chain reaction (PCR) and agglutination latex, especially in the case of *S. pneumoniae* [30]. Procedures based on PCR techniques can be applied to noninvasive samples; sensitivity remains high, in spite of antibiotic treatment. In addition, the results are available in only a few hours. The high cost of these procedures and the lack of well-prepared laboratories preclude their world-wide use.

In our view, in severe CAP, a basic etiologic investigation should be performed, including at least two blood cultures, a respiratory sample (obtained by means of bronchoscope or simple trackeal aspirate) and urinary antigen detection for *Legionella*. Other tests can be performed depending on the equipment available at the center in question. In our opinion, establishing the etiology is recommended whenever possible.

Mortality – Prognostic Factors

In spite of advances in antibiotic treatments and the technical improvements in ICU, severe CAP mortality remains unacceptably high. In different studies of SCAP that require ICU admission, crude mortality is around 20–54% [9, 12–17]. In a recent meta-analysis undertaken by Fine *et al.* [31] these data on mortality are confirmed. In that study 33,148 patients were evaluated from 127 publications. Thirteen of these studies were of patients admitted to ICU. Mortality in hospitalized patients was 14%, and 36.5% in those admitted to ICU.

Mortality from respiratory infection is due to a combination of microbial virulence, bacterial burden and the patient's defensive system. For its part the immune system is conditioned by underlying disease, immunosuppressive treatments and other factors. In this section we will review the factors associated with worse outcome.

HOST CHARACTERISTICS

Age: This factor has been considered for a long time as a risk factor for the development of pneumonia and a factor associated with worse outcome. Mufson *et al.* [32], reported that the incidence of pneumococcal bacteremia increased with advancing age. In the 34–44 year-old group the incidence was 1/100,000, whereas in the 65–74 year group it was 25/100,000. Furthermore, in a study from Canada undertaken by Marrie [33] in a population older than 65, it was concluded that the mortality rate increased with the age, reaching 61% in those over 71.

Although it is true that pneumonia incidence and mortality rate are higher in senior citizens, the population older than 65 years is a mixture of healthy people and others with devastating underlying diseases. Age itself is not a factor of bad prognosis. In a case-control study (older than 65) performed in 101 pneumonia patients, Riquelme *et al.* [34] concluded that risk factors for CAP in this group of people were gastric aspiration and malnutrition (albumin less than 30 mg/dl) (the two groups were similar in relation with age, gender, and day of admittance). The significant prognostic factors were bedridden patients (RR 10.7), deglutition impairment (RR 7.3), lack of fever (RR 10.5), respiratory rate >30/min (RR of 5.2) and bilateral and multilobar involvement in chest radiography (more than three lobules) (RR 2.33).

In a study performed in patients older than 65 requiring ICU admission for SCAP [17], the mortality rate was 40%; however, in patients younger than 65 it was 31%. Nonetheless, in multivariate analysis, of the 23 variables studied, only the initial degree of severity of pneumonia, radiologic progression, septic shock and immunosuppression (corticoids included) were significantly related with bad outcome.

Underlying diseases: In most studies of severe pneumonia, a significant percentage of patients are reported to be affected by one or several underlying diseases. COPD is the most prevalent disease, reaching 50% of patients [12–17]. Furthermore, in epidemiological studies of pneumonia performed in general population [35], 39% of patients had some comorbidity, COPD accounting for 40% of them. In another study undertaken in the general population by Lange *et al.* [36], age and low FEV_1 were related with increased risk of death and hospital admittance. In view of these results, it is not surprising that COPD is a risk factor of poor outcome, and hospital admission is recommended in most guidelines. However, in a prospective multicenter study performed in COPD patients admitted for CAP [37], mortality was only 23% in the 22 patients who required ICU admission. This percentage of mortality is similar to the rate in COPD patients undergoing intubation for exacerbation.

In a multicenter study performed in ICUs in the USA [38], crude mortality in exacerbated COPD patients was 24%. This level of mortality was not related to COPD status but to multiorganic failure. When mortality was evaluated at 180 days, underlying disease was clearly related with mortality; severe COPD patients had fewer possibilities of survival than less severe COPD patients.

In another prospective study performed in the ICU (including patients with SCAP and severe nosocomial pneumonia) Almirall *et al.* [39] evaluated 127 patients, finding no relationship between mortality and underlying disease. The most closely related variables were age older than 70, a *simplified acute physiology score* (SAPS) higher than 12, septic shock, radiological bilateral involvement and *Pseudomonas aeruginosa* infection.

Likewise, in the meta-analysis by Fine *et al.* [31], neither COPD nor alcoholism were among the eleven prognostic significant factors. These findings agree with Rello *et al.*'s findings in elderly patients [17]; in that study, comorbidities were not related with pneumonia outcome, excepting immunosupresion.

Although patients affected by AIDS, transplantation or chemotherapy are excluded in most studies, their relative importance is growing. In a general population study, 57% of 385 evaluated patients were affected by some degree of immunocompromise (mainly HIV infection). This is why *S. pneumoniae* and *Pneumocystis carinii* were the most isolated microorganisms [40].

The type of underlying disease clearly affects the prognosis of these patients. For example, HIV infected patients suffering from pneumococcal bacteremia are six times more likely to die than HIV infected patients without pneumonia [41]. In severe neutropenia (<500 cells) due to chemotherapy, bacteremia is frequent, the most commonly isolated microorganisms being *P. aeruginosa* and *S. pneumoniae* [42].

RADIOLOGIC AND LABORATORY FACTORS

Septic shock, infiltrate progression, need for mechanical ventilation and multilobar involvement in initial chest x-ray are well established prognostic factors. In contrast, hypoxemia *per se* is not a risk factor, although it is mentioned in most guidelines.

MICROBIAL CHARACTERISTICS

The isolation of a microorganism in blood has been considered as a factor of poor prognosis. The most frequently isolated microorganism is *S. pneumoniae*. In spite of the use of newer antibiotics, mortality due to pneumococcal bacteremia remains unchanged (20–45%), reflecting perhaps the existence of a subgroup of patients with frail immunological defense. Marfin *et al.* [43] tried to identify risk factors of mortality in 102 patients with pneumococcal pneumonia and bacteremia. By means of multivariate analysis they found that age >50 years, lack of fever and nosocomial acquisition were the most important factors. Hypothermia is probably a marker of WBC activity or of reduced interleukin production.

In several studies, the isolation of *Pseudomonas aeruginosa* has been identified as a risk factor for death. The mortality rate was 100% in one study [13], although the incidence was only 1%. Fine *et al.* [31] reported *P. aeruginosa*-attributable mortality to be 63%, the highest among a range of causative agents.

Treatment

Treatment of SCAP involves a number of aspects that will be reviewed in this section: adequate antibiotic spectrum, shock management, and ventilatory support. It is important to remember that mortality is due to septic shock (particularly within the first four days) and refractory hypoxemia (ARDS and MOF) despite adequate antibiotic treatment [14].

IMPACT OF TREATMENT ON MORTALITY

Several studies using multivariate analysis have shown that inadequate antibiotic treatment is associated with a significant increase in mortality [12, 13, 16]. In a multicenter, retrospective study [44] of more than 14,000 patients older than 65 years with CAP, the authors reported that delay in starting antibiotic treatment (>8 hours) and non-performance of blood cultures in the first 24 hours were associated with increased mortality at 30 days of admission. In spite of these findings, other studies specifically addressed to SCAP in ICU admissions reported that the correct adherence to guidelines did not increase survival. In one study of 57 SCAP patients, mortality was 58%, the most frequently isolated microorganisms being *S. pneumoniae*, *Legionella pneumophila* and *Staphylococcus aureus*. Ten years earlier (before guidelines were extensively used), the same authors reported a similar level of mortality (54%) [9, 10]. These findings suggest that some unknown host-dependent factor of severity is present. Perhaps improvement of ICU management with newer therapies and identification of new prognostic factors would lower the mortality rate

SHOCK MANAGEMENT

Hemodynamic instability is defined by the need for vasoactive drugs, once the hydroelectrolytic dysfunction has been corrected, in order to achieve an arterial blood pressure sufficient to preserve peripheral perfusion. 25–50% of patients meet shock septic criteria when admitted to ICU. Currently, management of these patients is based on adequate hydration followed by norepinephrine administration. The specific approach of patients with pneumonia and septic shock does not differ from the general population with septic shock and it is discussed in detail in Chapter 6. Rescue therapy with vasopresine is a promising alternative in patients with refractory shock.

TREATMENT OF REFRACTORY HYPOXEMIA

Among patients admitted to the ICU for SCAP, between 58–88% need mechanical ventilation [21]. In patients undergoing mechanical ventilation, the goal is to improve gas interchange maintaining plateau pressures low in order to avoid acute lung injury.

The main drawback of intubation is that it increases the possibility of superinfections. New forms of ventilation that avoid intubation have been promoted in recent years, known generically as noninvasive ventilation. Noninvasive forms of ventilation have been tested in several diseases, and are very useful in COPD patients. As regards respiratory failure in SCAP, Confalonieri *et al.* [45] concluded that noninvasive ventilation was associated with a significant reduction in the rate of endotracheal intubation and duration of ICU stay. In more than 50% of enrolled patients (33/56 patients), COPD was the main underlying disease. Moreover, in this subgroup, a significant reduction of mortality was achieved when noninvasive ventilation was applied.

In general, our policy is to implement noninvasive ventilation whenever possible in order to avoid endotracheal intubation. When the level of consciousness is depressed or the ability to clear secretions is impaired, we avoid their use. The success of this approach depends mainly on training of nurses and respiratory therapists. Regardless of the population evaluated, the performance of these techniques seems to be useful to reduce the rate of nosocomial respiratory infection, to shorten hospital stay and to reduce mortality rate [46].

SCAP is associated with ARDS in about 10% of cases [21]. In general, when ARDS is developed, mechanical ventilation is needed, requiring high level O_2 delivery as well as high levels of PEEP, to ensure venous oxygen saturation of 90%. Two important goals in this context are the maintenance of low FiO_2 and tidal volume. In general, it is desirable to achieve a level of PEEP that maintains FiO_2 below 0.6 whenever possible. A protective ventilatory strategy using tidal volume below 6 ml/kg improves survival in patients with ARDS and increases the number of days without ventilator use [47].

In very severe cases, nitric oxide (NO), alveolar recruitment maneuvers and placement of patient in prone position as rescue adjunctive therapy have all been tested. The two last maneuvers are employed for alveolar reopening of collapsed areas of lung. Sometimes these approaches can achieve a dramatic reduction in the level of FiO_2 and PEEP.

ANTIBIOTIC TREATMENT

Usually, antibiotic treatment is started empirically, trying to cover the most frequent microorganisms and taking into account the risk factors for specific microorganisms. For an accurate treatment, it is critical to identify whether the pulmonary infection is due to *P. aeruginosa*, *Legionella* or penicillin-resistant pneumococci (PRP). Given that clinical differentiation is usually inaccurate, most guidelines recommend expanded-spectrum antibiotherapy. A combination of two antibiotics is generally preferred. For example, the ATS guidelines [3] recommend in 1993 a combination of a third generation cephalosporine with antipseudomonal activity plus a macrolide. This recommendation is based on the high mortality level reported for *P. aeruginosa*, but it does not take into account the low incidence of this pathogen in the community. Furthermore, activity of cefoperazone or ceftazidime against PRP is poor [48]. When it is necessary to expand coverage to *P. aeruginosa* (for example, in a patient with bronchiectasis), beta-lactam antibiotics such as cefepime or carbapenems are suitable because they maintain good activity against PRP. Table 3 shows some antibiotics with a good alveolar penetration and

TABLE 3. Antibiotics with acceptable activity against PRP and good alveolar penetration

a) Cephalosporines
   - Ceftriaxone
   - Cefotaxime
   - Cefepime

b) Beta-lactam/beta-lactamase inhibitors

c) Third generation fluoroquinolones

d) Linezolid

e) Carbapenems

Modified from [49–52].

activity against PRP. Among new fluoroquinolones, none have greater antipseudomonal activity than ciprofloxacin. As for aminoglycosides, their poor lung penetration, the fact that they can be inactivated when pH is low and the risk of severe renal toxicity all advise against their use.

In the IDSA guidelines [23] for ICU patients, third generation cephalosporine such as cefotaxime or ceftriaxone (or beta-lactam/beta-lactamase inhibitors) plus a macrolide or a fluoroquinolone are recommended. The use of a macrolide is due to the high incidence of *Legionella* infection. Although the standard treatment has classically included erythromycin, the need for large volume infusion, the better *in vitro* activity and the uncomfortable side effects (epigastric pain, transitory deafness) has led to the progressive introduction of newer macrolides. Both fluoroquinolones and newer macrolides present better activity against *Legionella* than erythromycin. Table 4 presents the different MIC of most significant macrolides and other antibiotics against *Legionella sp*. When *Legionella sp* infection is confirmed, combination therapy with rifampin is recommended in the first three days of treatment.

In some geographic areas PRP has become an important problem. In a multicenter Spanish study [54], 95 isolates of *S. pneumoniae* were analyzed. Half showed penicillin resistance, 24% intermediately resistant (MIC: 0.1–1 μgr/ml) and 25.2% highly resistant (MIC >1 μgr/ml). All isolates were susceptible to ceftriaxone and cefotaxime. The prior use of beta-lactam antibiotics (OR 2.8; 95% CI 1.4–1.9) and alcohol consumption (OR 5.2 95% CI 0.9–8 2) were independent risk factors for penicillin resistance. The same study reported that 30% of PRP strains were resistant to macrolides. Using multivariate analysis, it was detected that age under five years (OR 16.7, 95% CI 1.6–176.3) or above 65 (OR 4.3; CI 1.4–13.2), as well as previous use of beta-lactam antibiotics in patients with non-invasive pneumococcal infection (OR 7.9; 95% CI 1.8–34) were associated with a higher risk of multiple antibiotic resistance.

TABLE 4. Activities of antimicrobial agents against *Legionella spp.*

Antimicrobial	MIC 90 (μg/ml)
Rifampin	0.002–0.008
Erythromycin	0.12
Roxithromycin	0.03–0.12
Clarithromycin	<0.004
Linezolid	4–8
Ciprofloxacin	≤0.01–0.06
Grepafloxacin	≤0.01
Trovafloxacin	≤0.01

Modified from [49, 53].

Whether or not these strains are associated with increased mortality remains a controversial issue. In a study reported in 1995, 504 pneumococcal episodes of pneumonia were evaluated [55]. Although in the univariate analysis mortality rate in patients affected by PRP was 38% and 24% in PSP, the multivariate analysis did not show any significant differences. In another study conducted by Einarrson *et al.* [56], no differences in mortality were shown, but hospital stay and pharmacy costs were both increased. In contrast, in another study [57], although no differences in mortality were observed between PRP and PSP, the authors found no differences in pharmacy costs or hospital stay either. Moreover, a further study [58] reported an excess of mortality among patients suffering from CAP by PRP. More important in clinical practice is that cefixime, cefoperazone, ceftazidime or macrolides alone, must be ruled out as first line therapy for SCAP.

Due to the world-wide increase in PRP and the high incidence of *Legionella sp* infection in SCAP, new antibiotics have been developed in order to cover both microorganisms. New fluoroquinolones (levofloxacin, grepafloxacin, moxifloxacin and trovafloxacin) seem to offer good coverage against PRP and *Legionella*, and excellent lung tissue levels have been reported. These antibiotics could be a good alternative to the combination therapy mentioned above.

Clinafloxacin, moxifloxacin and trovafloxacin are the most active against *S. pneumoniae*. Trovafloxacin has an expanded spectrum to anaerobes. The lack of clinical trials in SCAP patients admitted to ICU and the risk of emergence of resistances, makes the use of fluoroquinolones advisable only in patients allergic to beta-lactam antibiotics.

Finally, the new oxazolidines, such as lizenolid, may become an interesting alternative for resistant Gram-positive respiratory infections [59]. In contrast, the poor alveolar penetration of vancomycin is associated with significant low survival rates and should no longer be considered as first line therapy [60]. Initial antibiotic therapy with a carbapenem should be considered if *Staphylococcus aureus* is a probable pathogen.

Conclusions

Severe community-acquired pneumonia is an important challenge for clinicians, due to the high rate of mortality despite the use of new antibiotics and the introduction of high technology in the ICU setting. Although risk factors of mortality are well known, pneumonia is a dynamic process that needs careful evaluation within the first hours after diagnosis has been established. In addition, given the relevance of pulmonary infections due to *Legionella sp* and PRP, we believe that antibiotic treatment must cover these microorganisms when the etiology is unknown. Antibiotic coverage for *P. aeruginosa* is necessary in selected patients at risk (bronchiectasis, neutropenia, HIV infection).

In general, a beta-lactam with PRP activity along with a new macrolide or a fluoroquinolone, administered intravenously, remains the preferred choice for initial treatment of patients with SCAP. Aminoglycosides and glicopeptides have poor alveolar penetration, exposing patients to an enormous risk of clinical failure. Fluoroquinolones represent an alternative for patients with beta-lactam allergy or pharmacologic interactions (transplant patient). Early recognition of severity and improvements in adjunctive therapy for shock and respiratory failure (noninvasive ventilation and a protective ventilatory strategy) are key elements to improve survival.

References

1. US Department of Commerce, Bureau of the Census: Statistical Abstract of the United States, edn 118. Washington, DC, US Government Printing Office, 1998.
2. Ewing S, Torres A. Severe community-acquired pneumonia. Clin Chest Med 20:575, 1999.
3. American Thoracic Society. Guidelines for the initial management of adults with community-acquired pneumonia: Diagnosis, assessment of severity and initial antimicrobial therapy. Am Rev Respir Dis 148:1418, 1993.
4. European study on community-acquired pneumonia (ESOCAP) committee. Guidelines for management of adult community-acquired lower respiratory tract infections. Eur Respir J 11:986, 1998.
5. Torres A, El-Ebiary M, Zavala E, Hernández C. Severe community-acquired pneumonia. Sem Respir Crit Care Med 17:265, 1996.
6. Vallés J. Severe pneumonia: sources of infection and implications for prevention. Sepsis 1:199, 1998.
7. Research Committee of the British Thoracic Society and the Public Health Laboratory Service. Community acquired pneumonia in adults in British hospitals in 1982–83: a survey of aetiology, mortality, prognostic factors and outcome. QJMed 62:195, 1987.
8. Ewig S, Ruiz M, Mensa J, Marcos M Angeles, Martínez JA, Arancibia F, *et al*. Severe community-acquired pneumonia: assessment of severity criteria. Am J Respir Crit Care Med 158:1102, 1998.
9. Hirani NA, Macfarlane JT. Impact of management guidelines on the outcome of severe community acquired pneumonia. Thorax 52:17, 1997.
10. Woodhead MA, Macfarlane JT, Rodgers FG, Laverick A, Pilkington R, Macrae AD. Etiology and outcome of severe community-acquired pneumonia. J Infect 10:204, 1985.
11. Rello J, Valles J, Jubert P, Ferrer A, Domingo C, Mariscal D, *et al*. Lower respiratory tract infections following cardiac arrest and cardiopulmonary resucitacion. Clin Infect Dis 21:310, 1995.

12. Pachón J, Prado MD, Capote F, Cuello JA, Garnacho J, Verano A. Severe community acquired pneumonia. Etiology, prognosis and treatment. Am Rev Respir Dis 142:369, 1990.
13. Torres A, Serra-Batlles J, Ferrer A, Jiménez P, Celis R, Cobo E, *et al.* Severe community acquired pneumonia. Epidemiology and prognostic factors. Am Rev Respir Dis 114:312, 1991.
14. Rello J, Quintana E, Ausina V, Net A, Prats G. A three-year study of severe community acquired pneumonia with emphasis in outcome. Chest 103:232, 1993.
15. Moine P, Vercken JB, Chevret S, Chastang C, Gajdos P, and the French Study Group for Community-acquired Pneumonia in Intensive Care Unit. Severe community-acquired pneumonia. Etiology, epidemiology and prognosis factors. Chest 105:1487, 1994.
16. Leroy O, Santré C, Beuscart C, Georges H, Guery B, Jacquier JM, *et al.* A five-year study of severe community-acquired pneumonia with emphasis on prognosis in patients admitted to an intensive care unit. Intensive Care Med 21:24, 1995.
17. Rello J, Rodriguez R, Jubert P, Alvarez B and the Study Group of Severe Community-acquired Pneumonia. Severe community-acquired pneumonia in the elderly: epidemiology and prognosis. Clin Infect Dis 23:723, 1996.
18. Grau I, Pallarés R. Neumonía neumocócica. En Infecciones Graves. Implicaciones terapeúticas de la Neumonía Extrahospitalaria Grave. Ed. Ecika Med 1:17, 1988.
19. El-Ebiary M, Sarmiento X, Torres A, Nogué S, Mesalles E, Bodí M, *et al.* Prognostic factors of severe Legionella Pneumonia requiring admission to ICU. Am J Respir Crit Care Med 156:1467, 1997.
20. Menéndez R, Córdoba J, de la Cuadra P, Cremades MJ, López-Hontagas JL, Salavert M, *et al.* Value of the polymerase chain reaction assay in noninvasive respiratory samples for diagnosis of community-acquired pneumonia. Am J Respir Crit Care Med 159:1868, 1999.
21. Leeper KV, Torres A. Community-acquired pneumonia in the intensive care unit. Clin Chest Med 16:155, 1995.
22. Vanders Els NJ, Stover DE. Approach to the patient with pulmonary disease. Clin Chest Med 17:767, 1996.
23. Barlett JG, Dowell SF, Mandell LA, File TM, Musher DM, Fine MS. Community-acquired pneumonia in adults: Practice guidelines for the management. Clin Infect Dis 31:347, 2000.
24. Domínguez J, Gali N, Pedroso P, Hernández A, Matas L, Manterola, *et al.* Evaluación del Binax Now[tm] Legionella urinary antigen test para la detección del antígeno de Legionella en muestras de orina. Estudio preliminar. [Abstract] Arch Bronconeumol 35:46, 1993.
25. Antonelli M, Conti G, Riccioni L, Meduri U. Noninvasive positive-pressure ventilation via face mask during bronchoscopy with BAL in high-risk hypoxemic patients. Chest 110:724, 1996.
26. Jiménez P, Saldías F, Meneses M, Silva ME, Wilson MG, Otth L. Diagnostic fiberoptic bronchoscopy in patients with community-acquired pneumonia. Comparison between bronchoalveolar lavage and telescoping plugged catheter cultures. Chest 103:1023, 1993.
27. Vivès L, Biel P, Maler G, Labonne F, Lecoules N, Dufour M, *et al.* Acute community-acquired pneumonia of moderate and grave severity investigated by bronchoscopy. Analysis of 193 cases hospitalized in a general hospital. Rev Mal Respir 13:175, 1996.
28. Örtqvist A, Kalin M, Lejdeborn L, Lundberg B. Diagnostic fiberoptic bronchoscopy and protected brush culture in patients with community-acquired pneumonia. Chest 97:576, 1990.
29. Zalacaín R, Llorente JL, Gaztelurrutia L, Pijoan JL, Sobradillo V. Influence of three factors on the diagnosis effectiveness of transthoracic needle aspiration in pneumonia. Chest 107:96, 1995.
30. García A, Rosón B, Pérez JL, Verdaguer R, Dorca J, Carratalà J, *et al.* Usefulness of PCR and antigen latex agglutination test with samples obtained by transthoracic needle aspiration for diagnosis of pneumococcal pneumonia. J Clin Microbiol 37:709, 1993.
31. Fine MJ, Smith MA, Carson CA, Mutha SS, Sankey SS, Weissfeld LA, *et al.* Prognosis and outcomes of patients with community-acquired pneumonia. A meta-analysis. JAMA 275:134, 1996.
32. Mufson MA, Oley G, Hughey D. Pneumococcal disease in a medium-sized community in the United States. JAMA 248:1486, 1982.
33. Marrie TJ. Epidemiology of community-acquired pneumonia in the elderly. Semin Respir Infect 5:260, 1990.
34. Riquelme R, Torres A, El-Ebiary M, Puig de la Bellacasa J, Estruch R, Mensa J, *et al.* Community-acquired pneumonia in the elderly. A multivariate analysis of risk and prognostic factors. Am J Respir Crit Care Med 154:1450, 1996.

35. Almirall J, Morató I, Riera A, Verdaguer A, Priu R, Coll P, *et al*. Incidence of community-acquired pneumonia and *Chlamydia pneumoniae* infection: a prospective multicenter study. Eur Respir J 6:14, 1993.
36. Lange P, Vestbo J, Nyboe J. Risk factors for death and hospitalization from pneumonia. A prospective study of a general population. Eur Respir J 8:1694, 1995.
37. Torres A, Dorca J, Zalacaín R, Bello S, El-Ebiary M, Molinos L, *et al*. Community-acquired pneumonia in chronic obstructive pulmonary disease. A Spanish Multicenter Study. Am J Respir Crit Care Med 154:1456, 1996.
38. Seneff MG, Wagner DP, Wagner RD, Zimmerman JE, Knaus WA. Hospital and 1-year survival of patients admitted to intensive care units with acute exacerbation of chronic obstructive pulmonary disease. JAMA 274:1852, 1995.
39. Almirall J, Mesalles E, Klamburg J, Parra O, Agudo A. Prognostic factors of pneumonia requiring admission to the intensive care unit. Chest 107:511, 1995.
40. Mundy LM, Auwaerter PG, Oldach D, Warner ML, Burton A, Vance E, *et al*. Community-acquired pneumonia: Impact of immune status. Am J Respir Crit Care Med 152:1309, 1995.
41. Hirschtick RE, Glassroth J, Jordan MC, Wilcosky TC, Wallace JM, Kvale PA, and the Pulmonary Complications of HIV infection study group. Bacterial pneumonia in persons infected with the human immunodeficiency virus. N Engl J Med 333:845, 1995.
42. Carratalà J, Rosón B, Fernández Sevilla A, Alcaide F, Gudiol F. Bacteriemic pneumonia in neutropenic patients with cancer: causes, empirical antibiotic therapy, and outcome. Arch Intern Med 158:868, 1998.
43. Marfín AA, Sporrer J, Moore PS, Siefkin AD. Risk factors for adverse outcome in persons with pneumococcal pneumonia. Chest 107:457, 1995.
44. Meehan TP, Fine MJ, Krumholz HM, Scinto JD, Galusha DH, Mockalis JT, *et al*. Quality of care, process, and outcome in elderly patients with pneumonia. JAMA 278:2080, 1997.
45. Confalonieri M, Potena A, Carbone G, Della Porta R, Tolley EA, Meduri GU. Acute respiratory failure in patients with severe community-acquired pneumonia. A prospective randomized evaluation of noninvasive ventilation. Am J Respir Crit Care 160:1585, 1999.
46. Antonelli M, Conti G, Rocco M, Bufi M, De Blasi RA, Vivino G, *et al*. A comparison of noninvasive positive-pressure ventilation and conventional mechanical ventilation in patients with acute respiratory failure. N Engl J Med 339:429, 1998.
47. The Acute Respiratory Distress Syndrome Network. Ventilation with lower tidal volumes as compared with traditional tidal volumes for acute lung injury and the acute respiratory distress syndrome. N Engl J Med 342:1301, 2000.
48. Rello J. Therapy for severe community-acquired pneumonia. Clin Infect Dis 25:160, 1997.
49. Cantón R, Loza E, Valdezate S, Baquero F. Otros patógenos respiratorios de la comunidad and nuevas fluorquinolonas. Enf Infec Microbiol Clin 16(Supl.):12, 1998.
50. Martín M, Gómez-Lus ML, Aguilar L, Martínez P, Giménez MJ, Prieto J. Effect of clavulanic acid and/or polymorphonuclear neutrophils on amoxicillin bactericidal activity against Streptococcus pneumoniae. Eur J Clin Microbiol Infect Dis 16:512, 1997.
51. Liñares J, Pallarés R, Alonso T, Pérez JL, Ayats J, Gudiol F, *et al*. Trends in antimicrobial resistance of clinical isolates of *Streptococcus pneumoniae* in Bellvitge Hospital, Barcelona, Spain (1979–1990). Clin Infect Dis 15:99, 1992.
52. Gallego M, Rello J. Neumonía extrahospitalaria grave. Arch Bronchoneumol 36(suppl 4):61, 2000.
53. Schülin T, Wennersten CB, Ferraro MJ, Moellering RC, Eliopoulos GM. Susceptibilities of Legionella spp. to newer antimicrobials in vitro. Antimicrob Agents Chemother 42:1520, 1998.
54. Clavo AJ, Girón JA, López D, Canueto J, Sanchez A, Vergara A, *et al*. Multivariate analysis of risk factors for infection due to penicillin-resistant and multidrug-resistant *Streptococcus pneumoniae*: a multicenter study. Clin Infect Dis 24:1062, 1997.
55. Pallarés R, Liñares J, Vadillo M, Cabellos C, Manresa F, Viladrich P, *et al*. Resistance to penicillin and cephalosporin and mortality from severe pneumococcal pneumonia in Barcelona, Spain. N Engl J Med 333:474, 1995.
56. Einarsson S, Kristjanson M, Kristinsson K, Kjartansson G, Johnsson S. Pneumonia cause by penicillin-non-susceptible and penicillin-susceptible pneumococci in adults: a case-control study. Scand J Infect Dis 30:253, 1998.
57. Ewing S, Ruiz M, Torres A, Marco F, Martínez JA, Sanchez M, *et al*. Pneumonia acquired in the community through drug-resistant *Streptococcus pneumoniae*. Am J Respir Crit Care Med 159:1835, 1999.

58. Metlay JP, Hofmann J, Cetron MS, Fine MJ, Farley MM, Whitney C, *et al*. Impact of penicillin susceptibility on medical outcomes for adult patients with bacteremic pneumococcal pneumonia. Clin Infect Dis 30:520, 2000.
59. Bodí M, Ardanuy C, Rello J. Resistant Gram positive cocci as cause of respiratory infection in crtically ill patients. Crit Care Med 29(In Suppl.):N82, 2001.
60. Rello J, Bodí M, Díaz E. Appropiate antibiotic therapy for Staphylococcal pneumonia (letter). Clin Infect Dis 31:1314, 2000.

38. SEVERE LEGIONELLOSIS

María Bodí and José Antonio Porras

Introduction

Legionnaires' disease is a form of pneumonia, caused by bacteria of the genus *Legionella*. In contrast, Pontiac fever is a self-limited influenza-like illness, without pneumonia, that is associated with *Legionella* spp too. The name of this infection is in reference to an outbreak of pneumonia that affected 221 people and caused 34 deaths during the 58th American Legion Convention celebrated in Philadelphia during the summer of 1976 [1]. Epidemiologically, the Philadelphia outbreak was similar in many aspects to two large outbreaks of febrile disease, one in 1965 (District of Columbia) and the other in 1968 (Pontiac, Michigan). The Columbia outbreak involved patients in a large psychiatric hospital in which there were 81 cases and 12 deaths [2]. The Pontiac outbreak was very different, of the 144 documented cases neither death nor pneumonia were demonstrated. Pontiac fever is an acute febrile illness, self-limited and with minor respiratory symptoms [3]. In reality, the first isolation of this organism (OLDA agent) was made in 1947 by Jackson from a sick guinea pig that had been inoculated with the blood of a patient with a febrile respiratory illness [4].

Today, we know that legionella is a common cause of community-acquired and nosocomial pneumonia. The incidence of legionella as a cause of sporadic community-acquired pneumonia varies, but in studies from Europe and North America, it ranged from 2 to 15 per cent of all community pneumonias that require hospitalization [5]. But the most relevant factor is the role of Legionnaires' disease as a frequent cause of severe community-acquired pneumonia (when shock or acute respiratory failure is present), although this is not a universal finding. In some studies, *Legionella* ranks second, after pneumococcus, in the list of causes of pneumonias that are severe enough to require admittance in ICU and that show a high mortality (Table 1) [6–14]. In the nosocomial setting, legionellosis may also appear sporadically or, sometimes, in real outbreaks. In general, the true prevalence of legionellosis has probably been underestimated, since specific diagnostic methods are not routinely used in the initial diagnostic approach. Then, diagnosis is commonly performed retrospectively and we know that the delay in the initiation of adequate treatment due to diagnostic tardiness negatively influences the prognosis of the disease [15–19].

Etiology

Since the original isolation in 1977 of *L. pneumophila* by McDade [20] the number of different species and serogroups of the Legionellaceae family has been continually increasing. Currently there are more than 34 Legionella species and over 50 distinct serogroups. About half of those species have been proven to be pathogenic for humans [21] (Table 2). *Legionella pneumophila* serogroup 1 is responsible for more than 80% of these infections [22]. In general lines, the other species of the family, of which *Legionella micdadei* is the most frequent, tend to show clinical features and susceptibility patterns to antimicrobial agents similar to those shown by *L. pneumophila* [23].

TABLE 1. Characteristics of severe community-acquired pneumonia (SCAP) in the literature

Author (Ref)	Pachón (8)	Torres (9)	Rello (10)	Moine (11)	Leroy (12)	Rello (13)	Hirani (14)
Year	1990	1991	1993	1994	1995	1996	1997
Episodes	67	92	58	132	299	95	57
MV* (%)	–	61	72.4	61	48.9	87.3	96.4
Diagnosis of etiology (%)	48	52	60.3	72	65.9	39	67
S. pneumoniae (%)	37.5	15	37.1	45	30.8	29.4	67
Legionella spp (%)	21.8	14	22.8	4.2	0	3.1	16
Rank order Legionella SCAP	3rd	2nd	2nd	7th	–	3rd	2nd
Overall death ratio (%)	20.8	22	22.4	24	28.5	40	56
Legionella Mortality (%)	–	15	20	25	–	66	58

* Mechanical ventilation.

TABLE 2. *Legionella spp.* that have been linked to well-documented human infection

L. pneumophila	L. oakridgensis
L. bozemanii	L. wadsworthii
L. dumofii	L. birminghamensis
L. miccdadei	L. cincinnatiensis
L. longbeache	L. anisa
L. jordanis	L. cherrii
L. gormanii	L. sainthelensi
L. feeleil	L. lansingensis
L. hackeliae	L. parisiensis
L. maceachernii	

Legionella pneumophila is a small, aerobic, non-capsulated, Gram-negative bacilli. They are non-spore-forming, most are motile due to polar or subpolar flagellae, and electron microscopy reveals multiple fimbriae extending from the surface. These, in normal conditions measure 0.5–1 μm in width and 2–4 μm in length. The cell wall of all the species of the family shows a distintive fatty-acid profile and ubiquinone composition, different from other Gram-negative bacilli. Legionella have complex growth requirements and do not grow on standard bacteriologic media. All species require supplementation of growth media with L-cysteine and ferric salts and grow best at pH 6.8 to 7.0. So, in these conditions, the primary medium for isolation of *Legionella* is buffered charcoal yeast extract (BCYE) agar. Isolation of *Legionella* from contaminated specimens is enhanced both by acid pre-treatment and by multiple selective media obtained by the addition of antimicrobial agents [22].

Epidemiology

Legionnaires' disease occurs in sporadic, endemic and epidemic forms. To establish a link between the disease and a presumptive site of infection, an environmental investigation and the presence of clinical and environmental *Legionella* isolates are required.

SOURCES OF INFECTION

Water is the natural habitat of *Legionella*. The bacteria has been consistently isolated from a variety of man-made water reservoirs in most nosocomial outbreaks and in many community-acquired cases. The principal sources of nosocomial [24] and community-acquired [25, 26] Legionnaires' disease are the distribution systems for drinking water. The importance of air conditioning cooling towers, although they are undoubtedly a definitive disseminator at least in some outbreaks [27–29], has probably been overemphasized. Water temperature exerts a crucial influence on the growth of *Legionella*; it is favored in warm water [30, 31].

MODE OF TRANSMISSION

Legionnaires' disease can be fundamentally acquired by the inhalation of aerosols containing *Legionella*, such as cooling towers [32, 33], evaporative condensers [34], showers [35], faucets [31], whirlpool spa [36], saunas [37], humidifiers [38] and medication nebulizers [39]. Contaminated water may also be a mode of transmission after aspiration [40]. Nasogastric tubes have been implicated in several studies of nosocomial legionellosis; microaspiration of contaminated water was the presumed mode of transmission [41]. The patients with lowered consciousness, head and neck surgery, have a high propensity for aspiration, and these circumstances are risk factors for nosocomial pneumonia due to legionella [42]. Direct infection of surgical wounds after contact with contaminated water is also possible [43]. There is no evidence for person-to-person spread [44].

PATHOGENESIS VIRULENCE

The growth of *Legionella* organisms in water is favored by the fact that some algae may provide nutrients and by the role of amoeba; it preserves them in unfavorable environmental factors [45]. Thus, in infected patients, *Legionella* is an intracellular infectious agent and it replicates within the cells, avoiding intracellular destruction, by sophisticated mechanisms that inhibit phagosome-lysosome fusion [46]. In fact, cell-mediated immunity plays the critical role in the host's defence against this infection. There are many virulence factors involved in the intracellular multiplication of the organism: several genetic loci of *Legionella pneumophila* serogroup 1, the macrophage infectivity potentiator, lipopolysacharide endotoxins, or the "defect in organelle trafficking proteins" [47, 48]. The presence of flagella is also one phenotypic difference between avirulent and virulent strains of *Legionella pneumophila*: isogenic avirulent strains obtained by passage lose their flagella [49].

RISK FACTORS

Clinical diagnosis of the *Legionella* infection is difficult. Usually, the empirical treatment of severe community-acquired pneumonia [50, 51] includes specific antibiotics against *Legionella*, but that is different in nosocomial pneumonia [52]. Therefore, it would be useful to identify risk factors associated with *Legionella* pneumonia.

Virulent *Legionella* organisms are capable of causing pneumonia in a previously healthy individual. At least six per cent of nosocomial *Legionella* pneumonia occurs in previously healthy patients [22]. Cigarette smoking, chronic lung disease, diabetes, alcohol abuse, renal failure, immunosuppression and advanced age have been identified as general risk factors for *Legionella* infection, but also for other non-*Legionella* infections. The immunodepression has been consistently implicated as a risk factor (steroids, cytostatics) [53, 54].

The incidence of *Legionella* infections in patients with acquired immunodeficiency syndrome is low, and normally it doesn't occur among persons receiving prophylactic therapy with trimethoprim-sulfamethoxazole, and the clinical manifestations are more severe [55] but, usually they respond well to treatment. Surgery is a major predisposing factor in nosocomial infection, with transplant recipients at the highest risk [16, 56, 57]. Regional and seasonal differences in reported cases may be due to ecological factors [53].

Clinical Manifestations

Two clinical forms of *Legionella* infection have been described: Pontiac fever and Legionnaires' disease.

Pontiac fever is a non-pneumonic, usually self-limited, nonfatal influenza-like disease, with a short incubation period (36 h) and high attack rate (up to 95 per cent). Normally, it is caused by *L. pneumophila*, as well as other *Legionella spp*. It has recently been recognized that severe encephalopathy, due to acute disseminated encephalomyelitis, may rarely follow an allegedly benign Pontiac fever [58].

Pneumonia is the predominant clinical syndrome of Legionnaires' disease. The clinical manifestations of *Legionella* pneumonia are nonspecific. It is not possible to distinguish between Legionnaires' disease and other common causes of pneumonia on the basis of clinical findings [22, 59–61]. Demographic, clinical, laboratory, radiological and outcome data in nosocomial and community-acquired Legionella pneumonia are quite similar [62]. The disease presents itself with a broad spectrum of illness, ranging from a mild respiratory illness to a severe respiratory failure and multiorgan failure with fulminating course. Mild pneumonia generally occurs in young patients and those without underlying disease.

Initially, the patients present non-specific symptoms, including fever, malaise, myalgias, anorexia and headache. Although Legionellosis may behave as a multisystemic disease, fever (often exceeding 40°C) and non-specific respiratory manifestations are usually predominant. The frequency of cough, sputum production or purulence is variable. Chest pain, occasionally pleuritic, can be prominent. Progressive respiratory failure is the most common cause of death in Legionellosis [53, 63, 64].

Gastrointestinal symptoms are prominent, especially diarrhoea, which occurs in 20 to 40 per cent of cases [60, 65]. Neurologic symptoms are relatively common in Legionellosis, ranging from mild headache to severe encephalopathy [66].

The physical findings are those of pneumonia. Hyponatremia [63], elevated levels of serum transaminase and creatinine phosphokinase [65] are the most common types of non-specific laboratory abnormalities associated with Legionnaires' disease.

The chest radiograph of Legionellosis has been described in many reports [67–69]. Although some attempted to describe those which are specific for *Legionella*, chest radiographic findings are also non diagnostic. Initial focal infiltrates are the most frequent radiographic finding. The infiltrates often spread to contiguous lobes, eventually becoming bilateral. Recently, some authors have written that radiological findings are related to the outcome of Legionnaires disease. Thus, rapid progression of radiological infiltrates or multilobar lung involvement is an indication for admission in a critical care unit [50, 51]. Early, appropriate treatment against Legionella seems to decrease the incidence of radiological progression in about 30 per cent of cases [70]. Likewise, radiographic improvement is related to a better outcome [71].

The incidence of pleural effusions is about 30%, less frequent than other causes of severe pneumonia; and usually of moderate volume. Empiema is a rare complication of Legionellosis. Cavitation is a rare event, whereas, the immunocompromised host has a marked tendency to cavitation. Hiliar adenopathy is also seen in this subset of patients [68, 69]. A prolonged resolution phase of up four or six months is common in severe Legiontonaires' disease.

EXTRAPULMONARY LEGIONELLOSIS

Extrapulmonary *Legionella* infections are rare and normally occur through bacteremia. Bacteremia appears in the 20 per cent of severe legionnaires' disease. The extrapulmonary manifestations can be concomitant with the pulmonary infection or can become manifest weeks after the successful treatment of pneumonia. These are often dramatic [59, 60]. Most extrapulmonary infections develop in immunosuppressed patients [72].

A variety of locations of extrapulmonary Legionellosis have been reported. The most common site is the heart, especially pericarditis [73]. There are also described cases of myocarditis, post-cardiotomy syndrome and prosthetic-valve endocarditis [74, 75]. Some cardiac infections have been caused by direct contact with contaminated water, and normally were acquired in the hospital; there are reported cases of valvular infections, and thoracic aortic graft infection, usually it is through wound infection and is favoured by foreign bodies [43, 76].

Although neurologic symptoms are relatively common in legionellosis, CT shows no abnormality that can account for the symptoms; proving that neurologic infection is rare. A few brain abscesses have been reported [77]. Digestive legionella infections are not frequent; some reports have described perirectal abscess [78], peritonitis [79] and pancreatitis [80, 81]. Renal involvement is usually caused by hypotension and rhabdomyolisis [82]. Pyelonephritis with abscess formation is also described [83]. Other unusual clinical presentations of *Legionella* are: wound infections (hip, cardiothoracic surgery), sinusitis [84], hemodialysis fistula infections [85], and cellulitis [86].

Laboratory Diagnosis

It must be emphasized that prospective, well-designed comparative studies between Legionnaires' disease and those pneumonias that are caused by non-Legionella aerobic organisms have shown that a definite differential diagnosis based on clinical, analytical, and radiological signs is not possible [53, 63, 65, 87]. For this reason, specialized laboratory tests are necessary to establish the diagnosis (Tables 3 and 4) These tests must be specifically requested from the clinical microbiology laboratory because they are not routinely performed.

A variety of stains have been used to visualize the organisms in clinical samples, but they are not specific. Gimenez stain is a rapid and more effective technique than Gram stain and Dieterle silver-impregnation stain permits visualization in paraffin-fixed tissues [88].

Isolation of *Legionella* in culture is the definitive method for the diagnosis of legionellosis; however, *Legionella* does not grow on standard microbiologic medium [22, 59]. Investigators at the Centers for Disease Control ultimately grew legionella on a charcoal-containing medium (buffered-charcoal yeast-extract agar), which is the base formulation of the medium used today. Unfortunately, many laboratories either do not culture for legionella or do so inadequately. Anyway, *Legionella* usually takes three to five days to grow. Cultures should be held for many days so as not to miss some delayed isolations [64, 89, 90]. For maximal sensitivity, several types of dye-containing selective mediums with

TABLE 3. Usefulness of specialized laboratory test for the diagnosis of Legionnaires' disease

Test	Sensitivity (%)	Specificity (%)
Sputum culture*	80	100
Direct fluorescent-antibody stain of sputum	33–70	96–99
Urinary antigen assay**	70	100
Serologic tests for antibody***	40–60	96–99

*Multiple selective mediums that contain dyes and have been pretreated with acid or heat to minimize overgrowth of competing microorganims should be used.
**This test is useful only for L. Pneumophila serogroup 1.
***This approach requires IgG and IgM testing of serum samples obtained during both the acute phase and convalescence. A single titer of ≥1 : 128 in a patient with pneumonia is considered presumptive evidence of infection, and single titer of ≥1 : 256 or a fourfold increase in antibody titer is considered definitive evidence.
From: Stout JE, Yu VL. Legionellosis. New Engl J Med 337:682, 1997. (with permission).

TABLE 4. Laboratory criteria for diagnosis of Legionellosis

- Isolation of *Legionella* from respiratory secretions, lung tissue, pleural fluid, or other normally sterile fluids, or
- Demonstration of a fourfold or greater rise in the reciprocal immunofluorescence antibody (IFA) titer to greater than or equal to 128 against *Legionella pneumophila* serogroup 1 between paired acute- and convalescent-phase serum specimens, or
- Detection of *Legionella pneumophila* serogroup 1 in respiratory secretions, lung tissue, or pleural fluid by direct fluorescent antibody testing, or
- Demonstration of *Legionella pneumophila* serogroup 1 antigens in urine by radioimmunoasssay or enzyme-linked immunosorbent assay

CDC, Case Definitions for Infectious Conditions Under Public Health Surveillance. MMWR 46 (No.RR–10):20, 1997.

acid or heat pre-treatment to minimize overgrowth of competing microorganisms must be used. In patients with severe Legionellosis which have a productive cough, sputum is a good non-invasive sample for isolating the organism. Interestingly, sputum from patients suspected of having Legionnaires' disease should be cultured regardless of quality, since in one study specimens that did not meet the classical criteria of Murray and Washington and had more than 25 squamous epithelial cells and fewer than 25 leukocytes per low-power field often yielded the organism [64, 91]. Sputum culture sensitivity estimates increase in parallel with the severity of the disease by about 60% in severe community-acquired pneumonia due to *Legionella pneumophila* [64]. The isolation rate increases slightly when combining cultures from both sputum and other respiratory specimens obtained from more invasive methods [64].

Direct fluorescent-antibody (DFA) staining is a rapid diagnostic test that permits a quick diagnosis of severe legionellosis but requires skilled microbiology technicians to interpret the test [92]. Its sensitivity, regardless of the type of respiratory sample, is less than that of culture because large numbers of organisms need to be present before they can be readily visualized [22, 59]. The specificity has been determined to be about 95% [22]. For detecting *L. pneumophila* in respiratory specimens, it has been found that the monoclonal-antibody direct fluorescent-antibody reagent (Genetic Systems, Sanofi Diagnostics Pasteur, Chaska, Minn.) is superior to polyclonal reagents because there is less background fluorescence [59]. In addition, false positive results due to cross-reactions with nonlegionella bacteria do not occur. The average time for the DFA test to become negative is after four to six days of appropriate antibiotic therapy [89, 93].

In severe legionellosis, serologic tests are only useful for epidemiologic studies and are less valuable to physicians, given the requirement for measurement during convalescence [22, 59]. Immunofluorescent antibody (IFA) detection, ELISA, and microagglutination are the most commonly used serologic tests [92]. The IFA test is the most sensitive and widely employed serologic method. The diagnosis is based on a fourfold increase in the antibody titer to 1:128 or more. The period of time needed to obtain a four-fold rise in the antibody titer usually ranges from four to eight weeks after the onset of the illness. However, seroconversion may even take many months, specially in the elderly [94] and about 30% of patients suffering from Legionnaires' disease will never develop an antibody increase [89]. Single titers of 1:256 or more during convalescence in a patient with pneumonia are suggestive of Legionellosis. To improve the sensitivity, antibody screening should include both IgG and IgM because some patients will only have an IgM response [22, 59]. A high specificity of 95% is restricted to *L. pneumophila* serogroup 1 infection. When other *Legionella* species antigens are used, the IFA test clearly decreases its specificity [22, 59, 95].

The legionella urinary antigen test is a rapid test that detects antigens of *L. pneumophila* in urine. This test is commercially available as both a radioimmunoassay and an enzyme immunoassay, has a sensitivity of 56 per cent and a specificity that approaches 100 per cent [96]. Sensitivity can be further improved if the urine is concentrated by ultrafiltration [97], and today the new EIA test, (Biotest AG, Dreieich, Germany; Binax, Portland, Marine) can offer sensitivity in non-concentrated and concentrated urine of more than 83 per cent with a specificity of 100% [98, 99]. More recently, a novel 15 minute rapid *Legionella* urinary antigen test (Binax Now, Portland, Maine) has been presented with very high specificity and sensitivity [100]. Radioimmunoassay (RIA) does not seem to show any advantage over the more simple, non-isotopic, enzyme immunoassay (EIA) tests [101]. Moreover, it is often easier to obtain a urine sample than an adequate sputum specimen, since many patients have a nonproductive cough. Finally, unlike culture, the test results will remain positive for weeks despite antibiotic therapy. Although *Legionella* antigen has been reported to persist in a patient's urine for as long as one year [102], less than 10 per cent of culture-confirmed cases were positive for urinary antigen more than 60 days after the onset of disease. The chief drawback is that this test detects only *L. pneumophila* serogroup 1. However, serogroup 1 accounts for the large majority of cases of legionnaires' disease.

Genus-specific hybridation of *Legionella* spp. by a commercially available radiolabeled DNA probe test (Gen Prove Inc., San Diego, California) can be performed in a few hours. Once more, a good correlation between *Legionella* organism concentration and DNA probe activity has been observed. In contrast with the DFA test, the DNA probe does not depend on the operator's skill. The test may remain positive in the respiratory secretions for up to eight days after beginning proper therapy [103, 104]. Again, the sensitivity is less than that of culture and quite similar to that of the DFA test and specificity approaches 99% [22].

Several molecular systems have been developed for the detection of *Legionella* species using the polymerase chain reaction (PCR). Assays based on the PCR have been used to detect *Legionella* on clinical specimens, such as bronchoalveolar lavage fluid (BAL) [105–108], intratracheal aspirates [109], sputum [108], urine [110, 111], throat swabs [112] and serum [111, 113]. Although PCR-based assays for the detection of *Legionella* in clinical samples are highly specific (approach 99%), they show a clearly lower sensitivity than that of culture [107, 110]. However, a recent study has shown a better than usual sensitivity of 73% if testing was restricted to urine and/or serum samples taken within four days of the onset of the symptoms [111]. The advantages of PCR in urine and serum over conventional methods for the detection of *Legionella* DNA are evident. Urine and serum samples are readily obtainable and can be processed within a single working day, thereby providing a rapid result for the clinician. In one more recent study with respiratory specimens, such as sputum and BAL, the sentitivity of PCR was near to 100%, when the PCR inhibition that produces the group hem of the hemoglobin [114] was eliminated by the inclusion of a preliminary wash and centrifugation step in distilled water [108]. Finally, another important factor is that PCR of *Legionella* is not restricted to specific serogroups or species [59].

Finally, it is obvious that if Legionellosis is suspected in a critically ill patient, clinicians have to give priority to the laboratory diagnostic techniques that confirm, in a simple, fast, and reliable way, that *Legionella* is the etiology agent of the pneumonia. Along these lines, the last generation test for detection of urinary antigen and/or the news assays based on the polimerase chain reaction, seem to be the most important future diagnostic options.

Treatment

Since *Legionella pneumophila* is an intracellular pathogen, only antimicrobial agents that are concentrated in cells are effective. These agents must maintain biological activity against *Legionella*. Standard *in vitro* susceptibility testing is not reliable for study of antibiotic activity, as it does not measure the ability of the drug in the intracellular compartment. This fact can explain the *in vitro-in vivo* dichotomy (i.e. with imipenem or amoxicillin-clavulanic acid). Susceptibility of *Legionella* agents to new antimicrobial drugs is based on the intracellular infection and experimental guinea pig infection models. It has been postulated that the guinea pig is the animal model that offers the most similarities with Legionnaires' disease in humans [115]. In spite of this, conclusions derived from an animal model cannot be directly extrapolated to humans [22].

The most effective therapy in Legionnaires' disease must combine the highest activity against *Legionella* spp., the ability to enter and concentrate within phagocytic cells, and the ability to achieve high concentrations in lung tissue and alveolar exudate.

Normally, the best utility of extracellular susceptibility testing is as a screening test to determine which drugs are inactive. There are exceptions; β-lactam antibiotics are active against extracellular *Legionella*, but they have no activity against the intracellular bacterium. However, some antibiotics are less active in extracellular testing than they are in animal models and intracellular testing (doxicycline, azithromycin).

As expected, in most acute lung infections, early appropriate treatment usually implies the best outcome. Mortality of Legionnaires' disease is correlated with both delay in the initiation of specific treatment and the total delay in starting of specific treatment [19]. In endemic areas, the non-specific presentation of Legionnaires' disease obliges clinicians to include effective treatment against Legionellosis in all episodes of pneumonia, in which diagnosis remains uncertain. Specific treatment against *Legionella* infections is recommended by different guidelines on severe community-acquired pneumonia [50, 51, 116]. The recommendations for nosocomial pneumonia are highly dependent on every hospital epidemiology (water colonization) [52].

ANTIBIOTIC CHOICE

Erythromycin has historically been the drug of choice [22, 59, 117]. A number of clinical studies have proven that it is highly effective against *Legionella* spp. The intravenous route in severe pneumonia is recommended. The optimal dose is 4 g/d. Gastrointestinal intolerance, volume overload and ototoxicity have made this drug less attractive. Other side effects less well-known are prolongation of the Q-T interval and "torsades de pointes". Erythromycin can rarely be arrythmogenic, especially when given rapidly intravenously or to patients with a myocardial infarction. The existence of metabolic interactions between erythromycin and cyclosporine, at the cytochrome P-450 level, makes close monitoring of serum cyclosporine levels mandatory to avoid toxicity in organ transplantation recipients.

Many clinical and bacteriologic failures of erythromycin treatment have been reported, as might be expected by the fatality rates of 10%–40% reported in retrospective studies. In none of these instances "*in vitro*" resistance to erythromycin was demonstrated [118]. The accumulated clinical experience in favour of erythromycin as the treatment of choice for Legionnaires' disease has to be balanced against the appearance of new antibiotics that offer many theoretical and practical advantages. These new antibiotics, are especially the new macrolides (clarithromycin and azithromycin), and more recently third and fourth generation fluoroquinolones. These antibiotics have greater *in vitro* activity and better intracellular penetration than erythromycin [119]. There are studies which support the effectiveness or clarithromycin in severely ill patients with chest infections due to *Legionella pneumophila*. Azithromycin has been efficacious in some reports [120]; it offers advantages over the other macrolides due to its unique pharmacokinetics, high and sustained tissue penetration, and spectrum of activity [121]; with its intravenous formulation now available in some countries, it may displace erythromycin as the macrolide of choice [59].

As a class, fluoroquinolone antimicrobials have the greatest activity against *L. pneumophila* in experimental models and animal studies [118]. The bactericidal activity of the new quinolones (ciprofloxacin, levofloxacin and trovafloxacin) could make them the most effective treatment in the severest cases. Some guidelines have recommended quinolones as alternative therapy (as sole therapy) in severe community-acquired pneumonia [50]. In contrast with erythromycin, relatively little is known about these new drugs in large series of severely ill patients. These are the treatments of choice for *Legionella* infections in immunocompromised patients, based on the lack of pharmacologic interactions in this special group of patients. Probably these are the antibiotics of choice for severe Legionnaires' disease [122]; this affirmation needs future clinical studies for its confirmation. Rifampicin is highly active *in vitro* and *in vivo* against *Legionella* spp. [123, 124]. Its induction of rifampicin-resistant mutants argues against its use as sole therapy [117]. It can be added to the treatment regimen with macrolides in cases of more severe disease.

More recently, combination of macrolides with quinolones has shown promising preliminary results [125]. That must be confirmed with future clinical trials. At the moment no good clinical data exists confirming the superiority of combination therapy over single-antibiotic treatment. Some of these combination therapies can be selected if a lack of clinical response is observed after 3–5 days of therapy in an attempt to obtain synergy.

Trimethroprim-sulfamethoxazole has generally appeared inactive against extracellular *L. pneumophila*. It has been effective in the treatment of *legionella* pneumonia and *legionella* peritonitis in guinea pigs [126]. There is relatively little information regarding the clinical outcome for patients with Legionnaires' disease who have been treated with co-thrimoxazole. Again on the basis of a few uncontrolled studies, it has been suggested that it could be especially effective against *L. micdadei* [23].

TABLE 5. Recommended antibiotic dosage for severe Legionellosis

Erythromycin	1 g every 6 hours
Clarithromycin	500 mg every 12 hours
Azithromycin	500 mg every 24 hours
Ciprofloxacin	400 mg every 8 hours
Levofloxacin	500 mg every 12 hours
Trovafloxacin	200 mg every 12 hours
Rifampicin	600 mg every 12 hours
Trimetoprim/ Sulfamethoxazole	160/800 mg every 8 hours

Tetracycline therapy was apparently as effective as erythromycin therapy in the epidemic of Legionnaires' disease in Philadelphia in 1976 [1]. Tetracycline has apparently been effective as treatment for patients for whom erythromycin therapy failed [127]. Successes with minocycline and doxycicline have also been documented [59].

Several streptogramin drugs have been shown to be active *in vitro* against *L. pneumophila*. There is no clinical experience with these antibiotics for the treatment of *legionella* infections [118]. There is no good evidence that any of the β-lactam or aminoglycoside antimicrobials are effective treatments for Legionnaires' disease. Imipenem and clindamycin have proved efficacious in isolated reports. The recommended dosage of the different antibiotics for severe Legionellosis is shown in Table 5.

DURATION OF TREATMENT

Parenteral therapy should be given until there is an objective clinical response; normally within 3–5 days of treatment. This can then be switched to oral therapy. It is recommended that a full three week course of treatment be given to patients who are immunocompromised hosts, and patients with serious underlying disease, in severe cases of Legionnaires' disease. A recrudescence of the disease has been reported in patients with shorter courses of therapy [128].

OTHER MEASURES

Respiratory failure with progressive hypoxemia is the most important mechanism of death. Marked increases in intrapulmonary shunt combined with mild to moderate ventilation-perfusion inequalities are the predominant mechanisms of abnormal gas exchange in patients with pneumonia [129]. In addition, hypoxic pulmonary vasoconstriction is associated with an adaptative response. Recent studies have evaluated new strategies to improve oxygenation, including the administration of inhaled nitric oxide or body position changes. Elevated positive end-expiratory pressure (PEEP) with low tidal volume protect the lung in ARDS. FiO_2 should be minimized to target an acceptable SaO_2 (usually ≥90%).

The failure to improve survival rates in humans using a variety of adjunctive immunologic therapies, such as monoclonal antibodies directed against bacterial endotoxin or cytokins, means that current therapeutic options are based on standard supportive therapy with vasoactive drugs. Hemodynamic control is a priority when Legionnaires' disease evolves with severe sepsis or septic shock. Renal failure can be present, can be secondary to rhabdomyolysis; controlled treatment with fluids and electrolytes is very important, in this case. An optimal management of shock and renal failure may improve outcome [71, 82].

In purulent collection due to *Legionella* infection, drainage is required. Thus, prosthetic heart valve replacement is reguired in endocarditis.

Prognostic Factors and Mortality

The mortality rate of patients with *L. pneumophila* pneumonia who require admission to ICUs is 25–30% [71]. Delay in appropriate therapy of *Legionella* pneumonia is associated with increased mortality [19, 22, 59, 71]. Our group defined the prognostic factors in 84 cases of severe *Legionella* pneumonia [71]. Logistic regression analysis suggested that an initial APACHE II score greater than 15 and/or serum sodium level less than 136 mEq/l were the only independent factors related to death. Univariate analysis of the data also identified additional comorbid diseases and acute biochemical abnormalities, including renal failure, as significant contributors to mortality. The triad of *L. pneumophila* pneumonia, rhabdomyolysis, and renal failure is associated with a 40% mortality [130]. Bilateral chest x-ray involvement, ARDS, the need for mechanical ventilation, development of pulmonary complications (cavitation, lung abscess and pleural effusion), advanced age and septic shock, are major factors influencing outcome.

The majority of studies support hospital acquisition of Legionellosis as a factor that increases the likelihood of a fatal outcome [53].

Summary

L. pneumophila is an important cause of severe community- and hospital-acquired pneumonia, with a high mortality rate. The clinical and radiological presentations are not specific. These are the reasons for including an effective treatment against *Legionella* empirically in SCAP. The new macrolides and new quinolones have a relevant role in *Legionella* pneumonia treatment. We need new diagnostic methods, more sensitive, more specific and with quicker results. Currently, detection of urinary antigen and/or PCR are the most important diagnostic tools.

References

1. Fraser DW, Tsai T, Orenstein W, *et al.* Legionnaires' disease: description of an epidemic of pneumonia. N Engl J Med 297:1189, 1977.
2. Thacker SB, Bennet JV, Tsai T, *et al.* An outbreak in 1965 of severe respiratory illness caused by legionnaires' disease bacterium. J Infect Dis 238:512, 1978.
3. Kaufmann AF, McDade JE, Patton CM, *et al.* Pontiac fever: isolation of the etiologic agent

(*Legionella pneumophila*) and demonstration of its mode of transmission. Am J Epidemiol 114: 337, 1981.
4. McDade JE, Brenner DJ, Bozeman M. Legionnaires' disease bacterium isolated in 1947. Ann Intern Med 90:659, 1979.
5. Muder RR, Yu VL, Fang GD. Community-acquired Legionnaires' disease. Semin Respir Infect 3:32, 1989.
6. Woodhead MA, Macfarlane JT, Rodgers FG, Laverick A, Pilkintong R, Macrae AD. Aetiology and outcome of severe community-acquired pneumonia. J Infect 10:204, 1985.
7. Sorensen J, Cederholm I, Carlsson C. Pneumonia: a deadly disease a despite intensive care treatment. Scand J Infect Dis 18:329, 1986.
8. Pachón J, Prados MD, Capote F, Cuello JA, Garnacho J, Verano A. Severe community-adquired pneumonia: etiology prognosis and treatment. Am Rev Respir Dis 142:369, 1990.
9. Torres A, Serra-Batlles J, Ferrer A, Jimenez P, Celis R, Cobo E, *et al.* Severe community-adquired pneumonia: epidemiology and prognostic factors. Am Rev Respir Dis 144:312, 1991.
10. Rello J, Quintana E, Ausina V, Net A, Prats G. A three-year study of severe community-acquired pneumonia with emphasis on outcome. Chest 103:232, 1993.
11. Moine P, Vercken JB, Chevret S, Chastang C, Gajdos P, ICU French Study Group for SCAP. Severe community-acquired pneumonia. Etiology, epidemiology and prognosis factors. Chest 105:1487, 1994.
12. Leroy O, Santré C, Beuscart C, Georges H, Guery B, Jacquier JM, Beucaire G. A five-year study of severe community-acquired pneumonia with emphasis on prognosis in patients admitted to an intensive care unit. Intensive Care Med 21:24, 1995.
13. Rello J, Rodriguez R, Jubert P, Álvarez B Study Group for Severe community-acquired pneumonia. Severe community-acquired pneumonia in the elderly. Epidemiology and prognosis. Clin Infect Dis 23:723, 1996.
14. Hirani NA, Macfarlane JT. Impact of management guidelines on the outcome of severe community acquired pneumonia. Thorax 52:17, 1997.
15. Redón J, Borrás R, Vila B, Garcia de Lomas J, Pascual JM, Prat J, Uriel B, Perez M. A prospective study of nosocomial pneumonia by *Legionella pneumophila*. Med Clin (Barc) 87:363, 1986.
16. Kirby BA, Snyder KM, Meyer RD, Finegold SM. Legionnaires' disease: report of sixty-five nosocomially acquired cases and review of the lierature. Medicine 59:188, 1980.
17. Redón J, Pascual JM, Vila B, *et al.* A comparative adquired *Legionella pneumophila* pneumonia and pneumonia by other microorganisms. Med Clin (Barc) 88:349, 1987.
18. Woodhead MA, Macfarlane JT. Legionnaires' disease: a review of 79 community-acquired cases in Nottingham. Thorax 41:635, 1986.
19. Heath CH, Grove DI, Looke DFM. Delay in appropriate therapy of Legionella pneumonia associated with increased mortality. Eur J Clin Microbiol Infect Dis 15:286, 1996.
20. McDade JE, Shepard CC, Fraser DW, *et al.* Legionnaires' disease: isolation of a bacterium. N Engl J Med 297:1197, 1977.
21. Thacker WL, Dyke JW, Benson RF, *et al.* *Legionella lansingensis* sp. isolated from a patient with a pneumonia and underlying chronic lymphocytic leukemia. J Clin Microbiol 30:2389, 1992.
22. Roig J, Domingo C, Morera J. Legionnaires' disease. Chest 105:1817, 1994.
23. Fang GD, Yu VL, Vickers RM. Disease due to the Legionellaceae (other than Legionella pneumophila). Historical, microbiological, clinical, and epidemiolgical review. Medicine 68:116, 1989.
24. Joseph CA, Watson JM, Harrison TG, Barlett CLR. Nosocomial Legionnaires' disease in England and Wales, 1980–92. Epidemiol Infect 112:329, 1994.
25. Leverstein-van Hall M, Verbon A, Huisman MV, Kuijper EJ, Dankert J. Reinfection with *Legionella pneumophila* documented by pulsed-field gel electrophoresis. Clin Infect Dis 19: 1147, 1994.
26. Stout JE, Yu VL, Muraca P, Joly J, Troup N, Tompkins LS. Potable water as a cause of sporadic cases of community-acquired legionnaires' disease. N Engl J Med 326:151, 1992.
27. Muder RR, Yu VL, Woo AH. Mode of transmission of *Legionella pneumophila*: a critical review. Arch Intern Med 146:1607, 1986.
28. Addiss DG, Davis JP, La Ventura M, Wand PJ, Hutchinson MA, Mckinney RM. Community-acquired Legionnaires' disease associated with cooling tower: evidence for longer-distance transport of *Legionella pneumophila*. Am J Epidemiol 130:557, 1989.

29. Keller DW, Hajjch R, DcMaria A, *et al.* Community outbreak of Legionnaires' disease: an investigation confirming the potential for cooling towers to transmit *Legionella* species. Clin Infect Dis 22:257, 1996.
30. Stout JE, Yu VL, Yee YC, Vaccarello S, Diven W, Lee TC. *Legionella pneumophila* in residential water supplies: environmental surveillance with clinical assessment for Legionnaires' disease. Epidemiol Infect 109:49, 1992.
31. Straus WL, Plouffe JF, File TM Jr, *et al.* Risk factors for domestic acquisition of legionnaires disease. Ohio legionnaires Disease Group. Arch Intern Med 156:1685, 1996.
32. Garbe PL, Davis BJ, Weisfeld JS. Nosocomial legionnaires' disease: epidemiological demonstration of cooling towers as a source. JAMA 254:521, 1985.
33. Dondero TJ, Rentdorff RC, Mallison GF. An outbreak of legionnaires' disease associated with a contaminated air-conditioning cooling tower. N Engl J Med 302:365, 1980.
34. Breiman RF, Cozen W, Fields BS. Role of air-sampling in an investigation of an outbreak of legionnaires' disease associated with exposure to aerosols from an evaporative condenser. J Infect Dis 161:1257, 1990.
35. Breiman RF, Fields BS, Sanden GN, Volmer M, Meier A, Spika JS. An outbreak of legionnaires' disease associated with shower use: possible role of amoebae. JAMA 263:2924, 1990.
36. Jernigan DB, Hofmann J, Cetron MS, *et al.* Outbreak of Legionnaires' disease among cruise ship passengers exposed to a contaminated whirlpool spa. Lancet 347:494, 1996.
37. Den Boer JW, Yzerman E, Van Belkum A, Vlaspolder F, Van Breukelen FJM. Legionnaire's disease and saunas. Lancet 351:114, 1998.
38. Woo AH, Goetz A, Yu VL. Transmission of Legionella by respiratory equipment and aerosol generating devices. Chest 102:1586, 1992.
39. Mastro TD, Fields BS, Breiman RF, Campbell J, Plikaytis BD, Spika JS. Nosocomial Legionnaires' disease and use of medication nebulizers. JID 163:667, 1991.
40. Blatt SP, Parkinson MD, Pace E. Nosocomial Legionnaires' disease: aspiration as a primary mode of disease acquisition. Am J Med 95:16, 1993.
41. Venezia RA, Agresta MD, Hanley EM, Urquhart K, Schoonmaker D. Nosocomial legionellosis associated with aspiration of nasogastric feedings diluted in tap water. Infect Control Hosp Epidemiol 15:529, 1994.
42. Johnson JT, Yu VL, Best MG. Nosocomial legionellosis in patients with head-and-neck cancer: implications for epidemiological reservoir and mode of transmission. Lancet 2:298, 1985.
43. Lowry PW, Blankenship RJ, Gridley W, Troup NJ, Tompkins LS. A cluster of Legionella sternal-wound infections due to postoperative topical exposure to contaminated tap water. N Engl J Med 324:109, 1991.
44. Yu VL, Zuravleff JJ, Gavlik L, Magnussen MH. Lack of evidence for person-to-person transmission of Legionnaires' disease. J Infect Dis 147: 362, 1983.
45. Barker J, Brown MR, Collier PF, Farrell I, Gilbert P. Relationship between *Legionella pneumophila* and *Acanthamoeba polyphaga*: physiological status and susceptibility to chemical inactivation. Appl Environ Microbiol 58:2420, 1992.
46. Vogel JP, Andrews HL, Wong SK, Isberg RR. Conjugative transfer by the virulence system of *Legionella pneumophila*. Science 279:873, 1998.
47. Miyamoto H, Maruta K, Ogawa M, Beckers MC, Gros P, Yoshida S. Spectrum of *Legionella* species whose intracellular multiplication in murine macrophages is genetically controlled by Lgn1. Infect Immun 64:1842, 1996.
48. Andrews HL, Vogel JP, Isberg RR. Identification of linked *Legionella pneumophila* genes essential for intracellular growth and evasion of the endocytic pathway. Infect Immun 66:950, 1998.
49. Pruckler J, Benson R, Martin W, Fields B. Association of flagella and intracellular growth of *L. pneumophila*. In: Abstracts of the 95th General Meeting of the American Society for Microbiology, Washington, D.C., May 21–25, 7:7, 1995.
50. American Thoracic Society. Guidelines for the initial management of adults with community-acquired pneumonia: Diagnosis, assessment of severity, and initial antimicrobial therapy. Am Rev Respir Dis 148:1418, 1993.
51. Barlett JG, Dowell SF, Mandell LA, File TM. Musher DM, Fine MS. Community-acquired pneumonia in adults. Practice guidelines for the management of CID 31:347, 2000.
52. American Thoracic Society. Hospital-acquired pneumonia in adults: Diagnosis, assessment of severity, initial antimicrobial therapy, and pre-

ventive strategies. A consensus statement. Am J Respir Crit Care Med 153: 1711, 1995.
53. Roig J, Aguilar X, Ruiz J, *et al.* Comparative study of *Legionella pneumophila* and other nosocomial-aquired pneumonias. Chest 99:344, 1991.
54. Carratala J, Gudiol F, Pallares R, *et al.* Risk factors for nosocomial *Legionella pneumophila* pneumonia. Am J Respir Crit Care Med 149:625, 1994.
55. Blatt SP, Dolan MJ, Hendrix CW, Melcher GP. Legionnaires' disease in human immunodeficiency virus-infected patients: eight cases and review. Clin Infect Dis 18:227, 1994.
56. Korvick JA, Yu VL. Legionnaires' disease: an emerging surgical problem. An Thorac Surg 43:341, 1987.
57. Chow JW, Yu VL. Legionella: a major opportunistic pathogen in transplant recipients. Semin Respir Infect 13:132, 1998.
58. Spieker S, Petersen D, Rolfs A, *et al.* Acute disseminated encephalomyelitis following Pontiac fever. Eur Neurol 40:169, 1998.
59. Stout JE, Yu VL. Legionellosis. New Engl J Med 337:682, 1997.
60. Edelstein PH. Legionnaires' disease. CID 16: 741, 1993.
61. Hoge CW, Breiman RF. Advances in the Epidemiology and control of Legionella infections. Epid Rev 13:329, 1991.
62. Pedro-Botet ML, Sabria-Leal M, Haro M, *et al.* Nosocomial and community-acquired Legionella pneumonia: clinical comparative analysis. Eur Respir J 8:1929, 1995.
63. Yu, VL, Kroboth FJ, Shonnard J, Brown A, McDearman S, Magnussen M. Legionnaires' disease: new clinical perspective from a prospective pneumonia study. Am J Med 73:357, 1982.
64. Falco V, Fernández de Sevilla T, Alegre J, Ferrer A, Martínez Vázquez JM. Legionella pneumophila: a cause of severe community-acquired pneumonia. Chest 100:1007, 1991.
65. Sopena N, Sabrià-Lal M, Pedro-Botet ML, *et al.* Comparative study of the clinical presentation of Legionella pneumona and other community-acquired pneumonias. Chest 113:1195, 1998.
66. Johnson JD, Raff M, VanArsdall J. Neurologic manifestations of legionnaires' disease. Medicine 63:303, 1984.
67. Kirby BD, Peck H, Meyer RD. Radiographic features or legionnaires' disease. Chest 76 562, 1979.
68. Roig J, Martinez-Benitez J, Salvador J. Radiologic features of legionellosis. Curr Top Radiol 1:101, 1998.
69. Coletta FS, Fein AM. Radiological manifestations of Legionella/Legionella-like organisms. Semin Respir Infect 13:109, 1998.
70. Domingo C, Roig J, Planas F, Bechini J, Tenesa M, Morera J. Radiographic appearance of nosocomial legionnaires' disease after erythromycin treatment. Thorax 46:663, 1991.
71. El-Ebiary M, Sarmiento X, Torres A, *et al.* Prognosis factors of severe Legionella pneumonia requiring admission to ICU. Am J Respir Crit Care Med 156:1467, 1997.
72. Pedro-Botet ML, Sabria-Leal M, Sopena N, *et al.* Role of immunosppression in the evolution of Legionnaires' disease. CID 26:14, 1998.
73. Nelson D, Rensimer E, Raffin T. Legionella pneumophila pericarditis without pneumonia. Arch Intern Med 145:926, 1985.
74. White HJ, Felton WW, Sun CN. Etrapulmonary histopathologic manifestations of Legionnaires' disease. Arch Pathol Lab Med 104:287, 1980.
75. Tompkins LS, Roessler BJ, Redd SC, Markowitz LE, Cohen ML. Legionella prosthetic-valve endocarditis. N Engl J Med 318:530, 1988.
76. Brabender W, Hinthorn DR, Asher M, *et al.* *Legionella pneumophila* wound infection. JAMA 250:3091, 1983.
77. Andersen BB, Sogaard I. Legionnaires' disease and train abscess. Neurology 37:333, 1987.
78. Arnow PM, Boyko EJ, Friedman EL. Perirectal abscess caused by *Legionella pneumophila* and mixed anaerobic bacteria. Ann Intern Med 98: 184, 1983.
79. Dournon E, Bure A, Kemeny JL, *et al.* *Legionella pneumophila* peritonintis (Letter). Lancet 1: 1363, 1982.
80. Westblom TU, Hamory BH. Acute pancreatitis caused by *Legionella pneumophila*. South Med J 81:1200, 1988.
81. Parenti DM, Steinberg W, Kang P. Infectious causes of acute pancreatitis. Pancreas 13:356, 1996.
82. Byrd RP, Fields CL, Roy TM. Prognostic factors in Legionella pneumonia. Am J Respir Crit Care Med 159:342, 1999.
83. Dorman SA, Hardin NJ, Winn WC. Pyelonephritis associated with Legionella pneumophila, serogroup 4. Ann Intern Med 93:835, 1980.

84. Schlanger G, Lutwick LI, Kurzman M, *et al.* Sinusitis caused by *Legionella pneumophila* in a patient with the acquired immune deficiency syndrome. Am J Med 77:957, 1984.
85. Kalweit WC, Winn WC Jr, Rocco TA Jr, *et al.* Hemodialysis fistula infections caused by Legionella pneumophila. Ann Intern Med 96: 173, 1982.
86. Waldor MK, Wilson B, Swartz M. Cellulitis caused by *Legionella pneumophila*. Clin Infect Dis 16:51, 1993.
87. Fang GD, Fine M, Orloff J, *et al.* New and emerging etiologies for community-acquired pneumonia with implications for therapy: a prospective multicenter study of 359 cases. Medicine 69:307, 1990.
88. Chandler FW, Hicklin MD, Blackmon JA. Demostration of the agent of Legionnaires' disease in tissue. N Engl J Med 297:1218, 1977.
89. Edelstein PH, Meyer RD, Finegold SM. Laboratory diagnosis of Legionnaires disease. Am Rev Respir Dis 121:317, 1980.
90. Ruf B, Schürman D, Horback I, Fehrenbach FJ, Pohle HD. Prevalence and diagnosis of Legionella pneumonia: a 3-year prospective study with emphasis on application of urinary antigen detection. J Infect Dis 162:1341, 1990.
91. Ingram JG, Plouffe JF. Danger of sputum purulence screens in culture of Legionella species. J Clin Microbiol 32:209, 1994.
92. Edelstein PH. Laboratory diagnosis of infections caused by Legionellae. Eur J Clin Microbiol 6:216, 1987.
93. Kohorst WR, Schonfeld SA, Macklin JE, Whitcomb ME. Rapid diagnosis of legionnaires' disease by bronchoalveolar lavage. Chest 84: 186, 1983.
94. Monforte R, Estruch R, Vidal J, Cervera R, Urbano-Márquez A. Delayed seroconversion, Legionnaires' disease, and age. Lancet 2:1190, 1988.
95. Wilkinson HW, Reingold AL, Brake BJ, McGiboney DL, Gorman GW, Broome CV. Reactivity of serum from patients with suspected legionellosis against 29 antigens of legionellaceae and Legionella-like organisms by indirect immunofluorecent assay. J Infect Dis 147:23, 1983.
96. Plouffe JF, File TM Jr, Breiman RF, *et al.* Reevaluation of the definition of Legionnaires' disease: use of the urinary antigen assay. Clin Infect Dis 20:1286, 1995.
97. Dominguez JA, Manterola JM, Blavia R, *et al.* Detection of Legionella pneumophila serogroup 1 antigen in nonconcentrated urine and urine concentrated by selective ultrafiltration. J Clin Microbiol 34:2334, 1996.
98. Dominguez JA, Gali N, Pedroso P, *et al.* Comparison of the Binax Legionella urinary antigen enzyme immumoassay (EIA) with the Biotest Legionella urin antigen EIA for detection of Legionella antigen in both concentrated and nonconcentrated urine samples. J Clin Microbiol 36:2718, 1998.
99. Kazandjian D, Chiew R, Gilbert GL. Rapid diagnosis of Legionella pneumophila serogroup 1 infection with the Binax enzyme immunoassay urinary antigen test. J Clin Microbiol 35: 954, 1997.
100. Wever PC, Kuijper EJ, Yzerman EPF, Speelman P, Dankert J, Van Ketel RJ. Significance of the *Legionella* urinary antigen test during an outbreak. Abstracts of the 39th Interscience Conference on Antimicrobial and Chemotherapy, September 1999; Abstract 226:195, 1999.
101. Dominguez JA, Matas L, Manterola JM, *et al.* Comparison of radiommunoassay and enzyme immunoassay kits for detection of *Legionella pneumophila* serogroup 1 antigen in both concentrated and nonconcentrated urine samples. J Clin Microbiol 35:1627, 1997.
102. Kohler RB, Winn WC Jr, Wheat LJ. Onset and durating of urinary antigen excretion in Legionnaires disease. J Clin Microbiol 20:605, 1984.
103. Pasculle AW, Veto GE, Kristofiak S, McKelvey K, Vrsalovic K. Laboratory and clinical evaluation of a commercial DNA probe for the detection of *Legionella spp*. J Clin Microbiol 27:2350, 1989.
104. Pelloux I, Croize J, Hirtz P, Comet M, Le Noc P. Evaluation d'une tecnique de détection de *Legionella spp* par sonde nucléique. Pathol Biol 39:150, 1991.
105. Jaulhac B, Nowicki M, Bornstein N, *et al.* Detection of Legionella spp in bronchoalveolar lavage fluids by DNA amplification. J Clin Microbiol 30:920, 1992.
106. Kessler HH, Reinthaler FF, Pschaid A, *et al.* Rapid detection of *Legionella species* in bronchoalveolar lavage fluids with the EnviroAmp Legionella PCR amplification and detection kit. J Clin Microbiol 31:3325, 1993.
107. Matsiota-Bernard P, Pitsouni E, Legakis N, Nauciel C. Evaluation of commercial amplification kit for detection of *Legionella pneumophila*

in clinical specimen. J Clin Microbiol 32:1503, 1994.
108. Weir SC, Fischer SH, Stock F, Gill VJ. Detection of *Legionella* by PCR in respiratory specimens using a commercially available kit. Am J Clin Pathol 110:295, 1998.
109. Koide M, Saito A. Diagnosis of *Legionella pheneumophila* infection by polymerase chain reaction. Clin Infect Dis 21:199, 1995.
110. Maiwald M, Schill M, Stockinger C, *et al.* Detection of Legionella DNA in human and guinea pig urine samples by the polymerase chain reaction. Eur J Clin Microbiol Infect Dis 14:25, 1995.
111. Murdock DR, Walford EJ, Jenneings LC, *et al.* Use of the polymerase chain reaction to detect *Legionella* DNA in urine and serum samples from patients with pneumonia. Clin Infect Dis 23:475, 1996.
112. Ramirez JA, Ahkee S, Tolentino A, Miller RD, Summergill JT. Diagnosis of *Legionella pheumophila*, *Mycoplasma pneumoniae*, or *Chamydia pneumoniae* lower respiratory infection using the polymerase chain reaction on a single throat swab specimen. Diagn Microbiol Infect Dis 24:7, 1996.
113. Lindsay DS, Abraham WH, Fallon RJ. Detection of mip gene by PCR for diagnosis of Legionnaires' disease. J Clin Microbiol 32: 3068, 1994.
114. Akane A, Matsurbara K, Nakamura H, *et al.* Identification of the heme compound copurified with deoxyribonucleic acid (DNA) from bloodstains: a major inhibitor of polymerase chain reaction (PCR) amplification. J Forensic Sci 39:362, 1994.
115. Edelstein PH, Calarco K, Yasui VK. Antimicrobial therapy of experimentally induced Legionnaires' disease in guinea pigs. Am Rev Respir Dis 130:849, 1984.
116. Ewing S, Torres A. Severe community-acquired pneumonia. Clin Chest Med 20:575, 1999.
117. Roig J, Carreres A, Domingo C. Treatment of Legionnaires' disease. Drugs 46:63, 1993.
118. Edelstein PH. Antimicrobial chemotherapy for Legionnaires' disease: a review. CID 21(Suppl 3):S265, 1995.
119. Klein NC, Cunha BA. Treatment of Legionnaires' disease. Semin Respir Infect 13:140, 1998.
120. O'Doherty B, Muller O. Randomized, multicentre study of the efficacy and tolerance of azithromycin versus clarithromycin in the treatment of adults with mild to moderate community-acquired pneumonia. Eur J Clin Microbiol Infect Dis 17:823, 1998.
121. Garey KW, Amsden GW. Intravenous azithromycin. Ann Pharmacother 33:218, 1999.
122. Edelstein PH. Antimicrobial chemotherapy for Legionnaires' disease: time for a change. Ann Intern Med 129:328, 1998.
123. Reda C, Quaresima T, Pastoris MC. In-vitro activity of six intracellular antibiotics against *Legionella pneumophila* strains of human and enviromental origin. J Antimicrob Chemother 33:757, 1994.
124. Baltch AL, Smith RP, Ritz W. Inhibitory and bactericidal activities of levofloxacin, ofloxacin, erythromycin and rifampicin used singly and in combination against *Legionella pneumophila*. Antimicrob Agents Chemother 39: 1661, 1995.
125. Martin SJ, Pendland SL, Chen C, Schreckenberg P, Danzinger LH. In vitro sinergy testing of macrolide-quinolone combination against 41 clinical isolates of Legionella. Antimicrob Agents Chemother 40:1419, 1996.
126. Plouffe JF, Para MF, Bollin GE. Sulfamethoxazole-trimethoprim treatment of guinea pigs infected with *Legionella pneumophila*. J Infect Dis 150:780, 1984.
127. Ruiz-Santana S, Aguado-Bourrey JM, Narvaez-Bermejo JM, Gonzalez-Mediero G. *Legionella bozemanii* pneumonia and tetracycline [letter]. Ann Intern Med 105:969, 1986.
128. Morely JN, Smith LC, Baltch AL, Smith RP. Recurrent infection due to *Legionella pneumophila* in a patient with AIDS. Clin Infect Dis 19:1130, 1994.
129. Rello J, Valles J. Hospital-acquired pneumonia in the ICU patient. Semin Respir Crit Care Med 18:133, 1997.
130. Byrd RP, Roy TM. Rhabdomyolisis and bacterial pneumonia. Respir Med 92:358, 1998.

39. ADJUNCTIVE AND SUPPORTIVE MEASURES FOR COMMUNITY-ACQUIRED PNEUMONIA

Grant W. Waterer and Richard G. Wunderink

The widespread introduction of penicillin in the 1940s resulted in a substantial reduction in mortality from community-acquired pneumonia (CAP). However, despite significant advances in medical science, only a small improvement has occurred since, particularly in patients with bacteremic pneumococcal pneumonia [1, 2]. Even modern intensive care has only made a small difference to the mortality in patients with severe pneumonia [3, 4]. While the aging population, increased number of patients with severe co-morbid illnesses, and the human immunodeficiency virus (HIV) epidemic have certainly contributed to the persistently high mortality rate [2, 5, 6], apparently healthy, immunocompetent patients continue to die from CAP.

While some causative microorganisms, such as *Pseudomonas*, and some strains of common causative microorganisms appear to be more virulent, the majority of CAP patients who die are infected with organisms sensitive to commonly prescribed antibiotics. Even the recent emergence of high level penicillin-resistant strains of *S. pneumoniae* has not significantly increased the mortality of CAP. Given that most CAP patients die despite microbiological confirmation that they received appropriate antibiotic therapy, the introduction of new antibiotic classes is unlikely to reduce mortality further. For this reason, research has been directed into non-antibiotic therapeutic measures.

Generally, supportive measures for CAP can be separated into two categories – 1) immunomodulatory therapy for the systemic inflammatory response induced by pneumonia and 2) support for the gas exchange abnormalities unique to a pulmonary source of sepsis. This chapter will review the immunomodulatory therapies that have been studied in animal and human subjects with pneumonia. Advances in the intensive care management of patients with severe CAP, such as differential lung ventilation and extracorporeal membrane oxygenation (ECMO) will also be discussed.

Therapies Directed at the Immune Response

Patients who succumb to CAP seem to fall into two broad groups. The first group can be loosely categorized as having an excessive immune response to infection, including those who develop septic shock, acute respiratory distress syndrome (ARDS) and multiorgan failure. The second group is patients who can be categorized as having an inadequate host response to infection, including the elderly, alcoholics, diabetics and patients with significant co-morbid illnesses, such as cardiac failure or cirrhosis. Any immunomodulation strategy is likely to have different effects on the two populations. Even when patients are overtly similar, marked variability in the clinical response to the same causative organism is seen. The cause(s) of this significant variability in response to CAP is multifactorial but may have a genetic basis [7], similar to bacterial meningitis [8].

Immune Suppression

CORTICOSTEROIDS

With their potent anti-inflammatory action and proven efficacy in a variety of autoimmune diseases, glucocorticoids are an obvious choice of agent to try in patients thought to have an excessive, and deleterious, immune response to CAP.

The best evidence of benefit for corticosteroids comes from studies in specific, narrowly defined groups of CAP patients caused by less common agents. Randomized, controlled trials have shown corticosteroids reduce mortality in AIDS patients with *Pneumocystis carinii* pneumonia and significant hypoxia, if instituted at or prior to the onset of anti-pneumocystis therapy [9, 10]. Based on a small, retrospective study of 15 subjects, corticosteroids may also improve the outcome of severe *Varicella* pneumonia [11]. Anecdotally, corticosteroids are frequently used in the setting of severe fungal pneumonia, particularly due to *Histoplasmosis* [12, 13], and a small controlled trial of 55 patients supported their use in miliary tuberculosis [14].

Following the success of pre-antibiotic corticosteroids in children with meningitis [15], Marik and colleagues [16] studied the effect of a single dose of hydrocortisone (10 mg/kg) 30 minutes prior to antibiotic therapy in a small randomized placebo controlled trial of 30 adult patients with severe CAP (SCAP). Hydrocortisone had no detectable effect on tumor necrosis factor alpha (TNFα) production in the following 12 hours, mortality (only four deaths) or length of stay in the ICU. While not encouraging, the small number of subjects studied (14 received hydrocortisone), the use of only a single dose and the measurement of only a single pro-inflammatory cytokine for only 12 hours does not qualify this study to be a definitive statement on the role of corticosteroids in CAP. An important finding of this study was that beta-lactam antibiotics did not result in a significant increase in serum TNFα levels, as rapid antigen release due to bacterial lysis has been postulated as a potential cause of deterioration in patients with severe CAP [17].

Also supporting a possible role for corticosteroids in severe CAP, Montón and co-workers [18] studied the effect of intravenous methylprednisolone on bronchoalveolar lavage fluid (BALF) and serum cytokines in 20 patients with severe nosocomial pneumonia or CAP. The eleven patients who received methylprednisolone had significantly lower serum and BALF TNFα, interleukin (IL)-1β, IL-6 and C-reactive protein. There was also a non-significant trend to lower mortality in the steroid treated group (36% vs 67%). As higher TNFα [19–21] and IL-1β [10] concentrations in serum are known to correlate with greater mortality, this pilot study supports further research into the potential role of corticosteroids in severe CAP.

More damaging evidence for the potential role of corticosteroids as immunomodulatory agents in severe CAP are the unfavorable results from studies of septic shock. Pooled analysis of nine randomized, controlled trials showed no beneficial effect of corticosteroids in patients with septic shock [22]. Even more disturbing was a trend to greater mortality in patients receiving corticosteroids, particularly in those who developed secondary infections. The difficulty in balancing beneficial and detrimental effects is a common theme for all immunomodulatory therapy. Continuing research will hopefully define those subgroups most likely to benefit from corticosteroids, for example patients with refractory septic shock [23], or with specific pathogens, such as has already been demonstrated with *P. carinii* [9, 10].

ANTI-CYTOKINE THERAPIES

Anti-TNFα monoclonal antibodies [24–26], interleukin 1 receptor antagonist (IL1-Ra)

[27, 28], soluble TNFα receptors [29, 30], prostaglandin antagonists [31, 32], bradykinin antagonists [33] and platelet activating factor antagonists [34, 35] have all been assessed in patients with sepsis and septic shock. Pneumonia was the primary source of sepsis in a significant number of these trials. Despite promising initial studies, large, multicenter, phase III randomized controlled trials have failed to demonstrate any net beneficial effect from any of these agents [36].

When initial enthusiasm and promising phase I and II trials did not translate into successful phase III trials, the complexity of the system of pro- and anti-inflammatory agents became more apparent than had been appreciated previously [36]. While investigators often felt that individual patients clearly benefited from intervention, the observation of no net benefit in large studies implies that some patients had a detrimental effect from the intervention. Until our ability to clearly define the patients most likely to benefit, this experience is likely to be repeated with other anti-sepsis drugs.

PROSTAGLANDIN INHIBITORS

Prostaglandin antagonists are worth special comment as they have been studied in animal and human patients with pneumonia. Ibuprofen reduced the intrapulmonary shunt fraction from 29% to 21% in dogs with lobar pneumonia [37], with a corresponding decrease in the consolidated area of lung. Acetylsalicylic acid had a similar effect, reducing the shunt fraction from 38% to 23% [37]. The mechanism is unclear but may be due to reversal of prostaglandin inhibition of the hypoxia-induced pulmonary vasoconstriction.

In a small study of 10 subjects with pneumonia requiring mechanical ventilation, Hanley *et al.* [38] studied the effect of indomethacin (1 mg/kg oral or rectal) on arterial oxygenation. Five subjects had substantial improvement in oxygenation with a small improvement in three additional patients. Improvement tended to occur in the patients with the greatest degree of hypoxemia. As ibuprofen administration appears to be relatively safe even in the setting of sepsis [39], further studies are warranted.

In contrast, Ferrer *et al.* found a 2 g infusion of acetylsalicylic acid (ASA) had no effect on arterial oxygenation in seven patients with severe unilateral pneumonia [40]. Although intrapulmonary shunting did reduce by a small amount (28% ± 17% vs 23.5% ± 13%), the lack of clinically apparent benefit was discouraging. Several possible explanations were advanced to explain the discrepancy between this study and that of Hanley *et al.* Clearly, a difference in efficacy between ASA and indomethacin may be the cause. However, the subjects in the study by Hanley *et al.* were also more severely hypoxic, with a mean $Pa0_2/Fi0_2$ of 138 compared to 168. In any event, it would seem reasonable for future studies to use indomethacin in preference of ASA.

Immune Stimulation

IMMUNOGLOBULIN ENHANCEMENT

Before the advent of antibiotic therapy, passive immunization with serum was used with some success in patients with pneumonia [41]. Mortality was reduced by approximately 10% in most age groups with a diminishing effect in patients over the age of 60. With the exception of patients with specific immunoglobulin deficiencies, this therapy has largely been abandoned due to the much greater efficacy of antibiotics in addition to the difficulty, and cost, of obtaining sufficient serum. The development of new antiviral drugs has also largely obviated the anecdotal use of hyper-immune serum in cytomegalovirus and varicella pneumonitis.

While the overall efficacy of pneumococcal immunization is unclear, especially in the elderly with some comorbid illnesses, several studies and a meta-analysis have suggested that even if pneumococcal pneumonia is not prevented, the incidence of invasive pneumococcal disease is decreased.

The use of specific anti-Pseudomonal exotoxin antibodies have been tried as an adjunct to antibiotics with some success in mice [42] and guinea pigs [43], and pseudomonas specific vaccines have enhanced antibiotic response in guinea pigs [44]. Anti-Pseudomonal antibodies appeared safe in human subjects with evidence of increased opsonophagocytic activity in a small phase I study of 20 subjects [45], but further studies are required to determine whether they have any clinically relevant effect. In human sepsis studies, generic anti-endotoxin strategies have so far been disappointing [46, 47]. Although they have not specifically been studied in pneumonia, the primary site of sepsis in many of the patients in these studies was the lung, indicating a low likelihood of benefit.

NEUTROPHIL ENHANCEMENT

The neutrophil, or polymorphonuclear leukocyte (PMN), is a key cell in the host defense against microbial pathogens, particularly against bacteria and fungi. This includes the major pathogen in CAP, *S. pneumoniae* [48–54]. Both alcohol and diabetes, known risk factors for CAP [54, 55], have been shown to impair PMN function [56, 57]. A logical hypothesis following from this is that improving PMN function may improve the outcome of CAP.

Granulocyte colony stimulating factor (G-CSF) is one of a family of glycoproteins that control hematopoiesis [58]. G-CSF has significant effects on PMN function, increasing the response to chemotaxins, enhancing phagocytosis, increasing the respiratory burst, delaying neutrophil apoptosis and increasing bactericidal and fungicidal activity [58–60]. G-CSF also accelerates the development of PMNs leading to an increased rate of release from the bone marrow [59]. One further potential benefit of G-CSF is the enhancement of antibiotic uptake by phagocytic cells [61]. Due to these properties, G-CSF it is an attractive candidate for study in patients with pneumonia.

Since PMNs have been implicated in the development of multiorgan dysfunction, including ARDS [62, 63], the potential for harm from G-CSF therapy in some patients also exists. PMNs newly released from the bone marrow appear to preferentially sequester in the lung microvasculature [64], raising concern about an increased risk of ARDS. The effect of G-CSF in an individual CAP patient may also depend on the pathogen.

Animal pneumonia models demonstrate both potentials of GCSF treatment. Karzai and colleagues [65] used an endobronchial instillation model to demonstrate that G-CSF had a beneficial effect in *S. aureus* infected rats while *E. coli* infected rats had increased pulmonary injury and mortality with GCSF treatment. A significantly greater drop in peripheral PMN counts in *E. coli* infected rats was consistent with neutrophil mediated lung injury secondary to adherence to endothelium and subsequent degranulation, to which the lung is particularly susceptible [66, 67]. The dose of *E. coli* given was five-fold greater than the dose of *S. aureus*, raising the possibility that the *E. coli* arm actually produced a model of acute lung injury rather than pneumonia [68]. In other non-neutropenic animal models of pneumonia, G-CSF administration improved survival for both Gram-negative [69] and Gram-positive pathogens [70].

Initial studies of G-CSF in non-neutropenic human patients with pneumonia were encouraging [71]. In the most extensive trial published to date, Nelson *et al.* [72] conducted a prospective, multicenter, randomized, placebo controlled trial of G-CSF 300 μg/day (for up to 10 days) in 756 CAP patients, 380 of whom received active drug. G-CSF appeared to be safe in this population, with even a trend to less ARDS and disseminated intravascular coagulation (DIC), although the numbers of each complication was small. Overall, no significant benefit was demonstrated, although a trend to better outcome in patients with multilobar pneumonia was found. The similar trend was found in a recently completed multicenter trial [72b].

The likelihood is that G-CSF will not benefit all patients. GCSF does not appear to improve outcome in severe pneumonia with septic shock. Further research into both pathogen specific responses and specific patient subgroups, such as the elderly, diabetics and alcoholics, is needed before final conclusions on the role of G-CSF in pneumonia can be made. One important consideration will be the cost-benefit ratio, which has been questioned for G-CSF as therapy for neutropenia in patients receiving chemotherapy [73]. G-CSF clearly reduces the duration of neutropenia but no reduction in mortality or morbidity has been demonstrated in clinical trials in these patients.

MACROPHAGE ENHANCEMENT

Legionella pneumophila is consistently identified as a leading cause of CAP, particularly in patients with severe CAP [49, 50, 74–77]. Unlike pneumococcal pneumonia, the immune response to Legionella infection is predominantly of a TH1 type [78] and bacterial killing is predominantly by macrophages [79]. Skerrett and Martin studied the effect of interferon gamma (IFNγ), a potent stimulator of macrophage function [80, 81], given as an intratracheal bolus in rats with experimental *L. pneumophila* pneumonia [82]. Intratracheal IFNγ markedly reduced the replication of *L. pneumophila* in corticosteroid treated rats, but had no detectable effect in immunocompetent rats or when given intraperitoneally.

The ability to give IFNg by aerosol is particularly appealing as it not only avoids the systemic side effects, but also has a much greater effect on intrapulmonary macrophage function than systemic administration [83]. Aerosolized IFNγ has also been shown to be safe in patients with drug resistant tuberculosis [84], and may have a role in treatment of this condition. Further studies of nebulized IFNγ, especially in patients with pulmonary Legionellosis, are awaited.

Other Supportive Measures

The main additional supportive therapy unique to CAP is improved oxygenation and secretion clearance. The remainder of supportive care is not different than that of other critically ill patients with infection.

Improving Oxygenation

POSITIONING THERAPY

CAP is one of the more common causes of severe hypoxic respiratory failure. A common method to improve oxygenation, the addition of positive end expiratory pressure, may actually make oxygenation worse in patients with severe asymmetrical lung disease like CAP. The PEEP will tend to overdistend the unaffected lung, increasing pulmonary vascular resistance on the local area. This overdistension may then direct greater blood flow to the pneumonic area, especially if hypoxic vasoconstriction has been blocked by some bacterial product.

With extensive unilateral pneumonia, positioning the ventilated patient in the lateral decubitus position with the affected lung up has been demonstrated to improve oxygenation [85]. Positioning increases perfusion to the dependent, non involved lung, increases secretion clearance from the affected lung, and may allow addition of PEEP without increasing shunt because the dependent lung is now less compliant and less likely to become overdistended. The combination of positioning and prostaglandin inhibitors is usually adequate to temporarily improve oxygenation until hypoxic vasoconstriction is restored.

DIFFERENTIAL LUNG VENTILATION

Differentially ventilating each lung by means of a dual lumen endotracheal tube may also be beneficial [86, 87]. This allows the use of higher levels of PEEP in the affected, less compliant, lung and lower levels of PEEP in the normal lung, thus reducing the risk of barotrauma. A study by Ranieri *et al*. showing a correlation between the level of PEEP and pro-inflammatory cytokine production further supports this approach to protect the "normal" lung [88]. The point at which differential ventilation is worth commencing is not clear, but Carlon and colleagues [86] suggest optimal benefit occurs when there is a 200 ml or greater difference in distribution of tidal volume between each lung.

EXTRACORPOREAL MEMBRANE OXYGENATION

ECMO, a modification of cardiopulmonary bypass, was designed to provide oxygenation in patients with severe respiratory failure. Although available since the 1970s, initial poor results from a National Institutes of Health sponsored prospective, multicenter randomized trial [89] limited the use of ECMO to research centers. However, a significant reduction in complications has led to resurgence in interest in ECMO as a means of providing oxygenation when all other means have failed.

The role of ECMO has most extensively been studied in neonates. In newborn infants with respiratory failure unresponsive to other therapy it has proven highly effective, having an overall survival of 80% in over 10,000 neonates where nearly 100% mortality would be expected [90]. Modification of the neonatal ECMO technique has also been effective in some pediatric patients with respiratory failure [91], including those with pneumonia from both bacterial [92] and viral [93] pathogens. As would be expected, as the duration of ECMO required increases, the prognosis decreases [92].

In the NIH-sponsored ECMO trial, adults with viral pneumonia did particularly poorly. In a retrospective review of 100 adults with severe acute respiratory failure supported with ECMO by Kolla and colleagues [94], a 53% survival rate was found in the 49 patients with a primary diagnosis of pneumonia. Although this mortality seems high, patients selected for ECMO had an expected mortality in excess of 90%. Predictors of poor response to ECMO were increasing age, days of ventilation prior to commencement of ECMO and the degree of respiratory failure as measured by the PaO_2/FiO_2 ratio. Cases of successful intervention in adults with severe *Legionella* [95, 96], pneumococcal [97] and *Varicella* pneumonia [98] have all been reported.

The clearest indication for ECMO in adults may be the recently described Hantavirus Pulmonary Syndrome (HPS). With no effective antiviral therapy, care is entirely supportive. In a small series of three cases the dramatic but time-limited cardiovascular and pulmonary hemorrhagic manifestations of HPS appeared to be well supported by ECMO [99].

ECMO would appear to have a role in some patients with severe respiratory failure secondary to pneumonia. The timing, duration and patient selection for what is an expensive, labor intensive therapy remains to be determined by prospective studies.

OTHER THERAPIES

Liquid ventilation with volatile hydrocarbons has been studied in the management of ARDS. Little data is currently published on its use specifically in human subjects with pneumonia. In rats given lethal doses of pneumococci, partial liquid ventilation in combination with perfleurocarbon doubled survival compared to antibiotics alone [100].

Nitric oxide (NO) inhalation has also been studied as adjunctive therapy of ARDS, as well as some other forms of severe pulmonary hypertension. While there are no studies specifically addressing human patients with pneumonia, in dogs with *Eschericia coli* pneumonia, inhaled NO had a minimal effect on oxygenation and no effect on sepsis induced pulmonary hypertension [101].

Since NO is one of the effector molecules released by macrophages to kill bacteria [102], inhaled NO has a potential antibacterial effect. Hoehn and colleagues studied the bacteriostatic effect of NO on bacterial cultures from neonates [103]. At 120 ppm (greater than the usual dose range of 40–80 ppm) NO inhibited the growth group B Streptococcus, *Staphylococcus epidermidis* and *E coli* but not *Pseudomonas aeruginosa* or *Staphylococcus aureus*. Further studies will be required to determine whether inhaled NO has any real bacteriostatic effect *in vivo*, particularly as it may have deleterious effects on the function of neutrophils [104].

Aerosolized prostacyclin has also been shown by Walmrath *et al.* to improve oxygenation by reducing shunt and pulmonary hypertension in patients with pneumonia [105]. Twelve patients with severe pneumonia ($PaO_2/FiO_2 < 150$), six of whom had interstitial lung disease (ILD), received varying doses of prostacyclin. Patients with ILD required substantially larger doses of prostacyclin to produce a clinical effect. Although its efficacy has not been compared to NO in patients with pneumonia, its greater cost is a significant disadvantage.

CLEARANCE OF SECRETIONS

Significant accumulation of mucopurulent secretions can occur in CAP, particularly in patients on mechanical ventilation. Mucus impaction can lead to obstruction, ranging in severity from linear atelectasis to lobar collapse.

Physical Removal. Clearly the most effective secretion clearance is a spontaneous cough. However, the respiratory compromise often attendant to severe CAP may prevent an effective cough. Support with noninvasive ventilation (NIV) may benefit the patient by both improving respiratory mechanics while allowing the patient to spontaneously expectorate [106]. However, retained secretions are also one of the causes of failure of NIV. An important strategy to avoid this complication is to avoid continuous application of NIV and actively encourage the patient to cough during periods off NIV.

In mechanically ventilated CAP patients, removal of secretions by regular suctioning is essential. The use of percussion or vibration in ventilated patients has been associated with worsening of gas exchange and the benefit in CAP patients in general is unclear.

The benefit of bronchoscopy for secretion removal is also poorly supported. Bronchoscopy for secretion removal has been associated with an increased risk of development of subsequent nosocomial pneumonia [107]. Therefore its therapeutic use should be limited. One of the few studies in this area has suggested that if lobar atelectasis is accompanied by an air bronchogram, bronchoscopy is unlikely to find a mucus plug or benefit the patient.

Mucolytics. Changing the rheologic properties of thick tenacious mucus is often attempted with little scientific support. Avoidance of dessication and inspissation of secretions does appear to be important. Adequate hydration may be the most effective therapy. Intubated CAP patients with significant secretions are poor candidates for heat and moisture exchangers and should usually have ventilation initiated with heated humidification.

The pharmacologic intervention most often ordered is N-acetylcysteine. Most support for this therapy is an extension of results in some cystic fibrosis patients. Whether the same benefit can be achieved in CAP patients is unclear as there is no published data of n-acetylcysteine use in this setting. The potential benefit is also partially offset by induction of bronchial irritation and bronchospasm in some patients. Preliminary data on agents with more physiologic support, such as UTP [108], are encouraging but need further study. Guafenesin has limited data in non-pneumonia patients and is unlikely to have a major benefit in intubated CAP patients. Although a variety of other mucolytic agents are available, including bromohexine, rhDNase and polymixin B, there is no data to support their use in patients with pneumonia.

Conclusion

CAP remains a significant health problem and patients continue to die despite receiving appropriate antibiotic therapy. Modification of the host immune response, both anti and pro-inflammatory approaches, has yet to live up to the promise of improved outcome. Despite this, there is significant reason for optimism. Some immunomodulatory therapies clearly have efficacy in some patients. As our understanding of the immune response to pneumonia improves our ability to tailor specific therapies for individual patients will also improve, hopefully avoiding the deleterious effects that have so far prevented the development of an effective immune based therapy. The possibility of delivering cytokines directly to the lung, such as with nebulized IFNγ, is a particularly promising way of achieving the desired pulmonary effect without systemic side effects.

Corticosteroids are currently unique in that they have a proven role in the therapy of pneumonia due to *P carinii*. The development of pathogen specific therapies, such as INFγ for *L pneumophila*, based on an improved understanding of host-pathogen interactions, are awaited.

Once respiratory failure has ensued supportive measures such as patient positioning and differential lung ventilation can improve oxygenation at no additional risk in some patients, particularly those with severe unilateral pneumonia. In facilities where ECMO is available it may be beneficial in selected patients when all other means of providing respiratory support have failed. The role of inhaled NO and partial liquid ventilation is also currently unclear and awaiting further study.

The past 20 years has seen an explosion in our knowledge of human immunology and we are only now beginning to explore the therapeutic possibilities this has made available. The next 10 years promises to finally provide a significant advance in the therapy of pneumonia, the first substantial gain since penicillin.

References

1. Burman LA, Norrby R, Trollfors B. Invasive pneumococcal infections: incidence, predisposing factors and prognosis. Rev Infect Dis 7:133, 1985.
2. Watankunakorn C, Bailey TA. Adult bacteremic pneumococcal pneumonia in a community teaching hospital, 1992–1996. Arch Intern Med 157:1965, 1997.
3. Hook EW, Horton CA, Schaberg DR. Failure of intensive care unit support to influence mortality from pneumococcal bacteremia. JAMA 249:1055, 1983.
4. Franklin C, Henrickson K, Weil MH. Reduced mortality of pneumococcal bacteremia after early intensive care. J Intensive Care Med 6:302, 1991.
5. Torres JM, Cardenas O, Vasquez A, Schlossberg D. *Streptococcus pneumoniae* bacteremia in a community hospital. Chest 113:387, 1998.
6. Plouffe JF, Breiman RF, Facklam RR, Franklin County Pneumonia Study Group. Bacteremia with *Streptococcus pneumoniae*. Implications for therapy and prevention. JAMA 275:194, 1996.
7. Waterer GW, Quasney MW, Zhang Q, Jones CB, Wunderink RG. The impact of the TNFb + 250 gene polymorphism on the severity of community-acquired pneumonia. Chest 116:265S Abstract, 1999.
8. Westendorp RGJ, Langermans JAM, Huizinga TWJ, Elouali AH, Verweij CL, Boomsma DI, *et al.* Genetic influence on cytokine production and fatal meningococcal disease. Lancet 349:170, 1997.
9. Gagnon S, Ahmad M, Boota ND, *et al.* Corticosteroids as adjunctive therapy for severe *Pneumocystis carinii* pneumonia in the acquired immunodeficiency syndrome. N Engl J Med 323:1444, 1990.
10. Bozette SA, Sattler FR, Chiu J, *et al.* A controlled trial of early adjunctive treatment with corticosteroids for *Pneumocystis carinii* pneumonia in the acquired immunodeficiency syndrome. N Engl J Med 323:1451, 1990.
11. Mer M, Richards GA. Corticosteroids in life-threatening varicella pneumonia. Chest 114:426, 1998.
12. Goldman M, Johnson PC, Sarosi GA. Fungal pneumonias. The endemic mycoses. Clin Chest Med 20:507, 1990.
13. Bradsher RW. Histoplasmosis and blastomycosis. Clin Infect Dis 22:S102, 1996.

14. Togman S, Jiayu Y, Liye Z, Weiwu D, Zhaoying S. Chemotherapy and its combination with corticosteroids in acute miliary tuberculosis in adolescents and adults: analysis of 55 cases. Chin Med J 94:309, 1981.
15. Lebel MH, Freij BJ. Dexamethasone therapy for bacterial meningitis: results of two double-blind, placebo controlled trials. N Engl J Med 319:964, 1988.
16. Marik P, Kraus P, Sribante J, Havlik I, Lipman J, Johnson DW. Hydrocortisone and tumor necrosis factor in severe community-acquired pneumonia. Chest 104:389, 1993.
17. Klugman K. Pneumococcal resistance to antibiotics. Clin Microbiol Rev 3:171, 1990.
18. Torres A, Ewig S, El-Ebiary M, Filella X, Xaubet A. Role of glucocorticoids on inflammatory response in nonimmunosuppressed patients with pneumonia: a pilot study. Eur Resp J 14:218, 1999.
19. Casey LC. Plasma cytokine and endotoxin levels correlate with survival in patients with the sepsis syndrome. Ann Intern Med 119:771, 1993.
20. Puren AJ, Feldman C, Savage N, Becker PJ, Smith C. Patterns of cytokine expression in community-acquired pneumonia. Chest 107:1342, 1995.
21. van Dissel JT. Anti-inflammatory cytokine profile and mortality in febrile patients. Lancet 351:950, 1998.
22. Cronin L, Cook DJ, Carlet J, Heyland DK, King D, Lansang MAD, *et al.* Corticosteroid treatment for sepsis: a critical appraisal and meta-analysis of the literature. Crit Care Med 12:1439, 1995.
23. Bollaert PE, Charpentier C, Levy B, Debouverie M, Audibert E, Larcan A. Reversal of late septic shock with supraphysiologic doses of hydrocortisone. Crit Care Med 26:645, 1998.
24. Reinhart K, Wiegand-Lönhart C, Grimminger F, *et al.* Assessment of the safety and efficacy of the monoclonal anti-tumor necrosis factor antibody-fragment, MAK 195F, in patients with sepsis and septic shock: a multi-center, randomized, placebo-controlled, dose-ranging study. Crit Care Med 24:733, 1996.
25. Abraham E, Wunderink R, Silverman H, *et al.* Efficacy and safety of monoclonal antibody to human tumor necrosis factor-alpha in patients with sepsis syndrome: a randomized, controlled, double-blind, multicenter clinical trial. TNF-alpha MAb Sepsis Study Group. JAMA 273:934, 1995.
26. Cohen J, Carlet J, INTERSEPT: an international, multi-center, placebo-controlec trial of monoclonal antibody to human tumor necrosis factor-alpha in patients with sepsis. Crit Care Med 24:1431, 1996.
27. Opal SM, Fisher CJ, Dhainault JF. Confirmatory interleukin-1 receptor antagonist trial in severe sepsis: a phase III, randomized, double-blind, placebo-controlled, multicenter trial. Crit Care Med 25:1115, 1997.
28. Fisher CJ, Dhainault JF, Opal SM, *et al.* Recombinant human interleukin-1 receptor antagonist in the treatment of patients with sepsis syndrome. Phase III rhIL-1ra Sepsis Syndrome Study Group. JAMA 271:1836, 1994.
29. Fisher CJJ, Agosti JM, Opal SM, *et al.* Treatment of septic shock with the tumor necrosis factor receptor: Fc fusion protein. N Engl J Med 334:1697, 1997.
30. Abraham E, Glauser MP, Butler T, *et al.* p55 tumor necrosis factor receptor fusion protein in the treatment of patients with severe sepsis and septic shock. Ro 45-2081 Study Group. JAMA 277:1531, 1997.
31. Haupt MJ, Jastremski MS, Clemmer TP, Metz CA, Goris GB. Effect of ibuprofen in patients with severe sepsis: a randomized, double-blind, multicenter study. Crit Care Med 19:1339, 1991.
32. Bernard GR, Reines HD, Halushka PV. The effects of ibuprofen on the physiology and survival of patients with sepsis. N Engl J Med 336:912, 1997.
33. Fein AM, Bernard GR, Criner GJ, *et al.* Treatment of severe systemic inflammatory response syndrome and sepsis with a novel bradykinin antagonist, deltibant (CP-0127): results of a randomized, double-blind, placebo-controlled trial. JAMA 277:482, 1997.
34. Dhainault JF, Tenaillon A, Le Tulzc Y, *et al.* Platelet-activating factor receptor antagonist BN 52021 in the treatment of severe sepsis: a randomized, double blind, placebo-controlled, multicenter clinical trial. Crit Care Med 22:1720, 1994.
35. Dhainault JF, Tenaillon A, Hemmer M, *et al.* Confirming phase III clinical trial to study the efficacy of a P.A.F. antagonist, BN 52021, in reducing mortality of patients with severe gram-negative sepsis. Am J Respir Crit Care Med 151:A47, 1995.
36. Bone RC. Immunologic dissonance: a continuing evolution in our understanding of the systemic inflammatory response syndrome (SIRS)

and multiple organ dysfunction syndrome (MODS). Ann Intern Med 125:680, 1996.

37. Light RB. Indomethacin and acetylsalicylic acid reduce intrapulmonary shunt in experimental pneumococcal pneumonia. Am Rev Respir Dis 134:520, 1986.
38. Hanley PJ, Roberts D, Dobson K, *et al.* Effect of indomethacin on arterial oxygenation in critically ill patients with severe pneumonia. Lancet 1:351, 1987.
39. Bernard GR, Reines HD, Halushka RV, Higgins SB, Metz CA, Swindell BB, *et al.* Prostacyclin and thromboxane A_2 formation is increased in human sepsis syndrome. Am Rev Respir Dis 144:1095, 1991.
40. Ferrer M, Torres A, Bauer R, Hernández C, Roca J, Rodriguez-Roisin R. Effect of acetylsalicylic acid on pulmonary gas exchange in patients with severe pneumonia: a pilot study. Chest 111:1094, 1997.
41. Dowling HF, Lepper MH. The effect of antibiotics (penicillin, aureomycin, and terramycin) on the fatality rate and incidence of complications in pneumococcic pneumonia. A comparison with other methods of therapy. Am J Med Sci 222:396, 1951.
42. Kohzuki T, Eguchi Y, Kato M, Irie K, Ohtsuka H, Higuchi A, *et al.* Protective activity of anti-exotoxin A monoclonal antibody against mice infected with toxin-producing *Pseudomonas aeruginosa*. J Infect Dis 167:119, 1993.
43. Hector RF, Collins MS, Pennington JE. Treatment of experimental *Pseudomonas aeruginosa* pneumonia with a human IgM monocolonal antibody. J Infect Dis 160:483, 1989.
44. Pennington JE, Hickey WF, Blackwood LL, *et al.* Active immunization with lipopolysaccharide *Pseudomonas* antigen for chronic Pseudomonas bronchopneumonia in guinea pigs. J Clin Invest 68:1140, 1981.
45. Saravolatz LD, Markowitz N, Collins MS, Bogdanoff D, Pennington JE. Saftey, pharmokinetics, and functional activity of human anti-*Pseudomonas aeruginosa* monoclonal antibodies in septic and nonseptic patients. J Infect Dis 167:784, 1991.
46. Greenman RL, Schein RMH, Martin MA, *et al.* A controlled trial of E5 murine monoclonal IgM antibody to endotoxin in the treatment of gram-negative sepsis. JAMA 266:1097, 1991.
47. Ziegler EJ, Fisher CJ, Sprung CL, *et al.* Treatment of gram-negative bacteremia and septic shock with HA-1A human monoclonal antibody against endotoxin: a randomized, double blind, placebo-controlled trial. N Engl J Med 324:429, 1991.
48. Bates JH, Campbell GD, Barron AL, McCracken GA, Morgan PN, Moses EB, *et al.* Microbial etiology of acute pneumonia in hospitalized patients. Chest 101:1005, 1992.
49. Blanquer J, Blanquer R, Borrás R, Nauffal D, Morales P, Menéndez R, *et al.* Aetiology of community acquired pneumonia in Valencia, Spain: a multicentre prospective study. Thorax 46:508, 1991.
50. Macfarlane JT, Finch RG, Ward MJ, Macrae AD. Hospital study of adult community-acquired pneumonia. Lancet 2:255, 1982.
51. Marrie TJ, Durant H, Yates L. Community-acquired pneumonia requiring hospitalization: 5-year prospective study. Rev Infect Dis 11:586, 1989.
52. Marston BJ, Lipman HB, Breiman RF. Surveillance for Legionnaires' disease. Risk factors for morbidity and mortality. Arch Intern Med 154:2417, 1994.
53. Moldawer LL. Biology of proinflammatory cytokines and their antagonists. Crit Care Med 22:S3, 1994.
54. Bartlett JG, Mundy LM. Community-acquired pneumonia. N Engl J Med 333:1618, 1995.
55. Musher DM. Infections caused by *Streptococcus pneumonia*: clinical spectrum, pathogenesis, immunity and treatment. Clin Infect Dis 14:801, 1992.
56. Repine JE, Clawson CC, Goetz FC. Bactericidal function of neutrophils from patients with acute bacterial infections and from diabetes. J Infect Dis 142:869, 1980.
57. Brayton RG, Stokes PE, Schwartz MS, Louria DB. Effect of alcohol and various diseases on leucocyte mobilization, phagocytosis and intracellular bacterial killing. N Engl J Med 282:123, 1970.
58. Welte K, Gabrilove J, Bronchud MH, Platzer E, Morstyn G. Filgrastim (r-metHuG-CSF): The first 10 years. Blood 88:1907, 1996.
59. Dale DC, Liles WC, Summer WR, Nelson S. Granulocyte colony-stimulating factor-role and relationships in infectious diseases. J Infect Dis 172:1061, 1995.
60. Roilides E, Walsh TJ, Pizzo PA, Rubin M. Granulocyte colony-stimulating factor enhances the phagocytic and bactericidal activity of normal and defective human neutrophils. J Infect Dis 163:579, 1991.
61. McKenna PJ, Nelson S, Anderson J. Filgastrim

(rhuG-CSF) enhances ciprofloxacin uptake and bactericidal activity of human neutrophis *in vitro*. Am J Respir Crit Care Med 153:A535, 1996.

62. Fujishima S, Aikawa N. Neutrophil-mediated tissue injury and its modulation. Intensive Care Med 21:277, 1995.
63. Weiss SJ. Tissue destruction by neutrophils N Engl J Med 320:365, 1989.
64. Sato Y, van Eeden SF, English D, Hogg JC. Bacteremic pneumococcal pneumonia: bone marrow release and pulmonary sequestration of neutrophils. Crit Care Med 26:501, 1998.
65. Karzai W, von Specht BU, Parent C, Haberstroh J, Wollersen K, Natanson C, *et al*. G-CSF during *Escherichia coli* versus *Staphylococcus aureus* pneumonia in rats has fundamentally different and opposite effects. Am J Respir Crit Care Med 159:1377, 1999.
66. Bersten A, Sibbald WJ. Acute lung injury in septic shock. Crit Care Clin 5:49, 1991.
67. Repine JE, Bechler CJ. Neutrophils and adult respiratory distress syndrome: two interlocking perspectives in 1991. Am Rev Respir Dis 144:251, 1991.
68. Nelson S. A question of balance. Am J Respir Crit Care Med 159:1365, 1999.
69. Smith WS, Sumnicht GE, Sharpe RW, Samuelson D, Millard FE. Granulocyte colony-stimulating factor versus placebo in addition to penicillin G in a randomized blinded study of gram-negative pneumonia sepsis: analysis of survial and multisystem organ failure. Blood 86:1301, 1995.
70. Preheim LC, Snitily MU, Gentry MJ. Effects of granulocyte colony-stimulating factor in cirrhotic rats with pneumococcal pneumonia. J Infect Dis 174:225, 1996.
71. de Boisblanc BP, Summer WR, Mason C, Shellito J, Logan E, Bear M, *et al*. Phase 1 trial of granulocyte-colony stimulating factor in severe community acquired pneumonia. Am J Respir Crit Care Med A204, 1998.
72. Nelson S, Belknap SM, Carlson RW, Dale D, BeBoisblanc B, Farkas S, *et al*. A randomized controlled trial of filgrastim as an adjunct to antibiotics for treatment of hospitalized patients with community-acquired pneumonia. J Infect Dis 178:1075, 1998.

72b. Nelson S, Heyder AM, Stone J, *et al*. A randonited controlled trial of filgastrim for the treatment of hospitalized patients with multilobar pueumonia, J Infect Dis 182:970, 2000.

73. Urban T, Lebeau B. Colony-stimulating factor therapy and febrile neutropenia induced by chemotherapy: need for economical studies. Eur Resp J 13:1228, 1999.
74. Klimek JJ, Ajemian E, Tontecchio S, Gracewski J, Klemas B, Jiminez L. Community-acquired bacterial pneumonia requiring admission to hospital. Am J Infect Control 11:79, 1983.
75. Aubertin J, Dabis F, Fleurett J, Bornstein N, Salamon R, Brottier E, *et al*. Prevalence of legionellosis among adults: a study of community-acquired pneumonia in France. Infection 15:328, 1987.
76. Fang GD, Fine MJ, Orloff J, Arisumi D, Yu VL, Kapoor W, *et al*. New and emerging etiologies for community-acquired pneumonia with implications for therapy. A prospective multicenter study of 359 cases. Medicine 69:307, 1990.
77. Lieberman D, Schlaeffer F, Boldur I, Horowitz S, Friedman MG, Leiononen M, *et al*. Multiple pathogens in adult patients admitted with community-acquired pneumonia: a one year prospective study of 346 consecutive patients. Thorax 51:179, 1996.
78. Tateda K, Matsumoto T, Ishii Y, Furuya N, Ohno A, Miyazaki S, *et al*. Serum cytokines in patients with Legionella pneumonia: relative predominance of Th1-type cytokines. Clin Diag Lab Immunol 5, 1998.
79. Friedman H, Yamamoto Y, Newton C, Klein T. Immunologic response and pathophysiology to *Legionella* infection. Semin Resp Infect 13:100, 1998.
80. Murray HW. Interferon-gamma, the activated macrophage, and host defense against microbial challenge. Ann Intern Med 108:608, 1989.
81. Nathan CF, Prendergast TJ, Wiebe ME, Stanley ER, Platzer E, Remold HG, *et al*. In vivo and in vitro activation of alveolar macrophages by recombinant interferon-γ. J Exp Med 160:600, 1984.
82. Skerrett SJ, Martin TR. Intratracheal interferon-γ augments pulmonary defenses in experimental legionellosis. Crit Care Med 149:50, 1994.
83. Jaffe R, Buhl R, Mastrangeli A, Holroyd KJ, Saltini C, Czerski D, *et al*. Organ specific cytokine therapy. J Clin Invest 88:297, 1991.
84. Condos R, Rom WN, Schluger NW. Treatment of multidrug-resistant pulmonary tuberculosis with interferon-gamma via aerosol. Lancet 349:1513, 1997.
85. Remolina C, Khan AU, Santiago TV *et al*. Posi-

tional hypoxemia in unilateral lung disease. N Engl J Med 304:523, 1981.

86. Carlon GC, Ray CR, Klein R, *et al.* Criteria for selective positive end-expiratory pressure and independent synchronized ventilation of each lung. Chest 74:501, 1978.
87. Hillman KM, Barber JD. Asynchronous independent lung ventilation (AILV). Crit Care Med 8:390, 1980.
88. Ranieri VM, Suter PM, Tortorella C, De Tullio R, Dayer JM, Brienza A, *et al.* Effect of mechanical ventilation on inflammatory mediators in patients with acute respiratory distress syndrome: a randomized controlled trial. JAMA 282:77, 1999.
89. Zapol WM, Snider MT, Hill JD. Extracorporeal membrane oxygenation in severe acute respiratory failure. A randomized prospective study. JAMA 242:2193, 1979.
90. ECMO Registry of the Extracorporeal Life Support Organization (ELSO). ECMO Quarterly Report (January) 1997.
91. Green TP, Timmons OD, Fackler JC, Moler FW, Thompson AE, Sweeney MF, *et al.* The impact of extracorporeal membrane oxygenation on survival in pediatric patients with acute respiratory failure. Crit Care Med 24:323, 1996.
92. Masiakos PT, Islam S, Doody DP, Schnitzer JJ, Ryan DP. Extracorporeal membrane oxygenation for nonneonatal acute respiratory failure. Arch Surg 134:375, 1999.
93. Meyer TA, Warner BW. Extracorporeal life support for the treatment of viral pneumonia: collective experience from the ELSO registry. J Pediatr Surg 32:232, 1997.
94. Kolla S, Awad SS, Rich PB, Schreiner RJ, Hirschl RB, Bartlett RH. Extracorporeal life support for 100 adult patients with severe respiratory failure. Ann Surg 226:544, 1997.
95. Ichiba S, Jenkins DR, Peek GJ, Brennan KJ, Killer HM, Sosnowski A, *et al.* Severe acute respiratory failure due to legionella pneumonia treated with extracorporeal membrane oxygenation. Clin Infect Dis 28:686, 1999.
96. Nakajima H, Kutsuwada T, Ohdaira T, Saito A, Satoh K, Igarashi K, *et al.* Extracorporeal membrane oxygenation for acute respiratory failure induced by *Legionella pneumophile.* Nihon Kyobu Shikkan Gakkai Zasshi 35:1363, 1997.
97. Codispoti M, Sanger K, Mankad PS. Successful extracorporeal membrane oxygenation (ECMO) support for fulminant community-acquired pneumococcal pneumonia. Thorax 50:1317, 1995.
98. Lee WA, Kolla S, Schreiner RJ, Hirschl RB, Bartlett RH. Prolonged extracorporeal life support for varicella pneumonia. Crit Care Med 25:997, 1997.
99. Crowley MR, Katz RW, Kessler R, Simpson SQ, Levy H, Hallin GW, *et al.* Successful treatment of adults with severe Hantavirus pulmonary syndrome with extracorporeal membrane oxygenation. Crit Care Med 26:409, 1998.
100. Dickson EW, Heard SO, Chu B, Fraire A, Brueggemann AB, Doern GV. Partial liquid ventilation with perfluorocarbon in the treatment of rats with lethal pneumococcal pneumonia. Anesthesiology 88:218, 1998.
101. Quezado ZM, Natanson C, Karzai W, Danner RL, Koev CA, Fitz Y, *et al.* Cardiopulmonary effects of inhaled nitric oxide in normal dogs and during *E. coli* pneumonia and sepsis. J Appl Physiol 84:107, 1998.
102. Anggard E. Nitric oxide: mediator, murderer, and medicine. Lancet 343:1199, 1994.
103. Hoehn T, Huebner J, Paboura E, Krause M, Leititis JU. Effect of therapeutic concentrations of nitric oxide on bacterial growth *in vitro*. Crit Care Med 26:1857, 1998.
104. Chollet-Martin S, Gatecel C, Kermarrec N, Gougerot-Pocidalo M, Payen DM. Alveolar neutrophil functions and cytokine levels in patients with the adult respiratory distress syndrome during nitric oxide inhalation. Am J Respir Crit Care Med 153:985, 1996.
105. Walmrath D, Schneider T, Pilch J, Schermuly R, Grimminger F, Seeger W. Effects of aeroslized prostacyclin in severe pneumonia. Am J Respir Crit Care Med 151:724, 1995.
106. Confalonieri M, Potena A, Carbone G, Della Porta R, Tolley EA, Meduri GU. Acute respiratory failure in patients with severe community-acquired pneumonia. A prospective randomized evaluation of noninvasive ventilation. Am J Respir Crit Care Med 160:1585, 1999.
107. Joshi N, Localio AR, Hamory BH. A predictive risk index for nosocomial pneumonia in the intensive care unit. Am J Med 93:135, 1992.
108. Olivier KN, Bennett WD, Hohneker KW, Zeman KL, Edwards LJ, Boucher RC, *et al.* Acute safety and effects on mucociliary clearance of aerosolized uridine 5′-triphospate +/− amiloride in normal human adults. Am J Respir Crit Care Med 154:217, 1996.

40. THERAPY OF HOSPITAL-ACQUIRED PNEUMONIA IN THE INTENSIVE CARE UNIT

Olimpia A. Radu and Michael S. Niederman

Nosocomial pneumonia (NP) is a substantial cause of morbidity and the leading cause of death from hospital-acquired infections (HAI) among critically ill patients. Pneumonia is the second most common nosocomial infection and it is more prevalent in patients on mechanical ventilation than in those treated without this modality. The National Nosocomial Infections Surveillance (NNIS) program collected data from 181,993 patients in 112 medical ICUs between 1992–1997 and found pneumonia as the second most frequent nosocomial infection (27%) after urinary tract infections. In 86% of patients, NP was associated with ventilatory support [1]. Hospital-acquired pneumonia (HAP) is defined as occurring 48 hours or more after admission, while ventilator associated pneumonia (VAP) is defined as pneumonia diagnosed 48 hours or more after intubation. The treatment of NP is challenging and the use of appropriate antibiotic therapy is crucial, as the outcome is significantly influenced by the timing and accuracy of this decision. The choice of antibiotics in HAP is necessarily empiric, targeted against the most likely pathogen in a given patient, and bacteriology is likely to vary from one hospital to another. This initial empiric therapy may need to be changed once results of diagnostic tests (i.e. respiratory tract secretion or blood cultures) are available, with the goal of using as focused and specific a regimen as possible.

Microbiology of Nosocomial Pneumonia

The microorganisms causing HAP are different from those responsible for community-acquired pneumonia. The most common mechanism for the development of HAP is the aspiration of colonized secretions from the upper airway (oropharynx) or stomach and so the etiology of HAP depends on the type of organisms colonizing these sites. Thus early in the hospital stay, before a change in oral flora to enteric Gram-negatives occurs, NP is usually due to "community pathogens", while later the enteric Gram-negatives and other nosocomial pathogens predominate. The enteric Gram-negative bacilli and *Staphylococcus aureus* are the leading etiologic agents for NP, although the etiology is polymicrobial in half of mechanically ventilated patients with NP. In the National Nosocomial Infections Surveillance System data, Gram-negative aerobic organisms were isolated from 64% of patients with NP, with *Pseudomonas aeruginosa* present in 21%. *Staphylococcus aureus* was isolated with a similar frequency (20%) [1].

As described above the bacterial cause of NP varies with the time of onset of infection, as well as the method of diagnosis and the type of patient population studied. Early onset pneumonia occurring within the first four days of hospital stay is mostly caused by "community pathogens" (referred to in treatment guidelines as "core pathogens") such as *Streptococcus pneumo-*

niae, methicillin-sensitive *Staphylococcus aureus* (MSSA), *Hemophilus influenzae*, and non-resistant enteric Gram-negatives. NP occurring more than four days after admission is usually caused by Gram-negative bacilli, particularly resistant organisms such as *Pseudomonas aeruginosa*, *Acinetobacter* species or *Enterobacter* species, as well as by methicillin-resistant *Staphylococcus aureus* (MRSA), or other drug-resistant pathogens. In a study by Prod'hom and colleagues, in 54% of patients with early onset VAP, *S. aureus*, *S. pneumoniae* and *H. influenzae* were identified while Gram-negative organisms were found in only 17% of patients with early onset VAP, but in 66% of patients with late onset VAP [2]. Cazzadori and colleagues [3] studied 158 patients with closed head injury receiving mechanical ventilation. Out of 65 patients with suspected VAP, 38 (58.5%) had a bacteriologic diagnosis made on the basis of cultures from respiratory specimens obtained by bronchoalveolar lavage or protected specimen brush. Patients were separated according to the time of onset of VAP, and 20 patients had early onset pneumonia (within four days of the initiation of mechanical ventilation), while 18 patients had late onset pneumonia (after the fourth day of intubation). In-patients with early onset VAP, Gram-positive bacteria (Staphylococcus spp and *Streptococcus pneumoniae*) were found to be predominant (72%), while among-patients with late onset pneumonia, Gram-negative organisms (including *Pseudomonas aeruginosa* and *Stenotrophomonas maltophilia*) were isolated in 82% of cases [3].

There are few data available about anaerobic pathogens in VAP, because anaerobic bacteria require adequate transport and growth media in order to be identified. In a study of 130 VAP patients, anaerobic bacteria were isolated from protected specimen brush (PSB) cultures of 30 patients (23%), but in 26 of these patients aerobes were also identified. The identified anaerobic species were of oropharyngeal or dental origin, making aspiration of oropharyngeal material the most likely pathogenic mechanism. Compared with the rest of the patients, those with anaerobic infections were younger, had a higher simplified acute physiologic score, altered level of conciousness, orotracheal intubation or tracheostomy. VAP with anaerobic bacteria occurred more often in the first five days (early onset) [4]. In another study, quantitative aerobic and anaerobic cultures of PSB and mini-BAL from 143 patients with 185 episodes of suspected VAP and 25 additional intubated patients with aspiration pneumonia (AP) identified only one anaerobic organism, which came from a patient with suspected aspiration [5]. The role of anaerobes in pathogenesis of NP is uncertain and the need for anaerobic coverage in suspected AP still needs to be further assessed.

Host Risk Factors Predisposing to Specific Pathogens

Certain co-existing illnesses, prior therapy (antibiotics), the nature of the underlying disease, the presence of invasive devices (nasogastric tubes, endotracheal tubes, central lines) and length of hospitalization predispose to infection with specific pathogens (Table 1). If the patient has no risk factors, the infection is likely caused by one of a group of core organisms, so named because they may be found in any patient with NP. These organisms include non-pseudomonal enteric Gram-negative organisms (Klebsiella species, *Escherichia coli*, *Enterobacter* species, *Proteus* species, and *Seratia marcescens*) *Hemophilus influenzae*, methicillin-sensitive *Staphylococcus aureus* and *Streptococcus pneumoniae*.

The presence of specific host risk factors increases the likelihood of infection by certain pathogens in addition to the core organisms. For instance, previous antimicrobial therapy use increases the risk of infection with multiresistant organisms as *Pseudomonas aeruginosa* or *Acinetobacter* spp [6–8]. One recent study by Husni and colleagues [8] suggests third generation cephalosporins as a risk for *Acinetobacter* infection, while other studies report vancomycin and third generation cephalosporins use as a risk for

TABLE 1. Organisms (other than core organisms) causing NP and their specific risk factors

- Anaerobes
  - recent abdominal surgery
  - aspiration of gastric contents
- *Staphylococcus aureus*
  - coma
  - head trauma
  - diabetes mellitus
  - recent influenza
  - renal failure
- MRSA
  - prior antibiotics use
  - prolonged ICU stay
- *Pseudomonas aeruginosa*
  - prolonged ICU stay
  - prior antibiotics
  - corticosteroid use
  - chronic stuctural lung disease (bronchiectasis)
  - prolonged mechanical ventilation
- *Legionella* spp
  - corticosteroid therapy
  - cytotoxic therapy
- *Acinetobacter* species
  - prior antibiotic use (third generation cephalosporin)
  - mechanical ventilation
  - neurosurgery, head trauma
  - ARDS
  - large volume aspiration

vancomycin resistant *Enterococcus* colonization of the gastrointestinal tract. The length of hospitalization and endotracheal intubation, the presence of chronic obstructive pulmonary disease and prior use of third generation cephalosporin less effective against *P. aeruginosa* are significant predictors for infection with *P. aeruginosa* [6]. *S. aureus* is more common in patients who have coma, head injury, diabetes mellitus or renal failure [3, 9]. Cortico-steroid use predisposes to infection with *Legionella* spp., *P. aeruginosa*, and *Aspergillus* species [10, 11]. Witnessed aspiration and thoracoabdominal surgery may add anaerobes as potential pathogens. It is difficult to distinguish chemical pneumonitis following aspiration of gastric acid from bacterial aspiration pneumonia. If the patient has poor dentition, then aspiration of anaerobes is possible.

Several studies have evaluated risk factors for infection with specific pathogens. In critically ill patients on mechanical ventilation, *P. aeruginosa*, especially resistant strains, become a concern. In a prospective study, specimens from 190 mechanically ventilated patients from a surgical ICU revealed that 44 patients were colonized with *P. aeruginosa* in the bronchopulmonary tract and 13 had pneumonia. The risk of bronchopulmonary tract colonization, with this pathogen, increased with the length of hospitalization in the unit, the use of third generation cephalosporins poorly active against *P. aeruginosa*, the presence of a surgical emergency, and the presence of alcoholism. However, the presence of COPD was the most significant predictor of infection with *P. aeruginosa* [6].

Acinetobacter species, though commensual pathogens, have been increasingly reported as a cause of VAP. In the study by Baraibar *et al.* [12], *Acinetobacter baumanii* was identified in 12 patients from 148 episodes of VAP in 707 ventilated patients. Risk factors associated with *A. baumanni* pneumonia were neurosurgery, ARDS, head trauma, large volume aspiration, which are different from risk factors for *P. aeruginosa* pneumonia [12]. Husni and colleagues performed a study to investigate an outbreak of *Acinetobacter baumanii* and identified prior use of ceftazidime as a risk factor for developing infection with a resistant strain [8].

In a study of 49 patients with *Staphylococcus aureus* VAP, Rello *et al.* [13] found that MRSA infected patients, compared to those with MSSA, were more likely to have received steroids or prolonged ventilation (i.e. late-onset), were older than 25 years and had underlying COPD. MSSA infected patients were more likely to have had head trauma (i.e. risk for early aspiration). All patients with MRSA VAP had previously been treated with antibiotics compared with only 21.1% of those with MSSA VAP, making prior antibiotic therapy the most important risk factor for MRSA infection [13].

Of increasing significance is the rising number of resistant strains of nosocomial pathogens (MRSA, *Acinetobacter baumani*, *Pseudomonas aeruginosa*, *Enterobacter* spp., *Stenotrophomonas maltophilia*), therefore antibiotic selection should take into account the local sensitivity patterns of these pathogens. Trouillet and colleagues [14] studied 135 patients with VAP who underwent bronchoscopy with bronchoalveolar lavage and protected specimen brush. "Potentially resistant" organisms (methicillin-resistant *Staphylococcus aureus*, *Pseudomonas aeruginosa*, *Acinetobacter baumannii*, *Stenotrophomonas maltophilia*) were isolated in 77 cases (57%). Prior use of broad-spectrum antibiotics (i.e. imipenem, third generation cephalosporin, and/or fluoroquinolone) and mechanical ventilation for more than one week were found to increase the risk of developing NP with multiresistant bacteria (OR = 4.1 and 6.0 respectively) [14]. Rello and coworkers [15] studied 260 cases of VAP from three different ICUs. The most frequently isolated organisms from culture of respiratory specimens obtained by bronchoalveolar lavage or protected specimen brush were: *Pseudomonas aeuruginosa*, methicillin-sensitive *Staphylococcus aureus*, *Acinetobacter baumannii*, *Hemophilus influenzae*, *Streptococcus pneumoniae* and MRSA. The distribution of causative bacteria varied significantly among the three treatment sites, and especially with *A. baumannii* and *S. maltophilia*. MRSA was identified only in patients who received antibiotics prior to inclusion in the study. *P. aeruginosa* was the most frequently documented pathogen. The study confirmed the prior findings of the major risk variables determining the causative pathogens: the presence of comorbidities, duration of intubation and antibiotic pressure. The most important finding of this study remains the observation that the local microbial flora is different from hospital to hospital, warranting specific modification in empiric therapy accordingly [15].

In another study, Rello and colleagues [16] followed 250 patients from ICU to identify risk factors for developing pneumonia within the first 48 hours post-intubation. Thirty-two (12.8%) patients developed pneumonia. Pneumonia was more frequently encountered in patients who were intubated due to cardio-respiratory arrest (23%) or altered consciousness (19%). In patients who were reintubated, 12% developed pneumonia within the following 48 hours. Cardiopulmonary resuscitation and continous sedation were identified as the most significant risk factors for pneumonia development 48 hours after intubation. Prior antibiotic use showed a protective effect for this form of pneumonia [16].

Diagnosis and Prevention of Nosocomial Pneumonia

The diagnosis of nosocomial pneumonia is puzzling and controversial, with no clear consensus on whether the decision to start antibiotic therapy, when infection is suspected, should be guided by clinical criteria or by microbiologic data collected by quantitative sampling of lower airway secretions [17]. This controversy exists because the clinical definition of pneumonia is sensititive, but not very specific, and there are non-infectious causes that can be responsible for findings that suggest pneumonia. Nosocomial pneumonia is classically diagnosed clinically in the presence of a new or progressive infiltrate on chest radiograph plus at least two or more of the following signs and symptoms: fever, purulent sputum or tracheal secretions, and leukocytosis.

Microbiologic diagnosis can be obtained by quantitative or qualitative culture of sputum, tracheal aspirate, or lower airway secretions collected bronchoscopically by broncho-alveolar lavage (BAL) or protected specimen brush (PSB) or non-bronchoscopically by mini-BAL. The available methods for sampling respiratory tract secretions vary in their invasiveness and thus their risk, cost and potential benefits. Quantitative culture of endobronchial aspirates (QEA) is simple, cheap, has minimal risks (can be associated with minimal bleeding) has a specificity of 90% and is considered positive when >100,000 CFU/ml are identified, but the down side is that its reliability depends on laboratory technique. Thus, some investigators use only qualitative results of endotracheal aspirates to guide antibiotic management. The more invasive methods of bronchoscopy with BAL or PSB, or the use of transthoracic FNA (fine needle aspiration) are highly specific but expensive and carry the risks of bleeding, pneumothorax and hypoxia. BAL is diagnostic for pneumonia when >10,000 CFU/ml are identified while PSB is considered positive when >1000 CFU/ml are recovered [18].

A number of studies have shown that the most important determinant of outcome in VAP is choosing the right antibiotic during initial empiric therapy. This can be verified by collecting respiratory tract samples for culture. In a study conducted by Sanchez-Nieto *et al.* [19], the mortality and morbidity of patients with VAP managed using the data from QEA was no different from that of patients who underwent brochoscopy with BAL and PSB, and were managed based on the data from these studies. In 71% of cases there was total agreement between cultures results of the three techniques, and in 21% QEA coincided with either BAL or PSB. Antibiotic changes were made in more patients in concordance with the findings of PSB i.e. and BAL and were mostly related to *Ps. aeruginosa* identification, but outcome was not improved by these manipulations. Thus we may conclude that invasive tests provide diagnostic information useful to change antimicrobial therapy, but these changes don't alter the outcome, probably because the data became available too late in the patient's course of illness [19].

Blood cultures should be done in patients with nosocomial pneumonia because of their prognostic and diagnostic value A recent study by Luna *et al.* [20] tried to define the value of the presence of bacteremia for the diagnosis, management and prediction of complications and outcome in VAP. Two previous studies described a high mortality in patients with nosocomial bacteremia. However, in Luna's study, 162 patients with clinically diagnosed VAP underwent both bronchoscopy with quantitative culture of BAL fluid and blood cultures. BAL fluid culture was considered positive (>10,000 CFU/ml) in 90 patients. Bacteremia was more frequently present in the BAL positive than BAL negative group (22/90 patients vs 5/72 patients). The predominant microorganisms in the blood cultures were the same as those identified by BAL fluid culture with a slight trend toward a higher prevalence of *Staphylococus epidermidis* in blood cultures. However, in six of 22 bacteremic BAL positive patients, the isolated bacteremic pathogens were not in concordance with BAL data and the organisms originated from extra-pulmonary sources. Thus the sensitivity of blood cultures for identifying the pathogenic microorganism in patients with VAP confirmed by BAL was low (26%) and the positive predictive value to detect the respiratory pathogen was 73%. The presence of bacteremia did not increase mortality in a multivariate analysis, but mortality was higher in those patients with VAP and extrapulmonary source of bacteremia (83% vs 56%) [20].

Prevention of VAP by antimicrobial prophylaxis remains controversial. The major concern is the selection of antibiotic resistant microorganisms by inappropriate use of antibiotics. A recent meta-analysis of selective digestive decontamination by D'Amico and colleagues [21] concluded that prophylactic use of topical (polymyxin, tobramycin and amphotericin or related compounds) and systemic antibiotics (non-antipseudomonal third generation cephalosporin), in combination, reduces the prevalence of respiratory infections (OR: 0.35) and overall mortality of critically ill patients (OR: 0.80). The use of topical antibiotics only was associated with a reduction in infection (OR: 0.56), but no significant effect on total mortality. The practical application of these results is obscured by the lack of data on the risk of development of antibiotic resistance [21]. However, prohylactic antibiotics may predispose to pneumonia with resistant Gram-negative bacteria.

The incidence of early-onset pneumonia being very high in comatose patients, Sirvent and colleagues [22] studied the effect of prophylactic administration of systemic antibiotics in pneumonia development. One hundred and five patients were enrolled in the randomized, controlled study. Cefuroxime 3 gr was administered in two doses 12 hours apart after intubation in the prophylaxis group. The incidence of microbiologically confirmed pneumonia was 37%, 24% in the cefuroxime group and 50% in the control group, respectively. Early-onset pneumonia developed in 70% of pneumonia cases, with a significantly lower frequency in the group receiving antibiotics. Mortality and morbidity were not changed by using the prophylactic antibiotic [22]. It can be postulated that systemic antibiotics when used early in the hospital stay, can prevent early-onset VAP, while more prolonged use can predispose to late-onset VAP, especially with resistant pathogens.

Antibiotic Issues

Depending on their mechanism of action, antibiotics are broadly classified as bactericidal or bacteriostatic. Some antibiotics are bactericidal to certain bacterial pathogens, but bacteriostatic to others. Bactericidal antibiotics kill bacteria, by inhibiting cell wall synthesis or by interrupting a key metabolic function of the organism. Bacteriostatic agents inhibit bacterial growth and rely on host defense to eliminate the organism.

The use of specific antimicrobial agents is dictated by the susceptibility of the causative organism in a given location to a particular antibiotic. There are circumstances in which the use of bactericidal antibiotics is warranted (endocarditis, meningitis, osteomyelitis, bacteremia, neutropenia), but this may not be needed in most patients with VAP [23].

The susceptibility of a pathogen to a given antibiotic can be assessed by determining the minimal inhibitory concentration (MIC) and minimal bactericidal concentration (MBC). MIC is defined as the minimum concentration of an antibiotic that inhibits the growth of a standard sized bacterial innoculum. MBC is defined as the minimum concentration of an antibiotic, which reduces the initial bacterial innoculum by at least 99.9%. MBC determination is important in severe and difficult to treat infection (endocarditis, meningitis, osteomyelitis) [18]. The measurement of serum concentration of antimicrobial agents may be performed to ensure adequate treatment and to prevent toxicity, especially when there is a narrow therapeutic-toxic levels window (as is the case with aminoglycosides or vancomycin) or in patients with impaired renal function.

The efficacy of antibiotics also depends on the distribution within the body, at the infection site. To be effective a drug must reach the site of infection in adequate concentration and must resist inactivation by physical or microbial factors. For example, an acidic pH in infected tissue (common in pneumonia) reduces the activity of aminoglycosides. The concentration of a drug at the site of infection depends on the permeability of the capillary bed, the degree of protein binding and the type of transport through the endothelium. Antibiotics which are lipophilic and thus not dependent on inflammation to penetrate into lung tissue include quinolones, azithromycin, clarithromycin, tetracyclines, clindamycin, trimethoprim/sulfamethoxizole. Antibiotics that are poorly lipid soluble, depend on the presence of inflammation for their penetration into lung parenchyma and include aminoglycosides and β-lactams (penicillins, cephalosporins, monobactams, and carbapenems) [23].

Knowing the pharmacodynamic characteristics is useful in the choice of specific antibiotics. Some antibiotics are bactericidal in relation to how long their serum concentration is above the MIC of the target organism (time-dependent killing), while others are effective in relation to the peak concentration achieved (concentration-dependent killing). Vancomycin and β-lactam antibiotics have a time-dependent killing action. For this reason, they have to be administered at short intervals, so the trough level does not fall below MIC for a long period. The aminoglycosides and fluoroquinolones have a concentration-dependent killing activity. Thus, optimal administration would be in high doses at less frequent intervals [23, 24]. In the case of concentration-dependent killing, the antibiotic activity correlates with the concentration at the site of infection and with the AUC (area under the curve) of the drug's concentration over time. The area under the serum inhibitory curve (AUIC), defined as AUC/MIC, is predictive of antibacterial killing rates and should be at least 125 for significant Gram-negative bacterial eradication to occur. The higher the AUIC, the more rapid bacterial eradication can be achieved. The AUIC values of two antibiotics is additive, and so when combination therapy is used; the AUIC achieved by both drugs together may allow eradication of difficult pathogens [24].

The PAE (post antibiotic effect) refers to persistent suppression of bacterial growth even after the antibiotic's serum concentration falls below the MIC of the target organism. Most antibiotics have a PAE against Gram-positive organisms. A prolonged PAE against Gram-negative bacteria can be achieved by the aminoglycosides and fluoroquinolones, agents that kill in a concentration-dependent fashion. No or little PAE against Gram-negative organisms is seen in agents which have a time-dependent killing mechanism. This is generally the case with β-lactam antibiotics (penicillins, cephalosporins, monobactams), but one exception is imipenem, which has a PAE against *Ps. aeruginosa* [23, 25]. Another effect similar to PAE is termed PALE (post-antibiotic leukocytes enhancement), which refers to the particular susceptibility of organisms in the post-antibiotic phase of growth to the antibacterial activity of leukocytes. When the patient has functioning white cells, the PAE of some agents is prolonged by their PALE.

Certain antibiotics lyse the bacterial cell wall and the released bacterial wall products can stimulate the cytokines producing cells to release inflammatory mediators. Theoretically this might lead to the development or worsening of the sepsis syndrome or shock after the initiation of appropriate antibiotic therapy for infection. The clinical significance of these observations and their implication in antibiotic selection has to be defined [23, 25].

Algorithm for Empiric Antibiotic Therapy of VAP

In 1996, the ATS defined guidelines to help in the diagnosis and initial treatment of HAP [26]. The severity of pneumonia, the presence of patient comorbidities and the time of pneumonia onset (early, less than five days of hospitalization, or late, five days or more since admission) were combined into an algorithm for classifying the patients with HAP into three distinct groups and for each group a specific therapy was recommended according with the most likely pathogens. The severity of pneumonia is a reflection of both host defense status and

The algorithm for classifying patients with HAP

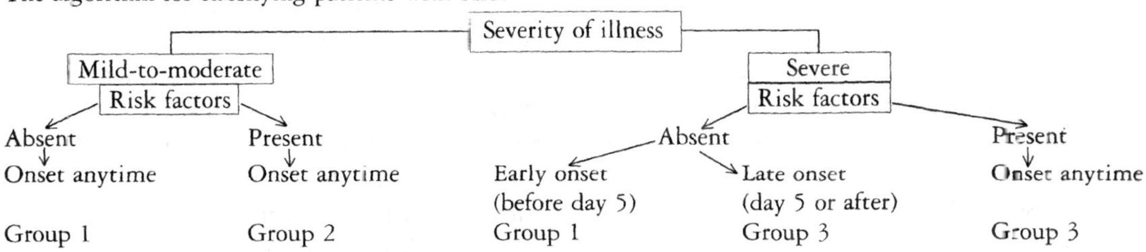

pathogen virulence. Patients with coexisting illnesses or those who received certain therapeutic interventions (which is often the case in the ICU patients) are predisposed to infection with highly virulent organisms (Table 1). On the other hand, certain pathogens induce a more severe disease, and so the severity of the disease may be a clue for the presence of organisms as *P. aeruginosa* or *Acinetobacter* species.

Severe HAP requires ICU admission and is associated with the presence of respiratory failure (i.e. mechanical ventilation or the need of >35% O_2 to maintain an arterial oxygen saturation of >90%), rapid radiographic progression, multilobar pneumonia, or cavitation of lung infiltrate. Other signs of severe HAP include evidence of severe sepsis with hypotension and/or end-organ dysfunction, as shock (systolic blood pressure <90 mm Hg or diastolic blood pressure <60 mm) or requirement of vasopressors for more than four hours, oliguria (urine output <20 ml/hr or total urine output <80 ml in four hours, with no other cause) or acute renal failure requiring dialysis [26].

Recommended Empiric Antibiotic Therapy Regimens

In a prospective study performed by Luna *et al.* [27] on a population of patients with VAP hospitalized in ICU, the use of inadequate initial empiric antibiotics was associated with increased mortality (91%) and subsequent change to the adequate antibiotic didn't substantially change the outcome. However, the administration of adequate antibiotic therapy early in the course of disease, at first signs of pneumonia seemed to improve the outcome (mortality 38%), emphasizing the need for accurate empiric therapy. In that study, even if bronchoscopy was able to accurately define the microbiologic etiology of pneumonia, its results were available too late to significantly alter the outcome [27]. In another study by Kollef and Ward [28] 130 patients with suspected VAP were evaluated with mini-BAL and changes in the antibiotic regimens were made according to the results of BAL culture, when necessary. In 51 (39.2%) patients the existing antibiotic regimen remained unchanged, because the mini-BAL cultures either didn't grow any pathogens or grew bacteria, which were sensitive to the prescribed regimens. In another 51 patients, the antibiotic regimen was changed because of either inadequate antibiotic use for the isolated pathogen, or identification of a pathogen in patients who were not receiving antimicrobial therapy. The most common indication for a change in antibiotic was the isolation of Gram-negative bacteria resistant to a prescribed third generation cephalosporin, followed by the need to add vancomycin to treat MRSA. In the remaining 28 patients, antibiotics were discontinued because there was no growth in the mini-BAL culture. There was no significant difference in mortality between patients with a positive mini-BAL culture and patients with a negative mini-BAL culture. However, the mortality rate of patients having antibiotic therapy started or changed following mini-BAL culture results (60.8%) was significantly greater than the mortality rate of patients having no change in their antibiotic regimens (33.3%) and patients having their antibiotic discontinued (14.3%). Thus, this study confirms that initial accurate empiric therapy is important for outcome and that inadequate initial antimicrobial therapy is associated with the highest risk of hospital mortality. These data also support the hypothesis that bacteriologic data from respiratory secretions are useful to confirm the diagnosis of VAP and focus the antibiotic regimen, but they don't change the outcome of patients with VAP [28].

In the ATS guidelines for HAP, by combining the severity of pneumonia with the presence of specific host risk factors and the time of onset of illness, three different patient groups emerged, each with their own specific antibiotic regimen targeting the most likely etiologic pathogens. The first group is composed of patients without specific risk factors who develop either mild-to-moderate NP occurring

TABLE 2. Group 1: Patients immunocompetent with no risk factors, with mild-to-moderate NP, onset any time; or early onset severe NP

Core organisms	Core antibiotics
Enteric non-Pseudomonal GNB	Cephalosporin
Escherichia. coli	second generation (Cefuroxime, Cefotetan)
Klebsiella species	non antipseudomonal third generation (Ceftriaxone, Cefotaxime)
Proteus species	Fourth generation cephalosporin (cefepime)
Serratia species	beta-lactam/beta-lactamase inhibitor combination (Ampicillin/Sulbactam)
Enterobacter species	
Hemophilus influenzae	Fluroquinolones (Ciprofloxacin, Levofloxacin)
Streptococcus pneumoniae	Clindamycin and Aztreonam-patient allergic to PCN
Staphylococcus aureus (methicillin-sensitive)	

at any time during hospitalization, or severe NP of early onset (within the first four days of admission) (Table 2). Group 2 includes patients who develop mild-to-moderate NP at any time while in the hospital and have specific patient risk factors (Table 3). The third group is comprised of patients with severe NP with risk factors beginning at any time and those patients with severe NP of late onset regardless of risk factors (Table 4) [25, 26].

Patients with NP, who do not have any unusual risk factors, but have mild-moderate HAP with onset at any time or severe HAP with early onset, will likely have infection with the core organisms and monotherapy with one of the antibiotics listed in Table 2 is usually appropriate. Antibiotics to be considered in this scenario are a second generation cephalosporin (such as cefuroxime), a non-antipseudomonal third generation cephalosporin (such as cefotaxime or ceftriaxone), a fourth generation cephalosporin (cefepime), and beta-lactam/beta-lactamase inhibitor combination (ampicillin/sulbactam, piperacillin/tazobactam) or a fluoroquinolone (ciprofloxacin or levofloxacin). If the patient is allergic to penicillin, a quinolone, alone, or aztreonam with clindamycin should be used. Therapy should be initiated intravenously and can be switched to oral administration in patients who improve. This switch to oral therapy is especially easy when using a quinolone, since these agents achieve a high serum and tissue levels after enteral or parenteral administration [25, 26].

TABLE 3. Group 2: Patients with risk factors, mild-to-moderate NP, onset any time

Core pathogens plus	Core antibiotics plus
Anaerobes	Clindamycin or beta-lactam/beta-lactamase inhibitor (alone)
Staphylococcus aureus	Vancomycin if MRSA likely, until ruled out
Legionella	Erythromycin/Clarythromycin +/− Rifampin Levofloxacin (alone)
Pseudomonas aeruginosa	Treat as severe HAP
Acinetobacter species	Treat as severe HAP

When specific risk factors for certain organisms are present in the setting of a mild-to-moderate clinical course the antibiotic choice should be extended accordingly to cover possible additional pathogens as outlined in Table 3. If the patient has witnessed aspiration or recent thoracoabdominal surgery, anaerobic pathogens should be covered by adding clindamycin or metronidazole to any of the antibiotics used against core organisms. Alternatively, a beta-lactam/beta-lactamase inhibitor combination (such as ampicillin/sulbactam, ticarcillin/clavulanic acid, piperacillin/tazobactam) can be used alone in patients with NP in whom anaerobic infection is a concern. If *Staphylococcus aureus* is suspected, a core antibiotic with good coverage of this organism should be

TABLE 4. Group 3: Patients with severe HAP, early onset with risk factors or late onset

Core pathogens plus	Aminoglycoside or Ciprofloxacin plus
Ps. aeruginosa	Antipseudomonal penicillins
Acinetobacter spp.	Beta-lactam/beta-lactamase inhibitor (Piperacillin/tazobactam, Ticarcillin/clavulanate)
	Third generation cephalosporin (Ceftazidime or Cefoperazone)
	Fourth generation cephalosporin (Cefepime)
	Carbapenemes (Imipenem, Meropenem)
	Monobactam (Aztreonam)
MRSA (methicillin-resistant *S. aureus*)	+/– Vancomycin or alternatives (Linezolid, Quinopristin/Dalfopristin)

used, reserving vancomycin for the situations in which MRSA is likely. The role of new agents such as quinopristin/dalfopristin and linezolid in this setting remains to be defined. If the patient has received high-dose corticosteroids and is not intubated at the time of pneumonia onset, Legionella infection is possible, and a macrolide (such as erythromycin or clarythromycin) or a quinolone should be considered in addition to therapy directed at the core organisms [25, 26]. When severe pneumonia is present, along with multiple risk factors and in patients with severe NP of late onset regardless of risks, *Pseudomonas aeruginosa* and other resistant bacteria are a concern and so, empiric antipseudomonal antibiotics are recommended (Table 4). In these patients, combination anti-pseudomonal agents should be used in the beginning and once respiratory tract cultures or blood cultures results become available, one of the antibiotics can be discontinued if *Pseudomonas aeruginosa* or other drug-resistant organisms are not identified. Antibiotics which can be used as monotherapy in severe VAP, in the absence of *Ps. aeruginosa* include: ciprofloxacin, imipenem, meropenem, cefepime, and piperacillin/tazobactam. Antibiotics active against *P. aeruginosa* include: the antipseudomonal penicillins (piperacillin, mezlocillin), the antipseudomonal betalactam/betalactamase inhibitor combinations (piperacillin/tazobactam, ticarcillin/clavulanate), some third generation cephalosporins (ceftazidime, cefoperazone), the fourth generation cephalosporin (cefepime), the carbapenemes (imipenem, meropenem), a monobactam (aztreonam), the aminoglycosides and one fluoroquinolone (ciprofloxacin). Combinations of anti-Pseudomonal antibiotics should also provide coverage for the core organisms. Several combination regimens are recommended. The combination of a beta-lactam with an aminoglycoside offers the advantage of anti-Pseudomonal synergy with all the limitations of aminoglycoside toxicity and possible reduced efficacy in the low pH environment of infected endobronchial areas, and with a poor penetration in lung tissue. The use of two beta-lactam agents does not achieve synergy and is limited by the possibility of the induction of a bacterial beta-lactamase which might inactivate both drugs and by the concern of competition of the agents for the same bacterial binding site. Another choice is the use of a beta-lactam with an quinolone active against *P. aeruginosa*, which does not achieve synergy but has the advantage of good lung penetration and reduced toxicity offered by the quinolones, compared to the aminoglycosides. In some severely ill patients, MRSA is a possible pathogen and adding vancomycin or an alternature aqent (linezolid, quinopristin/dalfopristin) should be considered if Gram stain of endotracheal aspirate shows Gram-positive cocci.

Monotherapy versus Combination Therapy in the Treatment of Nosocomial Pneumonia

Combination therapy has a number of advantages and disadvantages. Its advantages may include (1) broader spectrum of activity, than can be achieved with a single antimicrobial agent; (2) antibacterial synergy, achieved when a beta-lactam is combined with an aminoglycoside which can be beneficial in the presence of neutropenia or bacteremic *Ps. aeruginosa* infection; (3) prevention of the emergence of resistance that can develop when only one agent is used, especially in infections caused by *Ps. aeruginosa* and *Acinetobacter* spp. Combination therapy has a proven mortality benefit only in the presence of bacteremic *Ps. aeruginosa*, but critically ill patients should be treated with combination therapy if *Ps. aeruginosa* is a suspected pathogen, because of the high likelihood of resistance developing with monotherapy.

One study designed to compare the efficacy and safety of imipenem versus imipenem and netilmicin in the treatment of NP, showed that monotherapy was as effective and less nephrotoxic than the combination therapy, using an aminoglycoside [29]. The addition of an aminoglycoside did not prevent the emergence of imipenem resistant *Ps. aeruginosa* strains during therapy and did not add to efficacy and it caused renal toxicity [29]. In the case of infection with *Enterobacter* spp., a third generation cephalosporin should not be used alone, since resistance caused by bacterial beta-lactamase induction can develop during therapy.

A number of studies have been conducted using monotherapy for VAP, and these studies have defined several effective agents. Joshi *et al.* [30] found that piperacillin/tazobactam had increased efficacy, compared with ceftazidime, (clinical cure or improvement and eradication of baseline pathogens), especially against *Hemophilus influenzae*, *Staphylococcus aureus*, *Pseudomonas aeruginosa* (though the only statistically significant difference was in the eradication rate of *Hemophilus influenzae*). These results may be influenced, in part, by the growing number of beta-lactamase producing pathogens, for which using the beta-lactam/beta-lactamase inhibitor combination is a better choice. The extended spectrum of antimicrobial activity against anaerobic pathogens (not identified in performed cultures) may explain the higher clinical success of piperacillin/tazobactam [30].

Another study evaluated 154 patients with nosocomial pneumonia randomized to piperacillin-tazobactam treatment or imipenem-cilastatin treatment. Clinical success was achieved in 83% of patients treated with piperaillin-tazobactam versus 71% in those treated with imipenem-cilastatin ($p = 0.09$). When pneumonia was caused by *Ps. aeruginosa*, clinical failure was present more often in patients treated with imipenem-cilastatin than in those treated with piperacillin-tazobactam (50% vs 10% $RR = 0.19$, $p = 0.004$). Clinical failures were mainly related to the development of resistance during therapy or initial resistance to therapy [31].

In a large prospective, randomized, double-blind, multicenter trial, high-dose ciprofloxacin (400 mg every 8 h) was compared with high-dose imipenem (1000 mg every 8 h) in the treatment of severe pneumonia (compromised respiratory function requiring an FIO_2 of at least 35% to maintain an arterial pO_2 of at least 60 mm Hg, or mechanical ventilation). A total of 405 patients were enrolled, 78% with NP, 79% on mechanical ventilation and with a mean APACHE II score of 17.6; 205 patients met the criteria for being bacteriologically or clinically evaluable for efficacy endpoints. The primary and secondary endpoints were eradication of the pretreatment respiratory pathogen(s) and clinical response. Patients treated with ciprofloxacin had a significantly higher clinical response rate (69% vs 56%) and a higher bacteriologic response (69% vs 59%), especially against organisms from the *Enterobacteriaceae* family (93% vs 65%). Seizures occurred significantly more frequently among patients receiving high-dose imipenem. In both treatment groups, bacteriologic failure and development of resistance were more common in patients with *Ps. aeruginosa* infection, which was isolated in 23% of cases. The mortality rate was similar in both groups. Drug resistance emerged in 33% of patients on ciprofloxacin and 53% of patients on imipenem, after at least three days of treatment. The conclusion was that antibiotic monotherapy was successful in NP treatment, unless the responsible pathogen was *P. aeruginosa*, in which case a second agent should be added. This can be safely done in first 72 hours, once cultures results are available [32]. However, in clinical practice, as discussed above, most of these patients should initially receive combination therapy, but this can be reduced to monotherapy if non-resistant organisms are identified in culture.

Sieger and colleagues [33] compared meropenem with ceftazidime-tobramycin in the treatment of hospital-acquired pneumonia. Meropenem 1000 mg q8hs was administered to 104 patients with NP while the others received ceftazidime 2 g/tobramycin 1 mg/kg q 8 hs. The protocol allowed tobramycin to be discontinued if the first pretreatment culture was susceptible to ceftazidime (55% received more than six doses of tobramycin).

Only 63 patients on meropenem and 58 patients on ceftazidime were evaluable. Satisfactory clinical response to treatment was observed in 56 (89%) of meropenem treated patients and 42 (72%) of ceftazidime/tobramycin treated patients. Bacterial eradication was achieved in 56 (89%) of patients on meropenem and 39 (67%) of patients on ceftazidime/tobramycin. Meropenem was more effective than ceftazidime both clinically and microbiologically [33].

Antibiotic Rotation in Nosocomial Pneumonia Treatment

Of increasing interest is the concept of using a scheduled antibiotic rotation for the empiric therapy of NP, in an attempt to reduce the emergence of antibiotic resistant pathogens. Previous studies have showed that NP and bacteremia caused by resistant Gram-negative bacteria are related to prior antibiotic use, and changing the antibiotics used for empiric therapy may avoid the development of resistance to a specific agent because bacteria are exposed to different antibiotics over time.

Kollef and colleagues [34] performed a prospective before-after study to determine the impact of rotation of antibiotic classes (from ceftazidime to ciprofloxacin) used for the empiric treatment of suspected Gram-negative bacteria infection in the form of either VAP or nosocomial bacteremia. Six hundred and eighty eight patients undergoing cardiac surgery were evaluated. During a six-month period (the before period) ceftazidime was used for the empiric treatment of suspected Gram-negative bacteria infection, followed by a six-month period (the after period) during which ciprofloxacin was used. The incidence of VAP (11.6% vs 6.7%) microbiologically confirmed VAP using mini-BAL (9.6% vs 5.5%), and VAP caused by antibiotic resistant Gram-negative bacteria (4% vs 0.9%) was significantly lower during the after period. This was also true for the incidence of bloodstream infections caused by antibiotic resistant Gram-negative bacteria, although not statistically significant (1.7% vs 0.3%). There was also a decrease in the incidence of antibiotic-resistant Gram-negative pathogens associated with either VAP or bacteremia in the after period compared with before-period (48.8% vs 20%). There was no significant difference in the mortality rate among patients from both groups [34]. The findings in this study are provocative and raise important questions. If scheduled changing of antibiotics has favorable impact on the incidence and microbiology of nosocomial infections, then what classes of antibiotics should be used and how often should the switch take place? Are these data true for medical patients and for all classes of antibiotics? Should rotation also involve empiric therapy of suspected Gram-positive infection? Further studies are needed to explore this issue and find the answers to these questions, before this practice enters routine clinical use.

In conclusion, nosocomial pneumonia is a frequent infection in ICUs, and its diagnosis and treatment requires careful analysis of the available data. Prompt and accurate antibiotic therapy is a cornerstone in its management, and the most important determinant of the outcome. Guidelines for treatment are useful but they should be modified according to the particularity of the patient and the individual hospital setting. Infections with multidrug resistant organisms are of increasing incidence and concern, especially in the ICU environment. It remains for the future to determine if new antibiotics, more appropriate use or scheduled use of the available ones, or all of these strategies together will be the best approach to the antibiotics resistant problem.

References

1. Richards MJ, Edwards JR, Culver DH, Gayness RP. Nosocomial infections in medical intensive care units in the United States. National Nosocomial Infections Surveillance System. Crit Care Med 27:887.
2. Prod'hom G, Leuenberger P, Koerfer J, Blum A, Chiolero R, *et al.* Nosocomial pneumonia in mechanically ventilated patients receiving antacid, ranitidine or sucralfate as prophylaxis for stress ulcer. Ann Intern Med 120:653, 1994.
3. Cazzadori A, Di Perri G, Vento S, Boncra S, *et al.* Etiology of pneumonia following isolated closed head injury. Respir Med 91:193, 1997.
4. Dore P, Robert R, Grollier G, Rouffineau J, *et al.* Incidence of anaerobes in ventilator-associated pneumonia with use of protected specimen brush. Am J Respir Crit Care Med 153:1292, 1996.
5. Marik PE, Careau P. The role of anaerobes in patients with ventilator-associated pneumonia and aspiration pneumonia. Chest 115:178, 1999.
6. Talon D, Mulin B, Rouget C, Bailly P, Thouverez M. Risks and Routes for Ventilator-associated Pneumonia with *Pseudomonas aeruginosa*. Am J Respir Crit Care Med 157:978, 1998.
7. Rello J, Ausina V, Ricart M, *et al.* Impact of previous antimicrobial therapy on the etiology and outcome of ventilator-associated pneumonia. Chest 104:1230, 1993.
8. Husni RN, Goldstein LS, Arroliga AC, *et al.* Risk factors for an outbreak of multi-drug-resistant *Acinetobacter* nosocomial pneumonia among intubated patients. Chest 115:1378, 1999.
9. Rello J, Quintana E, Ausina V, *et al.* Risk factors for *Staphylococcus aureus* nosocomial pneumonia in critically ill patients. Am Rev Respir Dis 142: 1320, 1990.
10. Carratala J, Gudiol F, Pallarés R, *et al.* Risk factors for nosocomial Legionella pneumophila pneumonia. Am J Respir Crit Care Med 149: 625, 1994.
11. Rodrigues J, Niederman MS, Fein AM, Pai PB. Nonresolving pneumonia in steroid-treated patients with obstructive lung disease. Am J Med 93:29, 1992.
12. Baraibar J, Correa H, Mariscal D, *et al.* Risk factors for infection by Acinetobacter baumannii in intubated patients with nosocomial pneumonia. Chest 112:1050, 1997.
13. Rello J, Torres A, Ricart M, Valles J, *et al.* Ventilator-associated pneumonia by *Staphylococcus aureus*. Comparison of methicillin-resistant and methicillin-resistant episodes. Am J Respir Crit Care Med 150:1545, 1994.
14. Trouillet J, Chastre J, Vuagnat A, Joly-Guillou M, Combaux D. Ventilator-associated pneumonia caused by potentially drug-resistant bacteria. Am J Respir Crit Care Med 157:531, 1998.
15. Rello J, Sa-Borges M, Correa H, *et al.* Variations in etiology of ventilator-associated pneumonia across four treatment sites; implications for antimicrobial prescribing practices. Am J Respir Crit Care Med 160:608, 1999.
16. Rello J, Diaz E, Roque M, Valles J. Risk factors for developing pneumonia within 48 hours of intubation. Am J Respir Crit Care Med 159: 1742, 1999.
17. Niederman MS, Torres A, Summer W. Invasive diagnostic testing is not needed routinely to manage suspected ventilator-associated pneumonia. Am J Respir Crit Care Med 150:555, 1994.
18. Baughman RP, Tapson V, McIvor A. The diagnosis and treatment challenges in nosocomial pneumonia. Diagn Microbiol Infect Dis 33:131, 1999.
19. Sanchez-Nieto JM, Torres A, Garcia-Cordoba F, El-Ebiary M, Carrillo A, *et al.* Impact of invasive and noninvasive quantitative culture sampling on outcome of ventilator-associated pneumonia. A pilot study. Am J Respir Crit Care Med 157: 371, 1998.
20. Luna CM, Videla A, Mattera J, Vay C, Famiglietti A, *et al.* Blood cultures have limited value in

predicting severity of illness and as a diagnostic tool in ventilator-associated pneumonia. Chest 116:1075, 1999.

21. D'Amico R, Pifferi S, Leonetti C, Torri V, Tinazzi A, *et al*. Effectiveness of antibiotic prophylaxis in critically ill adult patients: Systematic review of randomised controlled trials. BMJ 316:1275, 1998.
22. Sirvent JM, Torres A, El-Ebiary M, *et al*. Protective effect of intravenously administered cefuroxime against nosocomial pneumonia in patients with structural coma. Am J Respir Crit Care Med 155:1729, 1997.
23. Niederman MS. Principles of antibiotic use and the selection of empiric therapy for pneumonia; Fishman's pulmonary diseases and disorders; 1939–1951.
24. Schentag JJ, Strenkoski-Nix LC, Nix DE, Forrest A. Pharmacodynamic interactions of antibiotics alone and in combination. Clin Infect Dis 27:40, 1998.
25. Niederman MS. An approach to empiric therapy of nosocomial pneumonia. Med Clin N Am 78:1123, 1994.
26. Hospital-acquired Pneumonia in adults: Diagnosis, assessment of severity, initial antimicrobial therapy and preventative strategies. A consensus statement. Am J Respir Crit Care Med 153: 1711, 1996.
27. Luna MC, Vujacich P, Niederman MS, Vay C, Gherardi C. Impact of BAL data on the therapy and outcome of ventilator-associated pneumonia. Chest 111:676, 1997.
28. Kollef MH, Ward S. The influence of mini-BAL cultures on patient outcomes. Chest 113:412, 1998.
29. Cometta A, Baumgartner JD, Lew D, Zimmerli W, Pittet D, *et al*. Prospective randomized comparison of imipenem monotherapy with imipenem plus netilmicin for treatment of severe infections in nonneutropenic patients. Antimicrob Agents Chemo 38:1309, 1994.
30. Joshi M, Bernstein J, Solomkin J, Wester BA, Kuye O, Piperacillin/Tazobactam Nosocomial Pneumonia Study Group. Piperacillin/tazobactam plus tobramycin versus ceftazidime plus tobramycin for the treatment of patients with nosocomial lower respiratory tract infection. J Antimicrob Chemo 43:389, 1999.
31. Jaccard C, Troillet N, Harbarth S, Zanetti G, Aymon D, *et al*. Prospective randomised comparison of imipenem-cilastatin and piperacillin-tazobactam in nosocomial pneumonia or peritonitis. Antimicrob Agents Chemo 42:2966, 1998.
32. Fink MP, Snydman DR, Niederman MS, Leeper KV, Johnson RH, *et al*. Treatment of severe pneumonia in hospitalized patients: Results of a multicenter, randomized, double-blind trial comparing intravenous ciprofloxacin with imipenem-cilastatin. Antimicrob Agents Chemo 38:547, 1994.
33. Sieger B, Berman SJ, Geckler RW, Farkas SA. Empiric treatment of hospital-acquired lower respiratory tract infections with meropenem or ceftazidime with tobramycin: A randomized study. Crit Care Med 25:1663, 1997.
34. Kollef MH, Vlasnik J, Sharpless L, Pasque C, Murphy D, Fraser V. Scheduled change of antibiotic classes: a strategy to decrease the incidence of ventilator-associated pneumonia. Am J Respir Crit Care Med 156:1040, 1997.

41. RESPIRATORY INFECTION IN IMMUNOCOMPROMISED NEUTROPENIC PATIENTS

Stephen W. Crawford

Scope of Problem

Neutropenia is increasingly common in the hospital. The rise in incidence is due to proliferation of indications for and centers performing hematopoietic stem cell transplantation, hematologic effects of AIDS, and myelosuppressive side-effects of anti-viral and cancer chemotherapies [Table 1]. As a result, these neutropenic patients are increasingly common in ICUs. These patients are often lymphopenic, anemic, and thrombocytopenic. They are at risk for multiple organ failures and various infections. This chapter will focus on respiratory infections in the neutropenic patient.

Neutropenia and the Risk Factor for Infection

The neutrophil plays a key role in host defense of extracellular bacteria (especially encapsulated organisms affected by opsonizing antibodies) and the molds and yeasts. The incidence of serious infection in neutropenic patients increases with the depth, rapidity of onset, and duration of neutropenia. The risk of infection increases with an absolute neutrophil count (ANC) <1000 cells/mm^3, and is significantly higher with an ANC <500 cells/mm^3. A rapid decline in ANC and duration of neutropenia >7 to 10 days is associated with increase in serious, life-threatening infection. Likewise, morbidity and mortality are increased in patients with profound neutropenia (ANC <100/mm^3) [1–3].

A study of severe, short-duration neutropenia demonstrates that fungal infections are rare when the ANC is reduced for less than five days. Neutropenic fever developed in 94% of patients after peripheral stem cell transplantation [4]. Profound neutropenia was short-lived (average five days) and most patient's fever defervesced in median of four days. Although bacteremia developed in 39% (predominately Gram-positive cocci), only 5% had pulmonary infiltrates and there were no fungi identified and no infection-related deaths.

Neutrophil function before chemotherapy to treat leukemia influences infection rates [5]. Patients with a significant decrease in phagocytic activity of neutrophils developed more severe infection or died more often compared to those with no infection. Study of the neutrophil oxidative burst capacity suggested that the neutrophils may have been pre-activated and have reduced function prior to the initiation of chemotherapy.

Neutropenia associated with myelosuppression, as occurs after chemotherapy, rarely occurs in isolation from other defense defects. Lymphopenia, decreased humoral immunity, and mucosal barrier defects invariably contribute to the defense abnormalities that predispose to infection in these settings.

TABLE 1. Some causes of neutropenia

- Drug myelosuppression
  - Chemotherapy
  - Ganciclovir
  - Trimethaprim-sulfamethoxazole
- Viral infection
  - Late stages of AIDS
  - Herpes viruses
- Congenital deficiency
  - Inherited cyclic neutropenia
- Functional defects
  - Corticosteroids
  - Chediak-Higashi syndrome
  - Myeloperoxidase deficiency
  - Chronic granulomatous diseases

Both tumors and chemotherapy contribute to infection among neutropenic patients. Obstruction of the lymphatic, biliary tract, gastrointestinal or urinary systems by tumors or as a result of surgical procedures is a common cause of infections. Chemotherapy not only decreases the number of neutrophils, but also results in chemotactic and phagocytic defects. Chemotherapy, radiation, peripheral and central intravenous lines, surgery, or tumor invasion can induce breakdown of skin and mucosal barriers and can result in bacteremia. Mucositis may occur throughout the gastrointestinal system. Translocation of endogenous flora in the GI tract may explain a majority of febrile neutropenic episodes.

Trends in Infection in the Neutropenic Patient

Historically, Gram-negative bacilli, particularly *P. aeruginosa*, were the most commonly identified pathogens. Data from several sources attest to a decrease in the incidence of pseudomonal bacteremia and an increase in Gram-positive infections. The use of long-term indwelling lines accounts for some of the appearance of Gram-positive infections; the empiric antibiotic regimens that were designed to cover *P. aeruginosa* may be an additional factor. For example, the incidence of bacteremia due to Gram-negative bacilli in Japan decreased (40% to 64%) and infections due to Gram-positive bacteria increased (51% to 24%) in 1991 to 1996 compared to the prior 15 years [6].

In the last decade there has been an increasing incidence of Gram-positive cocci infection in the neutropenic population. Foremost among these organisms are viridans streptococci, vancomycin-resistant enterococci, and coagulase-negative staphylococci. In addition, there is an alarming trend toward increasing fungal infections. Notably, reports of *Candida* species isolates are up 20-fold since the 1980s. *Aspergillus* reports have increase 14-fold. In addition, the number of "unusual" fungal species (*Trichosporon*, *Fusarium*, *Mucor*) has also increased.

Importantly, there has been an alarming increase in the frequency of antibiotic resistant organisms isolation. These pathogens include coagulase-negative staphylococci, methicillin-resistant *Staphylococcus aureus* (MRSA), vancomycin-resistant enterococci (VRE), and penicillin (ceftriaxone)-resistant *S. pneumonia*.

Sites and Causes of Infections

Mortality in the febrile, neutropenic population is high, in the range of 30 to 50 per cent. Early studies of empiric antibiotics in febrile neutropenia suggested that a majority of patients had occult bacterial infections. However, an infectious source is identified in only approximately 30 per cent of febrile neutropenic episodes. Often the only evidence of infection is bacteremia, which occurs in over 20 per cent of patients. Approximately 80 per cent of identified infections are believed to arise from patient's own endogenous flora. The most commonly identified sources of infection in febrile neutropenic patient with leukemia are the perineal and perirectal areas, followed by the urinary tract, skin (including intravenous lines and wounds) and the lungs. However, among non-hematopoietic cancer patients pulmonary infections predominate. Many infections are detected only at autopsy, particularly disseminated fungal or combined fungal and bacterial infections.

There are numerous infections that cause pneumonia in cancer patients [7–9]. Typical bacteria are most common, accounting for over one-third of infections. Fungi, viruses, *Pneumocystis carinii* (PCP), *Nocardia asteroides*, and *Mycobacterium tuberculosis* account for a measurable number of cases each. Compounding the difficulty in establishing an etiologic agent, mixed infections may be present in up to 20 per cent of cases.

Evidence suggests that fungal infection is a common component of neutropenic fever after chemotherapy. Pneumonia tends to develop several days after the onset of fever. Only 27% of febrile neutropenic patients with pneumonia respond without addition of anti-fungal agents. Over half of documented lower respiratory infections are due to fungi. Therefore, it is not surprising that the prognosis is worse for febrile neutropenic patients who develop pneumonia.

Noninfectious etiologies are common for immunocompromised patients with pulmonary infiltrates. Causes include pulmonary embolus, tumor, radiation pneumonia, atelectasis, pulmonary hemorrhage, and drug allergy or toxicity. Aspiration remains an important source of pulmonary infection in all compromised patients.

Bacterial Pathogens

Viridans streptococci (both *mitis* and *sanguis*) have become of major concern in the neutropenic host. These organisms are associated with 39% of neutropenic bacteremia after chemotherapy [10]. The complications associated with these organisms are: ARDS, shock, and endocarditis. An ANC $<100/mm^3$ is among the strongest risk factors.

Institutional infection patterns impact the frequency and type of organisms isolated and a variety of nosocomial outbreaks in cancer patients have been reported. Some centers have reported an increased incidence of resistant pathogens such as *Candida krusei* with the routine use of prophylactic antibiotics and antifungals [11, 12]. Antibiotic history, recent culture results, exposure to prophylactic antibiotics, and the susceptibility patterns for organisms in the institution should be used to help guide selection of initial antibiotic therapy.

Fungal Pathogens

Fungal infections probably represent the greatest infectious risk to neutropenic patients. Fungal infections are common among neutropenic patients, and usually arise after prolonged neutropenia and antibiotic use. Empiric antibiotics promote oral and vaginal colonization with yeast, most commonly *Candida albicans*. Hepato-splenic involvement is common in patients with disseminated candidiasis after chemotherapy. Often, symptoms are absent until the neutropenia resolves. Current diagnostic tests lack sufficient sensitivity to distinguish invasive yeast infection from colonization [13].

The incidence of nosocomial candidal infections continues to rise in the United States, and *C. albicans* is the most commonly identified species. Candidal infections are associated with the highest mortality rates of all hospital-acquired bloodstream infections, with substantial related increases in hospital costs, particularly length of stay. The three most common pathogens causing nosocomial bloodstream infections in US hospitals are cocci: coagulase-negative staphylococci, 31.9% of isolates; Staphylococcus *aureus*, 15.7%; and Enterococci, 11.1%. According to these Surveillance and Control of Pathogens of Epidemiologic Importance Program data from 1995–1998 the fourth most common pathogens were *Candida* species, representing 7.6% of all isolates [14]. Clearly, *Candida* species are increasing in importance in the ICU as well. According to recent data from Pfaller *et al.*, *Candida albicans* accounts for just over half of candidal species isolated. *C. tropicalis*, *C. glabrata*, and *C. parapsilosis* contribute 44% of isolates [15]. Speciation is important since *C. tropicalis* and *C. krusei* are resistant to fluconazole, the agent more commonly used to treat yeast infection in the ICU. The crude mortality associated with these pathogens increases with decreasing prevalence. Mortality with the most common, coagulase-negative staphylococci, is 21% and rises to 40% with the *Candida* species infections. The mortality attributable to *Candida* has been estimated at 70–88% [16, 17]. Diagnosis of candidiasis in the neutropenic host should be considered an indication for urgent therapy. The death rates among neutropenic patients with candidiasis are as high 24% with a week of diagnosis and 63% within three month [18]. Although lower among patients without neutropenia, the rates are still high.

Candida is a common infection among neutropenic patients but a rare cause of pneumonia. Haron *et al.* reported that there were only 31 cases documented at autopsy over 20 years at the MD Anderson Cancer Center [19]. The clinical and radiographic presentation of these cases was that of bronchopneumonia. There were no distinguishing features of the infection to identify the organism. Of note, most of the patients were not neutropenic at time of onset of pneumonia.

Candidiasis is rare in the absence of colonization of the skin, rectum or throat. Gut translocation may account for a substantial proportion of cases. The major threat to life is associated with disseminated, invasive candidiasis. Candidal invasion is associated with identified risk, and thus these are also risks for mortality. The reported risks include:

- Use of three or more antibiotics
- Neutropenia
- Immunosuppression (due to cancer/chemotherapy, steroids, other therapies)
- Concomitant infection
- Spending more than four days in ICU
- Mechanical ventilation >48 hours
- An elevated APACHE II score
- Abdominal surgery
- Central venous catheterization
- Total parenteral nutrition (TPN)
- Diabetes mellitus
- *Candida* colonization of more than 3 sites
- Candiduria (>100,000 colonies/ml)
- Thrush

The therapeutic choices for treatment of systemic candida infections include fluconazole, conventional amphotericin B, liposomal amphotericin B, and lipid-complex amphotericin B. All of these are available intravenously. Only fluconazole is available orally, however this is rarely an issue in the ICU population. Fluconazole has been shown recently to be comparable to conventional amphotericin b for treatment of candidemia in patients without neutropenia [20]. In this study, fluconazole was associated with less renal dysfunction, hypokalemia, and lower liver enzymes than amphotericin B. It is likely that the same pattern of efficacy and toxicity would be found among neutropenic patients.

Infections with molds, such as *Aspergillus* sp, vary from localized skin ulcers and invasive pneumonia, to fulminant disseminated disease. *Fusarium* sp. infections have been increasingly reported in immunocompromised host [21–25]. Reactivation of endemic fungi (histoplasmosis, blastomycosis, and coccidiodomycosis) or tuberculosis mimics the radiographic presentation of invasive fungal pneumonia and should be considered in appropriate patients with prolonged steroids or immune suppression.

Kaiser *et al.* recently reviewed the clinical presentations of invasive pulmonary aspergillosis (IPA) in a study of 35 confirmed cases [26]. The diagnosis of IPA was not suspected in 40% of the cases. The lungs were involved in 94% and the infection was limited to lungs in 74%. Other sites of infection were the heart, CNS, liver, spleen, and skin. Only 40% were neutropenic at the time of diagnosis but 91% had used steroids in the recent past. Of importance to the management of IPA, concurrent infections were found in 83% of cases. The mortality rate was 94%.

Viral Pathogens

Viral infections, especially human herpes viruses, are common in the neutropenic population. However, neutropenia *per se*, is not the primary risk factor for viral infection. Cell-mediated immunity (CMI) is the most important host defense against most respiratory viral pathogens. Since many patients with neutropenia also have concomitant defects in CMI they are at risk. Herpes simplex viruses, HSV-1 and HSV-2, while common causes of skin eruptions, can also cause a wide variety of clinical syndromes, including: encephalitis, meningitis, myelitis, esophagitis, pneumonia, hepatitis, erythema multiforme, and ocular syndromes. Immunocompromised patients with disseminated varicella zoster virus (VZV) infection can have pulmonary involvement and should be placed on respiratory precautions to prevent aerosolized transmission to susceptible individuals. Cytomegalovirus remains a significant cause of diffuse pneumonia and respiratory failure among transplant recipients.

Of great concern is the emergence of respiratory viral infections including Respiratory Syncytial Virus (RSV) as significant causes of nosocomial pneumonia. Outbreaks of infection resulting in diffuse pneumonia and respiratory failure have been reported among severely myelosuppressed patients after chemotherapy [27]. These infections should be suspected during winter and spring months, if there is associated airflow obstruction, or if upper respiratory tract symptoms preceded the onset of infiltrates. Many outbreaks reported appear to have been nosocomial. Visitors and hospital staff are likely responsible for transmission of the virus. Prompt treatment with ribavirin (with or without immunoglobulin) has been reported as beneficial. There are few data from large series to support that these are effective treatments in severely ill neutropenic patients.

Radiographic Diagnosis

The radiographic appearance of pneumonia in the neutropenic patient carries important diagnostic information as to the possible etiology of infection. A focal or multifocal consolidation of acute onset is most commonly caused by a bacterial infection. However, similar multifocal lesions with a subacute to chronic progression may be due to fungal, tuberculous, or nocardial infections. Large nodules are usually a sign of fungal or nocardial infection in this patient population, particularly if they are subacute to chronic in onset. Viruses (especially CMV) or *P. carinii* usually cause subacute disease with diffuse abnormalities, either peribronchovascular or small miliary nodules. The presence of cavitation suggests a necrotizing infection that can be caused by fungi, *Nocardia*, and certain Gram-negative bacilli (most commonly *Klebsiella pneumoniae* and *Pseudomonas aeruginosa*) [8].

Chest computed tomography of the chest can help to assess the extent of the disease process and more completely define its characteristics. The morphology of the abnormalities found on CT scan can also be very useful in developing a differential diagnosis in the individual patient. Cavitary mass lesions are suggestive of infections with *Nocardia*, *Cryptococcus*, or invasive fungus, such as *Aspergillus*. The invasive fungal pneumonias classically develop cavitation and a surrounding zone of radiographic attenuation. This zone is presumably due to associated edema and hemorrhage. However, this finding is nonspecific. Any process or infection resulting in lung infarction can yield similar CT findings (Table 2) [28]. In contrast, dense regional or lobar consolidation on CT is suggestive of bacterial pneumonia.

Chest CT scanning may identify the site for optimal sampling and assist in defining the most appropriate invasive procedure. Thus, CT can provide precise guidance for needle biopsy or for thoracoscopic or open lung excision in the case of peripheral lung nodules [29, 30]. CT can also

TABLE 2. Radiographic mimics of invasive pulmonary Aspergillosis

- *Mucor*, *Fusarium*, *Scedosporium*, etc.
- Legionella
- Nocardia
- Rhodococcus
- Gram-negative enterics
- Pulmonary embolism
- BOOP

help to predict whether bronchoscopy is likely to be useful. As an example, the demonstration of a feeding bronchus in association with a pulmonary nodule greatly increases the diagnostic yield when bronchoscopy is performed (60 versus 30 per cent when the feeding bronchus is not visible). If CT demonstrates centrally located diffuse opacifications, a bronchoscopic approach is the procedure of choice.

Treatment

Antibacterial drugs. None of the numerous antibiotic regimens studied as initial empiric therapy in febrile neutropenia have been shown to be clearly superior. The majority of the tested regimens provide coverage targeted at Gram-negative bacilli, especially *P. aeruginosa*. The most common empiric treatment approaches include either "monotherapy" (with agent such as, ceftazidime, imipenem, meropenem, or cefepime) or "double coverage" (with a beta-lactam and an aminoglycoside, or double beta-lactams).

Double beta-lactams are generally avoided due to the concern of overlapping toxicities. However, double coverage with the aztreonam and a beta-lactam in patients unable to tolerate an aminoglycoside may be a reasonable alternative. Two drug regimens for empiric therapy of febrile neutropenia are widely used. Clinical trials with monotherapy, either ceftazidime or imipenem cilastatin or meropenem, have demonstrated equal efficacy compared to two drug regimens [31, 32]. In one study treatment with meropenem was compared to ceftazidime in 187 patients; the number of patients on the therapy at 72 hours and the completion of treatment was equivalent between the groups (50% versus 56% and 46% versus 49%, respectively) [33]. However, changes in the antibiotic regimen are more common when monotherapy is used [2, 31].

The French Febrile Aplasia Study Group report is one of the few studies to show a difference in empiric antibiotic regimen [34]. The empirical use of a pipercillin/tazobactam and amikacin combination had superior response rates compared to ceftazidime and amikacin (48% versus 29%). Notably, the response rates to ceftazidime and amikacin decreased over time as the incidence of Gram-negative infections declined from 22% to 17.5%. The incidence of Gram-positive infections increased from 20% to 28%. This study provides increasing evidence of the fungal infection problem in neutropenic hosts. There was an increase in *Aspergillus*-related deaths (from 1.8% to 5.4%), while the overall infection-related mortality remained unchanged over time. It remains important to continue to monitor microbiology regardless of initial antibiotic choices.

Vancomycin is frequently considered in patients who present with hypotension, mucositis, skin or catheter site infection, a history of MRSA colonization, recent quinolone prophylaxis or persistent fever despite empiric antibiotics. However, addition of vancomycin to the initial empiric antibiotic regimen has not been shown to decrease mortality [2]. The addition of empiric vancomycin did not improve outcome among febrile neutropenic patients with skin and soft tissue infections despite a higher incidence of proven Gram-positive bacteremia compared to patients with other infections (31% versus 17%), [35].

Antifungal drugs. The incidence of fungal infection (especially *Candida* or *Aspergillus*) rises after patients have experienced more than seven days of persistent fever and neutropenia [36]. Antifungal therapy is routinely added at five to seven days of neutropenia in patients with persistent fever. While amphotericin B has been used for empiric therapy the longest, there is growing experience with fluconazole and lipid formulations of amphotericin B. For example, in one study fluconazole prophylaxis reduced the number of and mortality from invasive fungal infections compared to placebo in one multicenter trial in Canada [37]. The effect was greatest in patients with acute myelogenous leukemia and those receiving autologous bone marrow; both groups received the most intensive chemotherapeutic regimens. Another small study found empiric fluconazole equivalent in outcome to amphotericin B (at the relatively low dose of 5 mg/kg per day) in neutropenic patients who remained febrile after one week of broad-spectrum antibiotics; adverse effects were higher in the amphotericin group [38].

Fluconazole is well tolerated but is ineffective against *Aspergillus* and some yeast (e.g., *C. krusei* and *C. glabrata*). A retrospective study of hematogenous candidiasis from the M. D. Anderson Cancer Center found a shift toward *C. krusei* and *C. glabrata* infection and away from *C. tropicalis* and *C. albicans*; fluconazole prophylaxis appeared to be significant in promoting this trend [39].

Fluconazole prophylaxis is frequently used in populations at risk for *Candida* infection, such as neutropenic chemotherapy or organ transplant recipients. A review of 355 autopsies after marrow transplantation detected a disturbing trend among those patients who received fluconazole prophylaxis [40]. The treatment was effective in decreasing both *Candida* infections (from 27% to 8%) and fungal liver infection (from 16% to 3%). However, *Aspergillus* infections increased from 18% to 29%. Duration of survival increased but overall mortality was unchanged. The authors surmised that the fluconazole prophylaxis increased duration of survival by decreasing early infection with Candida and thus, increased the exposure to *Aspergillus* infections.

Recent trials suggest that lipid formulations of amphotericin B are better tolerated and offer similar efficacy. In one large randomized, multicenter trial, 343 neutropenic patients received liposomal amphotericin B (3 mg/kg per day) and 344 amphotericin B (0.6 mg/kg per day) as empiric therapy after at least five days of fever and broad-spectrum antibiotics [41]. The outcomes were comparable for the two therapies for overall success (50 versus 49 per cent), resolution of fever during neutropenia (58 versus 58 per cent), absence of documented fungal infection (90 versus 89 per cent), and cure of fungal infection (82 versus 73 per cent). The liposomal preparations were better tolerated than conventional amphotericin with fewer infusion related symptoms including rigors and less nephrotoxicity. However, these new forms of amphotericin are significantly more expensive. Recent studies suggest that itraconazole in daily dose of 200 mg to 400 mg also may be effective treatment for aspergillosis in patients refractory or intolerant to amphotericin B. Itraconazole is available both in oral and intravenous formulations. The precise role of this agent in the management of invasive fungal disease in the neutropenic ICU patient is undefined.

Colony stimulating factors. The role of colony stimulating factors (CSF) continues to expand. In some clinical settings, CSF has been reported to decrease the duration of neutropenia, fever and hospitalization [42–44]. However, CSF has not been shown to decrease mortality, and is not considered routine at this time [45]. It may be appropriate to consider their use in critically ill patients such as those with pneumonia, hypotension, or organ dysfunction or in patients whose bone marrow recovery is expected to be especially prolonged.

References

1. Hathorn JW, Lyke K. Empirical treatment of febrile neutropenia: evolution of current therapeutic approaches. Clin Infect Dis 24(Suppl 2): S256, 1997.
2. Pizzo PA. Management of fever in patients with cancer and treatment-induced neutropenia. N Engl J Med 328:1323, 1993.

3. Rubin RH, Ferraro MJ. Understanding and diagnosing infectious complications in the immunocompromised host. Current issues and trends. Hematol Oncol Clin North Am 7:795, 1993.
4. Kolbe K, Domkin D, Derigs HG, Bhakdi S, Huber C, Aulitzky WE. Infectious complications during neutropenia subsequent to peripheral blood stem cell transplantation. Bone Marrow Transplant 19:143, 1997.
5. Hubel K, Hegener K, Schnell R, *et al.* Suppressed neutrophil function as a risk factor for severe infection after cytotoxic chemotherapy in patients with acute nonlymphocytic leukemia. Ann Hematol 78:73, 1999.
6. Funada H, Matsuda T. Changes in the incidence and etiological patterns of bacteremia associated with acute leukemia over a 25-year period. Intern Med 37:1014, 1998.
7. Ramsey PG, Rubin RH, Tolkoff-Rubin NE, *et al.* The renal transplant patient with fever and pulmonary infiltrates: Etiology, clinical manifestations, and management. Medicine 59:206, 1980.
8. Rubin RH, Greene R. Clinical approach to the compromised host with fever and pulmonary infiltrates. In Rubin RH, Young LS (eds). Clinical Approach to Infection in the Compromised Host, 3rd edn. New York: Plenum Press, 1994: 121.
9. Chanock S. Evolving risk factors for infectious complications of cancer therapy. Hematol Oncol Clin North Am 7:771, 1993.
10. Bochud PY, Eggiman P, Calandra T, Van Melle G, Saghafi L, Francioli P. Bacteremia due to viridans streptococcus in neutropenic patients with cancer: clinical spectrum and risk factors. Clin Infect Dis 18:25, 1994.
11. Goodman JL, Winston DJ, Greenfield RA, *et al.* A controlled trial of fluconazole to prevent fungal infections in patients undergoing bone marrow transplantation. N Engl J Med 326:845, 1992.
12. Oppenheim BA. The changing pattern of infection in neutropenic patients. J Antimicrob Chemother 41:S7, 1998.
13. Sugar AM. Empiric treatment of fungal infections in the neutropenic host: review of the literature and guidelines for use. Arch Intern Med 150:2258, 1990.
14. Edmond MB, Wallace SE, McClish DK, Pfaller MA, Jones RN, Wenzel RP. Nosocomial bloodstream infections in United States hospitals: a three-year analysis. Clin Infect Dis 29:239, 1999.
15. Pfaller MA, Messer SA, Hollis RJ, Jones RN, Doern GV, Brandt ME, Hajjeh RA. Trends in species distribution and susceptibility to fluconazole among blood stream isolates of *Candida* species in the United States. Diagn Microbiol Infect Dis 33:217, 1999.
16. Digiovine B, Chenoweth C, Watts C, Higgins M. The attributable mortality and costs of primary nosocomial bloodstream infections in the intensive care unit. Am J Respir Crit Care Med 160:976, 1999.
17. Fraser VJ, Jones M, Dunkel J, Storfer S, Medoff G, Dunagan WC. Candidemia in a tertiary care hospital: epidemiology, risk factors, and predictors of mortality. Clin Infect Dis 15:414, 1992.
18. Anaissie EJ, Rex JH, Uzun O, Vartivarian S. Predictors of adverse outcome in cancer patients with candidemia. Am J Med 104:238, 1998.
19. Haron E, Vartivarian S, Anaissie E, Dekmezian R, Bodey GP. Primary *Candida* pneumonia. Experience at a large cancer center and review of the literature. Medicine 1993.
20. Rex JH, Bennett JE, Sugar AM, Pappas PG, van der Horst CM, Edwards JE, Washburn RG, Scheld WM, Karchmer AW, Dine AP, *et al.* A randomized trial comparing fluconazole with amphotericin B for the treatment of candidemia in patients without neutropenia. Candidemia Study Group and the National Institute. N Engl J Med 331:1325, 1994.
21. Richardson SE, Bannatyne RM, Summerbell RC, *et al.* Disseminated fusarial infection in the immunocompromised host. Rev Infect Dis 10: 1171, 1988.
22. Boutai EI, Anaissie EJ. *Fusarium*, a significant emerging pathogen in patients with hematologic malignancy: ten years' experience at a cancer center and implications for management. Blood 90:999, 1997.
23. Krcmery V Jr, Kunova E, Jesenska Z, *et al.* Invasive mold infections in cancer patients: Five years' experience with *Aspergillus*, *Mucor*, *Fusarium* and *Acremonium* infections. Support Care Cancer 4:39, 1996.
24. Martino P, Gastaldi R, Raccah R, *et al.* Clinical patterns of *Fusarium* infections in immunocompromised patients. J Infect 28:7, 1994.
25. Walsh TJ, Hiemenz JW, Seibel NL, *et al.* Amphotericin B lipid complex for invasive fungal infections: Analysis of safety and efficacy in 556 cases. Clin Infect Dis 26:1383, 1996.
26. Kaiser L, Huguenin T, Lew PD, Chapuis B, Pittet D. Invasive aspergillosis. Clinical features

of 35 proven cases at a single institution. Medicine 77:188, 1998.
27. Whimbey E, Couch RB, Englund JA, Andreeff M, Goodrich JM, Raad II, Lewis V, Mirza N, Luna MA, Baxter B, *et al.* Respiratory syncytial virus pneumonia in hospitalized adult patients with leukemia. Clin Infect Dis 21:376, 1995.
28. Won HJ, *et al.* Invasive pulmonary aspegillosis: Prediction at thin-section CT in patients with neutropenia – A prospective study. Radiology 208:777, 1998.
29. Jamzen DL, Adler BD, Padley SPG, *et al.* Diagnostic success of bronchoscopic biopsy in immunocompromised patients with acute pulmonary disease: Predictive value of disease distribution as shown on CT. Am J Roentgenol 160:21, 1993.
30. Scott WW, Kuhlman JE. Focal pulmonary lesions in patients with AIDS: Percutaneous transthoracic needle biopsy. Radiology 180:419, 1991.
31. Pizzo PA, Hathorn JW, Hiemenz J, *et al.* A randomized trial comparing ceftazidime alone with combination antibiotic therapy in cancer patients with fever and neutropenia. N Engl J Med 315:552, 1986.
32. Cometta A, Calandra T, Gaya H, *et al.* Monotherapy with meropenem versus combination therapy with ceftazidime plus amikacin as empiric therapy for fever in granulocytopenic patients with cancer. The International Antimcrobial Therapy Cooperative Group of the European Organization for Research and Treatment of Cancer and the Gruppo Italiano Malattie Ematologiche Maligne dell'Adulto Infection Program. Antimicrob Agents Chemother 40:1108, 1996.
33. Lindblad R, Rodjeer S, Adriansson M, *et al.* Empiric monotherapy for febrile neutropenia – A randomized study comparing meropenem with ceftazidime. Scand J Infect Dis 30:237, 1998.
34. Marie JP, *et al.* Neutropenic infections: Review of the French Febrile Aplasia Study Group trials in 608 febrile neutropenic patients. J Antimicrob Chemo 41(Suppl D):57, 1998.
35. Dompeling EC, Donnelly JP, Deresinski SC, *et al.* Early identification of neutropenic patients at risk of gram-positive bacteraemia and the impact of empirical administration of vancomycin. Eur J Cancer 32:1332, 1996.
36. Kibbler CC. Empirical antifungal therapy in febrile neutropenic patients: Current status. Current Topics in Medical Mycology 8:5, 1997.
37. Rotstein C, Bow EJ, Laverdiere M, *et al.* Randomized placebo-controlled trial of fluconazole prophylaxis for neutropenic cancer patients: Benefit based on purpose and intensity of cytotoxic therapy. Clin Infect Dis 28:331, 1999.
38. Malik IA, Moid I, Aziz Z, *et al.* A randomized comparison of fluconazole with amphotericin B as empiric anti-fungal agents in cancer patients with prolonged fever and neutropenia. Am J Med 105:478, 1998.
39. Abi-Said D, Anaissie E, Uzun O, *et al.* The epidemiology of hematogenous candidiasis caused by different Candida species. Clin Infect Dis 24:1122, 1997.
40. Einsele H, Hebart H, Roller G, Loffler J, Rothenhofer I, Muller CA, Bowden RA, van Burik J, Engelhard D, Kanz L, Schumacher U. Detection and identification of fungal pathogens in blood by using molecular probes. J Clin Microbiol 35:1353, 1997.
41. Walsh TJ, Finberg RW, Arndt C, *et al.* Liposomal amphotericin B for empirical therapy in patients with persistent fever and neutropenia. N Engl J Med 340:764, 1999.
42. Maher DW, Lieschke GJ, Green M, *et al.* Filgrastim in patients with chemotherapy-induced febrile neutropenia. A double-blind placebo-controlled trial. Ann Intern Med 121:492, 1994.
43. Rowe JM. Treatment of acute myeloid leukemia with cytokines: Effects on duration of neutropenia and response to infections. Clin Infect Dis 26:1290, 1998.
44. Rodriguez-Adrian LJ, Grazziutti ML, Rex JH, Anaissie EJ. The potential role of cytokine therapy for fungal infections in patients with cancer: Is recovery from neutropenia all that is needed? Clin Infect Dis 26:1270, 1998.
45. Hughes WT, Armstrong D, Bodey GP, *et al.* 1997 Guidelines for the use of antimicrobial agents in neutropenic patients with unexplained fever. Clin Infect Dis 25:551, 1997.

42. RESPIRATORY INFECTIONS IN IMMUNOCOMPROMISED NON-NEUTROPENIC PATIENTS

David L. Paterson and Nina Singh

Respiratory infections are a major cause of morbidity and mortality in immunocompromised non-neutropenic patients. For some respiratory infections in this patient group, mortality exceeds 80% (for example, invasive pulmonary aspergillosis in liver transplant recipients) [1]. The incidence of respiratory infections in immunocompromised patients is considerable; 15% of solid-organ transplant recipients and greater than 50% in patients with advanced human immunodeficiency virus (HIV) infection will develop pneumonia [2].

In recent years there have been a number of advances in the diagnosis and management of severe respiratory infection in immunocompromised patients. In addition, advances in the treatment of HIV infection and advances in immunosuppressive protocols have led to changes in the epidemiology of pneumonia in immunocompromised patients.

This chapter reviews the epidemiology, diagnostic approach and management of respiratory infections in immunocompromised patients.

The Pathogenesis of Respiratory Infection in Immunocompromised Patients

Immunocompromise can be broadly defined as a state in which the response of the host to a foreign antigen is subnormal. Neutropenia following treatment of hematologic or other malignancy is a major form of immunocom-promise but will be discussed in another chapter (pages 667–676). Numerically, solid organ transplant recipients (receiving tacrolimus, cyclosporine or other agents), patients with autoimmune disorders (also receiving immunosuppressive therapy) and patients with advanced human immunodeficiency virus infection form the major groups of patients with immunocompromise.

Much less common causes of immunocompromise include the congenital (primary) immunodeficiencies. These conditions usually produce specific defects in the host defenses against respiratory disease (Table 1). These defects in host defense are relatively "pure" and as a result susceptibility exists to limited classes of organisms. For example, Bruton's X-linked agammaglobulinemia is associated with a block in the normal maturation of immunoglobulin-producing B cells resulting in an absence of circulating mature B cells, plasma cells and serum immunoglobulin. It is not surprising therefore that organisms which are normally dealt with by immunoglobulin, such as *S. pneumoniae* and *H. influenzae*, are common in patients with agammaglobulinemia.

A vast array of defenses protect the lungs from environmental exposure to invading pathogens (Table 2). At a most basic level, mechanical defenses remove the bulk of potentially harmful agents from the lung. Aerodynamic filtration and impaction of large particulates (greater

TABLE 1. Primary immune defects and their relationship to different etiologies of respiratory infection

Condition	Defect	Description of respiratory infection
Phagocytic defects		
Kostmann's syndrome, Shwachman-Diamond syndrome and cyclic neutropenia	Low PMN counts	Pneumonia due to *S. aureus*, *P. aeruginosa* and Enterobacteriaceae
Chronic granulomatous disease	Defect in NADPH oxidase in phagocytic cells	Pneumonia and pulmonary abscess due to *S. aureus*, *E. coli*, *Klebsiella*, *Enterobacter*, *Serratia*, *Pseudomonas* and *Aspergillus*
Complement Disorders		
C3 deficency	Congenital absence of C3 or consumption of C3 due to deficiency of C3b inactivator	Recurrent pneumonia due to *S. pneumoniae*, *H. influenzae* or Enterobacteriaceae
Chediak-Higashi syndrome	Impaired micro-bicidal activity of phagocytes	*S. aureus* and *H. influenzae* pneumonia, less commonly *Aspergillus*
B lymphocyte deficiencies		
X-linked agammaglobulinemia (Bruton's)	Absence of B cells, plasma cells and antibody	Recurrent *H. influenzae*, *S. pneumoniae*, *S. aureus*, *P. aeruginosa*, *M. pneumoniae* and *P. carinii* pneumonia occurring after maternal antibody is consumed (ie, after the first 4–6 months of life)
Selective IgG subclass deficiencies	Selective deficiencies of IgG	Wide spectrum from recurrent severe bacterial pneumonias to close to normal
Selective IgA deficiency	Serum IgA less than 5 mg/dL (severe deficiency)	Wide spectrum from recurrent *S. pneumoniae* and *H. influenzae* pneumonia to close to normal
Hyper-IgM immuno-deficiency	Elevated IgM but reduced IgG, IgA	Recurrent bacterial pneumonia (usually not overwhelming); sometimes *P. carinii*
T lymphocyte deficiencies		
DiGeorge's syndrome	Thymic aplasia with reduced CD4 and CD3 cells (CD8 cells normal)	Severe viral pneumonias (herpes, measles), sometimes *P. carinii*, fungal and Gram negative bacterial etiologies
Purine nucleoside phosphorylase deficiency	Marked T cell depletion (CD4:CD8 ratio normal)	*P. carinii* and viral pneumonia
Mixed T and B cell deficiencies		
Common variable immunodeficiency	Various B cell activation or differentiation defects plus gradual deterioration of T cell number and function	Recurrent pneumonia or chronic bronchiectasis presenting in childhood or adulthood. Organisms include *P. carinii*, CMV, VZV, *S. pneumoniae*, *H. influenzae*

TABLE 1 (Continued)

Condition	Defect	Description of respiratory infection
Severe combined immunodeficiency	Severely reduced IgG and absent T	*P. carinii* within first 9 months of life; subsequent viral and Legionella pneumonia
Wiskott-Aldrich syndrome	Decreased T cell number and function; low IgM and sometimes IgG	*S. pneumoniae*, *H. influenzae*, herpesvirus, *P. carinii* pneumonia usually by age 6
Ataxia-telangiectasia	Decreased T cell number and function; IgA, IgE IgG2 and IgG4 deficiency	*S. aureus*, *S. pneumoniae*, *H. influenzae* recurrent pneumonia, leading to bronchiectasis

TABLE 2. Compromises of host defense against respiratory infection

Host Defense	Defects	Consequence of defect
Mechanical Defense		
Nasopharyngeal filtration	Intubation of the trachea	Aspiration and subsequent infection with mouth or stomach flora
Mucociliary clearance	Poor nutrition leading to impaired integrity of mucosal epithelial cells	Bacterial and fungal colonization of lower respiratory tract
Cough reflex	Altered neurologic function leading to diminished cough	Bacterial and fungal colonization of lower respiratory tract; Legionella infection
Epithelial barriers	Mechanical disruption by invasive procedures	Bacteria and fungal colonization of lower respiratory tract and skin
Alveolar Defense		
Alveolar macrophages	Disrupted function induced by corticosteroids and other immunosuppressive drugs	Propensity for intracellular microbes; poor containment of mycobacteria
Inflammatory Response		
Polymorphonuclear neutrophils	Diminished number because of cytotoxic chemotherapy or marrow aplasia/invasion	Infection with gram negative bacilli or *Aspergillus*
Specific T and B Cell Immune Responses		
CD4+ T lymphocytes	Diminished number due to HIV infection	Infection with *Pneumocystis carinii* mycobacteria, fungi, herpesviruses
B lymphocytes	Diminished function due to multiple myeloma, CLL or hypogammaglobulinemia	Infection with *Streptococcus pneumoniae* or *Haemophilus influenzae*

* HIV = human immunodeficiency virus, CLL = chronic lymphocytic leukemia.

than 10 μm) by the nasopharynx, mucociliary clearance and coughing are the principal means of mechanical defense. Only particles smaller than 3 μm are deposited on the alveolar surface.

Many immunocompromised patients, as well as having systemic immunosuppression, also have disruption of the local mechanical factors which prevent respiratory tract infection. Most prominent amongst these is the presence of invasive medical devices such as nasogastric and endotracheal tubes, which are frequently present in the postoperative period after solid organ transplantation. Endotracheal tubes eliminate the cough reflex, cause local mucosal injury and allow pooling of contaminated secretions above the tube's cuff [3]. All of these factors facilitate bacterial colonization of the tracheobronchial tree and lead to lower-airway aspiration of contaminated secretions. Nasogastric tubes also increase the potential for aspiration [3]. In the alveoli, defense against respiratory infection can be divided into three areas: Firstly, resident alveolar defense mechanisms are the primary line of defense against alveolar invasion. Extracellular surfactant has antibacterial activity against Staphylococci and some Gram-negative bacilli and fungi [4]. Alveolar macrophages are the resident cellular defenders of the lung. Derived from monocyte precursor cells and undergoing differentiation within the lung, they are involved in the clearance of particulates, macromolecular debris and organisms from the lung's epithelial surfaces. In order to do this the macrophage must recognize the foreign material and then destroy it. The recognition process can be nonspecific, but more often is a specific process as a result of specific antibody or complement. Phagocytosis follows recognition of the material. If it is an organism that is engulfed, killing takes place within a phagolysosome by way of oxidative and nonoxidative mechanisms. Oxidative mechanisms within alveolar macrophages can kill Staphylococci but not Gram-negative bacilli, *Cryptococcus* or *Toxoplasma*. Nonoxidative mechanisms include use of proteases, lysozyme and defensins (broad-spectrum cytotoxic peptides).

Secondly, an inflammatory response is necessary for effective clearance of most organisms. Although alveolar macrophages are important, if the microbial burden is large or more virulent, a dual phagocytic system involving polymorphonuclear neutrophils (PMNs) from the systemic vasculature is crucial. Important chemotaxins involved in attracting PMNs include the complement 5 molecule and its fragments, leukotriene B_4 and numerous chemotactic cytokines including interleukin 8. Directed migration of the PMNs into the alveolar space is the end-result of a complex cytokine mediated process involving endothelial cells, cell adhesion molecules, alveolar epithelial cells and mononuclear phagocytes.

Thirdly, specific pulmonary immune responses are essential for defense of the lung against certain pathogens such as virulent encapsulated bacteria, viruses and intracellular organisms that survive inside alveolar macrophages such as mycobacteria and fungi. Antigen specific T and B lymphocytes need to proliferate and differentiate in order to hold in check such organisms. An early event in this process is activation of T lymphocytes [5]. Activation of T lymphocytes requires an interaction between the T cell and an antigen presenting cell, a cell which can present the antigen on its surface in association with the major histocompatibility complex (MHC). Alveolar macrophages are ineffective antigen presenting cells; dendritic cells in the interstitium, alveolar septum and throughout the columnar epithelium of the bronchi are the major antigen presenting cells of the lung. Activation of both CD4 and CD8 T lymphocytes have key roles in pulmonary defenses against infection, particularly with mycobacteria, fungi and viruses. They produce high levels of interferon-gamma, granulocyte-macrophage colony stimulating factor and tumor necrosis factor, which recruit and activate monocytes from the circulation. Activated CD8 cytotoxic T lymphocytes can lyse virally infected cells. CD4

T lymphocytes contribute to the regulation of B cell expansion and differentiation. After migration from the bone marrow, B lymphocytes undergo differentiation in the lung to mature antibody producing plasma cells. Antibody gains access to the alveoli where it activates complement, neutralizes pathogens and their toxins and functions as opsonins to enhance macrophage recognition and ingestion of extracellular pathogens.

Several categories of immunosuppressive agents now exist. Corticosteroids broadly inhibit the immune response, including cellular immunity, innate inflammatory responses and to a lesser extent antibody formation. Methotrexate, cyclophosphamide and azathioprine are cytotoxic agents. Bone marrow depression is a risk with all of these agents. Mycophenolate mofetil, is a cytotoxic drug with an antiproliferative effect on T and B lymphocytes. Cyclosporine has a focused effect on T helper cell function; it inhibits cytokines (especially interleukin-2) normally produced when T helper cells are exposed to antigen. T-suppressor and B cells are relatively spared. It is interesting to note that patients with autoimmune diseases treated with cyclosporine alone have much lower rates of infection than solid-organ transplant recipients treated with combinations of cyclosporine and other immunosuppressive agents. Tacrolimus (FK-506) also inhibits production of interleukin-2 and other cytokines by T helper cells. Antilymphocyte serums, antithymocyte globulins and monoclonal anti-T-cell globulins are also used as prophylaxis or treatment of rejection.

The risk of infection in immunocompromised patients depends on not just the type but also the intensity and duration of the immunosuppression. For example, solid-organ transplant recipients, receiving tacrolimus and corticosteroids, who develop graft rejection refractory to a corticosteroid "recycle" and then receive OKT3, have a substantially high risk of cytomegalovirus (CMV) infection. In HIV infection, the likelihood of opportunistic pulmonary infection is inversely proportional to CD4 lymphocyte counts. Furthermore, HIV viral load measurements independently predict outcome in HIV [6–8]. Although protease inhibitors can dramatically diminish the amount of circulating human immunodeficiency virus, it is unlikely that total immune restoration occurs in patients who previously had low CD4 lymphocyte counts.

In patients with acquired immunocompromise, the risk of pneumonia is therefore related to the cumulative defects posed by different treatments and underlying disease processes. Thus, many patients have defects in all of the host defenses – disrupted mechanical barriers to pulmonary infection, decreased alveolar macrophage function, decreased neutrophil number or function and reduced T and B cell function.

It is also important to consider not just the immunosuppression present at the time of assessment but the immunosuppression which has occurred in the past. This could be likened to a shopping spree with a credit card. There is a risk of refusal of acceptance of the credit card during the spree because one has exceeded the credit limit (in this analogy, an infectious complication occurring at the time of heightened immunosuppression). However, there is also increased risk for several weeks after the spree and a final indignity when one receives the massive bill (in this analogy, an increased risk of infection even after the augmented immunosuppression has been discontinued). For example, corticosteroid boluses for graft rejection may not produce an immediate effect in terms of increased risk of infection; this continues for several weeks after the bolus.

Before leaving the area of host defense we must point out that in some instances pneumonia may be an immunopathological condition. For example, evidence from animal and limited human studies suggest that replication of CMV *per se* in the lung is unrelated to the development of pathological effects. Rather a host immune response is required for the induction of pneumonia. Cytomegalovirus may be found in the lungs of patients with advanced HIV infection without producing pneumonitis possibly because these patients can not mount a pathogenic T cell response. In contrast, in allogeneic bone marrow transplant recipients, the pneumonia may be due to uncontrolled accumulation and recruitment of host T cells in the lungs [9].

THE ROLE OF THE ENVIRONMENT IN CONTRIBUTING TO PNEUMONIA IN IMMUNOCOMPROMISED PATIENTS

The likelihood of a particular pathogen causing respiratory infection in an immunocompromised patient depends not only on the level and type of immunocompromise but also on environmental exposure to pathogens. Although some organisms which produce respiratory infections in the immunocompromised patient (for example, enteric Gram-negative bacilli) are endogenous, are harbored by most people and cause disease only when there is a breach in host defense, others are acquired from the environment, usually by the airborne route (Table 3). *Aspergillus* is a classic example. The organism is ubiquitous in the environment and is easily acquired by inhalation. Patients without immunosuppression who have functional alveolar macrophages and neutrophils can prevent vascular invasion by the organism. However, in immunocompromised groups of patients, outbreaks of invasive aspergillosis have been linked to construction activity within or near a transplant unit, *Aspergillus* proliferation on poorly maintained air conditioning units and exposure to large amounts of dust emanating from emptying vacuum cleaner bags [10–12].

There is debate over the modes of acquisition of *Pneumocystis carinii* and *Legionella* species. Some investigators hypothesize the *P. carinii* infection is acquired in childhood, becomes part of the host's residential microbial flora and remains quiescent, until the stimulus of immunosuppression results in replication of the organism. Others believe that *P. carinii* infections are transient and repeated, but can be held in check by an intact immune system. Although rare, there have been some clusters of infection in immunosuppressed hosts suggesting exposure from a common source patient [13]. A number of reports have linked outbreaks of *Legionella* infection to hospital cooling towers. However, more evidence supports aspiration of contaminated tap water as an important mode of transmission [14]. Hospital outbreaks of *Legionella* can be curtailed by disinfecting tap water distribution systems. In our unit, transplant patients are prohibited from consuming tap water.

TABLE 3. The environment as a source of infection in immunocompromised patients

Organism	Source
Legionella	Cooling towers, aspirated tap water
Aspergillus	Airborne, from construction work, dusty air conditioners etc
Cryptococcosis	Airborne, from soil or pigeon feces
Histoplasmosis, coccidioidomycosis, blastomycosis	Inhalation of organisms from within soil
Tuberculosis	Usually from person-to-person spread, rarely from milk (*M. bovis*)
Cytomegalovirus	Often endogenous (HIV patients), can be from donor organ or blood transfusions (transplant setting)
MRSA, VRE	Other patients via the hands of hospital staff members
Multiresistant gram negative bacilli	Other patients via the hands of hospital staff members

Legend: MRSA = methicillin resistant *Staphylococcus aureus*, VRE = vancomycin resistant enterococci.

The hospital environment is a more likely source of infection than the community. In addition to the infections detailed above, pulmonary infection with multiresistant bacteria are frequently spread within hospitals. Examples include methicillin resistant *Staphylococcus aureus* or extended spectrum beta-lactamase producing

Klebsiella pneumoniae. Spread of such multiresistant bacteria may occur from unsuspected colonized patients via the hands of hospital staff.

A number of causes of pneumonia in the immunosuppressed host can be acquired in the community. These include tuberculosis, the geographically restricted dimorphic fungi (histoplasmosis, coccidioidomycosis and blastomycosis), cryptococcosis and infection with the intestinal nematode, *Strongyloides stercoralis*. Each of these infections may occur in the transplant recipients by way of reactivation of previous infection, primary infection or reinfection. Primary community acquired pneumonia in the immunosuppressed host can occur with respiratory viruses such as respiratory syncytial virus, adenovirus and influenza.

Epidemiology and Diagnosis of the Causes of Respiratory Infection in the Immunocompromised Patient

GRAM-POSITIVE COCCI

Staphylococcus aureus. *S. aureus* pneumonia usually occurs as a result of intubation and aspiration, although septic pulmonary emboli from infected thrombotic material in the venous system (related to central venous catheters) sometimes occurs. Methicillin-resistant *S. aureus* now far exceeds more susceptible strains in isolates from immunosuppressed patients in tertiary referral centers. MRSA strains with reduced susceptibility to vancomycin and teicoplanin have now been recorded [15–17]. Like other forms of bacterial pneumonia, diagnosis rests on blood or respiratory specimen culture. A variety of patterns are seen on chest radiography, although rapid cavitation of a bronchopneumonia should increase suspicion of a staphylococcal cause. It has recently been reported that bacteremic MRSA pneumonia in liver transplant recipients has a mortality exceeding 80% [18].

Coagulase-negative staphylococci, although often cultured from respiratory specimens in immunosuppressed patients, are rarely a cause of significant pneumonia. Other diagnostic possibilities should be entertained in such patients.

Streptococcus pneumoniae. The pneumococcus is the most common cause of pneumonia in patients with normally functioning immune systems. However, all immunocompromised patients are also at risk, with some groups at higher risk than others. For example, serious pneumococcal infection occurs at a 200 fold increased rate for age-matched populations with HIV infection [19]. Pneumococcus is the most common bacterial pathogen in non-hospitalized patients with multiple myeloma, lymphoma or chronic lymphocytic leukemia. Patients who undergo splenectomy due to hematologic disease and other causes are at increased risk as are bone marrow transplant recipients with graft versus host disease and functional asplenia. Recurrent pneumococcal pneumonia is often the presentation of congenital immunodeficiencies. In all groups of immunosuppressed patients, *S. pneumoniae* may produce nosocomial pneumonia.

Diagnosis of pneumococcal pneumonia rests on culture from blood, sputum or other respiratory tract specimens. Segmental or lobar consolidation as seen on radiographic examination is present in only the minority of cases in immunosuppressed hosts.

Enterococci and Non-Pneumococcal Streptococci. Enterococcal pneumonia is exceedingly unusual, although enterococci (including vancomycin resistant *E. faecium* [20]) may sometimes be found in endotracheal aspirates or unprotected BAL specimens. Viridans streptococci are also much more likely to be contaminating mouth flora than true causes of pneumonia.

GRAM-POSITIVE BACILLI

Rhodococcus equi. *Rhodococcus equi* has long been recognized to be a cause of pneumonia in horses. It is now better known as a cause of pneumonia in HIV-infected patients, although transplant recipients are also at risk [21, 22]. Although exposure to horses is often recalled by the patient, the long-term survival of this organism in macrophages may account for exceptions to this rule. The clinical presentation tends to be insidious with fever, fatigue and nonproductive cough. Cavitary lesions (particularly in the upper lobes) with air-fluid levels are seen on chest roentgenograms. The organism may be grown from blood cultures, but biopsy and culture of the chest lesions can also differentiate this infection from tuberculosis (which it clinically resembles). Sometimes the organism is partially acid-fast, but culture reveals highly mucoid, salmon-pink colored colonies that grow well on ordinary media.

Nocardia. *Nocardia* species are an important cause of pulmonary nodules in immunosuppressed patients. Infections occur particularly in patients with lymphoreticular neoplasms and patients on chronic corticosteroid therapy. Solid-organ transplant recipients and patients with HIV infection are also at risk [23]. The infection tends to have a subacute or chronic onset. Sometimes subcutanous abscesses coexist with pneumonia. Unfortunately in the immunosuppressed host, dissemination can occur from the lungs via the blood to the brain.

The classical roentgenographic appearance is of single or scattered nodules or masses. Cavitation may occur. However, confluent bronchopneumonia, complete lobar consolidation, empyema and reticulonodular infiltrates can all be seen. Isolation of *Nocardia* from concomitant skin lesions greatly increases the chance that pulmonary lesions are due to the organism. Culture of specimens from percutaneous needle biopsy of lung nodules is a common mode of making the diagnosis, although sputum or bronchoscopic specimens occasionally yield the organism. Blood cultures are rarely positive. The laboratory should be alerted to the possibility of *Nocardia* since a modified Ziehl-Neelson stain that decolorizes with 1% sulfuric acid instead of acid alcohol is best for directly demonstrating the organism in clinical specimens. The organism is only weakly Gram-positive, so routine Gram stains may not be adequate. Culture can be performed on routine blood agar, although growth is not rapid.

GRAM-NEGATIVE BACILLI

Haemophilus influenzae. Splenectomized patients are at increased risk of serious type B *H. influenzae* infections as are patients with Hodgkin's disease and multiple myeloma. Congenital B cell deficiencies also place the patient at increased risk of recurrent *H. influenzae* pneumonia. The significance of *H. influenzae* in sputum is sometimes doubtful, since the organism, may be merely colonizing the airways. Occasionally serious *H. influenzae* pneumonia occurs in patients with advanced HIV infection and produces an interstitial pneumonia resembling that produced by *P. carinii*. The clinical picture also resembles *P. carinii* pneumonia with a subacute onset, non-productive cough, hypoxemia and increased lactate dehydrogenase levels [24, 25].

Enterobacteriaceae. Bacteria of the family *Enterobacteriaceae* include *Escherichia coli*, *Klebsiella pneumoniae*, *Serratia marcescens* and *Enterobacter cloacae*. These organisms are of gut origin but frequently colonize the mouth and upper respiratory tract of hospitalized patients. The majority of pneumonias caused by these organisms result from microaspiration of upper airway secretions that have been colonized with these bacteria. The classical lobar pneumonia of community-acquired *K. pneumoniae* infection is rarely seen in immunosuppressed patients. These patients typically have hospital-acquired bronchopneumonia (including ventilator-associated pneumonia). Immunocompromised patients are becoming increasingly likely to be colonized with strains of *Enterobacteriaceae* possessing extended spectrum beta-lactamases, which complicates treatment of pneumonia due to these organisms [26].

Acinetobacter species. Like the *Enterobacteriaceae*, *Acinetobacter* species colonize the respiratory tracts of hospitalized patients. Endotracheal intubation appears to be a significant risk. *Acinetobacter* pneumonia is frequently a multilobar bronchopneumonia. Multidrug resistance is frequent in many regions of the world.

Pseudomonas aeruginosa and Other Related Organisms. Bacteremic *P. aeruginosa* pneumonia occurs primarily in neutropenic patients after cancer chemotherapy, but may also be seen in patients with HIV infection. This is a fulminant disease associated with rapid onset of sepsis and respiratory failure. Radiographic appearance varies according to time since onset; early appearances are of pulmonary vascular congestion, interstitial edema and early pulmonary edema while after 2–3 days a more extensive mixture of alveolar and interstitial infiltrates are seen. Pathologically, necrotic nodules are observed, often with hemorrhage [27]. Cavitation may result from the necrosis. Ventilator-associated pneumonia due to *P. aeruginosa* may be less aggressive than primary bacteremic pneumonia, but is still associated with significant mortality. As with *Acinetobacter*, multidrug resistance is frequent in many regions of the world.

Burkholderia cepacia is a frequent colonizer of patients with cystic fibrosis and may cause pneumonia in lung transplant recipients. Bacteremia is common and is associated with high fever and severe progressive respiratory failure.

Stenotrophomonas maltophilia behaves in a similar manner to *P. aeruginosa*. It can cause bacteremic penumonia in neutropenic patients or ventilator-associated pneumonia in other immunosuppressed populations. It is intrinsically resistant to carbapenems, and frequently to many other drug classes.

Legionella. Legionella pneumonia occurs at increased frequency in transplant [28–30], but only sporadic reports have been received in other profoundly immunosuppressed populations. The incubation period for Legionnaires' disease is two to ten days, so most cases in transplant recipients are actually acquired in hospital. Early in the illness the patients experiences nonspecific symptoms only, with a mild cough. Diarrhea is present in up to 50% of cases, change in mental status may occur and hyponatremia (serum sodium less than 130 meq/l) may be noted on blood chemistry. Although a normal chest roentgogram may be seen if presentation is early, most cases have abnormal radiographic appearances when first assessed. The initial changes are often unilateral and have a lower lobe predominance but soon progress to multilobar disease. Cavitation and apparent abscess formation is not uncommon in the immunosuppressed host receiving corticosteroids [31].

Legionella pneumonia is almost certainly underdiagnosed since the organism does not grow on standard bacteriologic media. Microbiology laboratories should be requested to use specialized media (such as buffered charcoal yeast extract agar – BCYE) on bronchoalveolar lavage and sputum samples when the organism is suspected. Direct fluorescent antibody (DFA) tests have been used on respiratory specimens but probably have a sensitivity lower than culture. As mentioned previously, a test for detection of *L. pneumophila* serogroup 1 antigen in urine is available and has a sensitivity comparable to other methods. Serologic detection of antibodies is widely performed, but since it often takes 4–12 weeks for an antibody response to *Legionella* infection to develop, it only provides a diagnosis in retrospect.

Chlamydia pneumoniae and Mycoplasma pneumoniae. C. pneumoniae and *M. pneumoniae* are common causes of community-acquired pneumonia in the normal population. Their epidemiology in immunocompromised individuals has not been well established. Pneumonia usually has a subacute course. Initially the radiographic appearance is of unilateral interstitial or reticulonodular infiltrates, but may become bilateral with more advanced disease.

MYCOBACTERIA

Mycobacterium tuberculosis. Tuberculosis occurs with increased frequency in patients with T cell deficiencies (espeically HIV infection), transplant recipients, patients with neoplastic diseases (especially Hodgkin's disease) and any patient on prolonged corticosteroid therapy. Manifestations of tuberculosis vary with the intensity of immunosuppression. For example, HIV-infected patients with well-preserved CD4 lymphocyte counts have positive tuberculin skin tests, an upper lobe predisposition and frequently have cavitation. In contrast, HIV-infected patients with CD4 counts of less than 50 per mm^3, are usually anergic, may have lower and middle lobe involvement on chest radiography and rarely have cavitation. Disseminated extrapulmonary disease is also more common in those who are more heavily immunosuppressed.

Use of induced sputum should be considered in the patient who does not have a cough. Ziehl-Neelson or fluorochrome staining and culture of sputum or other respiratory secretions remains the cornerstone of diagnosis. Given the diversity of presentation of tuberculosis in immunocompromised patients, these tests should be considered routine in the evaluation of pneumonia in this patient population.

Nontuberculous Mycobacteria. Mycobacterium avium complex frequently produces disseminated disease in HIV-infected patients with CD4 counts of less than 50 per mm^3 who are not protected by azithromycin, clarithromycin or rifabutin prophylaxis. However, the lung is actually an unusual site of disease in HIV infected patients. When MAC is isolated from the sputum in HIV infected patients, it is usually a colonizer. Diagnostic confusion arises when acid-fast organisms are seen in sputum or BAL fluid, and culture results are not available. *M. tuberculosis* can not be accurately distinguished from MAC on the basis of stained smears. The BACTEC radiometric system for culturing mycobacteria, in combination with highly specific DNA probes to differentiate *M. tuberculosis* from MAC, can reduce the time for a definitive diagnosis to little more than 10–14 days. Depending on the local prevalence of *M. tuberculosis* compared to MAC, many clinicians opt to treat for tuberculosis on the basis of positive smears rather than wait for definitive speciation before initiating therapy.

Other mycobacterial species occasionally cause pneumonia in immunosuppressed hosts, including *M. kansasii*, *M. malmoense*, *M. haemophilum* and *M. fortuitum*. Treatment regimens vary so accurate speciation needs to be performed.

FUNGI

Pneumocystis carinii. *P. carinii* produces pneumonia in patients with a wide variety of immunosuppressive conditions, but most notably T lymphocyte deficiencies such as occur with HIV infection. The risk of *P. carinii* pneumonia increases when the CD4 count falls below 200 per mm^3. The infection is now rare in HIV-infected patients on protease inhibitors who have a significant reduction in HIV viral load, even if pre-therapy CD4 counts were less than 200 per mm^3. In solid organ transplant recipients, the risk of infection is greatest in the first six months after transplantation, although some risk probably persists for as long as the patient remains on immunosuppressive therapy. The risk increases when bolus corticosteroids or OKT3 are used to treat rejection. In either advanced HIV infection or the early months after solid organ transplant, failure to use prophylaxis (especially trimethoprim-sulfamethoxazole) is a risk factor for *P. carinii* pneumonia. Other immunosuppressed groups at risk of *P. carinii* pneumonia include those with collagen vascular diseases such as Wegeners granulomatosis [32] and less commonly patients with malignancy treated with chemotherapy or radiotherapy [33].

Occasionally the chest roentgogram is normal despite overt pulmonary symptoms due to *P. carinii*. In this circumstance, gallium scans will often be positive. More commonly, the chest roentgogram will be abnormal by the time the patient presents for medical attention. An interstitial alveolar butterfly pattern is most characteristic, but in the early stages of infection diffuse, fine, bilateral perihilar infiltrates are seen. Unusual patterns of infection (nodules, cysts, pneumothoraces, unilateral infiltrates, lobar consolidations) can be seen depending on factors such as sue of aerosolized pentamidine as prophylaxis, previous occurrence of the disease and time till presentation. Cystic changes or upper lobe involvement appear to be more common when aerosolized pentamidine is used as prophylaxis. Although an abnormal chest roentgogram is sufficiently prompt for further investigations to definitively diagnose *P. carinii* pneumonia, CT scanning may show interstitial and micronodular changes not visible by chest roentgography. Radiolabeled (^{111} indium) human immunoglobulin imaging may be useful in detecting superimposed focal infection due to other organisms in addition to the diffuse changes seen with *P. carinii*.

The diagnosis of *P. carinii* pneumonia depends on the finding of the organisms by use of a direct staining technique. Such stains include immunofluorescent staining using monoclonal antibodies to *P. carinii*, and less specifically by toluidine blue O or silver stains (which stain the cyst wall) or Giemsa or Diff-Quik stains (for sporozoites, trophozoites or intracystic bodies). Polymerase chain reaction has been used by some centers with high specificity and sensitivity.

The choice of specimen is important. Routine sputum examinations have a poor yield, but use of hypertonic saline for an induced sputum examination improves diagnostic abilities considerably (30–75% of cases positive). Bronchoalveolar lavage alone, or combined with transbronchial lung biopsy, when coupled with immunofluorescent staining will be positive in more than 95% of cases. Progress to open lung biopsy is rarely needed. It should be noted that patients will often have dead organisms in their respiratory secretions for many weeks after successful treatment of *P. carinii* pneumonia. This may confuse the diagnostic picture if new respiratory findings have developed.

In all cases of presumed or definite *P. carinii* pneumonia, arterial blood gases should be measured since corticosteroids are indicated in patients with marked hypoxemia. Finally it must be remembered that dual infection with other organisms may be present in the patient with *P. carinii* pneumonia and may account for delayed or poor response to anti-*Pneumocystis* therapy.

Aspergillosis. Invasive aspergillosis is an important cause of pneumonia in the immunosuppressed host by virtue of its high mortality. It occurs in the full spectrum of immunosuppressed populations including transplant recipients, neutropenic patients following treatment for hematologic malignancy, patients with advanced HIV infection and children with chronic granulomatous disease. It occurs with the following frequencies in the first year after transplantation: kidney transplant 0.7%, pancreas transplant 1.3%, liver transplant 1.7%, autologous hematopoietic stem cell 2.6%, heart transplant 6.2%, related donor allogeneic bone marrow transplant 6.7%, lung transplant 8.4% and unrelated donor allogeneic bone marrow transplant 10.3% [1]. Risk factors for invasive pulmonary aspergillosis include delayed recovery of neutropenia, severe graft versus host disease necessitating high dose steroid administration in bone marrow transplant recipients, and poor graft function, CMV infection, renal failure requiring hemodialysis and OKT3 use in solid-organ transplant recipients. Construction activity in or near the unit in which the immunosuppressed patient is housed is also a risk factor for [11].

Invasive pulmonary aspergillosis may have an insidious onset, but unsuspected dissemination of infection may occur contributing to a mortality of 92% for bone marrow transplant recipients, 87% for liver transplant recipients and approximately 75% for other immunosuppressed populations. In neutropenic patients this form of pneumonia may present as fever unresponsive to empirical antibiotic therapy, or much less commonly as an acute rapidly progressive pneumonia. Sometimes the disease clinically resembles pulmonary embolism and infarction with dyspnea, cough, pleuritic chest pain and hemoptysis occurring. Massive hemoptysis due to invasion of the infection into major vessels may occur.

Pulmonary nodules or areas of wedge-shaped consolidation are typical on chest roetgenography [34, 35]. Chest CT scan is more sensitive than chest roentgenography, and characteristically shows a halo of ground glass attenuation around focal nodules. This corresponds pathologically to hemorrhage around a focus of pulmonary infarction. Particularly upon return of neutrophils in neutropenic patients, cavitation occurs, being evident radiologically as an air crescent around a focal region of consolidation [34, 35]. *Aspergillus* tracheobronchitis can occur, characteristically in lung transplant recipients but sometimes in other populations; chest radiography is normal or unchanged from baseline films.

The finding of *Aspergillus* in culture from respiratory tract specimens in immunocompromised patients is highly predictive of invasive pulmonary aspergillosis, and is an indication for initiation of antifungal therapy. Unfortunately, *Aspergillus* is cultured from sputum in only 8–34% and from bronchoalveolar lavage fluid in 45–62% of patients with invasive pulmonary aspergillosis [36–38]. Although polymerase chain reaction of bronchoalveolar lavage fluid is potentially more sensitive than culture, in practice the risk of contamination of reaction buffers or patient samples with *Aspergillus* conidia is high, and reduces the positive predictive value of the test. Bronchoscopic or open lung biopsy is the gold standard of diagnosis, but waiting for this proof of infection before initiating therapy is frequently accompanied by treatment failure due to unsuspected disseminated disease. There is clearly a need for diagnostic tests which detect early *Aspergillus* infection before significant vascular invasion has occurred. Surveillance serological tests, performed twice a week during the at risk period, are emerging as a useful tool in early diagnosis. Enzyme linked immunoassay to detect the *Aspergillus* antigen, galactomannan, in serum has a sensitivity of 76% and a specificity of 85%. ELISA results can be available within four hours of collecting the sample and in some patients are positive as long as 28 days before symptoms or radiographic signs of invasive pulmonary aspergillosis become available [39]. Although less extensively studied, detection of IgG antibodies to *A. fumigatus* in serum may also predate radiographic signs of aspergillosis by several weeks. A management strategy based on use of serologic surveillance plus chest CT scanning or radiolabeled (^{111}indium) human immunoglobulin imaging has been proposed [40].

Cryptococcus neoformans. Although pulmonary Cryptococcal infection may occur in persons with intact immune systems, infection is more often found in the immunosuppressed patient. Well over 50% of cases now occur in HIV-infected patients, with solid-organ transplant recipients, patients with Hodgkin's disease and patients requiring chronic corticosteroid therapy sometimes being infected. Two varieties of *C. neoformans* can be cultured; *C. neoformans var. neoformans* grows best in composted bird droppings and is found in both immunocompetent and immunosuppressed patients, whereas *C. neoformans var. gattii* is found in association with certain eucalyptus trees, is almost exclusively found in immunocompetent patients and has a tendency to produce focal pulmonary or cerebral lesions (cryptococcomas).

Most immunosuppressed patients with pulmonary cryptococcosis have fever and cough, although the fever tends to be low-level. In transplant recipients, other patients receiving corticosteroid therapy, HIV-infected patients with relatively well preserved CD4 counts or patients with Hodgkin's disease, nodular or patchy alveolar infiltrates are seen. Sometimes masses (nodules greater than 6 cm) are seen. Cavitation is rare. In contrast, patients with HIV infection and low CD4 counts may have diffuse interstitial infiltrates or have alveolar consolidation.

The serum cryptococcal antigen is a useful, easily performed, non-invasive test which can provide rapid diagnostic information in the assessment of an immunosuppressed patient with pneumonia. However, several caveats need to be mentioned. In patients with cryptococcal pneumonia without dissemination beyond the lung, the serum cryptococcal antigen may be negative. In rare cases, infection with a nonencapsulated strain of *C. neoformans* will be accompanied by a false-negative test result. Infection with *Trichosporon beigelii* is a rare cause of a false-positive serum cryptococcal antigen.

Sputum cultures are positive for *C. neoformans* in up to 50% of patients with cryptococcal pneumonia. Cultures of bronchoalveolar lavage fluid are positive in 50 to 90% of cases. Staining BAL fluid with India Ink can provide a rapid diagnosis of infection. Cryptococcal antigen testing of BAL fluid can also been performed [41], although many laboratories do not regard this test as routine. Biopsy of nodules or mass lesions can provide definitive diagnosis; culture and pathologic examination of tissue can be performed. Cryptococci may be somewhat difficult to visualize on routine Hematoxylin-eosin staining, so request for the Mayers mucicarmine stain (which stains the fungal capsule) should be made.

In all immunosuppressed patients in whom a diagnosis of cryptococcal pneumonia is made, a search should be mounted for extrapulmonary sites of infection. In about 80% of cases of infection in the immunosuppressed patient, coexisting meningitis is uncovered by CSF examination. Cutaneous cryptococcosis is also sometimes observed, and may be clinically indistinguishable from bacterial cellulitis [2]. Therapy may need to be more intense and prolonged in those with meningitis than in those with pneumonia alone.

Histoplasma capsulatum, Coccidioides immitis *and* Blastomyces dermatidis. HIV-infected patients and solid-organ transplant recipients are numerically the most likely to present with these infections. These fungal infections have a geographically restricted distribution. Importantly, cases are often identified outside the endemic areas in immunosuppressed patients who travelled to or lived in the endemic regions even years before. Their previously dormant infections reactivated upon development of immunosuppression. However, new exogenous infection is also common in those presently living in the endemic regions.

Histoplasmosis is disseminated in more than 60% of immunosuppressed patients. Miliary or diffuse infiltrates may be seen on chest films. Occasionally a syndrome resembling septic shock is observed, with rapid development of respiratory failure and widespread pulmonary infiltrates. Rapid diagnostic methods include antigen detection in blood, urine or BAL fluid and methenamine-silver staining of peripheral blood or bone marrow. Results of these tests can be available within 24 hours. Fungal cultures provide the definitive diagnosis but take 2–4 weeks. Serologic tests may be falsely negative in acute infection or because of lack of antibody production in the immunosuppressed host, or be falsely positive from prior episodes of the disease. Histoplasmin skin tests are not recommended.

Coccidioidomycosis also is characterized by disseminated infection in the immunosuppressed host [42]. Characteristically spherules are seen in respiratory secretions or tissues. Cultures from sputum or other respiratory specimens can be positive in 3–5 days. Although serology in immunosuppressed patients has limitations, antibodies are detected in over 80% of HIV-infected patients. Skin tests are usually negative.

Blastomycosis is the least common of the endemic mycoses. Upper lobe nodular infiltrates are characteristic, but miliary or diffuse infiltrates associated with disseminated disease may occur. Fungal stains of respiratory secretions are usually positive and provide the most accessible means of rapid diagnosis. Blastomycosis antigen, which cross-reacts with *H. capsulatum*, may be detected in urine or blood. Culture is the only means of definitive diagnosis.

Mucormycosis, Pulmonary Candidiasis and Unusual Fungal Pathogens. *Mucormycosis* is seen in up to 8% of patients with leukemia who undergo autopsy. The infection occasionally occurs in solid-organ transplant recipients. Clinically, pulmonary mucormycosis resembles invasive pulmonary aspergillosis. The fungi have a distinctive appearance on tissue biopsy, but no other rapid diagnostic tests exist. Sputum or BAL specimens are rarely helpful. Definitive diagnosis relies on culture from biopsy specimens.

Candida albicans is often a colonizer found in sputum or BAL specimens. However, in lung transplant recipients, *Candida* can cause a fulminant pneumonia occurring within the first two weeks post-transplantation. The donor lungs are the most likely source of infection. Septic pulmonary emboli due to *Candida* may occur in immunosuppressed patients with infected central venous catheters. Disseminated candidiasis occurring in neutropenic patients or liver transplant recipients may also have pulmonary involvement, and will be indicated by culturing *Candida* at other sites.

Numerous other fungi can produce pneumonia in the immunosuppressed patient including *Pseudallescheria boydii* (producing a clinical appearance resembling invasive pulmonary aspergillosis especially in neutropenic patients), *Penicillium marneffei* (producing a patchy pneumonic process as part of disseminated infection in HIV-infected patients) and *Sporothrix schenckii* (producing cavitary lesions in patients chronically receiving corticosteroids).

VIRUSES

Cytomegalovirus. Cytomegalovirus pneumonia has traditionally been associated with a high mortality rate in immunosuppressed patients. For example, in bone marrow transplant recipients, CMV pneumonia was an inexorable process leading rapidly to death in at least 80% of patients with biopsy-proven disease. However, modern methods of pre-emptive treatment (particularly those based on antigen detection or PCR of peripheral blood) and, in selected situations, prophylaxis have markedly reduced the impact of this infection on the immunosuppressed population.

The clinical presentation of CMV pneumonia is not vastly different from other infectious entities that produce diffuse pneumonia. A gradual onset of nonproductive cough, dyspnea and fever are typical. Physical examination of the chest may be unrevealing. Chest roentgenography shows bilateral infiltrates, although sometimes in early stages of the infection unilateral, focal or nodular infiltrates are observed. As the infection progresses, diffuse consolidation and marked hypoxemia develop. Timing of the infection may give some clue as to its occurrence. In bone marrow transplant recipients the median time of onset is 60 days after transplant, and the disease is rare after 150 days post-transplant. Exceptions do occur – occasionally CMV pneumonia occurs before engraftment and in patients with chronic graft versus host disease the infection may occur from 6 to 12 months after transplant. Diagnosis from BAL fluid is considerably more reliable than in HIV-infected patients. Most cases of CMV pneumonia in bone marrow transplant recipients occur in patients seropositive for CMV prior to transplant. In contrast, in solid-organ transplant recipients, CMV pneumonia is most likely to occur in seronegative recipients of an organ from a CMV positive donor. In such patients, pneumonia is generally part of a clinical syndrome characterized by fever, constitutional symptoms and atypical lymphocytosis, occurring 1–4 months post transplant. Primary

CMV pneumonia in lung transplant recipients can be particularly severe and has been linked to acute graft rejection, invasive aspergillosis and bronchiolitis obliterans. True CMV pneumonia in HIV-infected patients only occurs when the CD4 count is less than 50 per mm^3.

Definitive diagnosis of CMV pneumonia requires demonstration of Cowdry type A intracytoplasmic inclusion bodies within areas of inflammation. Sometimes, even in true infection, the inclusion bodies can not be detected. Immunohistochemical markers may detect CMV-specific antigen in tissue in these cases of so-called "histologically occult" pneumonia.

Other Herpesviruses. The exact role of *human herpesvirus*-6 (HHV-6) in producing pneumonia in immunosuppressed patients remains to be determined [43]. It appears to be responsible for some cases of pneumonia in bone marrow transplant recipients [44]. Its role in HIV infection is controversial. Diagnosis is made by PCR or culture from BAL fluid, although the cutoff for true infection as opposed to asymptomatic shedding is not known. Growth from peripheral blood is probably indicative of active systemic infection. Serology is not helpful in ascribing pneumonia to this organism.

Pneumonia due to HSV undoubtedly occurs, although results from BAL specimens can be misleading due to contamination from the oropharynx. Hematogenous dissemination of HSV can produce a severe diffuse interstitial pneumonitis.

The lung is the major visceral target during chickenpox, and *varicella-zoster virus* (VZV) pneumonia usually occurs 3–7 days after onset of the skin lesions. Pneumonitis can be rapidly progressive over a few days. Disseminated zoster, involving the lung, can occur in those previously infected with VZV. During VZV pneumonia, the virus can be cultured from sputum or BAL fluid. Cytologic examination of sputum may show multinucleated giant cells with intranuclear inclusions. Not uncommonly, other causes of pneumonia may coexist with VZV, thereby complicating diagnosis and therapy.

Recent evidence suggests a new herpes virus, human herpesvirus 8, may be associated with development of Kaposi's sarcoma [45]. Although patients with HIV infection are most characteristically affected, Kaposi's sarcoma also occurs in solid-organ transplant recipients. Kaposi's sarcoma involves the lungs in up to 25% of those with skin involvement. Typical lesions can be visualized on bronchoscopy. Detection of HHV-8 DNA in the BAL fluid has recently been described [46], but it is not yet known how specific this test is for pulmonary Kaposi's sarcoma.

Respiratory Viruses (Influenza, Respiratory Syncytial Virus, Adenovirus). Over the last decade it has become increasingly recognized that common respiratory viruses are frequent causes of pneumonia in the immunocompromised patient. The pneumonia can be severe and has a mortality as high as 50% in bone marrow transplan [47]. In solid-organ transplant recipients these infections mainly affect children. Neutropenic patients with hematologic malignancies are also infected. Severely immunocompromised patients with upper respiratory tract symptoms should have nasopharyngeal aspirates or washes for viral detection by direct fluorescent antibody tests and viral culture. In more advanced cases, BAL fluid can also be subject to these tests and lung biopsy specimens examined for typical viral changes, such as multinucleated syncytial cells with intracytoplasmic viral inclusions, as is seen with respiratory syncytial virus pneumonia. Accurate serologic assessment usually requires acute and convalescent sera collected.

Respiratory syncytial virus is the most common community respiratory virus to cause pneumonia. Initial presentation is with rhinorrhea, nasal and sinus congestion, but quickly progresses to pneumonia especially if the patient is in the first month post-transplantation. Unless treatment is initiated rapidly, mortality is close to 100 [47].

Influenza pneumonia in the immunosuppressed patients also commences with upper respiratory symptoms. Both bone marrow transplant recipients and patients with hematologic malignancies can progress to life-threatening disease particularly if neutropenic [47, 48]. Mortality is highest in patients who remain neutropenic for a prolonged period. Secondary bacterial pneumonia is common.

Parainfluenza virus pneumonia in adult bone marrow transplant recipients has a 37% mortality [49]. Most develop the infection within 100 days of transplantation.

Picornavirus pneumonia also follows the typical pattern of upper respiratory tract symptoms followed by diffuse pneumonia, and has a mortality of 25% in bone marrow transplant recipients.

Adenoviruses are associated with hepatitis in transplant recipients, but can also cause pneumonia (either independently, or in conjunction with hepatitis). In contrast to the other respiratory viruses mentioned above, pneumonia is not usually preceded by upper respiratory tract symptoms. Usually the pneumonia is a bilateral, interstitial process, but pleural effusions occur in 20% of cases.

Polyoma Viruses. Fatal interstitial pneumonia due to BK virus has been described in a patient who underwent stem cell transplantation [50]. At autopsy, BK virus was detected in the lung tissue using immunofluorescence assays, cell culture and polymerase chain reaction (PCR).

HELMINTHS

Strongyloides stercoralis. S. stercoralis is an intestinal nematode (round worm) which can infect humans for years. Most cases are acquired in tropical regions (including southern parts of the United States) by skin contact with soil contaminated with the infective filariform larvae. Infection with *S. stercoralis* is potentially lethal because massive larval invasion of the lungs can occur in immunosuppressed hosts ("hyperinfection syndrome"). This has been described in patients with HIV infection, patients with hematologic malignancy, transplant recipients and others in receipt of corticosteroids. A cycle of autoinfection occurs when rhabditiform larvae penetrate into the vascular tree via the wall of the bowel or perianal skin. The larvae follow the venous circulation to the right heart and then to the pulmonary alveolar capillary bed, from where they penetrate into the alveolar space.

Diffuse pulmonary infiltrates occur which may cavitate. The pneumonia is frequently accompanied by severe abdominal pain. Polymicrobial bacteremia may occur from passenger bacteria which accompany the migrating nematodes into the blood. Peripheral eosinophilia while often observed is not universal. The diagnosis is based on demonstration of filariform larvae in sputum, BAL fluid or the stool. Formal-ether concentrates of sputum should be requested if the diagnosis is suspected. Serum antibody tests are available, but have diminished sensitivity in immunosuppressed patients. However, serology and stool examination should be performed in patients with a relevant geographical history before immunosuppressive therapy is commenced since treatment of uncomplicated gastrointestinal infection is far easier than treatment of the "hyperinfection syndrome".

Protozoa. Microsporidia have emerged as significant pathogens in patients with advanced HIV infection. Although these organisms usually produce diarrhea, disseminated infection can occur. Pulmonary involvement presents with small interstitial infiltrates. The laboratory should be alerted to the possibility of microsporidial pulmonary involvement in patients with advanced HIV infection who have had microsporidia detected in the stool. Sputum or BAL fluid can then be examined with Giemsa or modified trichrome stains in order to detect these tiny organisms. *Cryptosporidium*, an organism which also usually produces diarrhea, can occasionally produce respiratory infection and is detected by using modified acid-fast stains.

Toxoplasma pneumonia is rare, but can occur in HIV-infected patients or solid-organ transplant recipients. *Amebiasis*, *leishmaniasis* and *babesiosis* may all have pulmonary manifestations when disseminated infection occurs in the immunosuppressed host. Relevant exposure history should be sought.

A Diagnostic Approach to Respiratory Infections in Immunocompromised Pateints

Diagnosis of respiratory infection in the immunocompromised patient should follow the usual processes of history taking, physical examination, noninvasive tests and invasive procedures. The simple combination of history taking, physical examination and chest radiography can often dramatically narrow the differential diagnosis. Despite this an important caveat needs to be mentioned. Caution must be exercised in using the principle of Ockham's Razor, "Entities are not to be multiplied without necessity". In other branches of medicine, given all the patient's symptoms, signs and noninvasive laboratory tests, a physician will find that one unifying diagnosis can explain the illness. Pneumonia in the immunocompromised patient may be due to multiple simultaneous infections (or non-infectious conditions) occurring in the one patient at the one time. For example, an HIV patient may have simultaneous *P. carinii* pneumonia and pulmonary Kaposi's sarcoma causing pulmonary infiltrates or a transplant recipient have bacterial pneumonia and invasive pulmonary aspergillosis.

Nevertheless, there is no doubt that certain infectious processes are more likely to occur than others at various times from the transplant procedure. Bacterial pneumonia (due to Gram-negative bacilli or MRSA) is most likely to occur in the first month after transplantation when the patient may be intubated. Cytomegalovirus pneumonia is most likely to occur between four weeks and four months after transplantation. Invasive pulmonary aspergillosis can occur as early as 10–14 days after transplantation, and almost always occurs during hospital admission. Mycobacterial, cryptococcal or nocardial infections usually occur more than two months after transplantation.

In a similar manner, the etiologies of pneumonia in HIV-infected patients follows a somewhat pedictable course in terms of progression of decline of CD4 lymphocyte count. In patients with a CD4 count greater than 500 per mm^3, bacterial pneumonia (for example due to *S. pneumoniae* or *H. influenzae*) is the most likely diagnostic entity. Risk for bacterial pneumonia persists when CD4 count is from 200–500 per mm^3, but tuberculosis and cryptococcosis may occur at this time. These organisms may also be a cause of infection when the CD4 count is 50–200 per mm^3, but *Pneumocystis carinii* becomes the predominant pathogen then. Finally, when the CD4 count is less than 50 per mm^3, *Pneumocystis carinii*, CMV, *M. avium* and even *Aspergillus* become the major pathogens.

Despite these rules, in many cases an invasive procedure needs to be pursued in order to make an accurate diagnosis. Unfortunately, even in the most intensively investigated patient only nonspecific information may be forthcoming, leading to empiric treatment based on relevant epidemiologic information. In addition, to complicate the diagnosis of respiratory infection in the immunosuppressed patient, numerous noninfectious causes of pulmonary infiltrates exist.

Suspicion for these noninfectious entities must be raised by relevant exposure histories (chemotherapeutic agents, radiotherapy), history of malignancy (Kaposi's sarcoma, hematologic malignancy, hepatocellular carcinoma) and by nonspecific or negative findings on microbiologic workup. Early diagnosis by biopsy can allow effective therapy whether it be withdrawal of the inducing agent, corticosteroids or chemotherapy. Of all the noninfectious causes of pulmonary infiltrate, pulmonary edema, pulmonary embolism, adult respiratory distress syndrome and pulmonary hemorrhage are the most common. Septic shock, without lung infection, may produce diffuse pulmonary infiltrates. Aggressive therapy of pulmonary edema or septic shock is sometimes required before further assessment of infectious causes of pneumonia can be performed.

HISTORY AND PHYSICAL EXAMINATION

History-Taking: Assessing the patient's overall level, duration and type of immunosuppression can heighten suspicion of certain clinical entities. For example, the antiretroviral drug naive HIV-infected patient with a CD4 count of between 50 and 200 cells/mm^3 is highly likely to have *P. carinii* as the cause of pneumonia. Unfortunately the diagnostic possibilities rise with increasing immunosuppression and duration of time of the immunocompromised state. The tempo and mode of onset of pneumonia are also important. A rapidly progressive pneumonia of duration less than 24 hours in the neutropenic or ventilated patient usually suggests a bacterial (often Gram-negative) etiology. In contrast, viruses, *P. carinii* and *Aspergillus* have a subacute onset over several days to a week. Finally, a chronic course is more likely to suggest tuberculosis or infection with *Nocardia*, *Cryptococcus* or the geographically restricted fungi. A history of travel or residence in third world countries (tuberculosis) or south-Western United States (coccidioidomycosis) may further heighten clinical suspicion of these particular etiologies with a chronic course. Occupational and recreational history is sometimes important; *Rhodococcus equi* is sometimes (but not always) associated with exposure to horses. Finally, since pneumonia in the immunosuppressed patient may have noninfectious etiologies (such as drug-induced pneumonitis), a full knowledge of the patient's drug history is essential. The nature of the patient's symptoms can be important. Up to 50% of patients with legionellosis have gastrointestinal symptoms, especially watery diarrhea. Invasive pulmonary aspergillosis may present with symptoms mimicking pulmonary thromboembolism (pleuritic chest pain, dyspnea, hemoptysis) or occasionally massive hemoptysis.

Physical examination may also help narrow the infectious differential diagnosis. Patients with bacterial pneumonia are likely to be febrile, tachycardic and tachypneic, whereas patients with nocardiosis or cryptococcosis are often afebrile and maintain normal pulse and respiratory rates. Careful examination of the patient's skin for signs of cutaneous infection with *Nocardia* or *Cryptococcus* is also essential. Rarely, patients with invasive pulmonary aspergillosis have coexisting cutaneous infection around the insertion sites of long-standing central venous catheters.

RADIOLOGY

Chest roentgenograms and computed tomographic (CT) scans: Virtually all modern definitions of pneumonia include a necessity for pulmonary infiltrate to be visualized by radiologic assessment. In some circumstances, knowledge taken from history taking (particularly type and intensity of immunosuppression, and tempo of onset of pneumonic process) combined with the radiographic appearance can virtually ascertain a diagnosis. For example, an HIV-infected patient with CD4 count of less than 200 cells/mm^3 who is not taking prophylaxis against *P. carinii*, and who has a subacute pneumonic process visualized radiographically as an interstitial alveolar butterflypattern spreading from the hilar region should be treated empirically with high dose trimethoprim-sulfamethoxazole since *P. carinii* pneumonia is highly likely. Many times however, radiologic examination may simply narrow the diagnostic possibilities guiding empiric treatment before an invasive investigation can be performed (Tables 4–6).

Radiologic assessment is also necessary to guide choice of invasive investigation. If a pulmonary nodule is shown to be peripheral in location, percutaneous needle aspiration may

TABLE 4. Patterns of chest radiograph abnormality in acute onset pneumonia in the immunocompromised patient

Peribronchovascular infiltrate
Infective
: Gram-negative bacilli
: *S. aureus*
: *Legionella*
Non-infective
: Pulmonary edema
: Leukoagglutinin reaction
Consolidation
Infective
: Gram-negative bacilli
: *S. aureus*
: *Legionella*
: Anerobes (aspiration)
Non-infective
: Pulmonary hemorrhage
: Pulmonary thromboembolism
Nodular infiltrate
Infective
: *S. aureus*
: *Legionella*
Non-infective
: Pulmonary calcification
Cavitary lesions
Infective
: *S. aureus*
: *P. aeruginosa*

*Acute onset is defined as development of significant pneumonia within 24 hours.

be feasible. In contrast, radiologic assessment showing a peribronchovascular (interstitial) infiltrate may best be investigated by flexible fiberoptic bronchoscopy, allowing bronchoalveolar lavage and/or bronchoscopic biopsy.

Pneumonia in the immunosuppressed patient takes on the following clasical patterns, established by chest roentgenography. Unfortunately, although the following patterns are frequently seen, organisms may produce patterns outside that typically observed, especially if the patient is heavily immunosuppressed. Alveolar pneumonia (airspace or lobar pneumonia) classically occurs in pneumococcal pneumonia, and is characterized pathologically by presence of inflammatory exudate in peripheral alveoli. Air bronchograms are frequently present. While the process is typified by complete lobar involvement, often the process is not that extensive

TABLE 5. Patterns of chest radiograph abnormality in pneumonia developing over several days to weeks in the immunocompromised patient

Peribronchovascular
Infective
Pneumocystis carinii
Viruses (CMV, HHV-6, RSV, Influenza, Adenovirus)
Non-infective
Drug-induced
Radiation induced
Consolidation
Infective
Fungi, especially *A. fumigatus*
Nocardia
Tuberculosis
Non-infective
Drug-induced
Radiation induced
Pulmonary thromboembolism
Nodular
Infective
Fungi especially *C. neoformans*, *C. immitis*, *Aspergillus*
Nocardia
Tuberculosis
Rhodococcus equi
Bartonella
Non-infective
Adenocarcinoma
Squamous cell carcinoma
Post-transplant lymphoproliferative disorder
Cavitary
Infective
Legionella, especially *L. micdadei*
R. equi
M. tuberculosis
Aspergillus
Non-infective
Bronchogenic carcinoma

*Subacute-chronic onset is defined as a process developing over several days to weeks.

(although the pathology is the same). In the immunosuppressed patient, this form of consolidation is frequently multilobar, such as when due to *Legionella* species. Advanced infection with *Aspergillus*, *Nocardia* and *M. tuberculosis* may also produce this radiographic pattern, although discrete nodular infiltrates are more usual. Bronchopneumonia occurs when the inflammatory response is in the bronchi and surrounding parenchyma. Radiographically this produces a more patchy appearance than is seen with alveolar pneumonia. Segmental bronchopneumonia is commonly observed with *S. aureus*, *H. influenzae*, viral pneumonia, *Chlamydia pneumoniae* and *Mycoplasma pneumoniae*, and occasionally with pneumococcus.

Peribronchovascular infiltrates (interstitial pneumonia) are manifest radiographically as a reticular or reticulonodular pattern. Early *P. carinii* infection characteristically has this appearance, as does CMV, varicella-zoster and HSV. Nodular infiltrates are characteristically present in subacute or chronic fungal, mycobacterial or nocardial infections. Nodular infiltrates of more rapid onset can be the result of *S. aureus* or *P. aeruginosa* infection, either as a primary event or sometimes as a result of infected emboli originating from an infected intravascular catheter. Radiographically nodules can be defined as spherical or oval intrapulmonary opacities that are well enough circumscribed to permit measurement of their diameter [51]. Sometimes, multiple very small nodules can be seen. This may be due to miliary infection due to tuberculosis, histoplasmosis or blastomycosis, or if slightly larger due to varicella zoster or CMV infection. Masses are large nodules; sometimes defined as nodules greater than 6 cm in diameter. They are frequently due to *Cryptococcus* or *Nocardia*. Cavitation of nodules, masses or areas of consolidation occurs with *M. tuberculosis*, *R. equi*, *Legionella micdadei*, *P. aeruginosa*, *S. aureus*, *Aspergillus* and sometimes other fungi.

Although chest roentgenography is usually all that is necessary to establish a radiographic pattern, chest CT scanning plays an important role in diagnosis of pneumonia in the immunosuppressed patient. CT scanning of the chest can determine whether a pneumonia is necrotizing, whether mediastinal lymphadenopathy is present, whether and how many small granulomatous lesions or nodules are present and whether a pleural effusion or empyema

TABLE 6. Suggested diagnostic strategy for immunocompromised patient with pulmonary nodules (modified from Paterson *et al.* 1998) [51]

1. Chest CT scan (with contrast) to confirm roentographic diagnosis.
2. History
   - Type of immunosuppression – Transplant (PTLD), HIV (Kaposis sarcoma)
   - Underlying diseases – Prior history of carcinoma (metastatic hepatocellular carcinoma)
   - Geographic location – South-West USA (coccidiomycosis), developing nations (tuberculosis)
   - Previous positive PPD (tuberculosis)
   - Headache or neurologic symptoms (cerebral aspergillosis or nocardiosis)
   - Exposure to animals (horses – *Rhodococcus equi*, cats – *Bartonella*, dogs – *Echinococcus*)
3. Physical examination
   - Skin lesions (nocardiosis, crptococcosis, Kaposis sarcoma)
4. Non-invasive laboratory workup
   - Blood cultures (*Cryptococcus*, *Rhodococcus equi*)
   - PPD (tuberculosis)
   - Serology (*Cryptococcus*, *Aspergillus*, *Bartonella*, *Echinococcus*, EBV)
   - Tumor markers – Alpha Feto Protein (adenocarcinoma)
5. Tissue and microbiologic diagnosis
   - Punch biopsy of skin lesion if present
   - Thoracoscopic excision or percutaneous fine needle biopsy
     : Histology (all diagnoses)
     : Special stains (*Nocardia*, fungi, mycobacteria)
     : Culture, including specialized media (*Legionella*, *Nocardia*, *Bartonella*, mycobacteria, fungi, viruses)

accounts for part of the pulmonary density observed on chest roentgenograms. There is increasing evidence that high-resolution CT scanning is more sensitive than chest roentgenography in the detection of pneumonia in immunosuppressed [36, 52]. In a study of neutropenic patients who had fever for more than two days despite empiric antibiotic treatment, thin-section CT scans showed findings suggestive of pneumonia about five days earlier than chest roentgenograms [52]. This was particularly important for fungal pneumonia, because delay in diagnosis is associated with high mortality. Furthermore, a number of highly typical CT appearances can be seen with fungal (especially *Aspergillus*) pneumonia, especially in the neutropenic patient.

Nuclear medicine scans are generally nonspecific but may occasionally be useful in excluding certain infectious causes of pneumonia in immunosuppressed patients. For example, a normal ^{67}Gallium scan may exclude *P. carinii* infection. Similarly, radiolabeled (^{111}indium) human immunoglobulin may occasionally be useful in excluding invasive pulmonary aspergillosis in immunosuppressed patients with negative or nonspecific radiographic findings [53]. This scan may also be useful in assessing resolution of *P. carinii* infection, which is not possible with ^{67}Gallium scans.

SIMPLE NON-INVASIVE TESTS

Simple non-invasive tests may sometimes support the clinical impression gained by history-taking, physical examination and chest radiography and even obviate the need for an invasive procedure to establish the diagnosis. However, the cautions mentioned above about not assuming that only one pathology is present in the immunosuppressed patient at any one time must be remembered.

Arterial blood gas analysis should be performed on all immunosuppressed patients with significant pneumonia unless the patient has a bleeding diathesis. Pulse oximetry is a reasonable non-invasive alternative in selected patients, but in the patient with acute respiratory failure may be inaccurate owing to peripheral vasoconstriction from shock or the use of vasopressors. Severe anemia, onychomycosis, fingernail polish and presence of carboxyhemoglobin or methemoglobin may all cause falsely depressed measures of oxygen saturation when pulse oximetry is used. Significant hypoxemia is an indication to use corticosteroids in addition to antimicrobials in the treatment of *P. carinii* pneumonia. Well maintained oxygenation is almost always observed in chronic processes such as tuberculosis, nocardiosis and many fungal infections whereas hypoxemia is seen in acute bacterial and viral pneumonias.

Examination of sputum or respiratory secretions obtained through suction via an endotracheal tube can be of great value and should be attempted in all immunosuppressed patients with suspected pneumonia. A good quality sample is required – for sputum this entails collection of lower respiratory tract secretions produced by cough. Saliva is useless. Microscopically a good sample contains numerous polymorphonuclear neutrophils and few squamous cells. Laboratories which do not process such unsatisfactory specimens should be contacted if the patient is neutropenic. The value of Gram stain and routine bacteriologic culture of sputum in immunosuppressed patients is lower than in the immunocompetent individual. The finding of *S. pneumoniae*, *H. influenzae* or *Enterobacteriaceae* may represent bacterial pneumonia, but equally may represent colonization and mask another infectious process. In contrast, the finding of fungi such as *A. fumigatus* is of much more significance than in the immunocompetent host; positive predictive values of sputum culture for subsequent development of invasive aspergillosis are as high as 82% for bone marrow and 72% for liver transplant [11, 54]. Specialized media should be set up for culture of fungi, *Legionella* or mycobacteria from sputum. Culture of *Legionella*, *C. neoformans* or *M. tuberculosis* (but not necessarily other mycobacteria) is diagnostic and an indication to commence appropriate therapy.

Induced sputum samples are obtained by administration of aerosolized hypertonic saline. The applicability of the test is limited to alert, cooperative patients but provides a better alveolar sample than obtained by regular expectorated sputum. The test is of greatest use in diagnosing *P. carinii* pneumonia, where it has a diagnostic yield of up to 75%. The specimen can be stained with immunofluorescent monoclonal antibodies or Giemsa or silver stains. Induced sputum samples can also be used to obtain samples for mycobacterial smears and cultures in patients who do not have a cough, and can also be examined for fungi and cells with viral inclusions. While a positive test from induced sputum is an indication for specific antimicrobial treatment, a negative test does not rule out any of the above infections.

Serologic and other blood tests: Blood cultures should be performed in all patients and are most useful for detection of bacterial pathogens. Detection of CMV or HHV-6 in peripheral blood can be performed by way of cell culture of buffy coat, direct fluorescent antibody examination of buffy coat using the shell vial method, antigenemia assays (for example, PP65 antigen) and polymerase chain reaction (PCR) of peripheral blood. Antigenemia assays and PCR are becoming increasingly popular for detection of CMV as they represent a rapid accurate method of diagnosis of CMV infection. However, invasive CMV disease still needs to be verified by lung biopsy. Detection of serum cryptococcal antigen is a highly specific test which should be used in evaluation of pneumonia in HIV-infected patients and transplant recipients. Surveillance serology for the *Aspergillus* antigen, galactomannan, may also be useful in high-risk transplant recipients and neutropenic patients. Serology for detection of antibody against *Histoplasma capsulatum*, *Coccidioides immitis*, *Legionella* species, *Mycoplasma pneumoniae*, *Chlamydia pneumoniae* and respiratory viruses (Influenza A and B, Respiratory syncytial virus, adenoviruses and Parainfluenza virus) can also be performed in selected patients, but may rely on a convalescent sample to demonstrate a diagnostic rise in titre.

Miscellaneous non-invasive tests: Legionella pneumophila serogroup 1 infection can be diagnosed by way of antigen detection in urine [55]. While this serogroup is responsible for up to 80% of cases of *Legionella* pneumonia, other species or serogroups can not be detected by this method. The tuberculin skin test is often performed in assessment of pneumonia, but a negative result should never replace negative cultures in excluding the diagnosis of tuberculosis, since many immunosuppressed patients are anergic. Fungal skin tests suffer from the same problem.

FLEXIBLE FIBEROPTIC BRONCHOSCOPY

Fiberoptic bronchoscopy has become the cornerstone of assessment of pneumonia in the immunosuppressed patient and provides a diagnostic yield in 60–90% of patients with HIV infection and about 50% of patients with other forms of immunosuppression. Although all of the diagnostic techniques mentioned above can heighten clinical suspicion of certain diagnostic entities, requirement for tissue or at the very least a lower respiratory tract sample taken from the likely area of pathology is best approached by use of fiberoptic bronchoscopy. Bronchoalveolar lavage (BAL) is almost always performed; bronchoscopic biopsy improves the yield but can be risky in patients who have bleeding disorders not reversible with blood product support or in patients who are severely hypoxemic. Fiberoptic bronchoscopy also provides an opportunity to visually inspect the anatomy of the tracheobronchial tree (observing for infectious processes such as tracheobronchial aspergillosis, for example) and to perform bronchial washings and brushings, although these modalities have been largely replaced by BAL.

Bronchoalveolar lavage has proved to be of greatest use in diagnosing diffuse pulmonary infiltrates, particularly that due to *P. carinii* infection in HIV-infected patients or pulmonary hemorrhage in other immunosuppressed

TABLE 7. Noninfectious differential diagnoses of pneumonia in the immunosuppressed host

Transplant recipients
Pulmonary edema
Adult respiratory distress syndrome
Pulmonary calcification
Metastatic carcinoma
Post-transplant lymphoproliferative disorder
OKT3 administration
Drugs (azathioprine)
HIV infection
Kaposis sarcoma
Lymphoma
Bleomycin sulfate
Pulmonary alveolar proetinosis
Pulmonary emboli
Hematologic malignancies
Pulmonary edema
Radiation pneumonitis
Chemotherapeutic agents (bleomycin, busulfan, chlorambucil, cyclophosphamide, cytosine arabinoside, hydroxyurea, melphalan, methotrexate, mitomycin, nitrosurea, procarbazine)
Recurrent leukemia or lymphoma
Leukemic cell lysis pneumopathy
Pulmonary emboli
Pulmonary alveolar proteinosis

patients. In such cases it provides a diagnosis in up to 95% of cases. In part because of the success in diagnosing *P. carinii* pneumonia, BAL has become such a popular mode of investigating pulmonary infiltrates in immunosuppressed patients that its limitations are forgotten. For example, the significance of CMV identified in BAL in HIV-infected patients is unclear [56]. At least 50% of all severely immunosuppressed HIV-infected patients shed CMV in respiratory secretions. In one recent study, 72% of BAL samples from HIV-infected patients with pulmonary symptoms contained CMV, but pathologic evidence of CMV pneumonia was demonstrated in only 3% of these patients [56]. In contrast, the yield of any infectious diagnosis by using BAL in patients with hematologic malignancies is low, achieving a microbiologic diagnosis in only 28% of patients with symptoms consistent with pulmonary infection [57]. The yield of BAL in diagnosing invasive pulmonary aspergillosis is only 45–62%. BAL is of limited usefulness in evaluating nodular infiltrates and for diagnosing noninfectious processes such as drug toxicity, metastatic malignancy and the adult respiratory distress syndrome (Table 7).

Bronchoalveolar lavage is also critcized because of the high rate of false positive bacterial isolations due to contamination from the upper airway. Protected BAL is a variation of conventional BAL in which sealed probes or distally protected catheters are used, in order to avoid contact between the fluid used in BAL and mouth and upper airway organisms that may contaminate the suction channel of the bronchoscope [58]. This technique has been used to discriminate between upper airway colonizers and lower repsiratory tract pathogens, particularly in ventilator-associated pneumonia. Protected brushings can also be used. Quantitative culture has added a further level of sophistication to the procedure. At present, although widely used in some centers, the role of such techniques remains controversial because of questions of accuracy of the results and determining what is the threshold concentration of bacteria which can be defined as significant.

Transbronchial lung biopsy, although limited by the contraindications mentioned above, is particularly useful in definitively diagnosing viral pneumonia and noninfectious causes of pulmonary infiltrates in immunosuppressed populations. Transbronchial biopsy has found great impact in lung transplant recipients, where it can provide specimens for pathologic diagnosis of acute rejection and CMV pneumonia [59, 60]. In patients with hematologic malignancies the technique is useful for distinguishing leukemic infiltrates and radiation and drug-induced pneumonitis from infectious causes of pneumonia. Unfortunately, nonspecific or negative findings occur in a sizeable proportion of patients probably reflecting sampling error and the operator dependence of the procedure. Complications include hemorrhage, pneumothorax and transient hypoxemia.

NON-BRONCHOSCOPIC LUNG BIOPSY

Alternatives to bronchoscopic biopsies are potentially useful when a diagnosis can not be made by bronchoscopic techniques or when peripheral nodules or cavities are present.

Thoracoscopic transpleural lung biopsy is a useful and well-tolerated procedure for some patients. Excellent results have been obtained in patients with diffuse interstitial pulmonary disease [61]. The procedure is also of use in focal, pleural-based disease in the periphery of the lung. The procedure can be carried out under local analgesia but because a pneumothorax is created by virtue of the approach, a chest tube is needed for several days after the procedure.

Percutaneous needle biopsy of the lung is often the diagnostic procedure of choice for peripherally located nodules or cavities. The procedure is not appropriate for diffuse lung disease. CT guidance of the procedure greatly improves the diagnostic yield of the needle biopsy. Microscopy and culture for fungi, *Nocardia* and mycobacteria can be performed as can cytology for malignant cells. The specimen is usually insufficient for histopathological examination. Pneumothorax is the major complication, although its frequency has been reduced by using small gauge needles.

A combination of CT-guided needle localization of small nodules, with simultaneous injection of methylene blue to improve recognition of the nodule, followed by thoracoscopic resection of the localized nodule has been successfully used in transplant recipients (Schwarz 1994).

Open lung biopsy is regarded as the definitive procedure for diagnosing pneumonia in the immunosuppressed patient, because a large tissue sample (potentially from several different sites) can be obtained. Open lung biopsy provides a specific diagnosis is made in 60 to 90% of immunosuppressed patients in whom it is employed. It is most often used when previous diagnostic manoeuvres have been unsuccessful, pulmonary infiltrates are spreading rapidly, hypoxemia is worsening and the patient has a potentially treatable underlying condition. Thus it is rarely used in patients with advanced HIV infection or relapsing acute myelogenous leukemia, but is quite applicable in transplant recipients and those with collagen vascular disease. Like other diagnostic procedures it is less successful in patients with hematologic malignancy than patients with other forms of immunosuppression. It may however ascertain a diagnosis of non-infective causes of pulmonary infiltrate (for example, antineoplastic drug toxicity or lymphocytic interstitial pneumonia) which other diagnostic methods were unable to provide. An advantage of the procedure is that it offers the ability to control complications of the biopsy including bleeding and air leaks. Its disadvanatges include the need for intubation and a general anesthetic. Procedure-related mortality occurs in 1% of patients.

Therapy for Respiratory Infections in the Immunocompromised Patient

In many presentations if respiratory infection in the immunocompromised patient, antimicrobial therapy needs to be commenced empirically because of the risk of rapid progression of disease and worsening hypoxemia. The chronic progression of pulmonary nodules is one exception. Much of the decision as to whether empiric therapy be commenced rests with an assessment of the patient's clinical status. A frequent concern about empiric institution of antimicrobial agents is that they will prevent a precise microbiologic diagnosis being made. Certainly, before antimicrobial agents are commenced simple, but potentially very useful, tests such blood cultures should be collected.

The choice of empiric therapy depends on the stage of the immunosuppressive process, the use of prophylactic antimicrobial therapy as well as the radiologic and epidemiologic picture. For example, patients with granulocytopenia whose pneumonia develops with their initial fever usually require antibacterial therapy only. This should predominantly cover Gram-negative bacilli, including *Pseudomonas aeruginosa*. Traditionally an antipseudomonal beta-lactam antibiotic plus an aminoglycoside is chosen, although some advocate monotherapy with ceftazidime or a carbapenem. Local resistance patterns (for example, a high incidence of extended spectrum beta-lactamase producing *Enterobacteriaceae*) may call for modification of this approach. Only if no response occurs within 48 to 72 hours would more broad spectrum coverage be added or bronchoscopy be performed.

In contrast, persistently neutropenic patients who develop a new focal pulmonary infiltrate while already receiving antibiotic therapy have a much broader differential diagnosis. Such patients have such a high risk of fungal infection that we would advocate empiric use of aggressive antifungal therapy, including amphotericin deoxycholate in high dose (1–1.5 mg/kg/day) or a lipid formulation of amphotericin. Empiric addition of itraconazole or 5-flucytosine needs to be strongly considered. Traditionally, much lower doses of amphotericin (for example, 0.5 mg/kg/day) are used empirically, because of concerns that renal toxicity from higher doses can only be justified in microbiologically or histopathologically proven fungal infection. However, we believe the mortality of invasive fungal pneumonia in neutropenic patients is so high, that such concerns can be overridden. Empiric use of lipid preparations of amphotericin, when compared to amphotericin deoxycholate in a randomized controlled trial in neutropenic patients, is rarely associated with significant nephrotoxicity [62]. Invasive diagnostic procedures can be arranged, but only after aggressive empiric antifungal therapy has been instituted.

Choice of empiric treatment of severe pneumonia with diffuse or interstitial infiltrates in non-neutropenic patients depends on use of prophylaxis against *P. carinii*, time since transplant or CD4 lymphocyte count. Trimethoprim-sulfamethoxazole should be included in the empiric regimen if no *P. carinii* prophylaxis was being used. A macrolide or quinolone active against *Legionella* (for example, azithromycin, erythromycin, ciprofloxacin) should be included, especially if *Legionella* has been cultured from the hospital's water system. Ganciclovir may be used empirically in high-risk transplant recipients.

When specific organisms are known, targeted therapy should be initiated as outlined in Table 8.

Antimicrobial agents alone, however, may not suffice in the treatment of pneumonia in the immunosuppressed patient. Supportive therapy, preferibly including non-invasive mechanical ventilation, may need to be considered. Decreasing or eliminating immunosuppressive therapy and improving neutrophil number and function by use of granulocyte colony-stimulating factor is essential. Surgery may be useful, particularly in focal fungal infections such as aspergillosis or mucormycosis. Identification, and appropriate treatment, of extrapulmonary sites of infection is also important. Many antimicrobial agents have interactions with cyclosporine or tacrolimus; these can be avoided by careful antibiotic choice or dose adjustment [63]. Particular attention must be paid to duration of therapy, especially for organisms such as *M. tuberculosis*, *R. equi* and most of the fungi. In HIV-infected patients, maintenance therapy may need to be continued lifelong after the initial intense therapy has been given.

PREVENTION OF PNEUMONIA IN THE IMMUNOSUPPRESSED PATIENT

Much can be done to prevent pneumonia in immunosuppressed populations. This includes prevention of colonization, antimicrobial prophylaxis, surveillance with pre-emptive therapy and immunomodulation/immunoprophylaxis.

Prevention of colonization is probably the most important measure in preventing pneumonia. Its principles are relatively simple, but in

TABLE 8. Therapeutic options for respiratory infections in immunocompromised patients

Organism	Treatment of choice	Comments
Bacteria		
MRSA	Vancomycin	Removal of infected central venous lines may be important.
S. pneumoniae	Penicillin	High-level, but not intermediate, penicillin resistance may require cefotaxime or vancomycin.
R. equi	Azithromycin plus rifampin	Optimal regimen not yet determined, other possibilities include combinations with erythromycin, vancomycin, aminoglycosides or imipenem.
Nocardia	TMP/SMX	Ceftriaxone and imipenem also useful in some species
H. influenzae	Ampicillin	Ampicillin plus beta-lactamase inhibitor appropriate if beta-lactamase producer
Enterobacteriaceae	Ciprofloxacin or third generation cephalosporin	Extended spectrum beta-lactamase producers best treated with a carbapenem
Acinetobacter	Imipenem or ceftazidime	Ampicillin-sulbactam may be useful for resistant strains
P. aeruginosa	Ceftazidime, piperacillin or carbapenem plus aminoglycoside	High peaks of aminoglycoside required
B. cepacia	TMP/SMX	Imipenem, ciprofloxacin, minocycline or chloramphenicol may be alternatives
S. maltophilia	TMP/SMX	Ticarcillin/clavulanate may be an alternative or a useful addition
Legionella	Azithromycin or ciprofloxacin	Add rifampin in severe cases
C. pneumoniae	Azithromycin or doxycyline	Beta-lactams are not effective
M. pneumoniae	Azithromycin or erythromycin	Doxycyline is an alternative
M. tuberculosis	Isoniazid, rifampin, ethambutol and pyrazinamide	Must test susceptibilities
Fungi		
P. carinii	TMP/SMX	Add corticosteroids if hypoxemic
Aspergillus	Lipid preparation of amphotericin or high dose amphotericin deoxycholate (1–1.5 mg/kg)	Combination with G-CSF, GM-CSF, itraconazole or 5-flucytosine advised
C. neoformans	Amphotericin or fluconazole	Surgery should be considered for focal disease

TABLE 8 (Continued)

Organism	Treatment of choice	Comments
Mucormycosis	Lipid preparation of amphotericin or high dose amphotericin deoxycholate (1–1.5 mg/kg)	Surgery almost always needed for successful outcome
Viruses		
Cytomegalovirus	Ganciclovir	May need G-CSF to prevent neutropenia
Respiratory syncytial virus (RSV)	Ribavirin	Some use immunoglobulin in addition
Influenza	Amantadine or rimantidine	Resistance may emerge during treatment
HHV-6	Ganciclovir	May need G-CSF to prevent neutropenia
HSV	Acyclovir	Famciclovir an alternative
VZV	Acyclovir	Famciclovir an alternative

practice rarely performed well. Horizontal transmission of resistant bacteria from other patients via the hands of health care workers is a major problem and can be easily prevented by handwashing. Ingestion of water contaminated with *Legionella* can be prevented by disinfection of the hospital water distribution system. Risk of *P. aeruginosa* infection in neutropenic patients may be reduced by avoidance of fresh leafy vegetables. Respiratory transmission of mycobacteria, viruses and fungi within hospitals has been well demonstrated. In many institutions it is necessary to accommodate all HIV-infected patients with pneumonia in respiratory isolation until three smears of sputum samples are shown to be negative. Patients with VZV, influenza and RSV should also be accommodated in respiratory isolation. Accommodation of bone marrow transplant recipients in rooms with laminar air flow and high efficiency particulate air (HEPA) filtration reduces risk of invasive aspergillosis [11]. Construction activity within the hospital is also a risk factor for invasive pulmonary aspergillosis and should be appropriately contained.

In recent years there has been a tremendous vogue for use of widespread antimicrobial prophylaxis as a means of preventing pneumonia and other infections in the immunosuppressed patient. While strategies such as use of trimethoprim-sulfamethoxazole to prevent *P. carinii* pneumonia in HIV-infected patients and transplant recipients is clearly of benefit, prophylaxis against other fungi, bacteria and viruses is a less clearcut issue. Vancomycin resistance in enterococci and staphylococci, fluconazole resistance in yeasts and ganciclovir resistance in cytomegalovirus are becoming major concerns. Alternatives to widespread prophylaxis include selective use of prophylaxis in identified high-risk groups or pre-emptive use of antimicrobials [64]. The pre-emptive strategy is one of regular surveillance testing (usually by way of polymerase chain reaction or detection of antigen in blood) and then initiation of short-term therapy for asymptomatic or minimally symptomatic patients with positive surveillance results. Pre-emptive treatment has found widest use in management of cytomegalovirus and *Aspergillus* infections.

Immunomodulation/immunoprophylaxis is widely used. Inactivated vaccines (for example against influenza and pneumococcus) are indicated in virtually all immunosuppressed patients. In general, live vaccines should not be used. Intravenous pooled immunoglobulin is indicated in patients with immunoglobulin deficiencies.

References

1. Paterson D, Singh N. Invasive aspergillosis in transplant recipients. Medicine 78:123, 1999.
2. Singh N, Gayowski T, Wagener MM, Marino IR, Yu VL. Pulmonary infections in liver transplant recipients receiving tacrolimus. Transplantation 61:396, 1996.
3. Kollef MH. The prevention of ventilator-associated pneumonia. N Engl J Med 340:627, 1999.
4. Coonrod JD, Lester RL, Hsu LC. Characterization of the extracellular bactericidal factors of rat alveolar lung material. J Clin Invest 74:1269, 1984.
5. Croft M. Activation of naive, memory and effector T cells. Curr Opin Immunol 5:431, 1994.
6. Hughes MD, Johnson VA, Hirch MS, *et al.* Monitoring plasma HIV-1 RNA levels in addition to CD4 lymphocytes improves assessment of antiretroviral therapeutic response. Ann Intern Med 126:929, 1997.
7. O'Brien WA, Hartigan PM, Daar ES, *et al.* Changes in plasma HIV RNA levels and CD4+ lymphocyte count predicts both response to antiretroviral therapy and therapeutic failure. Ann Intern Med 126:939, 1997.
8. Mellors JW, Munoz A, Giorgi J, *et al.* Plasma viral load and CD+ lymphocytes as prognostic markers of HIV-1 infection. Ann Intern Med 126:946, 1997.
9. Grundy JE, Shanley D, Griffiths PD, *et al.* Is cytomegalovirus interstitial pneumonitis in transplant recipients an immunopathological condition? Lancet 2:996, 1987.
10. Weems JJ, David BJ, Tablan OC, Kaufman L, Martone WJ. Construction activity: an independent risk factor for invasive aspergillosis and zygomycosis in patients with hematologic malignancy. Infect Control 8:71, 1987.
11. Wald A, Leisenring W, van Burik J, Bowden RA. Epidemiology of *Aspergillus* infections in a large cohort of patients undergoing bone marrow transplantation. J Infect Dis 175:1459, 1997.
12. Anderson K, Morris G, Kennedy H, Croall J, Michie J, Richardson MD, *et al.* Aspergillosis in immunocompromised paediatric patients: associations with building hygiene, design, and indoor air. Thorax 51:256, 1996.
13. Chave J, David S, Wauters J, *et al.* Transmission of *Pneumocystis carinii* from AIDS patients to other immunosuppressed patients: A cluster of *Pneumocystis carinii* pneumonia in renal transplant recipients. AIDS 5:760, 1991.
14. Yu VL. Could aspiration be the major mode of transmission for Legionella? Am J Med 95:13, 1993.
15. Hiramatsu K, Hanaki H, Ino T, *et al.* Methicillin-resistant *Staphylococcus aureus* clinical strains with reduced vancomycin susceptibility. J Antimicrob Chemother 40:136, 1997.
16. CDC Update. *Staphylococcus aureus* with reduced susceptibility to vancomycin – United States. MMWR 46:813, 1997.
17. Paterson DL. *Staphylococcus aureus* with reduced susceptibility to vacncomycin – a review of current knowledge. Communicable Diseases Intelligence 23:69, 1999.
18. Singh N, Paterson D, Chang FY, Gayowski T, Squier C, Wagener MM, *et al.* Methicillin-resistant *Staphylococcus aureus*: the other emerging resistant gram-positive coccus among liver transplant recipients. Clin Infect Dis 30:322, 2000.
19. Redd SC, Rutherford GW, Sande MA, *et al.* The role of human immunodeficiency virus infection in pneumococcal bacteremia in San Francisco residents. J Infect Dis 162:1012, 1990.
20. Linden PK, Pasculle AW, Manez R. Differences in outcomes for patients with bacteremia due to vancomycin-resistant *Enterococcus faecium* or vancomycin-susceptible *E. faecium*. Clin Infect Dis 22:663, 1996.
21. Sane DC, Durack DT. Infection with *Rhodococcus equi* in AIDS. N Engl J Med 314:56, 1986.
22. Le Lay G, Martin F, Leroyer C, Abalain ML, Credoz L, Chastel C. *Rhodococcus equi* causing bacteremia and pneumonia in a pulmonary transplant patient. J Infect 33:239, 1996.
23. Forbes GM, Harvey FAH, Philpott-Howrd JN, *et al.* Nocardiosis in liver transplantation: variation in presentation, diagnosis and therapy. J Infect 20:11, 1990.
24. Moreno S, Martinez R, Barros C, *et al.* Latent *Haemophilus influenzae* pneumonia in patients infected with HIV. AIDS 5:967, 1991.
25. Schlmm HT, Yancovitz SR. *Haemophilus influenzae* pneumonia in young adults with AIDS. Am J Med 86:11, 1989.
26. Paterson DL, Ko WC, Mohaptra S, *et al.* *Klebsiella pneumoniae* bacteremia: impact of extended spectrum beta-lactamase (ESBL) production in a global study of 216 patients. Abstracts of the 37th Interscience Conference on Antimicrobial Agents and Chemotherapy, Toronto, Canada 1997: Abstract J–210.

27. Fetzer AE, Werner AS, Hagstrom JWC. Pathologic features of Pseudomonal pneumonia. Rev Respir Dis 96:1121, 1967.
28. Singh N, Muder RR, Yu VL, Gayowski T. Legionella infection in liver transplant reciepients: implications for management. Transplantation 15:1549, 1993.
29. Harrington RD, Woolfrey AE, Bowden R, McDowell MG, Hackman RC. Legionellosis in a bone marrow transplant center. Bone Marrow Transplantation 18:361, 1996.
30. Knirsch CA, Jakob K, Schoonmaker D, *et al.* An outbreak of *Legionella micdadei* pneumonia in transplant patients: education, molecular epidemiology, and control. Amer J Med 108:290, 2000.
31. Ebright JR, Tarakji E, Brown WJ, Sunstrum J. Multiple bilateral lung cavities caused by *Legionella pneumophila*: Case report and review. Infect Dis Clin Prac 2:195, 1993.
32. Ognibene FP, Shelhamer JH, Hoffman GS. *Pneumocystis carinii* pneumonia: a major complication of immunosuppressive therapy in patients with Wegener's granulomatosis. Respir Crit Care Med 151:795, 1995.
33. Arend SM, Kroon FP, van't Wout JW. *Pneumocystis carinii* pneumonia in patients without AIDS, 1980 through 1993. Ann Intern Med 155:2436, 1995.
34. Mori M, Galvin Jr, Barloon TJ, Gingrich RD, Stanford W. Fungal pulmonary infections after bone marrow transplantation: evaluation with radiography and CT. Radiology 178:721, 1991.
35. Logan PM, Muller NL. High-resolution computed tomography and pathologic findings in pulmonary aspergillosis: a pictorial easay. Can Assoc Radiol J 47:444, 1996.
36. Calliot D, Casasnovas O, Bernard A, Couaillier JF, Durand C, Cuisenier B, *et al.* Improved management of invasive pulmonary aspergillosis in neutropenic patients using early thoracic computed tomographic scan and surgery. J Clin Oncol 15:139, 1997.
37. Hopwood V, Johnson EM, Cornish JM, Foot ABM, Evans EGV, Warnock DW. Use of the Pastorex *Aspergillus* antigen latex agglutination test for the diagnosis of invasive aspergillosis. J Clin Pathol 48:210, 1995.
38. Guillemain R, Lavarde V, Amrein C, Chevalier P, Guinvarch A, Glotz D. Invasive aspergillosis after transplantation. Transplant Proc 27 1307, 1995.
39. Verweij PE, Stynen D, Rijs AJ, De Pauw BE, Hoogkamp-Korstanje JA, Meis JF. Sandwich enzyme-linked immunosorbent assay compared with Pastorex latex agglutination test for diagnosing invasive aspergillosis in immunocompromised patients. J Clin Microbiol 33:1912, 1995.
40. Severens JL, Donnelly JP, Meis JFGM, De Vries Robbe PF, De Pauw BE, Verweij PE. Two strategies for managing invasive aspergillosis: a decision analysis. Clin Infect Dis 25:1148, 1997.
41. Baughman RP, Rhodes JC, Dohn MN, *et al.* Detection of cryptococcal antigen in bronchoalveolar lavage fluid: a prospective study of diagnostic utility. Am J Respir Dis 145:1226, 1992.
42. Holt CD, Winston DJ, Kubak B, Imagawa DK, Martin P, Goldstein L, *et al.* Coccidioidmycosis in liver transplant patients. J Infect Dis 24:216, 1997.
43. Singh N, Carrigan DR. Human herpesvirus-6 in transplantation: an emerging pathogen. Ann Intern Med 124:1065, 1996.
44. Cone RW, Hackman RC, Huang M-L, *et al.* Human herpesvirus-6 in lung tissue from patients with pneumonitis after bone marrow transplantation. N Engl J Med 329:156, 1993.
45. Chang Y, Cesarman E, Pessin MS, *et al.* Identification of herpesvirus-like DNA sequences in AIDS-associated Kaposi's sarcome. Science 266: 1865, 1994.
46. Cathomas G, Tamm M, McGandy CE, Perruchoud AP, Mihatsch MD, Dalquen P. Detection of herpesvirus-like DNA in the bronchoalveolar lavage fluid of patients with pulmonary Kaposi's sarcoma. Eur Respir J 9:1743, 1996.
47. Whimby E, Champlin RE, Couch RB, *et al.* Community respiratory virus infections among hospitalized adult bone marrow transplant recipients. Clin Infect Dis 22:78, 1996.
48. Yousef HM, Englund J, Couch R, *et al.* Influenza among hospitalized adults with leukemia. Clin Infect Dis 24:1095, 1997.
49. Lewis VA, Champlin RE, Englund J. Respiratory disease due to parainfluenza virus in adult bone marrow transplant recipients. Clin Infect Dis 23:1033, 1996.
50. Sandler ES, Aquino VM, Goss-Shohet E, Hinrichs S, Krisher K. BK papova virus pneumonia following hematopoietic stem cell transplantation. Bone Marrow Transplant 20:163, 1997.
51. Paterson DL, Singh N, Gayowski T, Marino IR. Pulmonary nodules in liver transplant recipients. Medicine 77:50, 1998.
52. Heussel CP, Kauczor HU, Heussel G, Fischer B, Mildenberger P, Thelen M. Early detection of

pneumonia in febrile neutropenic patients: use of thin-section CT. AJR 169:1347, 1997.

53. Oyen WJ, Claessens RA, Raemakers JM, de Paux BE, van der Meer JW, Corstens FH. Diagnosing infection in febrile granulocytopenic patients with indium-111-labeled human immunoglobulin G. J Clin Oncol 10:61, 1992.
54. Kusne S, Torre-Cisneros J, Manez R, Irish W, Martin M, Fung J, *et al.* Factors associated with invasive lung aspergillosis and the significance of positive *Aspergillus* culture after liver transplantation. J Infect Dis 166:1379, 1992.
55. Stout JE, Yu VL. Current concepts: Legionellosis. N Engl J Med 337:682, 1997.
56. Mann M, Shelhamer JH, Masur H, *et al.* Lack of clinical utility of bronchoalveolar lavage cultures for cytomegalovirus in HIV infection. Am J Respir Crit Care Med 155:1723, 1997.
57. Eriksson B-M, Dahl H, Wang F-Z, *et al.* Diagnosis of pulmonary infections in immunocompromised patients by fiber-optic bronchoscopy with bronchoalveolar lavage and serology. Scand J Infect Dis 28:479, 1996.
58. Nieto JMS, Alearez AC. The role of bronchoalveolar lavage in the diagnosis of bacterial pneumonia. Eur J Clin Microbiol Infect Dis 14:839, 1995.
59. Chan CC, Abi-Saleh WJ, Arroliga AC, Stillwell PC, Kirby TJ, Gordon SM, *et al.* Diagnostic yield and therapeutic impact on flexible bronchoscopy in lung transplant recipients. J Heart Lung Transplant 15:196, 1996.
60. Boehler A, Vogt P, Zollinger A, Weder W, Speich R. Prospective study of the value of transbronchial lung biopsy after lung transplantation. Eur Respir J 9:568, 1996.
61. Dijkman JH, van der Meer JW, Bakker W, *et al.* Transpleural lung biopsy by the thoracopic route in patients with diffuse interstitial pulmonary disease. Chest 82:76, 1982.
62. Walsh T, Bodensteiner D, Hiemenz J, *et al.* Liposomal amphotericin B for empirical therapy in patients with persistent fever and neutropenia. N Engl J Med 340:120, 1999.
63. Paterson DL, Singh N. Interactions between tacrolimus and antimicrobial agents. Clin Infect Dis 25:1430, 1997.
64. Singh N, Yu VL, Mieles L, Wagener MM, Miner RC, Gayowski T. High-dose ayclovir compared with short-course preemptive ganciclovir therapy to prevent cytomegalovirus disease in liver transplant recipients, a randomized trial. Ann Intern Med 120:375, 1994.

43. PREVENTION OF VENTILATOR-ASSOCIATED PNEUMONIA

Marin H. Kollef

Introduction

Nosocomial infections add significant costs to individual hospitalizations. They are estimated to involve more than two million patients annually at a cost of more than 4.5 billion dollars [1]. The Centers for Disease Control estimated that an episode of nosocomial pneumonia added 5.9 days to the average hospital stay and $5683 dollars in excess costs [1]. Other estimates put the excess hospital costs associated with nosocomial pneumonia at $4947 with excess hospital stays ranging from 6.8 to 30 days per episode of nosocomial pneumonia or ventilator-associated pneumonia (VAP) [2]. Boyce and colleagues also reported that among 31 of 33 Medicare patients who developed nosocomial pneumonia, hospital costs for the entire admission exceeded reimbursements with a net loss of $5800 per case [3]. Therefore, the occurrence of nosocomial infections, including VAP, are associated with excess medical care costs which may, in part, be preventable.

Antibiotic-resistant nosocomial bacterial infections are an increasingly important subgroup of nosocomial infections associated with prolonged hospitalization and increased health care costs relative to antibiotic-sensitive bacterial infections [4–6]. Recently, a study from Beth Israel Deaconess Medical Center examined 489 inpatients with positive clinical cultures for Pseudomonas aeruginosa [7]. The emergence of antibiotic resistance in infections due to Pseudomonas aeruginosa was independently associated with greater hospital mortality and longer lengths of hospital stay. These authors estimated that the emergence of antibiotic resistance increased hospital charges by $611,981. Other authors have also reported increased medical care costs associated with antibiotic-resistant infections [8]. The overall national costs of antimicrobial resistance have been estimated to be between $100 million and $30 billion annually for the control and treatment of infections caused by antibiotic-resistant bacteria [6, 9]. The increased costs of infection due to antibiotic-resistant bacteria have been attributed to prolonged hospitalizations and higher antibiotic costs [10]. Additionally, the increasing emergence of antibiotic resistance results in the need to develop new antimicrobial agents [11, 12]. The costs required for the development of new antimicrobial agents, including the necessary clinical research to demonstrate their effectiveness and safety, has also increased in the last decade possibly explaining, in part, the slow development of new antimicrobial agents [13, 14].

Nosocomial pneumonia is a leading cause of death from hospital-acquired infections with an associated crude mortality rate of approximately 30% [15]. VAP specifically refers to nosocomial pneumonia developing in mechanically ventilated patients. VAP occurring within 48 to 96 hours of tracheal intubation is usually termed early-onset, often resulting from aspiration complicating the intubation process [16]. VAP occurring after this time period is considered late-onset. Early-onset VAP is most often due to antibiotic-sensitive bacteria including Oxacillin-sensitive *Staphylococcus aureus*, *Haemophilus influenzae,* and *Streptococcus pneumoniae*, while late-onset VAP is frequently caused by antibiotic-resistant pathogens (e.g., Oxacillin-resistant *Staphylococcus aureus*, *Pseudomonas aeruginosa*, *Acinetobacter* species and *Enterobacter* species) [17–19].

The pathogenesis of VAP usually requires the occurrence of two important processes: bacterial colonization of the aerodigestive tract and the aspiration of contaminated secretions into the lower airway [20]. Therefore, the individual strategies aimed at preventing VAP usually attempt to reduce the burden of bacterial colonization within the aerodigestive tract, to decrease the incidence of aspiration, or to accomplish both of these goals. The data describing the excess costs associated with VAP, particularly VAP attributed to antibiotic-resistant bacteria, suggests that infection control activities aimed at the prevention of this nosocomial infection could be cost effective in addition to potentially reducing patient morbidity.

Risk Factors and Treatment of VAP

The need for invasive medical devices during mechanical ventilation are important contributors to the pathogenesis and development of VAP. Many patients have nasogastric tubes in place which predispose to gastric reflux and increase the potential for aspiration to occur. Additionally, endotracheal tubes facilitate bacterial colonization of the tracheobronchial tree, as well as lower airway aspiration of contaminated secretions, due to associated mucosal injury, pooling of contaminated secretions above the endotracheal tube cuff, and elimination of the cough reflex [20]. The ventilator circuit and respiratory therapy equipment may also contribute to the pathogenesis of VAP when they become contaminated with bacteria which usually originate from the patient's secretions [20, 21].

The risk of VAP appears to be higher in patients with chronic lung disease and the acute respiratory distress syndrome, and as the duration of mechanical ventilation increases [22]. Manipulation of the airway and/or ventilator circuit may predispose to aspiration and subsequent VAP, as suggested by the following risk factors: reintubation, tracheostomy, frequent ventilator circuit changes, low intracuff pressure of endotracheal tubes, failed subglottic suctioning, and patient transport out of the ICU [22]. Other risk factors also emphasize the role of the gastrointestinal tract in the development of VAP, such as presence of a nasogastric tube, enteral feeding, supine positioning, witnessed aspiration, and stress ulcer prophylaxis with gastric pH-altering agents [22]. Antibiotic administration has been associated with both an increased and decreased risk of VAP [23, 24]. However, a recent study suggests that the prior administration of broad-spectrum antibiotics, particularly in patients requiring prolonged mechanical ventilation, is an important independent risk factor for VAP due to antibiotic-resistant bacteria [25].

Once VAP occurs, treatment is usually supportive along with the administration of antibiotics. Several studies have suggested that the attributable mortality of VAP, particularly late-onset infection due to antibiotic-resistant pathogens, is greater than 10% [18, 26, 27]. However, other investigations have not found an excess mortality while controlling for confounding factors [28]. More recently, the importance of adequate initial antibiotic treatment for this infection has become recognized and might influence the estimates of attributable mortality [29–32]. These studies suggest that patients with suspected VAP should initially be treated with a broad-spectrum antibiotic regimen aimed at covering all likely bacterial pathogens. This regimen should subsequently be narrowed based on the respiratory culture results and the bacterial antibiotic sensitivity profiles [32]. In addition to potentially increasing hospital mortality rates, the occurrence of VAP, especially VAP due to antibiotic-resistant bacteria, is associated with prolonged hospitalization and increased medical care costs which supports the need for dedicated prevention efforts [20, 28].

VAP Prevention Strategies

Clinicians caring for mechanically ventilated patients should participate in focused programs aimed at the prevention of VAP as well as other nosocomial infections. A VAP prevention program should incorporate readily available methods whose efficacy and cost-effectiveness are supported by clinical studies, local experience, and the input of experts in this field [21, 23]. Additionally, such efforts should be tailored to the characteristics and resource availability of individual hospitals in order to increase the likelihood of their acceptance and success. Several resources are available to assist in the development of this type of prevention program [21, 33–38]. The following clinical recommendations are presented to serve as a guide for the development of a VAP prevention program.

USE OF A QUALITY IMPROVEMENT TEAM OR PROTOCOL

The application of systematic efforts aimed at improving patient outcomes and the efficiency of the medical care provided to them, by identifying and implementing best available medical practices, is at the heart of the improvement process [39]. This usually requires measurement of a clinical outcome (e.g., occurrence of VAP) prior to and during the application of the improvement initiative aimed at that outcome [40]. Several clinical trials, and real world examples, have demonstrated the potential for practice guidelines to reduce the rates of VAP in the ICU setting [35–38, 41]. In addition to reducing infection rates, substantial cost savings were associated with the use of these guidelines which employed readily available infection control strategies for the prevention of VAP.

The duration of mechanical ventilation has been shown to be an important risk factor for the development of VAP, especially VAP due to antibiotic-resistant bacteria [22, 25]. Therefore, efforts aimed at reducing the duration of ventilatory assistance could also decrease the incidence of VAP. Unfortunately, specific clinical trials evaluating this preventive strategy have not been performed. Nevertheless, several clinical investigations have demonstrated the ability of weaning teams and protocol guidelines to reduce the length of mechanical ventilation compared to standard medical practices [41–43]. Similarly, the application of noninvasive mask positive pressure ventilation has been demonstrated to reduce the occurrence of VAP when systematically substituted for conventional mechanical ventilation with tracheal intubation [44–46]. Such efforts should probably be included in prevention guidelines developed for VAP. Additionally, animal data suggests that a strategy of mechanical ventilation which over distends the lung may result in iatrogenic lung injury predisposing to the development of nosocomial pneumonia with resultant blood borne dissemination of the infection [47]. These data lend support to the use of protocols aimed at providing mechanical ventilation which does not result in lung unit overdistension [48]

EFFECTIVE HAND WASHING, PROTECTIVE GOWNS, AND GLOVES

Hand washing is widely recognized as an important but underutilized measure for the prevention of nosocomial infections [49]. Unfortunately, increased numbers of patient contacts, as occurs in a busy ICU, can erode the efficiency with which hand washing occurs [50]. Therefore, alternative handwashing methods such as the use of alcohol foams or gels may improve handwashing compliance due to shorter durations of time needed for handwashing [51]. Failure of strict hand washing techniques, in combination with other infection control measures, to control an outbreak of ventilator-associated pneumonia attributed to a specific high-risk pathogen should suggest the presence of contaminated respiratory therapy equipment or aerosol solutions. The use of protective gowns and gloves has also been shown to reduce the rate of acquired nosocomial infections in pediatric populations [52]. However, their use appears to be most effective when directed at specific antibiotic-resistant pathogens, such as Vancomycin-resistant enterococci. Therefore, the routine use of protective gowns and gloves may not be cost-effective for the prevention of VAP. Gloves, and possibly gowns, should be worn when the risk of skin contamination is great such as during the removal of condensate from ventilator circuits.

SEMIRECUMBENT POSITIONING

Aspiration of upper airway secretions is a common event even in normal healthy adults. Positioning of mechanically ventilated patients in the semirecumbent position should be employed in all VAP prevention programs in order to reduce the occurrence of aspiration [53]. Additionally, measures aimed at reducing unplanned extubations (e.g., appropriate use of physical and chemical restraints, securing of the endotracheal tube to the patient) and reducing the need for subsequent reintubation performed in the supine position may also be beneficial [54].

AVOIDANCE OF LARGE GASTRIC VOLUMES

Although ventilator-associated pneumonia is commonly due to the aspiration of contaminated secretions into the lower airway, the origin of these infected inocula can be variable [20]. The stomach, upper airway, teeth, artificial airway, ventilator circuit condensate, and nasal sinuses have all been implicated as potential sources of origin for aspirated secretions. Unfortunately, the relative importance of these sites as a source for the causative agents of pneumonia, particularly the stomach, is not precisely known resulting in considerable controversy [55]. This is an important issue since providing adequate nutritional support to ventilated patients is also thought to prevent the occurrence of VAP [56]. Therefore, it seems reasonable to administer nutritional support in a manner which minimizes patient risks for bacterial colonization of the aerodigestive tract and subsequent aspiration. Gastric over distention should be avoided by reducing the use of narcotics and anticholinergic agents, monitoring gastric residual volumes following intragastric feedings, using gastrointestinal motility agents (e.g., metoclopramide), and when deemed necessary supplying enteral nutrition with smaller bore feeding tubes directly into the small bowel instead of the stomach. However, the effectiveness of such interventions await validation in clinical trials.

ORAL (NON-NASAL) INTUBATION

Prolonged nasal intubation (i.e., greater than 48 hours) should be avoided due to the association between the occurrence of nosocomial sinusitis and VAP [57]. Nosocomial sinusitis may predispose to the development of pneumonia via the aspiration of infected secretions from the nasal sinuses. Therefore, the preferred route of intubation should be the oropharynx. Additionally, nasal intubation may be associated with a greater need for antibiotics which can further increase medical care costs [58].

ROUTINE MAINTENANCE OF VENTILATOR CIRCUITS

Several clinical studies have demonstrated no benefit from routinely changing ventilator circuit tubing or any of their subcomponents (e.g., in-line suction catheters) [59, 60]. In large part, this appears to be due to the rapid bacterial colonization of this tubing, usually within 24 hours of its placement. Nevertheless, ventilator circuits will occasionally require replacement due to overt soilage (e.g., emesis, blood) or mechanical malfunction. Additionally, regular monitoring of ventilator circuits for the removal of accumulated tubing condensate should always be performed for the prevention of ventilator-associated pneumonia [61]. This is due to the high concentration of pathogenic bacteria found in condensate fluid which if aspirated may result in pneumonia. This condensate can also serve as a reservoir for the spread of nosocomial pathogens to other patients.

CONTINUOUS SUBGLOTTIC SUCTIONING

Several lines of investigation have suggested that secretions pooling above inflated endotracheal tube cuffs may be a source of aspirated material resulting in VAP. Endotracheal tubes manufactured with a separate dorsal lumen above the endotracheal tube cuff, in order to suction pooled secretions in the subglottic space, are now available for clinical use [62, 63]. Additionally, endotracheal tube cuff pressures should be adequately maintained to prevent the leakage of colonized subglottic secretions into the lower airway [64].

HUMIDIFICATION WITH HEAT AND MOISTURE EXCHANGERS

Heat and moisture exchangers are attractive alternatives to heated water humidification systems because of their passive operation (i.e., they do not require electricity or active heating elements) and their lower costs More recent improvements in the performance characteristics of heat and moisture exchangers have resulted in the development of safe and easily applied devices. In theory, heat and moisture exchangers should reduce the occurrence of VAP by minimizing the development of condensate within ventilator circuits [65]. However, they should primarily be considered a cost-effective alternative for providing humidification to ventilated patients when contraindications to their use are not present (e.g., hemoptysis, copious or tenacious secretions, difficulty weaning from mechanical ventilation due to increased airway resistance). Moreover, certain heat and moisture exchangers can be safely left in place for up to one week, further increasing their cost effectiveness relative to heated water humidification [66, 67].

POSTURAL OSCILLATION/ROTATION/ CHEST PHYSIOTHERAPY

It has long been appreciated that among patients confined to bed there is an increased frequency of pulmonary and nonpulmonary complications. Kinetic therapy (i.e., patient movement achieved with specialized beds medical devices) is hypothesized to be beneficial for the prevention of VAP by improving the drainage of pulmonary secretions. However, the added expense of such therapy and its lack of demonstrated effectiveness precludes recommending its routine use [21]. Similarly, the routine use of chest physiotherapy for the prevention of VAP should be avoided due to its lack of efficacy and associated risks (e.g., arterial oxygen desaturation) [68].

STRESS ULCER PROPHYLAXIS

Mechanically ventilated patients are at high-risk for upper gastrointestinal hemorrhage due to stress ulcer formation and thus require preventive therapy for this potential complication [69]. The importance of gastric pH in the pathogenesis of VAP is controversial. Bacterial colonization of the stomach, enhanced by the administration of pH altering drugs (e.g., histamine type-2 receptor antagonists and antacids), is thought to be an important source of pneumonia pathogens [20]. Sucralfate administration into the stomach has been demonstrated to prevent stress ulcer bleeding without lowering gastric pH. Several randomized trials have shown sucralfate to be associated with lower rates of VAP compared to the use of antacids or histamine type-2 receptor antagonists [70]. The choice of agent for stress ulcer prophylaxis should depend on patient factors (e.g., presence or absence of a nasogastric tube), the potential for unwanted drug interactions, and the local costs associated with providing the various forms of therapy [71].

ANTIBIOTIC ADMINISTRATION

Colonization of the lower respiratory tract by antibiotic-resistant organisms such as Pseudomonas aeruginosa and Oxacillin-resistant

Staphylococcus aureus has been shown to be closely correlated with the subsequent development of overt pneumonia [72, 73]. In an attempt to reverse the trend of increasing antimicrobial resistance among hospital-acquired infections, more effective antibiotic utilization strategies have been advocated which restrict antibiotic use or offer practice guidelines for their administration [34, 74]. Changing or rotating the use of antibiotic classes for the treatment of suspected bacterial infections (i.e., avoiding the use of a single class of antimicrobial agents in an ICU) may also be effective at reducing the rates of nosocomial pneumonia due to antibiotic-resistant pathogens [75, 76]. However, the elimination or reduction of the unnecessary use of antibiotics should be seen as the primary goal in preventing antibiotic-resistant nosocomial infections [34].

PROPHYLACTIC ANTIBIOTIC THERAPY

The use of aerosolized antibiotics for the prevention of VAP has been abandoned due to its lack of efficacy and the subsequent emergence of antibiotic-resistant infections [21]. Similarly, the routine use of selective digestive decontamination, with nonabsorbable antibiotics applied to the orodigestive tract, has not gained acceptance in the United States due to its lack of demonstrated impact on mortality, the emergence of antibiotic-resistant infections, and additional toxicity [77]. A recent metaanalysis of selective digestive decontamination did not demonstrate a survival advantage for selective digestive decontamination as compared with parenteral antibiotic prophylaxis which is commonly administered in the perioperative period [78]. Therefore, a definitive recommendation cannot be made on the cost effectiveness of routine selective digestive decontamination for the prevention of VAP.

The routine use of broad-spectrum parenteral antibiotics for the prevention of VAP also cannot be recommended at the present time due to concerns over increasing antibiotic resistance among subsequent hospital-acquired infections [25, 79]. Nevertheless, one recent investigation suggests that the administration of such therapy to patients with coma may reduce the incidence of VAP [80]. Further investigations are required to determine the general applicability of this observation. At present, antibiotics directed against specific infections for patients requiring mechanical ventilation may protect against the development of VAP [24].

CHLORHEXIDINE ORAL RINSE

Chlorhexidine is an antiseptic solution used by dentists since 1959 for the control of dental plaques. Bacteria accumulating in dental plaques have been implicated as a source of pathogens for VAP. Chlorhexidine has been shown to be effective in the control of ventilator circuit colonization and pneumonia due to antibiotic-resistant bacteria [81]. The use of oropharyngeal decontamination with chlorhexidine solution has also been shown to reduce the occurrence of VAP in patients undergoing cardiac surgery [82]. Preventative oral washes with chlorhexidine seems reasonable in selected high-risk patients given its ease of administration. However, overuse could result in patient colonization and superinfection with chlorhexidine-resistant pathogens [83].

VACCINES

Various vaccination programs in adults and children have been demonstrated to be successful in reducing the incidence of pneumonia due to specific pathogens including Haemophilus influenza type b strains, Streptococcus pneumoniae, and the influenza virus [84–86]. It would be expected that vaccination against infection with these pathogens may also prevent some hospital-acquired infections as well. Indeed, the difference between nosocomial and community-acquired infections is becoming "grayer", particularly in the era of managed care where patients with acute and chronic illnesses are often medically managed outside of the hospital setting. Therefore, pneumococcal vaccination and if indicated, influenza vaccination should be considered prior to hospital discharge or included in the discharge planning of all patients at risk for subsequent respiratory infections, including VAP.

Summary

The prevention of VAP appears to be a cost effective endeavor based on the healthcare costs and morbidity associated with this nosocomial infection. Infection control measures should be integrated into a systematic program for general application to all patients requiring mechanical ventilation at a particular hospital [36, 37]. Additionally, attention needs to be focused on the emergence of antibiotic-resistant bacterial infections in the ICU setting [87, 88]. The prevention of antibiotic-resistant bacterial infections should result in fewer overall nosocomial infections including VAP [75]. At present, VAP prevention programs should employ practices which are readily accepted by local practitioners, safe for patients, and associated with acceptable costs to the institution.

References

1. Public health focus: Surveillance, prevention, and control of nosocomial infections. MMWR 41:783, 1992.
2. Jarvis WR. Selected aspects of the socioeconomic impact of nosocomial infections: morbidity, mortality, cost, and prevention. Infect Control Hosp Epidemiol 17:552, 1996.
3. Boyce JM, Potter-Bynoe G, Dziobek L, Solomon SL. Nosocomial pneumonia in Medicare patients. Hospital costs and reimbursement patterns under the prospective payment system. Arch Intern Med 151:1109, 1991.
4. Ascar JF. Consequences of bacterial resistance to antibiotics in medical practice. Clin Infect Dis 24:S17, 1997.
5. Cohen ML. Epidemiology of drug resistance: implications for a post-antimicrobial era. Science 257:1050, 1992.
6. Impacts of antibiotic-resistant bacteria: Thanks to Penicillin – He will home! Washington, DC; Office of Technology Assessment, Congress; 1995. Publication OTC-H-629.
7. Carmeli Y, Truillet N, Karchmer AW, Somore MH. Health and economic outcomes of antibiotic resistance in *Pseudomonas aeruginosa*. Arch Intern Med 159:1127, 1999.
8. Holemberg SD, Solomon SL, Blake PA. Health and economic impact of antimicrobial resistance. Rev Infect Dis 9:1065, 1987.
9. Phelps CE. Bug-drug resistance: Sometimes less is more. Med Care 27:194, 1989.
10. Einarsson S, Kristjansson M, Kristinsson KG, Kjartansson G, Jonsson S. Pneumonia caused by penicillin-non-susceptible and penicillin-susceptible pneumococci in adults: a case-control study. Scand J Infect Dis 30:253, 1998.
11. Moellering RC. A novel antimicrobial agent joins the battle against resistant bacteria. Ann Intern Med 130:155, 1999.
12. Hancock RE. The role of fundamental research and biotechnology in finding solutions to the global problem of antibiotic resistance. Clin Infect Dis 24:S148, 1997.
13. Bax RP. Antibiotic resistance: A view from the pharmaceutical industry. Clin Infect Dis 24:S151, 1997.
14. Jones RN. The emergent needs for basic research, education, and surveillance of antimicrobial resistance. Problems facing the report from the American Society for Microbiology Task Force on Antibiotic Resistance. Diag Microbiol Infect Dis 25:153, 1996.
15. Leu HS, Kaiser DL, Mori M, Woolson RF, Wenzel RP. Hospital-acquired pneumonia. Attributable mortality and morbidity. Am J Epidemiol 129:1258, 1989.
16. Pingleton SK, Fagon JY, Leeper KV Jr. Patient selection for clinical investigation of ventilator-associated pneumonia. Criteria for evaluating diagnostic techniques. Chest 102:553S, 1992.
17. Niederman MS, Craven DE, Fein AM, Schultz DE. Pneumonia in the critically ill hospitalized patient. Chest 97:170, 1990.
18. Kollef MH, Silver P, Murphy DM, Trovillion E. The effect of late-onset ventilator-associated pneumonia in determining patient mortality. Chest 108:1655, 1995.
19. Rello J, Ausina V, Ricart M, Castella J, Prats G. Impact of previous antimicrobial therapy on the etiology and outcome of ventilator-associated pneumonia. Chest 104:1230, 1993.
20. Craven DE, Steger KA. Epidemiology of nosocomial pneumonia. New perspectives on an old disease. Chest 108:1S, 1995.
21. Tablan OC, Anderson LJ, Arden NH, Breiman RF, Butler JC, McNeil MM. Guideline for

prevention of nosocomial pneumonia. The Hospital Infection Control Practices Advisory committee, Centers for Disease Control and Prevention. Infect Control Hosp Epidemiol 15:587, 1994.

22. Cook DJ, Kollef MH. Risk factors for ICU-acquired pneumonia. JAMA 279:1605, 1998.
23. Kollef MH. Ventilator-associated pneumonia: a multivariate analysis. JAMA 270:1965, 1993.
24. Cook DJ, Walter SD, Cook RJ, Griffith LE, Guyatt GH, Leasa D, Jaeschke RZ, Brun-Buison C. Incidence and risk factors for ventilator-associated pneumonia in critically ill patients. Ann Intern Med 129:433, 1998.
25. Trouillet JL, Chastre J, Vuagnat A, Joly-Guillou ML, Combaux D, Dombret MC, Gibert C. Ventilator-associated pneumonia caused by potentially drug-resistant bacteria. Am J Respir Crit Care Med 157:531, 1998.
26. Fagon JY, Chastre J, Hance AJ, Montravers P, Novara A, Gibert C. Nosocomial pneumonia in ventilated patients: a cohort study evaluating attributable mortality and hospital stay. Am J Med 94:281, 1993.
27. Brewer SC, Wunderink RG, Jones CB, Leeper KV Jr. Ventilator-associated pneumonia due to Pseudomonas aeruginosa. Chest 109:1019, 1996.
28. Papazian L, Bregeon F, Thirion X, Gregoire R, Saux P, Denis JP, Perin G, Charrel J, Dumon JF, Affray JP, Gouin F. Effect of ventilator-associated pneumonia on mortality and morbidity. Am J Respir Crit Care Med 154:91, 1996.
29. Rello J, Gallego M, Mariscal D, Soñora R, Valles J. The value of routine microbial investigation in ventilator-associated pneumonia. Am J Respir Crit Care Med 156:196, 1997.
30. Luna CM, Vujacich P, Niederman MS, Vay C, Gherardi C, Matera J, Jolly EC. Impact of BAL data on the therapy and outcome of ventilator-associated pneumonia. Chest 111:676, 1997.
31. Kollef MH, Ward S. The influence of mini-BAL cultures on patient outcomes: implications for the antibiotic management of ventilator-associated pneumonia. Chest 113:412, 1998.
32. Kollef MH, Sherman G, Ward S, Fraser VJ. Inadequate antimicrobial treatment of infections: A risk factor for hospital mortality among critically ill patients. Chest 115:462, 1999.
33. Kollef MH. The prevention of ventilator-associated pneumonia. N Engl J Med 340:627, 1999.
34. Goldmann DA, Weinstein RA, Wenzel RP, Tablan OC, Duma RJ, Gaynes RP, Schlosser J, Martone WJ. Strategies to prevent and control the emergence and spread of antimicrobial-resistant microorganisms in hospitals. A challenge to hospital leadership. JAMA 275:234, 1996.
35. Boyce JM, White RL, Spruill EY, Wall M. Cost-effective application of the Centers for Disease Control Guideline for Prevention of Nosocomial Pneumonia. Am J Infect Control 13:228, 1985.
36. Joiner GA, Salisbury D, Bollin GE. Utilizing quality assurance as a tool for reducing the risk of nosocomial ventilator-associated pneumonia. Am J Medical Quality 11:100, 1996.
37. Kelleghan SI, Salemi C, Padilla S, McCord M, Mermilliod G, Canola T, Becker L. An effective continuous quality improvement approach to the prevention of ventilator-associated pneumonia. Am J Infect Control 21:322, 1993.
38. Gaynes RP, Solomon S. Improving hospital-acquired infection rates: the CDC experience. Joint Commission Journal on Quality Improvement 22:457, 1996.
39. Berwick DM. Continuous improvement as an idea in healthcare. N Engl J Med 320:53, 1989.
40. Booth FV. ABCs of quality assurance. Crit Care Clin 9:477, 1993.
41. Kollef MH, Horst HM, Prang L, Brock WA. Reducing the duration of mechanical ventilation: Three examples of change in the intensive care unit. New Horizons 6:52, 1998.
42. Ely EW, Baker AM, Dunagan DP, Burke HL, Smith AC, Kelley PT, Johnson MM, Browder RW, Bowton DL, Haponik EF. Effect on the duration of mechanical ventilation of identifying patients capable of breathing spontaneously. N Engl J Med 335:1864, 1996.
43. Kollef MH, Shapiro SD, Silver P, St. John RE, Prentice D, Sauer S, Ahrens TS, Shannon W, Baker-Clinkscale D. A randomized, controlled trial of protocol-directed versus physician-directed weaning from mechanical ventilation. Crit Care Med 25:567, 1997.
44. Nava S, Ambrosino N, Clini E, Prato M, Orlando G, Vitacca M, Brigada P, Fracchia C, Rubini F. Noninvasive mechanical ventilation in the weaning of patients with respiratory failure due to chronic obstructive pulmonary disease. A randomized, controlled trial. Ann Intern Med 128:721, 1998.
45. Antonelli M, Conti G, Rocco M, Bufi M, Deblasi RA, Vivino G, Gasparetto A, Meduri GV. A comparison of noninvasive positive-pressure ventilation and conventional mechanical ventilation in patients with acute respiratory failure. N Engl J Med 339:429, 1998.

46. Nourdine K, Combes P, Carton MJ, Beuret P, Cannamela A, Ducreux JC. Does noninvasive ventilation reduce the ICU nosocomial infection risk? A prospective clinical survey. Intensive Care Med 25:567, 1999.
47. Nahum A, Hoyt J, Schmitz L, Schmitz L, Moody J, Shapiro R, Marini JJ. Effect of mechanical ventilation strategy on dissemination of intratracheally instilled *Escherichia coli* in dogs. Crit Care Med 25:1733, 1997.
48. Amato MB, Barbas CS, Medeiros DM, Magaldi RB, Schettino GP, Lorenzi-Filho G, Kairalla RA, Deheinzelin D, Munoz C, Oliveira R, Takagaki TY, Carvalho CR. Effect of a protective-ventilation strategy on mortality in the acute respiratory distress syndrome. N Engl J Med 338:347, 1998.
49. Doebbeling BN, Stanley GL, Sheetz CT, Pfaller MA, Houston AK, Annis L, Li N, Wenzel RP. Comparative efficacy of alternative hand-washing agents in reducing nosocomial infections in intensive care units. N Engl J Med 327:88, 1992.
50. Pittet D, Mourouga P, Perneger TV, and the Members of the Infection Control Program. Compliance with handwashing in a teaching hospital. Ann Intern Med 130:126, 1999.
51. Pereira LJ, Lee GM, Wade KJ. An evaluation of five protocols for surgical handwashing in relation to skin condition and microbial counts. J Hosp Infect 36:49, 1997.
52. Klein BS, Perloff WH, Maki DG. Reduction of nosocomial infection during pediatric intensive care by protective isolation. N Engl J Med 320:1714, 1989.
53. Torres A, Serra-Batlles J, Ros E, Piera C, Puig de la Bellacasa J, Cobos A, Lomena F, Rodriguez-Roisin R. Pulmonary aspiration of gastric contents in patients receiving mechanical ventilation: the effect of body position. Ann Intern Med 116:540, 1992.
54. Torres A, Gatell JM, Aznar E, el-Ebiary M, Puig de la Bellacasa J, Gonzalez J, Ferrer M, Rodriguez-Roisin R. Re-intubation increases the risk of nosocomial pneumonia in patients needing mechanical ventilation. Am J Respir Crit Care Med 152:137, 1995.
55. Niederman MS, Craven DE. Devising strategies for preventing nosocomial pneumonia – should we ignore the stomach? Clin Infect Dis 24:320, 1997.
56. Niederman MS, Mantovani R, Schoch P, Papas, J, Fein AM. Patterns and routes of tracheobronchial colonization in mechanically ventilated patients. The role of nutritional status in colonization of the lower airway by *Pseudomonas* species. Chest 95:155, 1989.
57. Rouby JJ, Laurent P, Gosnach M, Cambau E, Lamas G, Zouaoui A, Leguillou JL, Bodin L, Khac TD, Marsault C. Risk factors and clinical relevance of nosocomial maxillary sinusitis in the critically ill. Am J Respir Crit Care Med 150:776, 1994.
58. Holzapfel L, Chastang C, Demingeon G, Bohe J, Piralla B, Coupry A. A randomized study assessing the systematic search for maxillary sinusitis in nasotracheally mechanically ventilated patients. Influence of nosocomial maxillary sinusitis on the occurrence of ventilator-associated pneumonia. Am J Respir Crit Care Med 159:695, 1999.
59. Kollef MH. Prolonged use of ventilator circuits and ventilator-associated pneumonia. A model for identifying the optimal clinical practice. Chest 113:267, 1998.
60. Kollef MH, Prentice D, Shapiro SD, Fraser VJ, Silver P, Trovillion E, Weilitz P, von Harz B, St. John R. Mechanical ventilation with or without daily changes of in-line suction catheters. Am J Respir Crit Care Med 156:466, 1997
61. Craven DE, Goularte TA, Make BJ. Contaminated condensate in mechanical ventilator circuits. A risk factor for nosocomial pneumonia. Am Rev Respir Dis 129:625, 1984.
62. Valles J, Artigas A, Rello J, Bonsoms N, Fontanals D, Blanch L, Fernandez R, Baigorri F, Mestre J. Continuous aspiration of subglottic secretions in preventing ventilator-associated pneumonia. Ann Intern Med 122:179, 1995.
63. Kollef MH, Skubas NJ, Sundt TM. A randomized clinical trial of continuous aspiration of subglottic secretions in cardiac surgery patients. Chest 116:1339, 1999.
64. Rello J, Soñora R, Jubert P, Artigas A, Rue M, Valles J. Pneumonia in intubated patients: role of respiratory airway care. Am J Respir Crit Care Med 154:111, 1996.
65. Kirton OC, DeHaven B, Morgan J, Morejon O, Civetta J. A prospective randomized comparison of an in-line heat moisture exchange filter and heated wire humidifiers: rates of ventilator-associated early-onset (community-acquired) or late-onset (hospital acquired) pneumonia and incidence of endotracheal tube occlusion. Chest 112:1055, 1997.
66. Kollef MH, Shapiro SD, Boyd V, Silver P, Von Harz B, Trovillion E, Prentice D. A randomized clinical trial comparing an extended-use hygro-

scopic condenser humidifier to heated water humidification in mechanically ventilated patients. Chest 113:759, 1998.

67. Djedaini K, Billiard M, Mier L, Le Bourdelles G, Brun P, Markowicz P, Estagnasie P, Coste F, Boussougant Y, Dreyfuss D. Changing heat and moisture exchangers every 48 hours rather than 24 hours does not affect their efficacy and the incidence of nosocomial pneumonia. Am J Respir Crit Care Med 152:1562, 1995.
68. Hall JC, Tarala RA, Tapper J, Hall JL. Prevention of respiratory complications after abdominal surgery: a randomized clinical trial. BMJ 312:148, 1996.
69. Cook DJ, Fuller HD, Guyatt GH, Marshall JC, Leasa D, Hall R. Risk factors for gastrointestinal bleeding in critically ill patients. Canadian Critical Care Trials Group. N Engl J Med 330:377, 1994.
70. Cook DJ, Reeve BK, Guyatt GH, Heyland DK, Griffith LE, Buckingham L, Tryba M. Stress ulcer prophylaxis in critically ill patients. Resolving discordant meta-analysis. JAMA 275:308, 1996.
71. Cook D, Guyatt G, Marshall J, Leasa D, Fuller H, Hall R, Peters S, Rutledge F, Griffith L, McLellan A, Wood G, Kirby A. A comparison of sucralfate and ranitidine for the prevention of upper gastrointestinal bleeding in patients requiring mechanical ventilation. Canadian Critical Care Trials Group. N Engl J Med 338:791, 1998.
72. Johanson WG Jr, Pierce AK, Sandford JP, Thomas GD. Nosocomial respiratory infections with gram-negative bacilli. The significance of colonization of the respiratory tracet. Ann Intern Med 77:701, 1972.
73. Garrouste-Orgeas M, Chevret S, Arlet G, Marie O, Rouveau M, Popoff N, Schlemmer B. Oropharyngeal or gastric colonization and nosocomial pneumonia in adult intensive care unit patients. A prospective study based on genomic DNA analysis. Am J Respir Crit Care Med 156:1647, 1997.
74. Evans RS, Pestotnik SL, Classen DC, Clemmer TP, Weaver LK, Orme JF, Lloyd JF, Burke JP. A computer-assisted management program for antibiotics and other antiinfective agents. N Engl J Med 338:232, 1998.
75. Kollef MH, Vlasnik J, Sharpless L, Pasque C, Murphy D, Fraser V. Scheduled change of antibiotic classes: a strategy to decrease the incidence of ventilator-associated pneumonia. Am J Respir Crit Care Med 156:1040, 1997.
76. Rahal JJ, Urban C, Horn D, Freeman K, Segal-Maurer S, Maurer J, Mariano N, Marks S, Burns JM, Dominick D, Lim M. Class restriction of cephalosporin use to control total cephalosporin resistance in nosocomial Klebsiella. JAMA 280:1233, 1998.
77. Gastinne H, Wolff M, Delatour F, Faurisson F, Chevret S. A controlled trial in intensive care units of selective decontamination of the digestive tract with nonabsorbable antibiotics. The French Study Group of Selective Decontamination of the Digestive Tract. N Engl J Med 326:594, 1992.
78. D'Amico R, Pifferi S, Leonetti C, Torri V, Tinazzi A, Liberati A. Effectiveness of antibiotic prophylaxis in critically ill adult patients: systematic review of randomized controlled trials. BMJ 316:1275, 1998.
79. Tenover FC, McGowan JE Jr. Reasons for the emergence of antibiotic resistance. Am J Med Sci 311:9, 1996.
80. Sirvent JM, Torres A, El-Ebiary M, Castro P, de Batlle J, Bonet A. Protective effect of intravenously administered cefuroxime against nosocomial pneumonia in patients with structural coma. Am J Respir Crit Care Med 155:1729, 1997.
81. Rumbak MJ, Cancio MR. Significant reduction in methicillin-resistant Staphylococcus aureus ventilator-associated pneumonia associated with the institution of a prevention protocol. Crit Care Med 23:1200, 1995.
82. DeRiso AJ II, Ladowski JS, Dillon TA, Justice JW, Peterson AC. Chlorhexidine gluconate 0.12% oral rinse reduces the incidence of total nosocomial respiratory infection and nonprophylactic systemic antibiotic use in patients undergoing heart surgery. Chest 109:1556, 1996.
83. Russell AD. Plasmids and bacterial resistance to biocides. J Appl Microbiol 83:155, 1997.
84. Herceg A. The decline of Haemophilus influenza type b disease in Australia. Communicable Dis Intell 21:173, 1997.
85. Gross PA, Hermogenes AW, Sacks HS, Lau J, Levandowoski RA. The efficacy of influenza vaccine in elderly persons. A meta-analysis and review of the literature. Ann Intern Med 123:518, 1995.
86. Nuorti JP, Butler JC, Crutcher JM, Guevara R, Welch D, Holder P, *et al*. An outbreak of multidrug-resistant pneumococcal pneumonia and bacteremia among unvaccinated nursing

home residents. N Engl J Med 338:1861, 1998.

87. Richards MJ, Edwards JR, Culver DH, Gaynes RP. Nosocomial infections in medical intensive care units in the United States. Crit Care Med 27:887, 1999.

88. Hanberger H, Garcia-Rodriguez JA, Gobernado M, Goossens H, Nilsson LE, Struelens MJ. Antibiotic susceptibility among aerobic gram-negative bacilli in intensive care units in 5 European Countries. JAMA 281:67, 1999.

SECTION 7: INFECTIONS OF THE DIGESTIVE, URINARY TRACT AND PELVIS

M. Kollef

44. ANTIBIOTIC INDUCED DIARRHEA

Omar J. Pérez Jiménez

Abstract

Antibiotic induced diarrhea is a spectrum of diseases compromising from asymptomatic colonization with *Clostridium difficile* to fulminant colitis. This chapter will cover the clinical presentation of antibiotic induced diarrhea with special attention to the critically ill patient. The pathophysiology, epidemiology and diagnosis will be reviewed. Treatment options including the treatment of relapsers will be covered.

Introduction

Antibiotic-induced diarrhea is a spectrum of diseases compromising from asymptomatic colonization with *Clostridium difficile* to fulminant colitis. The most common expression of this disease complex is antibiotic induced diarrhea without colitis. This chapter will cover the clinical and epidemiological manifestations of pseudomembranous colitis with special attention to the critically ill patient. Other causes of antibiotic induced diarrhea will be reviewed briefly.

Pseudomembranous colitis was initially described by Finney at the end of the nineteenth century [1]. The case was a 22 year old female with a gastric tumor who underwent resection, post-operatively the patient developed severe diarrhea. Post mortem examination showed the presence of a diphteric membrane in the small bowel [1]. With the advent of antibiotics a surge in cases of nosocomial diarrhea was noted. Even with only the use of antibiotic prophilaxis there is a rate of diarrhea of 14–27% [2, 3]. Earlier microbiological studies revealed the presence of *Staphylococcus aureus* in some patients and the fact that treatment with oral vancomycin improved the diarrhea supported the theory of *Staphylococcus aureus* as the etiologic agent.

In the 1950s the relationship of antibiotic use and the development of a syndrome of fever, diarrhea and colitis was clearly established. Anatomic studies specially in patients that received antibiotic prophylaxis prior to surgery show the presence of *Staphylococcus aureus*. This findings based on Gram's stain and stool culture. In 1970 a group from Barnes Hospital in Saint Louis performed the first prospective study of Clindamycin associated diarrhea. Ten per cent of the patients showed the presence of pseudomembranes in the colon at endoscopy [4]. *Staphylococcus aureus* was not isolated in any of these patients. Further studies on stool samples in the same group showed the presence of *C. difficile* and its cytopathic toxin in patients with colitis.

Several animal studies using rodents have shown that treatment with penicillin induced fulminant colitis. In 1974, while looking at the role of viruses in a guinea pig model of antibiotic induced diarrhea Green noted cytopathic changes in tissue cultured cells. This is probably the first report of the effect of *C. difficile* toxin in the literature [5]. Earlier reports noted that *C. difficile* produce a toxin that was lethal to guinea pigs and rabbits and that most strains of this bacteria produce this toxin. Attention was shifted to these bacteria and in 1977 the relationship between colitis, toxin and *C. difficile* was clearly elucidated [6].

CLINICAL PRESENTATION

The typical presentation for *Clostridium difficile* diarrhea is abdominal pain, profuse diarrhea, fever and leucocytosis after exposure to antibiotics. Symptoms can start 48 hours after antibiotic administration, but can be seen up to eight weeks after cessation of antibiotic therapy. The abdominal pain is crampy in nature, most frequently diffuse but can be localized to the left lower quadrant. Reports of patients with *C. difficile* colitis presenting with an acute abdomen have been noted especially in the elderly. Diarrhea is profuse, mucoid, green colored and watery with evidence of fecal leukocytes. Diarrhea can be severe with 15–30 bowel movements per day. The large volume loss can cause dehydration, electrolytic disturbances and hypotension. Bloody stools are unusual, but trace amounts of blood are frequently found. The fever is usually low grade but can be as high 40.7 °C. The leucocytosis, usually in the range of 10,000–20,000 per cubic millimeter, can reach counts greater than 40,000 cells per cubic millimeter. Hypoalbuminemia may be present early in the disease and is attributed to a protein-losing enteropathy. Polyarthritis involving large joints has been reported as a extraintestinal manifestation of pseudomembranous colitis [7].

PATHOPHYSIOLOGY

C. difficile diarrhea, colitis and pseudomembranous colitis are toxin mediated mucosal inflammatory processes that are usually characterized by the presence of grossly or microscopically visible pseudomembranes consisting of nodules or large plaques containing leukocytes, fibrin, mucus, and epithelial cells loosely adherent to the surface of the underlying inflamed and necrotic mucosa [7]. *Clostridium difficile* infection can manifest as asymptomatic carriage, diarrhea (secretory type), colitis with and without pseudomembranes, fulminant colitis with toxic dilatation of the colon, perforation, hypovolemia, shock and death.

C. difficile diarrhea is caused primarily by the elaboration within the intestinal lumen of both toxin A and B. These toxins bind to the colonic mucosa inducing mucosal damage and inflammation. Most toxigenic isolates produce both toxins. Toxin A is a 308 Kd protein that is a neutrophil chemoattractant, cytotoxic to certain cell lines, activates macrophages and mast cells. Cellular damage is induced by desegregation of actin and by release of intracellular calcium [8]. Recently direct damage to neurons has been reported.

Toxin B is a 270 KD protein that causes depolymerarization of filamentous actin. It is also a necrotizing enterotoxin 10 times more potent than toxin A in causing damage to colonic mucosa in cell culture lines [9]. The diarrhea is caused by the toxins in the intestinal lumen adhering to the mucosal surface and inducing a severe inflammatory response that causes disruption of cell integrity and fluid flux into the lumen.

Newborns present a high colonization rate with *Clostridium difficile*, up to 70% in the first eight months but a minimal rate of pseudomembranous colitis. Healthy adults show a prevalence of 2–3%, when there is a recent history of antibiotic use the prevalence of *C. difficile* increase to 15% to 30% [10].

Epidemiology

C. difficile is a sporulating organism that survives well in nature. Like most of the Clostridia species their distribution in the environment is wide. Evaluation of epidemics includes case surveillance, stool cultures to identify carriers, typing of strains and cultures of environmental sources. These epidemiological tools have shown that *C. difficile* is the most common cause of nosocomial diarrhea. Most cases occur in hospitals, nursing homes and chronic care facilities, where cases have been reported occurring sporadically as well as in outbreaks. On the other hand, community acquired diarrhea caused by *C. difficile* is less common.

C. difficile has been isolated from environmental samples in bed pans, toilets and floors of these facilities. Asymptomatic carriage of *C. difficile* has been reported in up to 30% of patients treated with antibiotics [10]. Transmission of *C. difficile* often occurs via the hands of hospital personnel and also by contact with contaminated surfaces and fomites [11, 12]. The frequency and incidence of *C. difficile* induced diarrhea varies widely not only geographically but within different institutions in the same geographic area. Risk factors for the development of *C. difficile* colitis other than antibiotic use are: colonic, gastric or pelvic surgery, spinal fracture, intestinal obstruction, colon carcinoma, leukemia, severe burns, uremia, heavy metal poisoning, hemolytic-uremic syndrome, ischemic vascular disease, shigellosis, severe infection, neonatal necrotizing enterocolitis, ischemic colitis, and Hirschprung's disease [13, 14]. Patients receiving postpyloric tube feeding have been noted to be at increased risk of acquiring *C. difficile* when compared to non-tube fed patients [15].

Almost every antibiotic on the market has been implicated in cases of antibiotic induced diarrhea. The most common agents are ampicillin/amoxicillin, other penicillin derivatives, cephalosporins and clindamycin; and less frequently macrolides, fluoroquinolones and aminoglycosides. Even the drugs of choice for treatment of this condition, metronidazole and vancomycin, have been implicated in some cases of *C. difficile* diarrhea. Tetracycline, chloramphenicol and sulfonamides are now rarely implicated [16, 17]. Drugs with limited data to support a relationship are urinary antiseptics, parenteral aminoglycosides, parenteral vancomycin, antifungals, antiparasitics and antimycobacterial agents.

Antibiotics are not the only agents associated with *C. difficile* infection. Cases of patients developing *C. difficile* infection after chemotherapy have been reported [18]. Most of chemotherapeutic agents also have antimicrobial activity that can alter gut flora and cause overgrowth of *C. difficile*.

Diagnostic Tests

ENDOSCOPY

Endoscopy is the most rapid way to establish the diagnosis, but because of its cost and invasiveness it is usually reserved for patients that are seriously ill or in-patients in which a non-invasive test has been negative. Endoscopy is also helpful when other disease processes are being considered in the differential diagnosis. Physicians should be aware of the possibility of bowel perforation and bleeding as complications of endoscopy.

Diagnosis can be confirmed when yellowish nodules or classic pseudomembranes are visualized. Lesions are more commonly found in the left colon, but a minority of patients will present only with right colonic lesions. Full colonoscopy should be performed especially if the left colon examination is unremarkable. Some patients may present with mild colonic erythema or patchy inflammation. Biopsies should be performed in cases with abnormal mucosa without the classic pseudomembranes to look for the microscopic changes suggestive of pseudomembranous colitis and to rule out other etiologies. The histologic features of pseudomembranous colitis are not pathognemonic and can be seen in patients with ischemic colitis and other disorders.

Non-Invasive Tests

There is yet no simple inexpensive, rapid, sensitive and specific test for the diagnosis of *C. difficult* diarrhea and colitis [6]. Not all laboratories provide all the tests available on the market. Most tests target the cytotoxins produced by the pathogenic strains of *C. difficile*. The two most common tests available are: cell culture assay for cytotoxin B and the enzyme immunoassay test for toxins A and B.

The cell culture assay is considered the gold standard for diagnosis of *C. difficile*. This assay detects toxin B by its cytopathic effect in monolayer cell culture, usually in HEp-2 cells. The specificity of this assay is verified by neutralization of the cytopathic effect when antitoxin to *C. difficile* or *C. sordelli* is added. The major drawbacks of this test are that most laboratories do not offer tissue culture, results takes 24–48 hrs and sensitivity and specificity can be affected by handling, storage of stool sample, stool sample dilution and cell culture line used. On average this test is positive in more than 90% of patients with pseudomembranous colitis. The result is usually reported as detection of cytotoxin in the assay. Quantification of this response does not correlate with severity of disease.

ENZYME IMMUNOASSAYS FOR TOXIN A AND B

Immunoassay is the most common and widely used test for the detection of *C. difficile*. It is rapidly performed and relatively inexpensive. It provides good specificity (95–100%) and sensitivity (63–89%) [19, 20]. On average EIA test for toxin A or B failed to detect about 10% (5–33%) of cases of *C. difficile* when compared to endoscopy or cell tissue culture assay. In cases of high clinical suspicion and a negative EIA, consideration for a more sensitive test like cell tissue culture assay or endoscopic evaluation should be performed to confirm the diagnosis. Sensitivity is rarely improved by sending more than one stool sample on the same day for EIA testing.

Latex Agglutination Test

This test detects the presence of the enzyme glutamate dehydrogenase produced by *C. difficile* and not toxin A as previously thought [20]. The sensitivity of this test is similar to the EIA assay, but with less specificity. The lack of specificity comes from the fact that glutamate dehydrogenase is expressed by some of the non toxigenic strains of *C. difficile*.

Other Available Tests

A test based on the immunobloting technique is commercially available (C. diff CUBE). This test is a rapid assay for the detection of toxin A, with similar sensitivity and specificity to the EIA [21]. New promising techniques includes: PCR-based detection of the toxin genes and culture on CCFA media. *C. difficile* culture is reserved for epidemiological studies when strain typing is necessary. Other tests like lactoferrin or fecal leukocytes are non-specific but if found positive should be used as a guide to early therapy specially in critically ill patients.

DIAGNOSTIC IMAGING

Plain abdominal films are usually unremarkable and should be reserved to rule out the late complications of this condition like toxic megacolon and bowel perforation. Barium studies provide little information and can cause bowel perforation.

Computed tomography can demonstrate colonic wall thickening, colonic inflammation and ascites, but these findings can be seen in other infectious processes and also with bowel ischemia. Up to 50% of patients with *C. difficile* colitis have normal imaging studies. In one study CT failed to detect which patients would benefit from surgical therapy or medical therapy [22]. Nuclear medicine studies are only used on a experimental basis.

Treatment

Therapy includes the discontinuation of the implicated antibiotic, supportive measures and, in some cases therapy with antimicrobial agents. Large volume diarrhea, when present, may be associated with fluid and electrolytic imbalances that need to be corrected with intravenous fluids and electrolyte replacement. Some cases may need hyperalimentation secondary to severe catabolism and the presence of protein loosing enteropathy. The administration of antiperistaltic agents and opiates should be avoided.

Opiates can mask the patients symptoms and the decreased motility can cause greater exposure to the toxin in the colonic lumen [23]. Antimicrobials are used frequently to treat pseudomembranous colitis. The most commonly used agents are metronidazole and vancomycin. Less frequently used are teicoplanin and bacitracin. Failure to respond to conservative treatment and a diagnostic test positive for *C. difficile* are indications for antibiotic therapy. In patients with severe symptoms empiric therapy may be started while waiting for the results of the diagnostic tests. If the patient is more than 10 years old and not pregnant, therapy with oral metronidazole should be given. An expert committee of hospital infection control practitioners has recently recommended that metronidazole is preferred for specific and empiric antimicrobial treatment of *C. difficile* diarrhea [24]. Vancomycin is an alternative with equal efficacy [25–28]. Response rates of 95–100% have been reported with Vancomycin.

Rationale for Metronidazole

The main reason for the preferential use of metronidazole is the concern about development of vancomycin resistance in strains of enterococci (VRE) and Staphylococcus (MRSA).

Metronidazole is very active *in vitro* against *C. difficile*. Metronidazole is rapidly and almost completely absorbed in the upper GI tract. Even though metronidazole levels in stool are low, therapeutic response is similar to vancomycin [29]. Metronidazole is also significantly less expensive than vancomycin.

Metronidazole is well tolerated in short therapy courses. Major side effects include: unpleasant metallic taste, nausea, vomiting, diarrhea, abdominal pain, pruritus, erythematous rashes, headache, confusion, dizziness, reversible neutropenia and neuropathy. Of importance is the development of disulfiran type reaction when the drug is mixed with alcohol. Use in pregnancy should be avoided because of potential carcinogenic risk. Metronidazole crosses the placental barrier and *in vitro* is fetotoxic.

Resistance to metronidazole has been reported. A report from the University of Michigan showed a 3% *in vitro* resistance [30]. All of the strains depicted as metronidazole resistant were highly sensitive to vancomycin. Clinical significance of this phenomena in terms of treatment failures have not been proven.

The dosing for treatment of *C. difficile* diarrhea is: metronidazole 250–500 mg four times a day or 500–750 mg three times a day for 7–10 days. Pediatric dosing is 35–50 mg/kg/day divided in three doses. In neonates and children less than 10 years old vancomycin should be the drug of choice. In patients with a nonfunctioning gut or the critically ill, metronidazole can be given intravenously at a dose of 500 mg four times a day. Efficacy of this route is decreased when compared to the oral route.

Use of Vancomycin

Oral vancomycin was originally the preferred treatment for *C. difficile* diarrhea, however concerns about the emergence of *Enterococcus faecium* resistant to vancomycin and the high cost made metronidazole the current treatment of choice. Some advantages of vancomycin use in this condition include poor systemic absorption, excellent bioavailability in the colonic lumen and high infection cure rate. Recent guidelines published by the American College of Gastroenterology recommend the use of vancomycin in the following circumstances [71]:

1. Failure to respond to metronidazole
2. Organism resistant to metronidazole
3. Patient unable to tolerate metronidazole or is allergic to medication
4. Pregnancy or children younger than 10 yr
5. Critically ill secondary to *C. difficile* colitis
6. Evidence suggesting that the diarrhea can be related to *Staphylococcus aureus*

It is important to mention that *Staphylococcus aureus* can cause antibiotic induced diarrhea, colitis, enteritis and even involvement of the stomach. This possibility should arise especially in patients with diarrhea, fever and negative *C. difficile* assay. At least one report mentioned methicillin resistant *Staphylococcus aureus* as the etiologic agent of a case of enteritis [31].

Vancomycin is given orally at a dose of 125 mg four times a day for 7–10 days, or 500 mg four times a day in critically patients ill, which impending ileus, colonic dilatation or perforation. Pediatric doses are based on the formula 500 mg/1.73 m^2 every six hours. If a patient can't tolerate oral vancomycin or if there is a paralytic ileus, direct instillation to the cecum should be performed using a tube or a pig tail catheter. Dosing for this regimen is 200 or 500 mg in 500 ml diluent given four times a day. Another alternative is to place a decompression or colonic tube and instill 2000 mg initially followed by 100 mg/500 ml diluent every four hours or every bowel movement [32].

Other Therapies

Other treatment alternatives includes non-absorbable oral antibiotics like bacitracin [28] and teicoplanin [33]. The dose for bacitracin is 25,000 U orally four times a day for 7–10 days. Clinical response to bacitracin is slower than conventional therapy. Teicoplanin availability is limited in the United States and concerns about the development of resistance to enterococci are present. Clinical experience with these antibiotics is limited and their use should be limited to cases where both vancomycin and metronidazole are contraindicated.

Anion binding resins such as cholestyramine binds toxin B of *Clostridium difficile*, but their capacity to do this is limited. The other potential problem when using cholestyramine or colestipol is binding of the resin to vancomycin if the two drugs are used in conjunction [34]. Their use should be limited to mild cases, if at all. Special interest in non-antibiotic alternatives to the treatment of colitis is an area of active research. Bacteriotherapy using rectal instillation of normal feces haven tried with some success [35]. In a recent report Goerg and Schlorer noted improved symptoms after gastrointestinal lavage followed with oral administration of live *E. coli* [36]. Other alternatives like fecal enemas, lactobacillus GG instillation and yogurt enemas have been tried with limited success [37–39].

In certain populations like children with immunodeficiencies, intravenous immune globulin infusion may be used with some benefits at least for the prevention of relapses [40, 41].

Surgery is considered when conservative measures fail to achieved clinical improvement and the patient has intractable symptoms [42]. Surgical management is also used for the late complications of the disease such as bowel perforation, peritonitis and toxic megacolon. Like any inflammatory bowel disorder there is an increased morbidity and mortality when patients are submitted to surgery. Resectional procedures carry a better prognosis than diversion procedures (colostomy) [43]. Less than half of a per cent of patients will need surgical management for the treatment of antibiotic induced colitis [44].

Treatment of Relapsers

Relapse of *C. difficile* related colitis is very common ranging from 5–50% of the cases with a mean frequency of 20% [45, 46]. Symptoms of recurrence usually occur 3–10 days after discontinuation of antibiotic therapy. The largest published series on relapses showed a 24% relapse rate. All patients responded to a second trial of the same antibiotic in this case vancomycin. Important in this study is the fact that 22 of the original 46 relapsers suffered a second relapse [47]. There is no difference in the relapse rate between metronidazole and vancomycin.

Relapse is probably related to sporulation of *C. difficile* and lack of antibiotic efficacy during this dormant stage. When antibiotics are discontinued, bacteria found in this vegetative stage are thought to reactivate and infection may recur. This theory is supported by the fact that strain typing of isolates from relapsers are the same as the one causing the original infection [48].

The current approach to the treatment of relapsers is retreatment with an antibiotic, metronidazole if possible, for 7–10 days [49]. Some advocate the use of tapered dosing for 2–3 months to promote low *C. difficile* count and reestablishment of the colonic flora. It is important to avoid antibiotic use for at least two months after treatment to decrease the chance of relapse.

Alternatives to decrease relapse have been described earlier, especially bacteriotherapy. Other alternatives includes: intermittent therapy with metronidazole or vancomycin, combination of vancomycin and rifampin. The administration of live yeast (*Saccharomyces boulardii*) to patients with history of relapse have decreased the recurrence rate in 50% [50].

Prevention of C. difficile *Diarrhea*

Exposure to antibiotics, hospitalization and enteral feedings are some of the risk factors for acquisition of this condition. Therefore, judicious use of antibiotics has been shown to decrease the incidence of *C. difficile*. One study restricting the use of clindamycin demonstrated a decreased incidence of antibiotic induced diarrhea [51].

Hospitalized patients are at risk to acquire the infection nosocomially. Strict hand washing, use of gloves while manipulating patients and disinfection of objects infected with *C. difficile* with sodium hypochlorite, glutaraldehyde or ethylene oxide are effective measures to control spread of the organism. Patients with colitis should be placed in rooms with private bathrooms at least during the diarrhea phase. Enteric isolation should be discontinued once the diarrhea resolves. Eradication of the carrier state is difficult, neither vancomycin nor metronidazole are reliably effective in eradicating the *C. difficile* carier state.

The most important measure is education of the medical and nursing staff about the epidemiology and pathophysiology of this condition. The importance of hand washing between contact with patients, the use of gloves when caring for a patient with *C. difficile* diarrhea and the judicious use of antimicrobials are simple measures that will decrease the incidence of this infection.

References

1. Finney JMT. Gastro-enterostomy for cicatrizing ulcer of the pylorus. Bull Johns Hopkins Hosp 4:53, 1893.
2. Hummel RP, Alteimer WA, Hill EQ. Iatrogenic staphylococcal enterocolitis. Ann Surg 160:551, 1964.
3. Wakefield RD, Sommers SC. Fatal membranous staphylococcal enteritis in surgical patients. Ann Surg 138:249, 1953.
4. Tedesco FJ, Barton RW, Alpers DH. Clindamycin-associated colitis: A prospective study. Ann Intern Med 81:429, 1974
5. Green RH. The association of viral activation with penicillin toxicity in guinea pigs and hamsters. Yale J Biol Med 47:166, 1974.
6. Bartlett JG, Chang TW, Gurthwith M, *et al.* Antibiotic-associated pseudomembranous colitis due to toxin producing clostridia. N Engl J Med 298:531, 1978.
7. Veillard E, Guggenbuhl P, Bello S, *et al.* Reactive oligoarthritis in a patient with Clostridium difficile pseudomembranous colitis, review of literature. Rev Rhum Engl Ed 65:795, 1998.
8. Fekety R. Guidelines for the diagnosis and management of Clostridium difficile diarrhea and colitis. Am J Gastroenterol 92:5, 739, 1997.
9. Riegler M, Sedivy R, Pothoulakis C, *et al.* Clostridium difficile toxin B is more potent than toxin A in damaging human colonic mucosa in vitro. J Clin Invest 95:2004, 1995.
10. Johnson S, Gerding D. Clostridium difficile. In Mayhall CG (ed). Hospital epidemiology and infection control. Baltimore: Williams & Wilkins, 1996: 399.
11. Kim K-H, Fekety R, Batts DH, *et al.* Isolation of Clostridium difficile from the environment and contacts of patients with antibiotic induced colitis. J Infect Dis 143:42, 1981.

12. Wilcox M. Cleaning up Clostridium difficile infection. Lancet 348:767, 1996.
13. Bartlett JG, Gorbach SL. Pseudomembranous enterocolitis (antibiotic-related colitis). In Stollerman GH (ed). Advances in Internal Medicine. Chicago, Year-Book Medical Publishers, 1995: 445.
14. Cudmore MA, Silva J, Feketey R, *et al. Clostridium difficile* colitis associated with cancer chemotherapy. Arch Intern Med 142:333, 1982.
15. Zimmaro D, Johnson S, Savik, K, *et al.* Acquisition of Clostridium difficile and Clostridium difficile-associated diarrhea in hospitalized patients receiving tube feeding. Ann Intern Med 129:1012, 1998.
16. Kelly CP, Pothoulakis C, LaMont TT. *Clostridium difficile* colitis. N Engl J Med 330:257, 1994.
17. Fekety R. Antibiotic-associated colitis. In Mandell G, Bennet JE, Dolin R (eds). Principle and Practices of Infectious Diseases, 4th edn. New York: Churchill Livingstone, 1996: 978.
18. Jarvis B, Shevchuk YM. Recurrent Clostridium difficile diarrhea associated with mitoxantrone and etoposide: a case report and review. Pharmacotherapy 17:606, 1997.
19. Merz CS, Kramer C, Forman, M, *et al.* Comparison of four commercially available rapid immunoassay with cytotoxin assay, and toxigenic culture for detection of Clostridium difficile toxin(s) from stool specimens. J Clin Microbiol 32:1142, 1994.
20. Barbut F, Kajzer C, Planas N, *et al.* Comparison of three enzyme immunoassays, a cytotoxicity assay and toxigenic culture for diagnosis of Clostridium difficile-associated diarrhea. J Clin Microbiol 31:963, 1993.
21. Kurzynski TA. Evaluation of C. difficile CUBE test for detection of Clostridium difficile-associated diarrhea. Diagn Micribiol Infect Dis 15:493, 1992.
22. Kawamoto S, Horton KM, Fishman EK. Pseudomembranous colitis: can CT predict which patients will need surgical intervention? J Comput Assist Tomogr 23:79, 1999.
23. Fekety R, Shah A. Diagnosis and treatment of C. difficile colitis. JAMA 269:71, 1993.
24. Hospital Infection Control Advisory Committee. Recommendations for preventing the spread of Vancomycin-resistant enterococci. Am J Infect Control 23:87, 1995.
25. Bartlett JG. Treatment of Clostridium difficile colitis. Gastroenterology 89:1192, 1985.
26. Fekety R, Silva J, Armstrong J, *et al.* Treatment of antibiotic-associated enterocolitis with vancomycin. Rev Infect Dis 3:S273, 1981.
27. Viscidi R, Willey S, Bartlett JG. Isolation rates and toxigenic potential for *Clostridium difficile* isolates from various patients populations. Gastroenterology 81:5, 1981.
28. Dudley MN, McLaughlin JC, Carrington G, *et al.* Oral bacitracin vs. Vancomycin therapy for Clostridium difficile-induced diarrhea. Arch Intern Med 146:1101, 1986.
29. Teasley DG, Olson MM, Gebhard RL, *et al.* Prospective randomized trial of metronidazole versus vancomycin for Clostridium difficile-associated diarrhea and colitis. Lancet 2:1444, 1983.
30. Fekety R. Unpublished data.
31. Takesue Y, Yokohama T, Kodama T, *et al.* Toxin involvement in methicillin resistant Staphylococcus aureus enteritis in gastroenterological surgery. Gastroenterol Jpn 26:716, 1991.
32. Pasic M, Jost R, Carell T, *et al.* Intracolonic vancomycin for pseudomembranous colitis. New Engl J Med 329:583 (letter), 1993.
33. de Lalla F, Nicolin R, Rinaldi E, *et al.* Prospective Study of oral teicoplanin versus oral vancomycin for therapy of pseudomembranous colitis and Clostridium difficile-associated diarrhea. Antimicrob Agents Chemother 36:2192, 1992.
34. Taylor NS, Bartlett JG. Binding of Clostridium difficile cytotoxin and vancomycin by anion exchange resins. J Infect Dis 141:92, 1980.
35. Schwan A, Sjolin S, Trottestan U, *et al.* Relapsing *Clostridium difficile* enterocolitis cured by rectal infusion of normal feces. Scand J Infect Dis 16:211, 1984.
36. Goerg KJ, Schlorer E. Probiotic therapy of pseudomembranous colitis combination of intestinal lavage and oral administration of *Escherichia coli.* Dtsch Med Wochenschr 123:1274, 1998.
37. Gorbach SL. Succesfull treatment of relapsing *Clostridium difficile* colitis with Lactobacillus GG. Lancet 2:1519, 1987.
38. Tvede M, Rask-Madsen J. Bacteriotherapy for Chronic relapsing *Clostridium difficile* diarrhea in six patients. Lancet 1:1156, 1998.
39. Siitonen S, Vapautalo H, Salminen S, *et al.* Effect of Lactobacillus GG Yogurt in prevention of antibiotic induced diarrhea. Ann Med 22:57, 1990.
40. Lung DY, Kelly CP, Boguniewicz M, *et al.* Treatment with intravenously administered gamma globulin of chronic relapsing colitis induced by

Clostridium induced toxin. J Pediatr 118:633, 1991.

41. Salcedo J, Keates S, Pothloulakis C, *et al.* Intravenous immunoglobulin therapy for severe *Clostridium difficile* colitis. Gut 41:366, 1997.
42. Synnott K, Mealy K, Merry C, *et al.* Timing of surgery for fulminant pseudomembranous colitis. Br J Surg 85:229, 1998.
43. Viswanath YK, Griffiths CD. The role of surgery in pseudomembranous enterocolitis. Postgrad Med J 74:216, 1998.
44. Lipsett PA, Samantaray DK, Tam ML, *et al.* Pseudomembranous colitis: A surgical disease? Surgery 116:491, 1994.
45. Bartlett JG. *Clostridium difficile* infection: Pathophysiology and diagnosis. Semin Gastrointest Dis 8:12, 1997.
46. Walters BAJ, Roberts R, Stafford R, *et al.* Relapse of antibiotic-associated colitis: Endogenous persistence of *Clostridium difficile* during vancomycin therapy. Gut 24:206, 1983.
47. Kelly CP, LaMont JT. *Clostridium difficile* infection. Annu Rev Med 49:375, 1988.
48. Bartlett JG. Treatment of antibiotic associated pseudomembranous colitis. Rev Infect Dis 6:S235, 1984.
49. Jobe B, Grasely A, Deveney K, *et al.* *Clostridium difficile* colitis: an increasing hospital acquired illness. Am J Surg 169:480, 1995.
50. McFarland LV, Surawicz CM, Greenberg RN, *et al.* A randomized placebo control trial of *Saccharomyces boulardii* in combination with standard antibiotics for Clostridium difficile disease. JAMA 271:1913, 1994.
51. Climo MW, Israel DS, Wong ES, *et al.* Hospital wide restrictions of clindamycin: effect on the incidence of *Clostridium difficile* associated diarrhea and cost. 128:989, 1998.

45. URINARY TRACT INFECTIONS

L. Alvarez-Rocha, P. Rascado-Sedes and M.J. Castro-Orjales

Urinary tract infections (UTI) as a whole are amongst the most habitual infectious diseases in everyday clinical praxis. They are traditionally classified into non-complicated and complicated UTIs. Although this classification has certain limitations [1], it relates acceptably well both to the complementary studies the patient will need and to the type and duration of the treatment. The first group refers to those which develop in healthy individuals with no risk factors likely to increase the possibilities of acquiring this type of infection; or increase their severity; or cause treatment to fail. In the second group, the patient will show one or more of the mentioned factors (structural anomalies, metabolic/hormonal changes, alterations of the immunity system, presence of non-habitual pathogens), which shall condition a greater severity in this type of pathology.

Complicated urinary tract infection is a common cause of severe sepsis as well as septic shock in intensive care patients [2–4]. Although this group of infections, and more specifically pyelonephritis, may determine a significant number of cases of hospitalization [5], in the Intensive Care Units (ICU) most UTI have a nosocomial origin. In a prevalence study carried out on a total of 1417 ICUs in Europe in 1992 [6], community-acquired infections were diagnosed in 13.7% of patients, and infections of nosocomial origin in 30.3% of the cases (9.7% extra-ICU; 20.6% intra-ICU). According to this study, nosocomial UTI affected 17.6% of the patients and occupied the third place of the intra-ICU nosocomial infections (NI) after pneumonia and other infections of the lower respiratory tract (46.9% and 17.8%, respectively), unlike what usually occurs in the other hospital departments, where it is the first or second most frequent NI, in competence with the infections of surgical wounds [7]. The numeric importance of these infections is confirmed also in other studies on different ICU, where UTI was the first/second NI before or after pneumonia, affecting 7.8% of the patients with urinary catheter [8] or representing 31% of the NI [9]. On the other hand, nosocomial UTI are often connected with the use of urologic devices, especially with urinary catheters. According to a number of authors, up to 95% of the episodes occur in catheterized patients [9]. These devices are widely used in ICU, with rates that go from 0.45 to 0.86, depending on the type of unit to be considered [9, 10]. In view of that, the onset of UTI has to be correlated with the time of catheterization in order to a better appraisal of the problem. Taking into account this fact, the incidence rate of this type of infection may be seen to vary from 3.3‰ catheter-days in a cardiothoracic ICU to 10‰ in a burn unit [8, 10]. These figures coincide with the findings of the National Survey on Nosocomial Infection Study carried out in the Spanish ICUs (ENVIN-UCI-study)[1], according to which the rate was 6.1‰ catheter-days in 1996 [11].

Furthermore, this group of infections may increase the morbidity/mortality of the patients, a fact that contributes to stressing its impor-

[1] ENVIN-UCI stands for Sp. "Estudio Nacional de Vigilancia de la Infección Nosocomial" and Unidad(es) de Cuidados Intensivos".

tance. Unlike bacteremia or pneumonia, a connection between UTI and patient mortality is not yet firmly established [12, 13]. However, UTIs do constitute a significant source of bacteremia and may contribute to the deterioration of the renal function; they also increase the hospital stay from 1–4 days, and mean a cost of $558–593 per episode [2, 14].

Finally, the clinical spectrum of UTI ranges from asymptomatic bacteriuria to pyelonephritis or renal/perirenal abscesses, comprising cystitis, uretritis and prostatitis. However, in the present chapter we shall only revise those clinical patterns which are more habitually found in the patients admitted to our ICUs.

Pathophysiology

The possibility of onset of UTI will be partly related to the virulence of the causing microorganism as well as with the size of the inoculum and the quality of the host's defense mechanisms. These factors will also have an influence on the anatomic location of the process.

INVASION PATHS OF THE URINARY TRACT

There are three possible paths for microorganisms to reach the urinary tract:

1. **Ascendent**: the urethra is the most common path germs have to access the urinary bladder. Most of the microorganisms causative of UTI come from the hands of hospital staff during some manipulation or, more frequently, from the fecal flora of the patients themselves and can be either habitual colonizers or be acquired during the patient's stay in hospital [15–17]. Furthermore, in later years the vagina has been observed to play an important role as a reservoir of uropathogens in the female patient [16]. The colonization of the perineal area and the distal urethra is the previous step to the access of the germs to the bladder and, in this sense, the intensity of the colonization of the urinary meatus seems to be directly connected with the hazard of developing bacteriuria [15].

Sexual activity, especially in women, helps the access of microorganisms to the urinary bladder because of the urethral massage produced during sexual intercourse. In fact, the smaller length of the female urethra favors a greater incidence of UTI in women. Once in the bladder, bacteria multiply and may reach the renal parenchyma through the ureters. This retrograde expansion is facilitated by vesicoureteral reflux, pregnancy or ureteral obstruction, and even by exotoxins from certain microorganisms, since all of these factors may have an antiperistaltic effect [16].

The ascendent path has also a major role in the catheter-associated UTIs. The access of the invading microorganisms to the urinary bladder may be either *Extraluminal*, through the space between the catheter and the urethral mucosa, or *Endoluminal*. The first type can in turn be early and be associated to noncompliance of the sanitary norms while passing the catheter, or delayed, if the germs expand from the perineum through the biofilm formed on the outer surface of the urinary catheter. Regarding the endoluminal path, this is associated to the reflux of organisms which reach the lumen of the catheter as a result of the disconnecting of the collector tube or the contamination of the drainage of the collector bag.

The presence of germs in the distal urethra causes a single catheterization maneuver with immediate removal to be accompanied by onset of UTI in about 1% of the healthy individuals and at least in 6% of the high-risk patients [15]. The importance of the bacterial colonization of the urinary meatus in relation to the possibility of onset of UTI has been confirmed in many studies [15].

Tambyah *et al.* [17], in their study on the pathogenesis of the catheter-associated UTIs, found that 66% of the cases have been acquired through the extraluminal path (18% early; 48% delayed) and 34% through the endoluminal path. Strikingly, these authors did not appreciate any difference in the pathogenic mechanism associated to the sex of the patients, unlike other studies, which found a higher significance of the extraluminal path in female patients [15]. Yet, they did observe a predilection of the Gram-positive microorganisms and fungi for the extraluminal path, whereas Gram-negative microorganisms may cause infection by either way.

The biofilm deposited on the surface of the catheter not only helps its obstruction but also protects the invading microorganisms from the action of antibiotics and the host's defenses Its growing is the result of adhering bacteria and their multiplication as well as extracellular secretion of polysaccharides which combine with urinary proteins and salty precipitates from the patient [18].

Finally, it is important to remember that, even after the urinary catheter has been removed, the patient continues to be exposed to a higher risk of developing bacteriuria for an undetermined length of time [19]. This fact is probably related to the urethral colonization caused by the catheter.

2. **Hematogenous**: UTIs caused through this path are infrequent. However, it is a well described possibility in male patients, especially for *Staphylococcus aureus* and *Candida spp.* [16, 20, 21]. On the contrary, Gram-negative bacilli, the main responsibles for UTIs, are unlikely to reach the urinary tract this way unless there exists an ureteral obstruction [20]. The hematogenous path is the habitual way of bacterial implantation for cortical renal abscesses, whereas in other cases it will represent the complication of an acute pyelonephritis or the extension of a neighboring pathology [22, 23].

3. **Lymphatic**: there is little evidence to date that this way has an important role in the genesis of pyelonephritis. It is possible that an increased intravesical pressure favors the lymphatic flux to turn to the kidneys, as has been seen in experiments on animals [22].

DEFENSE MECHANISMS OF THE HOST

The healthy urinary tract is resistant to bacterial colonization and, in most cases, rapidly eliminates any microorganism that has succeeded in enter it. There are several mechanisms available for reaching that purpose [16, 22].

First, urine possesses a bactericide activity due fundamentally to its urea content. A high osmolarity, a concentration of salts and organic acids, and a low pH also contribute to inhibit the growth of bacteria. Likewise, the maintenance of an adequate urinary flux and a normal voiding of the bladder are fundamental elements, as dilution and mechanical dragging prevent bacterial proliferation. Furthermore, the mucous membrane of the urinary tract, probably due to the presence of a glycosaminoglycan, maintains a natural resistance to adhesion of germs. The Tamm-Horsfall glycoprotein (uromodulin) produced by the cells of the ascending limb of Henle's loop and the distal convoluted tubule as well as other oligosaccharides with low molecular weight also have a role in limiting bacterial adhesion, acting as analogues of the bacterial receptors. In men, the prostatic secretion forms part of this defensive system.

Second, the inflammatory response itself is also a part of these defense mechanisms. The presence of polymorphonuclear leukocytes seems to play little part in the prevention of infection; however, it is important for its localization and for holding up its extension. The uroepitelial cells help the arrival of these leukocytes by producing chemotactic factors (IL-8) and expressing adhesion molecules (ICAM-1). Likewise, the cytoquines (IL-1, IL-1β, IL-6, IL-8 or TNF-α) produced both by the uroepitelial cells and the non-epithelial cells resident or recruited in the urinary tract (polymorphonuclear leukocytes, macrophages, lymphocytes) in response to the presence of the bacteria or their products, also take part in this defensive system [16].

Last, the activation of the humoral and/or cellular immunity system may also collaborate in the defense of the urinary tract [16, 22]. However, there is little evidence at present that the latter has an important function apart from the production by the T-cells of the immunoregulating cytoquines which take part in the inflammatory response [16]. On the contrary, a production of specific antibodies in the urine and serum 7–10 days after onset of a UTI has been observed. The rate of antibodies is higher in pyelonephritis than in cystitis in accordance with the severity of the process. In serum, immunoglobulines are made up fundamentally by IgM and IgG as opposed to the O and K antigens and the fimbria of the infecting organisms. In the urine, the predominance corresponds to IgA, either secretory or monomeric, and IgG as opposed to the same bacterial components. The main role of these antibodies consists in limiting the severity of the lesion. Their preventive function for UTI is controversial, although a potential usefulness might be derived from positive results obtained in animal experiments by means of vaccines and the increase of UTI hazard observed on individuals with low urinary levels of sIgA [16].

FACTORS OF BACTERIAL VIRULENCE

UTI may be caused by a large number of bacterial species, although in most of the cases the responsible agent is *Escherichia coli*. In fact, the number of serogroups of *E. coli* habitually involved in the appearance of UTI is rather small (01, 02, 04, 06, 07, 075, 0150) [22]. This gave rise to the emergence of the concept of the uropathogenic *E. coli*. Some strains of *E. coli*, selected from the fecal flora, show certain virulence factors that give them a higher capacity to invade, colonize and cause disease in the urinary tract. Among them, we can find adhesion factors (fimbria P, S, type 1), toxins (lipopolysaccharides, hemolysin), aerobactin and other elements that facilitate their invasivity or increase their resistance to the bactericide action of the serum.

The adhesion process is a result of the interaction between certain components of the bacterial surface (adhesins) and the receptors of the host cell. These adhesins may exist as filamentous surface organelle, called pili or fimbria, or as non-filamentous proteins of the outer membrane. The former are the most frequent and are able to recognize several glycoconjugates of the host cell. The fimbria P join to the globoseries of the glycolipids, whereas the fimbria S do it to the glycoconjugates with sialic acid, and the type 1 fimbria join to mannose residues [24]. Other adhesins known at present are the type 1c, the G, M or X, which have different serologic properties and specific joints [22].

These adhesion factors seem related both with the severity and the type of UTI to appear. As the serogroups of *E. coli* that have been isolated as causative agents of urinary infections were studied, a good capacity of adhesion was found in 80% of the cases of acute pyelonephritis, whereas it was in 40–50% of the cases of cystitis and in 20% of the cases of asymptomatic bacteriuria [24]. During the investigation of fimbria P, the most important adhesion factors, those strains of *E. coli* provided with them proved to be the responsibles of acute pyelonephritis and urosepsis, especially in individuals free from risk factors. This group of adhesins also helps the serogroups that have them colonize and persist in the large intestine as well as to invade the urinary tract, and increase the intensity of the inflammatory response. However, it is not clear whether they are necessary for a longer permanence of the invading microorganism in the urinary tract. On the other hand, the role of the type 1 fimbria in the increase of the severity of the infection is under discussion, though according to experimental models, they do contribute to the persistence of *E. coli* in the urinary tract [24].

Another well-known factor of virulence is the lipopolysaccharide present in the outer membrane of the Gram-negative bacilli. Its toxic and inflammatory properties cause many of the symptoms of sepsis by Gram-negative bacilli to reproduce after its administration. However, it is not well known to which extent it is accountable for the signs and symptoms of UTI [24]. Likewise, the presence of capsular polysaccharides increases the resistance to the defense mechanisms of the host. Thus, the encapsulated strains of *E. coli* have been observed to have a higher persistence *in vivo* in the kidneys than the unencapsulated ones [24]. On the other hand, the production of hemolysin, which has a cytotoxic activity not only on the erythrocytes but also on other cell families like the polymorphonuclear leucocytes, monocytes or the cells of the renal tubule, also participate in the development of the renal lesion. Aerobactin, a type of protein which gains iron for the metabolism and multiplication of *E. coli*, may also contribute to the onset of UTI.

Yet the presence of these factors is not indispensable for the development of infection. In a large number of studies investigating their importance in the presence of structural anomalies favoring UTI, they were not often identified [22]. Moreover, the size of the bacterial inoculum is directly related with the infection risk.

Risk Factors

There are various circumstances, which are either inherent to the patients or initially external to these, which may favor development of UTI (Table 1).

The *obstruction of the urinary flux* at any level, secondary to stenosis of multiple etiology or neurologic disfunction, is one of the most important ones. The resulting stasis compromises the defense mechanisms of the host, facilitating bacterial multiplication both in the urine and in the renal parenchyma. Furthermore, the secondary increase of the retrogradely transmitted pressure seems to alter the pattern of the renal blood flow. This hinders the arrival of the phagocytic cells, at the same time as the papillae and ischemic medulla become more vulnerable to bacterial invasion. The higher incidence of UTI seen on pregnant or elderly patients, as well as on patients with calculi, vesical neck stenosis, tumors, uterine prolapse, etc. stresses the importance of this problem [16].

TABLE 1. Risk factors in urinary tract infections

- Anatomic or functional obstruction of the urinary flow
- Diabetes Mellitus
- Advanced age
- Female sex
- Urological instrumentation

Diabetes Mellitus, fundamentally when accompanied of urologic instrumentation, neuropathy with vesical repercussion or a nephrosclerosis, the severity of which keeps a direct relation with the risk, is another favoring factor [16]. It will have a major role especially in the case of suppurated complications [25, 27].

Advanced age determines a greater incidence of UTI which, at the same time, tends to reach the same rate of incidence in both sexes [28]. In the first stages of adulthood the risk of bacteriuria is 30 times higher in women than in men. However, in individuals over 65 years of age, at least 10% of men and 20% of women present bacteriuria. The different degrees of obstruction, alteration of the defense mechanisms or instrumentation of the urinary system that appear in advanced ages, are the responsibles of the changes described [16]. Rosser *et al.*, in their study on urosepsis, find a correlation in multivariate analysis of its incidence with an age >60 years, a long hospital stay and the catheterization time [4].

The higher incidence rate of UTI in *women* may be partly associated to the anatomic fact of a shorter urethra. Yet, when female patients with repeating UTI despite a functional and structurally normal urinary tract were studied, this predisposition was found to be likely to correlate with a longer and more frequent colonization of the perineal area by pathogens. This fact is thought to be associated to genetic circumstances (individuals with a non-secretory phenotype of the blood groups A, AB or P; presence of subtype A3 HLA), to certain behavioral patterns (sexual activity, use of spermicides), or to the estrogenic deficit characteristic of menopause [16].

However, an important number of nosocomial UTIs are conditioned by several types of *urologic manipulations*. As has been mentioned above, up to a 95% of these infections in ICU are related

TABLE 2. Risk factors of catheter-associated urinary tract infections

- General risk factors of urinary tract infection
- Catheterization time
- Indications of catheterization other than monitoring of diuresis or drainage during surgery
- Errors in the maintenance of the closed drainage system
- Periurethral colonization by uropathogens
- Catheterization in an advanced stage of hospital stay
- High plasmatic creatinine rate

to urinary catheterization [15]. Between 1% and 6% of the individuals subjected to a single catheterization maneuver with immediate removal develop UTI [15, 18]. At the same time, the onset of a UTI associated to catheterization will be facilitated by the coincidence of several risk factors (Table 2). Sex (female), advanced age, Diabetes Mellitus, the absence of previous use of antibiotics, a high rate of plasmatic creatinine, not using the urinometer, catheterization indications other than drainage during surgery or diuresis monitoring, errors in the care of the catheter, microbial colonization of the collector bag, catheterization in an advanced stage of hospital stay, and periurethral colonization by uropathogens are some of the factors described in the literature [15, 18, 19]. However, the most important one is the catheterization time [4, 15, 19]. The incidence of bacteriuria in hospitalized patients ranges from 3% to 10% per catheterization day [15, 19]. In the ICUs, where the rate and time of use of indwelling catheters is higher than in other hospital departments, the incidence rate of UTI varies from 3.3 to 10 episodes/1000 catheter days [8, 10, 11].

Etiology

Escherichia coli continues to be the most important causative agent of UTI at present [22]. This is particularly true for community-acquired infections, since its relative importance diminishes in nosocomial or complicated UTI of any origin [18, 19, 22]. In the latter, the presence of other Gram-negative bacilli (*Proteus spp*, *Klebsiella spp*, *Pseudomona aeruginosa*, *Enterobacter spp*), Gram-positive cocci (*Staphylococcus epidermidis*, *Staphylococcus aureus*, *Enterococcus spp*) or fungi (*Candida spp*) is more important. *Staphyloccus aureus* usually appears through the hematogenous path, and thus determines the appearance of renal/perirenal abscesses. *Candida spp*, an agent of increasing importance, which can also appear by means of hematogenous dissemination, is identified principally in hospitalized patients with indwelling catheter who have received wide spectrum antibiotic therapy. However, an advanced age, female sex, Diabetes Mellitus and urologic anomalies have also been associated to the presence of *Candida spp* in urine [21, 29].

The anaerobic microorganisms are rare in UTI, although they may form part of the flora accountable for perinephric abscesses [23]. Other less habitual germs are group D2 *Corynebacterium*, *Ureaplasma urealyticum* and *Mycoplasma hominis*. *Providencia stuartii* has been associated to UTIs related to long catheterization time [19].

The majority of UTI are caused by a single organism. However, in complicated or nosocomial infections the percentage of polymicrobial episodes is higher. Thus, these can be observed in 15% of the episodes of UTI associated to short-time catheterization, in 95% of the UTIs associated to long-time catheterization, and around 25% of renal/perirenal abscesses [19, 23, 25]. In all of these cases, it is important that we learn both about the patient's characteristics and the habitual flora of our work environment in order to an accurate assessment of the etiology of UTIs, since there may exist notable etiologic differences between ICUs, especially as regards NI (Tables 3 and 4).

Diagnosis

1. **Clinical**: Typically, infections of the lower urinary tract characterize by the presence of

TABLE 3. Etiology of the urinary tract nosocomial infection

	Warren[19]				
	Short-time catheterization (n = 135)	Long-time catheterization (n = 1599)	NNISS[10] (n = 2321)	Richards[9] (n = 4956)	ENVIN-UCI[35] (n = 238)
S. coagulase-negative	8%	3%	3%	2%	8%
S. aureus			3%	2%	2%
Enterococcus sp.	7%	11%	14%	14%	20%
E. coli	24%	14%	28%	14%	27%
Enterobacter spp.			4%	5%	1%
C. albicans			10%	21%	18%
K. pneumoniae			6%	6%	4%
S. marcescens			1%	0.7%	1%
P. aeruginosa	9%	12%	7%	10%	10%
Other Candida spp.			4%	5%	
C. glabrata			3%	5%	1%
Acinetobacter spp.			0.2%	1%	4%
Other yeast			5%	8%	
Yeast (overall)	26%		22%	39%	19%
P. mirabilis	6%	15%	4%	2%	5%
Providencia stuartii		24%			

[n] Bibliographic reference number; short-time catheterization: <30 days; long-time catheterization: ≥30 days; n: number of isolated microbial serogroups; JW Warren: Patients admitted to one general hospital and to two nursing homes; NNISS (National Nosocomial Infection Surveillance System): Coronary ICUs in the USA: MJ Richards; Medical ICUs in the USA; ENVIN-UCI: 49 medical and surgical ICUs in Spain.

TABLE 4. Etiology of the renal abscess and the emphysematous pyelonephritis

	Renal Abscess	Emphysematous Pyelonephritis	
	Fowler[25] (n = 74)	Wan[26] (n = 35)	Shokeir[27] (n = 20)
E. coli	36%	63%	80%
Proteus mirabilis	18%		5%
Klebsiella pneumoniae	14%	26%	20%
Pseudomonas aeruginosa	11%		5%
Other enterobacteriaceae	8%		
Staphylococcus aureus	8%		
Enterococcus spp.	4%		
Candida albicans	1%		
Polymicrobial episodes	23% (14/60)	11%	10%

[n]: Bibliographic reference number, n: Number of microbiological isolates (Fowler), or episodes of infection (Wan, Shokeir).

pollakiuria, dysuria and, occasionally, fever. The clinical picture of the upper UTI usually comprises fever, chills, abdominal flank pain, and symptoms of the lower UTI. The pain is habitually stronger when there is an obstruction and, with calculi, it frequently irradiates to the groin. However, this pattern may be extremely variable, with a large number of asymptomatic upper UTI or those with just low symptoms [19, 22]. It is not unusual to see an atypical clinical picture in patients admitted to ICU. 37% to 44% of the nosocomial UTI manifest as asymptomatic bacteriuria [9, 10]. Catheterized patients do not usually manifest low symptoms [22]. Sedation, brain injury, advanced age or other circumstances may mask the picture and cause the general manifestations to predominate. Thus, Rosser *et al.* [4] found a urinary origin in 18.5% of ICU patients with a clinical picture of sepsis. Furthermore, bacteremia and shock are more frequent in elderly patients, especially if they are catheterized (up to 61% and 26%, respectively) [4, 19, 22]. On the other hand, bacteremia is a serious complication of UTI, with mortality rates of 16% to 30% in patients manifesting it [3, 30]. Both community-acquired and the nosocomial UTI are an important cause of bacteremia. However, in the group of the ICU nosocomial bacteremia, a urinary origin is infrequent (2%–6%), but up to 34% of these is accompanied by severe sepsis or septic shock, especially when caused by Gram-negative bacilli [2, 31]. The possibilities that this complication appears varies according to the population and the UTI studied. In patients with short catheterization time and bacteriuria, <5% manifested bacteremia [19]. In pyelonephritis, it can be seen in up to 61% of cases, especially in elderly individuals [22]. And 40% of the episodes of renal abscesses and emphysematous pyelonephritis are accompanied by bacteremia [3, 25–27].

In a large number (59%) of renal/perirenal abscesses, there are no low symptoms, and there is a possibility of an insidious clinical picture and persistent fever [22, 23, 25]. Furthermore, pain by compression of the eleventh rib or the presence of an abdominal mass on the flank can be observed. In their series, Fowler and Perkins find unilateral pain in 22% of the cases, and palpable abdominal mass in 36% of the cases [25]. Whereas they are, as a whole, more frequent in women (with a ratio of 3:2), some are more frequent in men (cortical abscess), or in patients with advanced ages (corticomedullar) [22, 23, 25].

Lastly, emphysematous pyelonephritis,though infrequent, is a critical form of necrotizing UTI, which is typified by the presence of gas in the renal parenchyma. It often extends to the perinephric area. It is prevalent in women (2–3 : 1) and affects especially the left kidney [27, 32]. Although not exclusive, 70–90% of the cases occur on diabetic patients [33]. The clinical picture is not very different from that of the other UTI. However, the severe presentation with shock and renal failure is frequent, whereas the occurrence of low symptoms is less habitual [27]. *E. coli* remains to be the first responsible organism (Table 4) [26, 27]. Three circumstances seem to determe its appearance: Presence of gas-forming bacteria, a high tissular glucose concentration, and bad perfusion of the parenchyma. Therefore, Diabetes Mellitus, an obstruction of the excretory tract and a previous renal infection are to be considered as the most habitual risk factors. Its prognosis relates to the level of renal disfunction and radiological extension, being more critical in individuals with levels of creatinine >2.4 mg/dl and in type I pyelonephritis [26].

2. **Laboratory**: Some of the results are not very specific or did not clearly demonstrate their clinical usefulness so far (leucocytosis, Limulus endotoxin test, α_2-microglobuline, antibody coating of bacteria) [22]. The presence of pyuria in the urinary sediment (more than 5–10 leucocytes/high power field) is not specific, and there are not yet enough studies which correlate it adequately with the presence of bacteriuria. However, it is useful to suspect the diagnosis of UTI, as it associates to most of them, despite the fact that it may not be present in 30% of the

cases of renal abscesses [22, 23]. Likewise, the leukocyte esterase test, a rapid urine test with high sensitivity, specificity and negative predictive value, excludes reasonably well the possibility of pyuria when negative [22, 32].

More useful in the presumptive diagnosis is the direct identification of bacteria in the urinary sediment by means of Gram's staining, or the direct identification by means of a nitrites urinary test. In the first, the presence of a bacterium/high power field correlates with $>10^5$ bacteria/ml of urine. In the second, the identification of the product of the nitrites reduction by the bacteria has a high sensitivity and yields a small number of false positives [22, 34].

However, in patients with UTI admitted to ICUs, it is necessary in the first place to identify the causative microorganism by means of a urine or blood culture, or other appropriate specimens. In this sense, we have to keep in mind some considerations. First, unlike non-complicated UTIs, there is a greater possibility that there exist a multiplicity of germs, that these are multiresistant, non-habitual, or of difficult growth, thus increasing the severity of the clinical picture or make the treatment more difficult [4, 18, 23, 25–27, 33, 35]. Second, on the background of studies on the female population, the presence of $\geq 10^5$ cfu/ml in urine culture is admitted as the limit of significant bacteriuria. However, UTIs with a lower rate may be seen, amongst other cases, in men, catheterized patients, presence of abscesses or diluted urine, and when the causative agent is not an enterobacteria [19, 22, 23, 25, 34]. Thus, Stark and Maki [36] found that the initial concentration of $<10^5$ cfu/ml observed in 41 out of 110 patients, increased to $\geq 10^5$ cfu/ml in a mean of three days, unless these were administered antibiotics. This was also appreciated in those patients with initial counting within the lowest detectable range (1–99 cfu/ml). On the other hand, even in 40% of the cases of renal abscesses, the urine culture may be negative [22]. Last, the urine culture with a growth of more than one single pathogen is usually considered to be contaminated, especially, when there is a presence of *Diphteroids* or coagulase-negative *Staphylococcus*. However, a confirmation and analysis of the context in which it occurs is indispensable, since, as mentioned formerly, an important number of times it will represent a true UTI. We can find it especially in elderly patients, in patients with a long catheterization time and in nosocomial infections [37].

3. **Radiologic**: In most UTIs, performing an imaging test is not necessary. However, for those cases of complicated infections which may make it necessary, we have the following possibilities at our disposal (Table 5):

- *Plain film of the Abdomen*. Of scant value for a diagnosis of pyelonephritis and its complications. It is very useful, however, for the detection of radio opaque calculi suggestive of an obstruction; it is also highly sensitive to emphysematous pyelonephritis [27, 33].
- *Intravenous urography (IVU)*: Results will be normal in 75% of the cases of non-complicated pyelonephritis [38]. In the rest, an increase of the focal or diffuse renal size with delayed appearance of the contrast in the calices, and attenuation of the nephrogram and the urogram can be appreciated [38, 39]. It is not very useful for the study of parenchymatous anomalies and perirenal extension [39]. A further disadvantage is that it requires the use of a contrast. The usefulness of IVU lies in the fact that it allows a knowledge on the exact location of obstructions and their extension.
- *Radionuclides*: Some of them, like Tc99m glycoheptanate, Tc99m mercaptoacetilglycine X3, or Tc99m DMSA, adhere specifically to the renal tissue. Thus, they allow good pictures of the renal anatomy to be obtained, at the same time they serve to assess its working. However, they do not adhere to the inflammated areas, because of the compromised blood flow and tissular destruction. Therefore, there is no indication for its use in the cases of acute pyelonephritis in adult patients.

Others, like Gallium Citrate (Ga-67) and Indium-111 combined with leucocytes (In-

TABLE 5. Imaging techniques in the diagnosis of urinary tract infection

	Advantages	Disadvantages
P.F. abdomen	No need of moving the patient No need of contrast High sensitivity to emphysematous pyelonephritis	No specific findings of pyelonephritis or complications
IVU	Exact assessment of the location and size of an obstruction	Contrast necessary Requires moving the patient No specific findings of pyelonephritis or complications
Radionuclides	Location of the infection in case of uncertain diagnosis	Requires at least 24 hours for obtention of the image No differentiation of acute pyelonephritis or abscesses No assessment of the extension of the disease
Echography	It can be done at the patient's bed Very good sensitivity for diagnosis of abscesses The technique of choice in hydronephrosis No need of contrast	No correct assessment of the extrarenal extension No assessment of renal functioning
CT	It is the most sensitive technique for the study of pyelonephritis and its complications	It needs contrast The patient has to be moved

P.F. abdomen: Plain film of the abdomen; IVU: Intravenous urography; CT: Computed tomography.

111-WBC) provide little information about the renal anatomy or function. They are useful to locate hidden infection sites, when the other techniques are not diagnostic [39]. However, the pictures are not available until after 24 hours (In-111-WBC), or 48–72 hours (Ga-67), and do not allow the differentiation between an abscesses and an acute pyelonephritis. Moreover, Ga-67 adheres to tumors (lymphoma) and non-infectious inflammatory processes (interstitial nephritis) [39]. Thus, its usefulness for a diagnosis and follow-up of UTI is rather limited.

– *Renal echography*: Its non-invasivity, absence of radiations and no need of using contrasts, as well as the possibility of being used at the patient's bed, allowing directed punctures at the same time, are some of the advantages of this technique. However, it is less sensitive than computed tomography (CT) [38].

In most cases of UTI, the echography will be normal [38, 39]. In acute pyelonephritis, the most typical finding is an increase in the size of the kidneys and the loss of corticomedullar differentiation, with a diminishing of the echogenicity of the organ caused by the presence of edema [38]. The presence of hyperechoic lesions is less frequent, and would represent areas of hemorrhage.

On the other hand, echography is highly sensitive for the diagnosis of complications: abscesses will be seen as thin-wall cystic lesions with echoes in their insides [39]. In their series, Fowler and Perkins [25] were able to locate abscesses with this technique in 92% of the cases. In pyonephrosis, the characteristic fact is the visualization of a swollen pyelocalyceal system, with echoes in the inside changing their location as the patient moves [38, 39].

However, it is little sensitive for a diagnosis of emphysematous pyelonephritis. Hyperechoic areas with posterior acoustic shade due to the presence of gas may be observed with echography [38], however it does not assess adequately the extension of the illness. In their study, Shokeir *et al.* [27], refer only a 10% of echographic diagnoses.

Other limitations of echography are that it does not asses the renal function and that it has a low sensitivity for a study of the extrarenal extension of the UTI [38, 39].

- *Computed tomography (CT)*: It is the most valuable technique for a study of acute pyelonephritis and its complications. It allows an assessment of the extension of the illness and the performing of directed punctures.

It is important to remember that a correct renal study with CT requires performing this technique both before and after administering a contrast [40]. Without the contrast, presence of gas, calculi, calcifications, hemorrhage and inflammatory mass can be appreciated. Between 20 seconds–2 minutes after injecting the contrast, the renal anatomy can be visualized; within 2–3 minutes, the contrast appears in the collector system, outlining accurately the extension of the disease and the presence of abscesses or obstructions [40].

In acute pyelonephritis, the most typical findings are the focal or diffuse increase of the renal size, associated to lesions with a wedge-shaped diminishing of the attenuation, which extends from the papilla to the cortical surface [39, 40].

CT is the most suitable technique for a diagnosis of the abscesses [40]. These usually appear as a well-defined mass of low attenuation, with a thin and irregular wall, or pseudocapsule. The presence of gas is very suggestive of abscesses. It is also the most sensitive test for a diagnosis of emphysematous pyelonephritis, with a sensitiveness of 100% in the series of Shokeir *et al.* [27]. Without the contrast, we can observe the presence of intrarenal or extrarenal gas, with or without liquid accumulation.

However, some disadvantages are that it needs the administration of contrasts and taking the patient out of the ICU.

- Taking into account the former, our view is that imaging tests should be performed on critically ill patients (septic shock), on those who present a higher risk of complications (improperly controlled Diabetes, or obstruction), or those with a bad clinical course (e.g., with symptoms like fever on the 72 hours after initiating antibiotic therapy), or relapse.

The customary techniques for that purpose should be echography and CT, with the choice depending both on their availability in the hospital and the possibility of moving the patient, and keeping in mind that CT provides a higher diagnostic reliability. A suspicion of emphysematous pyelonephritis should be confirmed with the performance of a CT. Although, where this is not possible, it should be remembered that abdominal radiography may diagnose between 55% [27] and 85% [33] of the cases. After diagnosis, the follow-up may be done by means of using echography, because of its low risks and good availability. The frequency of check-ups will depend on the type of treatment and the clinical course. In the cases of good clinical course we can perform a weekly check-up until resolution of the picture.

Treatment

Apart from the general supporting measures the patient may need (fundamentally, volume and inotropic agents or vasopressors), the treatment of the UTIs is directed towards controlling both the origin of the infection and the underlying pathology precipitating its onset. In relation to the first aspect of the treatment, we have at our disposal antibiotic therapy and percutaneous or surgical drainage, and even nephrectomy. As to the second aspect, we shall resort to an adequate metabolic control (Diabetes Mellitus), or solve the anatomic-functional problems that may exist (especially obstruction) by means of using a nephrostomy tube, surgery or other measures.

The antibiotic to be used has to have good renal elimination, so as to achieve appropriate levels both in the parenchyma and in urine. For most of the cases, the beginning of the treatment will be empiric, taking into account the characteristics of the patient and his clinical picture, as well as the usual flora of the environment. At this stage, a Gram's staining of the collected specimens may help us to select the pattern (presence/absence of Gram-negative bacilli, Gram-positive cocci, and their disposition). In the light or moderate infections, oral treatment may be started if the patient shows a good tolerance; as for the rest of cases we have to consider switching to this type of treatment for the moment of the deffervescence of the clinical picture.

The use of monotherapy is an appropriate way of initiating treatment of both light and moderate UTI. Trimethoprim-sulphametoxazole, ciprofloxacin, amoxicillin/clavulanic acid, an aminoglycoside, or aztreonam are some of the possible options.

However, it is necessary to know the level of sensitiveness of the *E. coli* in the environment, as resistance levels of >20% have been described, especially against the first three antibiotics mentioned [22, 34, 41, 42].

In severe infections, especially in patients with hemodynamic instability, we shall first resort to a combination of a betalactamic, or ciprofloxacin in the case of allergy, with a parenteral aminoglycoside. Aztreonam, a cephalosporin of the 3rd or 4th generation, piperacillin-tazobactam, or a carbapenem are possible alternatives for this combination. As mentioned above, nosocomial infection, urologic instrumentation, a previous use of antibiotics, or a long catheterization time are some of the risk factors for the appearance of non-habitual or resistant microorganisms. If we use a cephalosporin for these cases, we should choose those with antipseudomonal activity (ceftazidime, cefepime). The covering of *Enterococcus spp*, in the treatment patterns with aztreonam or cephalosporin, will be achieved by associating ampicillin, or vancomycin or teicoplanin for the case of allergy. Moreover, increasing importance of the betalactamase-producing microorganisms inside the ICU shall be taken into account by using those antibiotics which show a better stability against them (cefepime, piperacillin-tazobactam, carbapenem) [3].

The theoretical advantages of the inclusion of an aminoglycoside in the antibiotic pattern (wider antibacterial spectrum, antibiotical synergy and reduction of resistance) are not firmly established yet. With the antibiotics of wide spectrum available at present, good cure rates may be achieved [43, 44]. However, there are patients with severe infections, especially of bacteremic type caused by high-risk microorganisms (*Pseudomonas aeruginosa*, *Acinetobacter spp*, *Enterobacter spp*), who showed a better clinical course with the use of an associated aminoglycoside [44]. Thus, we advocate initiating empiric combination therapy with those patients who run a high risk of UTI caused by the mentioned microorganisms, and later adjust the treatment in line with the microbiological results.

For the case of renal abscesses, the relative importance of *Staphylococcus aureus* as an etiologic agent gets us to include cloxacillin in the initial covering or, in the case of allergy, vancomycin. Carbapenem, which shows a good activity against *S. aureus*, may be a good alternative to monotherapy in these cases, as long as these are methicillin-sensible. On the other hand, the anaerobicidal spectrum of this group of antibiotics and piperacillin-tazobactam will be useful in the treatment of those UTI with a risk of anaerobic microorganisms (perirenal abscess).

The management of *Candida spp* in urine is yet far from being solved. Most often, it represents a colonization that may be controlled just with the removal of the most habitual risk factors (urinary catheter, antibiotics). However, if symptomatic candiduria persists after the catheter has been replaced, we shall have to initiate treatment, the same as in the case of its pressence with Diabetes Mellitus, anomalies in the urinary tract, renal transplantations, or when it is symptomatic (with presence of accompanying pyuria) [45]. Likewise, initiation of treatment is indicated in this case, when there is a need of undertaking any urologic manipulation. The eradication rate of funguria is similar using vesical irrigation with anphotericin B, or fluconazol by systemic via. However, some authors observed a higher mortality rate with the first treatment pattern [29]. The cause of this is not clear yet, but it might relate to a higher rate of candidemia in the patients receiving local treatment. Thus, it is advisable to treat candiduria with fluconazol, unless there is a risk of resistance to that drug [45].

In 50% of the patients with candidemia there may exist candiduria, or *vice versa* [21, 29]. At the same time, the presence of *Candida spp* in urine may be a manifestation not only of a cystitis but also of other renal infections (obstructive uropathy by fungus balls, pyelonephritis, or abscesses). This shall force us to be alert to these possibilities and initiate the corresponding research, especially, if the candiduria persists despite the treatment. On the other hand, oral or endovenous fluconazol may be the first therapeutic option to be considered for the upper UTIs as long as the patient's condition is stable and the possibility of azoles-resistant *Candida spp* is low (not-previous use of these drugs, absence of No-*C. albicans*, especially *C. krusei*) [21, 45]. In the opposite case, we shall resort to systemic administration of anphotericin B. Furthermore, if there exists an obstructive uropathy or abscesses, an endoscopic or surgical correction is indicated.

There is no evidence that the treatment of asymptomatic bacteriuria, so frequent in elderly people and individuals with a long catheterization time, has a positive repercussion on the morbidity/mortality rate of the patients [22, 46]. Therefore, it might only be indicated in some special situations (as prior to genitourinary surgery or other, where a prosthesis is going to be implanted; after a renal transplantation; immunodepressed patients, patients with a prosthesis, pregnant women; or as a means of controlling an outbreak of nosocomial infections or bacterial resistance).

The antibiotic treatment of UTI in our unit has to be kept around 10–14 days [3, 19, 22, 34]. In normal cases, deffervescence of the clinical picture occurs rapidly. Thus, if fever persists more than 72 hours, it is necessary to initiate an investigation of the causes. An inadequate covering, insufficient renal concentration of the antibiotics (it is important to pay special attention to individuals with renal insufficiency), or the onset of complications (calculi, obstructions, abscesses) may be some of the possible causes. However, we have to be aware that a hyperthermia that lasts more than three days is not necessarily indicative of a negative course. Behr *et al.* [47] found a mean duration of the fever of 34 hours in a series of 70 patients hospitalized for acute pyelonephritis. In 13% of the cases, fever persisted more than 72 hours without any complications existing. Anyhow, although in most of the UTIs the mentioned time will be sufficient, in some more complicated infections (upper UTI for *Candida spp*, abscesses) we shall have to prolong the antibiotic treatment up to 4–6 weeks [21, 23].

On the other hand, in the case of emphysematous pyelonephritis, the exclusive medical treatment is accompanied by a mortality rate higher than 70% [32]. For that reason, a precocious nephrectomy is indicated once the patient has been stabilized. By this way, Shokeir *et al.* were able to reduce the mortality rate to 20% [27]. However, Chen *et al.* [32] reached a cure rate of 80% in a series of 25 patients by using antibiotic therapy associated to percutaneous drainage directed by CT. In another 12%, after an initial improvement with percutaneous drainage, it was necessary to carry out nephrectomy without ulterior complications. The final mortality rate was of 8%. Although further studies are necessary to obtain confirmation, this strategy might be indicated for those patients where bilateral nephrectomy is being considered, of for those ones who run a high risk if subjected to aggressive initial surgery.

Furthermore, in a number of renal abscesses antibiotic treatment shall be sufficient, although some patients will also require pus drainage. In this indication, percutaneous drainage, because of its better tolerance and good results, is gaining positions against surgery [23, 25]. The size of the collection is one of the most important factors in considering possible alternatives. On a total of 52 patients, Siegel *et al.* [48] resolved 100% of the abscesses just with antibiotic therapy, when the size was ≤3 cm. With abscesses of 3–5 cm, the success with percutaneous drainage was 92%. And in those of >5 cm, more than one percutaneous drainage procedure was necessary in 33% of the cases, being even necessary to perform open surgery in 37% of the cases.

Last, most of the UTIs cure without any consequence on the middle or long term under application of the appropriate treatment [18, 19, 22, 28]. It is the more complex infections (papillary necrosis, emphysematous pyelonephritis) which may cause them to occur most habitually, facilitated frequently by the accompanying pathology [21, 22, 27, 32, 33]. However, it is as well to remember that their mortality rate, although not always connected to the UTI itself [12], may be high. Mortality rates of 30% have been described for urinary catheter-associated bacteremia [3], of 15%–60% for sepsis of urinary origin [4], of 7%–50% for renal abscesses [23, 25], and of 8%–42% for emphysematous pyelonephritis [25, 32].

Prevention

As has been mentioned at the beginning of this chapter, catheter-associated NIs are the most frequent UTIs in ICUs. The efforts undertaken to reducing its incidence will affect positively in the rate of morbidity/mortality of our patients. Here, some of the most important aspects associated with their prevention shall be revised:

- *Catheterize patients only if necessary*: The best way of avoiding catheter-associated UTIs is by rationalizing the use of catheters.

  Routine or convenience of the sanitary staff shall not be accepted as a reason for catheterization. In ICUs, the most important indications for use of catheters are monitoring of diuresis in unstable patients and resolution of episodes of retention related to anatomic or functional alterations of the urinary tract. When it is not necessary any longer, the catheter has to be removed as soon as possible.

  Although reasonable, this policy is not always kept. Jain *et al.* [49] found that 21% of the indications were not appropriate, being the catheter was kept unnecessarily in 47% of the total of days studied. In patients admitted to ICUs, an excessive time of measurement of the diuresis determined 64% of the unjustified days with indwelling catheter. In other areas of the hospital, urinary incontinence was the most important cause for the unnecessary use of indwelling catheters.
- *Use closed drainage systems*: With their introduction, a reduction of the infection rate from 100% to 28% in short-time catheterization was achieved [18].

  However, it is necessary to observe a set of norms that contribute to keep the effectiveness of this system [18, 50, 51]. The passing of the catheter has to be done aseptically, and sterilized material has to be used. The collector bag must be situated below the level of the patient's bladder and without touching the floor. Urine specimens will be obtained aseptically by means of puncture on the indicated point. Likewise, the indispensable irrigation of the system shall be done aseptically. In the case of obstruction, disconnection, breaking of the asepsis, or leakage, the entire system must be replaced. Last, it is of the utmost importance that the clinical staff wash their hands before and after any manipulation of the device [52].
- *Other measures*: There are many methods under study to prevent or delay appearance of bacteriuria, but to date none of these has proved

to be totally efficient [18, 19, 51]. Latex, silicone, latex with a covering of silicone, and teflon are some of the materials used in the manufacture of urinary catheters. The silicone catheters seem to be more comfortable and have a lower tendency to get obstructed, a reason which makes them an appropriate alternative for long-term catheterization [18].

Likewise, several strategies designed to limiting bacterial adhesion and multiplication on the catheters are being studied (like impregnating them with antibiotics or antiseptics, or using silver-lined catheters, and application of substances produced by iontoforesis) [18, 19, 51]. Among all of these, the covering with silver alloys is the one showing better results, although the cost and other factors put limits to its use [53]. On the other hand, despite the fact that some authors refer benefits of the disinfection of the urinary meatus with povidone-iodine solution [54], a daily hygiene with water and soap still seems to be the most reasonable practice. Moreover, though several studies have correlated a lower incidence of UTI to a previous use of antibiotics, their systematic use as a prophylactic is not indicated because of its time-limited effectiveness and the possibility of appearance of resistant microorganisms [15, 18, 19]. However, it may be considered for those cases of short-term catheterization of high-risk patients, like those who have been subjected to renal transplantation, or the neutropenic patients.

Also, the use of antiseptics like oral Methenamine, was able to reduce the onset of bacteriuria in individuals subjected to intermittent catheterization [19, 51]. Other strategies, like the use of vaccines, of analogues of the bacterial receptors, bacterial interference, or immunotherapy are being explored at present [51].

– *Alternatives to the use of indwelling catheters*: The confirmation of risks derived from the use of indwelling catheters has brought about an increased concern about possible alternatives. The use of some of these in selected groups of patients seems to reduce both the incidence of UTI and other complications associated to indwelling catheters [55]. The options which seem to be more valuable with patients admitted to the ICU, are as follows:

a. *Condom collectors*: Placed on the penis, they drain urine to a collector bag to which they are connected. They are useful with men without obstructive problems and conserved vesical voiding reflexes. Although their use does not lack problems (cutaneous ulceration, gangrene of the penis because of excessive constriction, or removal of the device by agitated patients), several studies showed a reduction of the incidence of UTI [18, 19, 55]. Nevertheless, the urine collected may contain high concentrations of microorganisms that might colonize the urethra and the skin. In this sense, although with methodological limitations, some study has shown that these devices may become UTI-risk factors [56]. Thus, they have to be replaced every day, and special attention has to be devoted to the hygiene of the area.

b. *Intermittent catheterization*: This method has become the standard for the urinary care of the patients with medullar lesion. However, other patients with altered vesical functions are likely to benefit from this alternative even in critical situations [18, 19]. Despite the fact that, with a theoretical incidence of bacteriuria of 1%–3% per catheterization the patient will develop an episode of bacteriuria after 1–3 weeks, a number of studies proved that this method may have advantages with respect to permanent catheterization [19, 57, 58]. The use of low-friction hydrophilic catheters seems to diminish the complications with respect to the conventional catheters [57].

Indeed, the vesical voiding with a frequency enough as to allow the volume in each catheterization to be <400 ml, is a good way of minimizing the hazard of UTI [58]. Other complications associated to catheterization which have been described are: bleeding, urethral stenosis, urethral fistulae, vesical calculi, hydronephrosis and epididymitis [19].

c. *Suprapubic catheterization*: Used especially with individuals subjected to urologic or gynecologic surgery, there is still a lack of sufficient studies that compare the advantages of this technique over urethral catheterization [18, 19]. It is more comfortable for the patient, allowing to check their capacity of vesical voiding and, as has been shown in some studies, the lower bacterial density of the skin of the anterior abdominal wall helps the UTI risk to be kept down [18]. However, it has to be implanted by specialists and is not exempt of complications (hematoma, leakage, infections).
d. *Diapers*: It is an alternative which, in well selected patients, and with a proper hygiene, may be accompanied with a risk of UTI lower than with the use of urinary catheters, as Zimakoff *et al.* [56] have observed.

Summary

Urinary tract infections (UTI) are frequent in daily clinical practice. In ICU, most of them will be of nosocomial origin, fundamentally related to the use of a urinary catheter. The most habitual way of arrival of microorganisms is the ascendent path. The presence of obstruction of the urinary flow, Diabetes Mellitus, an advanced age, female sex and urologic instrumentation are the main risk factors. In the case of catheter-associated UTI, the most important factor is the catheterization time. *Escherichia coli* continues to be the first causative agent, though in nosocomial or complicated UTI the presence of other Gram-negative bacilli, *Staphylococcus aureus*, coagulase-negative *Staphylococcus*, *Enterococcus spp.* and *Candida spp.* is increasing. Polymicrobial etiology can be observed in ≥15% of the episodes. Several circumstances present in our patients (sedation, brain pathologies, advanced age, urinary catheter) may mask the typical clinical picture. It is not unusual that a bacteriuria $\leq 10^5$ cfu/ml represents a true UTI in our patients, especially if they are catheterized. In critically ill patients, as well as those with a high risk of complications, or those with a negative course, it is advisable to perform an imaging test (echography, computed tomography), in order to help us attain an overall knowledge of their clinical picture. Both in light and moderate infections, the application of monotherapy with trimethoprim-sulphametoxazole or ciprofloxacin will be sufficient, while in severe infections we find it more indicated to initiate treatment with an association of a betalactamic and an aminoglycoside, which shall be adjusted as we receive the microbiological results. The prevention of catheter-associated UTI by means of a correct indication and maintenance of the catheter, the use of closed systems and, in selected individuals, the use of alternatives to permanent catheterization, is indispensable if we are to reduce the morbidity/mortality of these infections.

References

1. Ronald A, Harding G. Complicated urinary tract infections. Infect Dis Clin North Am 11(3):583–592, 1997.
2. Vallés J, León C, Alvarez-Lerma F, Spanish Collaborative Group for Infections in Intensive Care Units. Nosocomial Bacteremia in Critically Ill Patients: A multicenter study evaluating epidemiology and prognosis. Clin Infect Dis 24:387–395, 1997.
3. Paradisi F, Corti G, Mangani V. Urosepsis in the critical care unit. Crit Care Clin 14:165–180, 1998.
4. Rosser C, Bare R, Meredith J. Urinary tract infections in the critically ill patient with urinary catheter. Am J Surg 177(4):287–290, 1999.
5. Nicole L, Friesen D, Harding GKM, Roos LL. Hospitalization for acute pyelonephritis in Manitoba, Canada, during the period from 1989 to 1992: Impact of diabetes, pregnancy and aboriginal origin. Clin Infect Dis 22:1051–1056, 1996.
6. Vincent J, Bihari DJ, Suter PM, Bruining HA, White J, Nicolas-Chanoin MH, Wolf M, Spencer RC, Hemmer M. The prevalence of nosocomial infection in Intensive Care Units in Europe. Results of the European Prevalence of Infection in Intensive Care (EPIC) Study. JAMA 274(8):639–644, 1995.

7. Vaqué J, Roselló J, Trilla A, Monge V, García-Caballero J, Arribas JL, Blasco P, Sáenz-Domínguez JR, Albero I, Calvo F, Barrio J, Herruzo R, Sáenz-González C, Arévalo JM. Nosocomial infections in Spain: Results of five nationwide serial prevalence surveys (EPINE project, 1990 to 1994). Infect Control Hosp Epidemiol 17(5):293–297, 1996.
8. Legras A, Malvy D, Quinioux AL, Villers D, Bouachour G, Robert R, Thomas R. Nosocomial infections: prospective survey of incidence in five French intensive care units. Intensive Care Med 24:1040–1046, 1998.
9. Richards M, Edwards JR, Culver DH, Gaynes RP. Nosocomial infections in medical intensive care units in the United States. Crit Care Med 27(5):887–892, 1999.
10. No authors listed. National Nosocomial Infections Surveillance (NNIS) System Report, Data Summary from October 1986–April 1998, issued June 1998. Am J Infect Control 26:522–533, 1998.
11. Alvarez-Lerma F, de la Cal MA, Palomar M, Insausti J, Olaechea P, Spanish Study Group Surveillance of ICU-acquired Infection. Nosocomial Infection Rates as an Indicator of Quality Care in Critically Ill Patients. in 10th Annual Congress of the European Society of Intensive Care Medicine. Paris (France). Intensive Care Med 23 (Suppl 1): Abstract 159, 1997.
12. Fagon J, Novara A, Stephan F, Girou E, Safar M. Mortality attributable to nosocomial infections in the ICU. Infect Control Hosp Epidemiol 15(7):428–434, 1994.
13. Platt R, Polk F, Murdock B, Rosner B. Mortality associated with nosocomial urinary-tract infection. N Engl J Med 307:637–642, 1982.
14. Jarvis W. Selected aspects of the socioeconomic impact of nosocomial infections: morbidity, mortallity, cost, and prevention. Infect Control Hosp Epidemiol 17(8):552–557, 1996.
15. Schaeffer A. Catheter-associated bacteriuria. Urol Clin North Am 13(4):735–747, 1986.
16. Sobel J. Pathogenesis of urinary tract infection. Infect Dis Clin North Am 11(3):531–549, 1997.
17. Tambyah P, Halvorson K, Maki D. A prospective study of pathogenesis of catheter-associated urinary tract infections. Mayo Clin Proc 74:131–136, 1999.
18. Sedor J, Mulholland S. Hospital-acquired urinary tract infections associated with the indwelling catheter. Urol Clin North Am 26:821–828, 1999.
19. Warren J. Nosocomial Urinary Tract Infections, in Mandell, Douglas and Bennett's Principles and Practice of Infectious Diseases. Mandell G, Bennett J, Dolin R (eds). Churchill Livingstone: New York, Edinburgh, London, Madrid, Melbourne, Milan, Tokyo. 1995: 2607–2616.
20. Measley R, Levison M. Host defense mechanisms in the pathogenesis of urinary tract infection. Med Clin North Am 75(2):275–286, 1991.
21. Wise G, Talluri G, Marella V. Fungal infections of the genitourinary system: manifestations, diagnosis and treatment. Urol Clin North Am 26(4):701–718, 1999.
22. Sobel J, Kaye D, Urinary Tract Infections, in Mandell, Douglas and Bennett's Principles and practice of Infectious Diseases. Mandell G, Bennett J, Dolin R (eds). Churchill Livingstone: New York, Edinburgh, London, Madrid, Melbourne, Milan, Tokyo. 1995: 662–690.
23. Dembry L, Andriole V. Renal and Perirrenal Abscesses. Infect Dis Clin North Am 11(3):663–680, 1997.
24. Svanborg C, Godaly G. Bacterial virulence in urinary tract infection. Infect Dis Clin North Am 11(3):513–529, 1997.
25. Fowler J, Perkins T. Presentation, diagnosis and treatment of renal abscesses: 1972–1988. J Urol 151:847–851, 1994.
26. Wan Y-L, Lo S, Bullard M, Chang P, Lee T. Predictors of outcome in emphysematous pyelonephritis. J Urol 159:369–373, 1998.
27. Shokeir AA, El-Azab M, Mosen T, El-Diasty T. Emphysematous pyelonephritis: a 15 year experience with 20 cases. Urology 49(3):343–346, 1997.
28. Bacheller C, Bernstein J. Urinary tract infections. Med Clin North Am 81(3):719–730, 1997.
29. Jacobs L, Eskidmore E, Freeman K. Lipschultz D, Fox N. Oral Fluconazole compared with bladder irrigation with Amphotericin B for treatment of fungal urinary tract infections in elderly patients. Clin Infect Dis 22:30–35, 1996.
30. Ackerman R, Monroe P. Bacteremic urinary tract infection in older people. J Am Geriatr Soc 44(8):927–933, 1996.
31. Edgeworth J, Tracher D, Eykyn S. A 25-year study of nosocomial bacteriemia in an adult intensive care unit. Crit Care Med 27(8):1421–1428, 1999.
32. Chen M, Huang ChN, Chou Y, Huang ChH, Chiang ChP, Liu G. Percutaneous drainage in the treatment of emphysematous pyelonephritis: 10-year experience. J Urol 157:1569–1573, 1997.

33. Patterson J, Andriole V. Bacterial urinary tract infections in diabetes. Infect Dis Clin North Am 11(3):735–750, 1997.
34. Hamilton-Miller J. Urinary Tract Infections. Curr Opin Infect Dis 10:66–69, 1997.
35. Palomar M, Alvarez-Lerma F, de la Cal MA, Insausti J, Olaechea P, ENVIN-UCI Study Group. Aetiology and sensitivity patterns of the ICU acquired infections in Spain. in 10th Annual Congress of the European Society of Intensive Care Medicine. Paris (France): Intensive Care Med 23 (Suppl 1): Abstract 655, 1997.
36. Stark R, Maki D. Bacteriuria in the catheterized patient. What quantitative level of bacteriuria is relevant? N Engl J Med 311:560–564, 1984.
37. Siegman-Igra Y. The significance of urine culture with mixed flora. Curr Opin Nephrol Hypertens 3:656–659, 1994.
38. Baumgarten D, Baumgartner B. Imaging and radilogic management of upper urinary tract infections. Urol Clin North Am 24:545–569, 1997.
39. Papanicolau N, Pfister R. Acute renal infections. Radiol Clin North Am 34:965–995, 1996.
40. Kawashima A, Sandler CM, Goldman SM, Raval BK, Fishman EK. CT of renal inflamatory disease. Radiographics 17:851–868, 1997.
41. Natsch S, Conrad C, Hartmeier C, Schmid B. Use of amoxicillin-clavulanate and resistance in Escherichia coli over a 4-year period. Infect Control Hosp Epidemiol 19:653–656, 1998.
42. Verzasconi R, Rodoni P, Monotti R, Marone C, Mombelli G. Amoxicillin and clavulanic acid versus amoxicillin plus gentamicin in the empirical initial treatment of urinary tract infections in hospitalized patients. Schweiz Med Wochenschr 125:1533–1539, 1995.
43. Sandberg T, Alesting K, Eliard T, Ek E, Hebelka M, Johanson E, Olinder-Nielsen AM. Aminoglycosides do not improve the efficacy of cephalosporins for treatment of acute pyelonephritis in women. Scand J Infect Dis 29:175–179, 1997.
44. Edson R, Terrell C. The Aminoglycosides. Mayo Clin Proc 74:519–528, 1994.
45. Edwards J, Bodey GP, Bowden RA, Buchner T, de Pauw BE, Filler SG, Ghannoum MA, Glauser M, Herbrecht R, Kauffman CA, Kohno S, Martino P, Meunier F, Mori T, Pfaller MA, Rex JH, Rogers TR, Rubin RH, Solomkim J, Viscoli G, Walsh TJ, White M. International Conference for the Development of a Consensus on the Management and Prevention of Severe Candidal Infections. Clin Infect Dis 25(1):43–59, 1997.
46. Reid G, Nicolle L. Asymptomatic bacteriuria in spinal cord patients and the elderly. Urol Clin North Am 26(4):789–795, 1999.
47. Behr M, Drummond R, Libman MD, Delaney JS, Dylewsky JS. Fever duration in hospitalized acute pyelonephritis patients. Am J Med 101:277–280, 1996.
48. Siegel J, Smith A, Moldwin R. Minimally invasive treatment of renal abscess. J Urol 155:52–55, 1996.
49. Jain P, Parada JP, David A, Smith LG. Overuse of the indwelling urinary tract catheter in hospitalized medical patients. Arch Intern Med 155:1425–1429, 1995.
50. Wong E. Guideline for prevention of catheter-associated urinary tract infections. Am J Infect Control 11:28–36, 1983.
51. Galloway A. Prevention of urinary tract infection in patients with spinal cord injury – a microbiológical review. Spinal Cord 35:198–204, 1997.
52. Goldman D, Larson E. Hand-washing and nosocomial infections. N Engl J Med 327:120–122, 1992.
53. Saint S, Elmore JG, Sullivan SD, Emerson SS, Koepsell TD. The efficacy of silver alloy-coated urinary catheters in preventing urinary tract infection: a meta-analysis. Am J Med 105:236–241, 1998.
54. Matsumoto T, Sakumoto M, Takahashi K, Kumazawa J. Prevention of catheter-associated urinary tract infection by meatal disinfection. Dermatology 195(Suppl 2):73–77, 1997.
55. Larsen L, Chamberlin DA, Khonsari F, Ahlerin TE. Retrospective analysis of urologic complications in male patients with spinal cord injury managed with and without indwelling urinary catheters. Urology 50:418–422, 1997.
56. Zimakoff J, Stickler DJ, Pontoppidan B, Larsen SO. Bladder management and urinary tract infections in danish hospitals, nursing homes, and home care: a national prevalence study. Infect Control Hosp Epidemiol 17:215–221, 1996.
57. Waller L, Jonsson O, Norlén L, Sullivan L. Clean intermittent catheteriaztion in spinal cord injury patients: long-term followup of a hydrophilic low friction technique. J Urol 153:345–348, 1995.
58. Bakke A, Digranes A, Hoisaeter P. Physical predictors of infection in patients treated with clean intermittent catheterization: a prospective 7-year study. B J Urol 79:85–90, 1997.

46. PANCREATIC INFECTION

Christopher P. Johnson and Charles E. Edmiston, Jr

Pancreatic infection occurs most often as a complication of acute pancreatitis. The unique aspects of pancreatic inflammation predispose to secondary bacterial infection, which occurs in approximately 5% of all cases of acute pancreatitis. This review focuses on the pathogenesis, microbiology and surgical management of pancreatic infections, which occur as a complication of acute pancreatitis.

Pathophysiology of Acute Pancreatitis

Acute pancreatic inflammation leads to a spectrum of pathologic conditions ranging from mild edematous pancreatitis which is usually self limited, to severe necrotizing pancreatitis, a fulminant illness associated with mortality rates approaching 50–70%. Clinical and pathological severity of acute pancreatitis correlate with the development of pancreatic and peripancreatic necrosis. The unique predilection of the pancreas to undergo necrosis during acute inflammation is due to the high content of lipolytic and proteolytic enzymes that are contained within this exocrine gland. Although these enzymes are normally stored in an inactivated precursor form, they may become activated following various physiologic stressors such as toxin exposure, direct trauma, viral infection and ischemia.

The two most common causes of acute pancreatitis are alcohol ingestion and biliary tract disease (gallstones). These two etiologies comprise over 90% of cases. The relative frequencies of alcohol and biliary disease vary depending on the population studied. In rural areas of the United States and in Europe, gallstone-pancreatitis predominates, while in large urban areas alcohol is the primary cause of acute pancreatitis [1].

Additional etiologies for acute pancreatitis include the postoperative state (following abdominal or thoracic operations, especially coronary bypass procedures), hypercalcemia, hypertriglyceridemia and drug-associated pancreatitis. Of the latter, azathioprine, sulfonamides, pentamidine and various nucleoside analogues used to treat the Human Immunodeficiency Virus are the most commonly implicated agents. Endoscopic retrograde cholangiopancreatography (ERCP) is the cause of acute pancreatitis in up to 5% of cases. Finally, in 10% of cases, no obvious inciting agent can be identified. However, about two-thirds of idiopathic pancreatitis has been shown to be due to microlithiasis of the biliary tract [2].

Pancreatitis also occurs as a result of ischemia – reperfusion injury in association with pancreas transplantation. The outcome in this situation may be loss of the allograft, as the management of peripancreatic infection in conjunction with immunosuppressive therapy is especially difficult.

The exact mechanisms by which various insults trigger pancreatic inflammation are not known. Regardless, the clinical and pathologic severity seem to be related to the extent of pancreatic enzyme activation and autodigestion which results in pancreatic and peripancreatic necrosis. In addition to local release of pancreatic enzymes and consequent tissue damage, significant systemic release (and toxicity) occurs as reflected by elevated serum levels of amylase,

TABLE 1. Ranson's early prognostic signs for acute pancreatitis

At admission:
Age older than 55 yrs
WBC > 16,000 cells/mm^3
Blood glucose > 200 mg/dl
Serum LDH > 350 lμ/l
AST > 250 μ/dl
During initial 48 hours:
Hematocrit fall > 10 points
BUN elevation > 5 mg/dl
Serum Ca^{++} fall to < 8 mg/dl
Arterial pO_2 < 60 mmHg
Base deficit > 4 mEq/l
Estimated fluid sequestration > 6 l

WBC, white blood cell, BUN, blood urea nitrogen, LDH, lactate dehydrogenese, AST, asparate amino transferase. (Data from [4]).

lipase and protease [3]. The clinical course in acute pancreatitis is typically not related to the magnitude of serum enzyme elevation, but rather other factors or criteria that may be present on admission to the hospital or develop within the first 48 hours of illness.

The most widely used classification system, initially presented by Ranson *et al.* [4] identified 11 factors that were predictive of poor outcomes for acute pancreatitis. Using the classification as presented in Table 1, patients with 0–2 criteria experienced almost no mortality. Patients with three or four signs had an expected mortality of 15% and approximately 40% require intensive care support. Patients with five or six criteria had mortality rates of approximately 50% and essentially all require intensive care support. Patients with seven or more criteria experienced mortality rates approaching 100%. It is important to recognize that these criteria were published in 1974. Modern day outcomes are expected to be better. Nonetheless, Ranson's criteria are useful because patients can be identified early on for more aggressive management which may include hemodynamic monitoring, frequent computed tomography (CT) scans and prophylactic antibiotics.

Other classification systems have been used in acute pancreatitis. These include the Glasgow (or Imrie) criteria [5], Acute Physiology and Chronic Health Enquiry (APACHE) [6] and the Atlanta Symposium criteria [7]. These criteria and classification systems all have similar predictive value for assessment of acute pancreatitis.

The complications of acute pancreatitis can be divided into two phases: early and late. In both phases the severity of complication is related to the intensity of inflammation and the associated development of pancreatic and peripancreatic necrosis.

Early complications are related to extravascular fluid shifts that are associated with edema in the peripancreatic region and intestinal ileus. Additional fluid shifts may occur in the form of pulmonary edema as the lung serves as a target organ in pancreatic inflammation. Pulmonary capillary dysfunction has been linked to abnormalities of circulating phospholipase A [8] to increased levels of free fatty acids generated from the action of pancreatic lipase [9] and to alteration of pulmonary surfactant [10]. Up to 50% of patients with acute pancreatitis show demonstrable impairment of pulmonary function, usually in the form of hypoxemia. This may be subtle and manifest only as tachypnea or may be dramatic as occurs in adult respiratory distress syndrome (ARDS). Despite advances in critical care medicine, patients with respiratory failure associated with acute pancreatitis experience a high mortality rate [11, 12].

Bacterial translocation and/or alteration of the gut mucosal barrier may be important in the pathophysiology of early organ dysfunction in acute pancreatitis. Endotoxin, a lipopolysaccharide derived from the outer membrane of Gram-negative bacteria and a potent activator of inflammation, can be detected in the serum of patients with severe pancreatitis [13]. Elevated endotoxin levels correlate with the syndrome of multiple organ failure. However, it is not known whether this relationship represents cause or effect.

Patients with severe acute pancreatitis may also experience renal insufficiency. In many cases this is due in part to hypovolemia. Acute renal failure, which does not respond to fluid replacement, is a grave complication generally associated with overwhelming illness and multiple organ failure. Mortality rates approach 100%.

Late complications of acute pancreatitis occurring after seven days are generally due to the development of secondary infection or pseudocyst formation. Of these, pancreatic infection is associated with much greater morbidity and will be the focus for the remainder of this review.

Pancreatic Infection – Definitions

Secondary pancreatic infections occur in 2% to 5% of all cases of acute pancreatitis and are responsible for more than 80% of the late deaths associated with this disease. The risk of infection is proportional to the severity of illness as determined by Ranson's or other criteria. Three kinds of pancreatic infection occur: pancreatic abscess, infected pancreatic necrosis and infected pancreatic pseudocyst. *Pancreatic abscess* is a discrete, often circumscribed collection of purulent material within or around the pancreas that contains little or no necrotic tissue. *Infected pancreatic necrosis*, on the other hand, is an infection within or around the pancreas that contains nonviable tissue of pancreatic or peripancreatic origin. Most commonly, it is the peripancreatic fat that undergoes necrosis in response to acute pancreatic inflammation. Infected necrosis is by far the most common form of infection accompanying acute pancreatitis, constituting approximately 90% of infections [14]. Pure pancreatic abscess is relatively rare.

Both pancreatic abscess and infected pancreatic necrosis occur as a progression or continuation of pancreatic inflammation and, therefore, develop within 2–4 weeks of the onset of initial illness. *Pancreatic pseudocyst* develops after resolution of the acute illness, usually after four weeks. By definition, pancreatic pseudocyst is a localized collection of pancreatic juice enclosed by a wall of fibrous granulation tissue and, thus, requires time to develop. Most pancreatic pseudocysts are sterile, but they may become secondarily infected either spontaneously or as a consequence of instrumentation.

Pathogenesis of Infection

The pathogenesis of pancreatic infection in acute pancreatitis may be multifaceted, as there are several potential pathways by which microorganisms can reach the pancreas or peripancreas tissue during acute inflammation. The most direct pathway is through the biliary ducts, which contain bacteria in up to 90% of cases of choledocholithiasis [3]. This would seem to be the most likely pathway in gallstone pancreatitis. Another pathway appears to be by way of translocation through the adjacent transverse colon, either through direct spread or via lymphatic channels [15]. Other possible routes include hematogenous [16, 17], via lymphatic channels to the circulation [18, 19] and via ascites to the pancreas [16, 18]. Experimental studies support both direct extension from the colon and transperitoneal migration. Widdison *et al.* demonstrated in a feline model of acute pancreatitis that radioactively labeled intestinal *E. coli* were not recovered from the site of acute necrotizing pancreatitis when the colon was enclosed in an impermeable plastic bag which prohibited direct bacterial translocation [15]. Using a model of caerulein-induced pancreatitis in rats, Medich *et al.* [20] concluded that bacterial translocation leads to transperitoneal infection of the pancreas. These authors suggested that selective decontamination of the gut and peritoneal lavage may prevent secondary pancreatic infection in acute pancreatitis. In contrast, Arendt *et al.*, using the same model of acute pancreatitis, found that bacteria did not spread through the peritoneal route [21].

In humans the mechanism for pancreatic and peripancreatic infection in acute pancreatitis is not known. However, the results of a prospective randomized trial by Luiten *et al.* suggests a prominent role for enteric organisms [22]. These investigators examined the use of selective gut decontamination in severe acute pancreatitis. Patients were entered into this trial according to clinical or radiographic criteria that placed them at high risk for development of secondary pancreatic infection. The treatment group received oral colistin sulfate 200 mg, amphotericin 500 mg and norfloxacin 50 mg every six hours until the episode of pancreatitis resolved clinically. The control group did not receive any prophylactic antibiotics. The groups were equally matched with respect to severity of pancreatitis as judged by clinical and CT criteria. Secondary pancreatic infection occurred in 20/52 (38%) of the control group vs 9/50 (18%) of the selective decontamination group ($p = 0.03$). Gram-negative infection predominated in the control group (33%) whereas only 8% of patients in the selective decontamination group developed Gram-negative pancreatic infection. Patients in the control group developed more frequent complications such as requirement for bowel resections and fistula formation and trended toward a higher mortality rate (35% vs 22%) although the latter difference did not reach statistical significance ($p = 0.19$). However, when early mortality (due to the initial phase of acute pancreatitis) was excluded, the difference in late mortality was impressive: 10/44 (23%) for control and 3/42 (7%) for selective decontamination. The authors of this study also demonstrated convincingly that Gram-negative pancreatic infection in the control group was preceded by intestinal colonization with the same Gram-negative organisms. The results from this multicenter trial reported by Luiten *et al.* provide strong evidence for the role of gut-derived organisms in the pathogenesis of secondary infection in acute pancreatitis.

The risk of pancreatic infection rises steadily during the course of illness from acute pancreatitis [23–25]. Beger *et al.* reported that 24% of patients undergoing surgery within the first week for severe acute pancreatitis were infected and this figure rose to 46% after the second week and 71% after the third week [23]. Similar rates

TABLE 2. Correlation of the extent of pancreatic necrosis (as determined from contrast enhanced CT scanning) and risk of infection in 226 patients with severe acute pancreatitis

Extent of necrosis	Sterile (n = 155)	Infected (n = 71)
<30%	57	35
30–50%	22	23
>50%	21	42

From [34].

of infection were reported by Gerzof *et al.* who performed CT-guided percutaneous aspirates [24] and by Bassi *et al.* who examined smears taken intra-operative [25].

The risk of secondary pancreatic infection in acute pancreatitis is clearly related to the extent of pancreatic and peripancreatic necrosis [26–28]. Using contrast-enhanced CT scanning, Berger *et al.* demonstrated that an increasing percentage of pancreatic necrosis was associated with an increasing risk of infection. Patients with more than 50% necrosis had a 66% incidence of infection, whereas patients with less than 30% necrosis had a 38% incidence of infection (Table 2).

Due to the association between pancreatic and peripancreatic necrosis, one of the therapeutic goals in the management of acute pancreatitis should be to decrease tissue necrosis. A variety of strategies have been tried, including the use of high molecular weight dextran [29], Somatostatin [30, 31] and protease inhibitors such as gabetate mesilate. The latter inhibits phospholipase A2 [32, 33]. Unfortunately, none of these agents have been found to be effective when administered in the clinical setting.

Microbiology of Pancreatic Infection

Pancreatic or peripancreatic infection in the setting of acute pancreatitis is most often caused by Gram-negative enteric bacteria [34–36]. As many as 50% of infections are polymicrobial [37]. Table 3 illustrates the spectrum of bacteria

TABLE 3. Bacteriology in severe acute pancreatitis (n = 87 patients)

Escherichia coli	25%
Staphylococcus aureus	17%
Pseudomonas spp	15%
Klebsiella spp	9%
Proteus spp	9%
Candida	4%
Streptococcus faecalis	3%
Enterobacter spp	3%
Anaerobes	16%
Monomicrobial	76%
Polymicrobial	24%

Adapted from [34].

involved. The most common organism isolated is *E. coli*, which occurs in 25–40% of cases. The next most common organisms tend to be Pseudomonas spp [22, 34], although in some studies Enterobacter spp are more common [35]. Klebsiella spp, Proteus spp, Acinetobacter spp and Citrobacter spp have also been noted [38]. Staphylococcus epidermidis and staphylococcus aureus are the most common Gram-positive organisms isolated. Enterococci are increasingly isolated as are Candida (usually Candida albicans) in more recent reports [22, 35]. Infections with Gram-negative organisms seem to carry a higher mortality rate than infections with Gram-positive organisms [38]. It should be noted that the preponderance of pseudomonas and staph infections in some series may be related to the use of percutaneous drainage catheters.

The use of selective gut decontamination may modify the bacterial flora found in secondary pancreatic infections. When a regimen of colistin, amphotericin and norfloxacin was used, the percentage of gram isolates decreased from 61% to 21% [22]. However, of four Gram-negative infections from 50 patients treated with this combination of antibiotics, three of these involved resistant strains of Pseudomonas aeruginosa or Klebsiella.

Anaerobic species have not been cultured frequently from infections complicating acute pancreatitis. This is perhaps surprising considering the close proximity of the colon and a postulated role for direct extension of organisms. The paucity of anaerobes could be in part related to technical difficulties in culturing anaerobes from intra-abdominal infections [39].

The Role of Prophylactic Antibiotics

The potential role of prophylactic antibiotics in preventing secondary pancreatic infections in acute pancreatitis has been demonstrated in experimental studies [13]. In a rat model of caerulein-induced pancreatitis, Foitzik *et al.* compared several prophylactic regimens: intravenous cefotaxime, intravenous imipenem, selective gut decontamination (with polymyxin E, tobramycin and amphotericin) and full gut decontamination (the same oral antibiotics plus intravenous cefotaxime). None of these regimens affected early mortality, but animals receiving imipenem or full gut decontamination demonstrated decreased bacterial counts in the pancreas relative to controls [40].

Additional studies with the rat caerulein-induced pancreatitis model have examined the prophylactic use of intravenous ciprofloxacin and imipenem [41]. At seven days, 75% of control rats (not receiving antibiotics) had developed pancreatic infection with organisms similar to those found in humans. Both ciprofloxacin and imipenem significantly reduced the incidence of secondary infection in these animals by roughly 50%. However, due to the low numbers of animals surviving, the authors were not able to show a difference in mortality.

In a feline model of pancreatic infection, Widdison *et al.* demonstrated that cefotaxime was effective in reducing bacterial counts in the pancreas when administered 12 hours after induction of pancreatitis [42]. However, this model is clearly different from other experimental models as pancreatitis is induced by ductal infusion of glycodeoxycholic acid and live E. coli. Animals in this study did not develop necrotizing pancreatitis and mortality did not occur in any of the groups. Therefore, the relevance to human pancreatitis is uncertain.

The efficacy of antibiotic prophylactics in acute pancreatitis is related to the properties of tissue penetration for specific agents. Trudel *et al.* demonstrated that ampicillin does not achieve adequate concentrations in pancreatic tissue in a model of canine pancreatitis [43]. Roberts and Williams also investigated penetration of ampicillin into pancreatic tissue by measuring ampicillin levels in pancreatic ductal fluid at the time of ERCP [44]. In six of seven subjects, ampicillin was undetectable in the fluid.

In contrast, ciprofloxacin and imipenem consistently achieve good penetration into pancreatic tissue. Buchler *et al.* examined pancreatic tissue levels for ten different antibiotics in patients undergoing elective pancreatic surgery [45]. They found that aminoglycosides consistently failed to achieve significant tissue levels in the pancreas. Extended-spectrum penicillins including mezlocillin, piperacillin and third generation cephalosporins such as ceftizoxime and cefotaxime achieved minimum inhibitory concentrations that inhibited most, but not all, of the common infecting organisms. Ciprofloxacin and imipenem achieved bactericidal levels against most organisms.

Acute inflammation may alter the penetration characteristics of antibiotics. Foitzik *et al.* demonstrated in a rat model of acute pancreatitis that cefotaxime tissue levels may vary according to changes in capillary blood flow and pancreatic edema [46]. Interestingly, tissue imipenem levels do not seem to be altered by changes in blood flow or inflammation. It has been shown, in addition, that ofloxacin (from the 4-Quinolone class) achieves bactericidal tissue levels in normal and inflamed pancreas, but, more importantly, in pancreatic necrosis.

In human studies, Drewelow *et al.* have shown that ceftazidime achieved adequate antimicrobial concentrations in both viable and necrotic pancreatic tissue in three human subjects with acute necrotizing pancreatitis [47]. Bassi *et al.* examined penetration of several antibiotics including aminoglycosides, perfloxacin, imipenem, mezlocillin and metronidazole into infected pancreatic necrosis [48]. These samples were collected by CT-guided needle aspiration or at the time of surgical intervention. The authors found that perfloxacin and metronidazole consistently attained levels greater than the MICs for the organisms found in necrotic tissue. Aminoglycoside levels were consistently inadequate. Mezlocillin and imipenem were intermediate, although imipenem tissue levels increased with time.

In summary, the third generation cephalosporins, piperacillin, mezlocillin, 4-quinolones, imipenem and metronidazole achieve adequate pancreatic tissue concentrations when given as prophylactic agents for acute pancreatitis. The aminopenicillins (ampicillin), first generation cephalosporins and aminoglycosides do not achieve effective concentrations in pancreatic tissue. It should be noted, however, that the relevance of pancreatic tissue penetration to clinical efficacy in acute pancreatitis is debatable since, in most cases, secondary infection occurs in peripancreatic necrosis.

Clinical Trials of Antibiotic Prophylaxis

The rationale for prophylactic antibiotic therapy in acute pancreatitis is based on the widely accepted premise that severe acute pancreatitis is commonly associated with pancreatic and peripancreatic necrosis, which is, in turn, susceptible to secondary infection. Thus, prevention of infection should have a measurable impact on clinical outcomes. Unfortunately, it has not been possible to demonstrate unequivocal benefit for the use of prophylactic antibiotics in acute pancreatitis. There are many reasons for this. Many cases of pancreatitis are mild and these patients are not at high risk for secondary infection. Studies which fail to include sufficient numbers of patients with severe pancreatitis as determined by clinical (Ranson, Imrie) or CT criteria may not show a difference in outcome with antibiotic prophylaxis. Furthermore, if enrollment criteria for antibiotic studies are based on CT criteria that require establishment of pancreatic or peripancreatic necrosis, it may be too late for antibiotics to alter the outcome. The failure of early trials may also have been related to use of ampicillin and similar drugs that do not achieve good tissue penetration. Recent studies provide stronger evidence for a beneficial role of prophylactic antibiotics.

In 1993, Pederzoli *et al.* from Italy reported the results of a multicenter randomized controlled trial [49]. Seventy-four patients with severe pancreatitis as judged by Ranson's criteria and with pancreatic necrosis proven by CT scan, were randomized to receive imipenem 0.5 g intravenously every eight hours for 14 days or to a control group receiving no antibiotics. Pancreatic infection was confirmed by fine needle aspiration or at operation. Imipenem reduced the incidence of secondary pancreatic infection from 30% in control to 12% in treated patients ($p < 0.001$). However, multiple organ failure, need for operative intervention and mortality were not reduced to an equal extent and none of the differences in these outcome measures achieved statistical significance. Of note, there was a trend toward decreased mortality in the imipenem group (7.3% vs 12.1%). Also, the rates of non-pancreatic infection were significantly reduced in the antibiotic treated group (14.6% vs 48.5%). A weakness of this study is the small number of patients overall and a selection bias whereby only two of 16 patients with extensive (>50%) pancreatic necrosis were randomized to the control group. Thus, infection and mortality in the control group were lower than expected making it difficulty to detect a difference between control and treatment arms.

In 1995, Sainio *et al.* from Finland reported a randomized controlled trial evaluating the use of cefuroxime, a second generation cephalosporin, for prophylaxis of pancreatic infection in patients with alcohol-induced severe pancreatitis [50]. Sixty patients were randomized to receive either intravenous cefuroxime 1.5 g three times daily or no antibiotics. Cefuroxime did not reduce the incidence of pancreatic sepsis, but significantly decreased both the number of surgical interventions (8 vs 36, $p = 0.012$) and mortality from 23% in the control group to 3% in the antibiotic group ($p = 0.028$). The reason for this dramatic effect on mortality is not clear, especially in view of the fact that cefuroxime did not alter the incidence of secondary pancreatic infection.

In another small study, Schwarz *et al.* in 1997 reported 26 patients with necrotizing pancreatitis proven by CT scan, randomized to a regimen of ofloxacin plus metronidazole versus no antibiotics [51]. The antibiotic regimen did reduce the number of Gram-negative pancreatic infections (1/13 vs 6/16), but the overall infection rate and mortality were not significantly different.

Several uncontrolled studies support the use of prophylactic antibiotics in severe acute pancreatitis. In the previously cited study [48] a series of 60 patients receiving either prophylactic perfloxacin or imipenem for severe pancreatitis were compared. Although perfloxacin more consistently penetrated pancreatic tissue and exceeded the MICs for commonly isolated organisms, imipenem was more effective at preventing pancreatic infections (10% vs 34%; $p < 0.05$) and lowering mortality (10% vs 24%) although the latter did not reach statistical significance.

A recent retrospective review by Ho and Frey [14] also supports the use of prophylactic antibiotics for severe acute pancreatitis. These authors reviewed 180 patients treated over 14 years and grouped them into three periods. During 1982–1989 (50 patients) no prophylactic antibiotics were used; during 1990–1992 (n = 55) patients were given antibiotics in a non-uniform manner. From 1993–1996, 75 patients with severe pancreatitis and APACHE II scores greater than six associated with abnormal CT findings were given a four-week course of intravenous imipenem. A progressive decrease in the incidence of secondary pancreatic infection was noted over the three time periods. During the most recent period 20 of 75 (27%) patients developed pancreatic infection. Moreover, mortality was progressively lowered from 16% during 1983–1989, to 7% during 1990–1992, to 5% during 1993–1996. Due to the increasing numbers of patients observed during these three time periods and use of the APACHE scoring system which may have included patients with slightly milder forms of pancreatitis, it is difficult to compare the results of this retrospective study to the prospective studies which have been based on Ranson or Imrie criteria. Also, these authors included significant numbers of patients with peripancreatic fluid collections only (without necrosis) whereas most of the randomized trials have included primarily patients with necrosis. Nonetheless, the overall results suggest a beneficial role for prophylactic antibiotics in severe acute pancreatitis.

Finally Golub *et al.* performed a meta-analysis of eight published trials of prophylactic antibiotics in acute pancreatitis [52]. Using an endpoint of death, their analysis revealed a positive benefit for prophylactic antibiotics when limited to cases of severe pancreatitis and using antibiotics that achieve therapeutic pancreatic tissue levels such as the 4-quinolones and imipenem. However, the validity of meta-analysis as used to define the role of prophylactic antibiotics in acute pancreatitis has been questioned [13] as varying antibiotic regimens have been used and the majority of studies have not been sufficiently powered to detect important clinical differences.

In summary, there is substantial evidence, experimental and clinical, to provide a rationale for prophylactic antibiotics in severe acute pancreatitis. The majority of published reports indicate a benefit and, to date, there are no reports to suggest a worse outcome due to infection with resistant strains. By using various clinical and radiographic criteria, it is relatively simple to identify subsets of patients who are at greatest risk for secondary pancreatic infection. It would seem prudent to identify these patients as early as possible and administer prophylactic antibiotics such as imipenem.

Clinical Management of Pancreatic Infections

PRESENTATION

Abdominal pain, tenderness and fever are the most common symptoms and signs of pancreatic infection. Unfortunately, these findings are neither sensitive nor specific. Fever may be absent in up to 35% of patients [53, 54]. Additional findings may include prolonged nausea or vomiting and a palpable mass. In general, patients who do not resolve their symptoms of acute pancreatitis within one week should be suspected of developing pancreatic infection.

DIAGNOSIS

There are no sensitive or specific laboratory markers for pancreatic infection. Leukocytosis to a variable degree is almost uniformly seen, but is certainly not pathopneumonic for infection. Amylase and lipase values may return to normal despite the presence of pancreatic infection. Elevated serum levels of C-reactive protein, phospholipase A_2 and trypsinogen activation peptides have been shown to correlate with the development of pancreatic and peripancreatic necrosis [55–60]. However, none of these assays are specific for infection nor are they readily available in most hospitals. Currently, the diagnosis of pancreatic infection requires radiologic imaging.

Contrast-enhanced computed tomography (CT scanning) has become the gold standard for evaluating the pancreas in acute pancreatitis. The value of CT scanning is greatly enhanced by intravenous injection of contrast. In certain situations there may be hesitancy to use intravenous contrast, but the information gained usually justifies its use. The contrast-enhanced CT scan delineates normal homogeneously perfused pancreatic tissue from under-perfused or

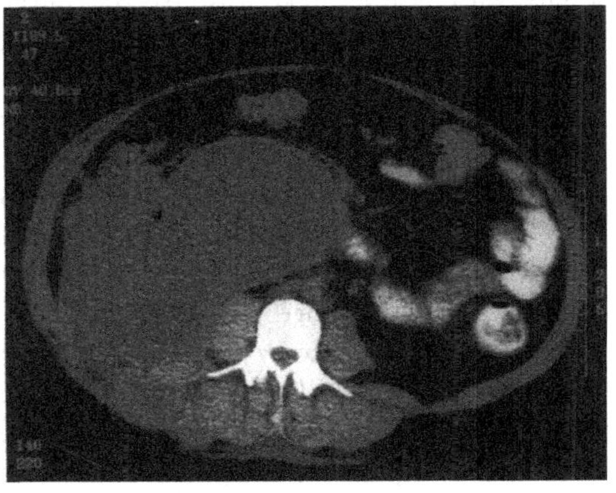

FIGURE 1. CT scan of a patient with severe pancreatitis and a large peripancreatic collection tracking behind the ascending colon. At operation, the collection contained a mixture of fluid and necrotic tissue.

nonviable pancreatic tissue. In addition, extension of inflammation, fluid and necrosis beyond the pancreas into retroperitoneal tissue planes can be appreciated with CT scanning. It is often not possible to distinguish peripancreatic fluid from necrosis and most often there is a combination of both (Figure 1).

Several investigators have developed scoring systems to characterize the CT findings of acute pancreatitis [61]. Balthazar and colleagues have reported a grading system which correlates well with clinical course and has predictive value similar to Ranson's criteria for assessing the risk of infection [62].

Definitive diagnosis of pancreatic infection requires percutaneous CT-guided aspiration or direct operative sampling of tissue or fluid. Blood cultures are often negative or may reflect alternate sites of infection such as pulmonary or central venous lines. Percutaneous CT-guided aspiration of suspicious fluid collections has been found to be safe and accurate for diagnosis but probably not 100% reliable in excluding pancreatic infection [63, 64].

The role of percutaneous CT-guided aspiration in clinical management of pancreatitis continues to be debated. The appearance of peripancreatic fluid collections or necrosis in a patient who is exhibiting recovery from acute pancreatitis does not mandate immediate intervention. Thus, percutaneous aspiration is less useful in this situation. At the other extreme, patients who are failing medical management in association with peripancreatic fluid collections and/or necrosis should probably undergo operation anyway. It is the patient in between the two extremes, with an unresolved illness and positive findings on CT scan, who may benefit from CT-guided aspiration. A positive aspirate mandates surgical intervention while a negative aspirate permits continued close observation. It is important to remember that patients should be re-aspirated if fluid collections or inflammatory masses persist and illness continues.

Gerzof and colleagues have reviewed the role of CT-guided aspiration in diagnosis and management of pancreatic inflammatory masses [65]. They evaluated the outcome of 92 aspirations in the setting of acute pancreatitis. Fifty of these aspirates were sterile. All of these were judged to be true negatives on the basis of cultures obtained at the time or surgery or by resolution of the pancreatic mass or fluid collection without surgery. Forty-two aspirates were judged to have been positive and all of these were confirmed by surgery or catheter drainage. Of these 42, six were initially negative but positive on reaspiration. These were no significant complications related to the procedure. The authors emphasized that CT appearance together with clinical findings cannot distinguish sterile vs. infected inflammatory masses. They also demonstrated that pancreatic infection occurs earlier than previously suspected, with 55% of infections occurring within 14 days of the onset of pancreatitis. Their study and others [66–69] emphasize the useful role of percutaneous aspiration in the evaluation and management of complicated pancreatitis.

MANAGEMENT OF STERILE PANCREATIC NECROSIS

Many patients with sterile pancreatic or peripancreatic necrosis can be managed nonoperatively. However, this assumes a negative CT-guided aspirate and a resolving clinical course. Repeated aspirates may be necessary in order to reduce the possibility of false negative results. Several authors have emphasized the need for operative débridement in selected cases of sterile necrosis [70–72]. There is clearly a subset of patients with sterile necrosis and clinical deterioration who probably benefit from an aggressive surgical approach as outlined in the next section on management of pancreatic infection. There is no role for percutaneous catheter drainage in sterile necrosis as this will serve only to provide a route for secondary bacterial infection.

MANAGEMENT OF INFECTED NECROSIS

The vast majority of secondary pancreatic infections are associated with pancreatic and peripancreatic necrosis. As a result, these infections are not managed adequately using percutaneous techniques. Surgical treatment requires adequate exposure of the pancreas through a generous incision – either midline or bilateral subcostal. Patients with wide costal angles may be easier to explore through subcostal incisions. The incision should be designed to achieve exposure of the pancreas and both paracolic gutters as directed by CT findings. The anterior surface of the pancreas should be visualized by entering the lesser sac, if possible. Also, the base of the transverse mesocolon should be examined as should the paraduodenal area, tail of the pancreas and the retroperitoneal spaces behind the ascending and descending colon. Resection and débridement should be limited to that which is easily performed by digital dissection, using blunt forceps or by gently pinching away necrotic tissue. Extensive resections with concomitant hemorrhage should be avoided. We believe a series of repeated gentle débridements is better tolerated (and more effective) than one or two major operations with heavy blood loss. At the initial operation, one should make a decision regarding number and frequency of re-explorations. Traditional management has consisted of a single extensive débridement and placement of closed-suction drains [70]. However, in recent years there has been increasing consensus about the merits of repeated laparotomies for management of necrotizing pancreatitis [71–75].

The repeated laparotomy approach involves a less extensive initial débridement but multiple re-operations at 24 to 48 hours apart. There are several advantages of this method. Pancreatitis is a unique inflammatory disease, which may persist over a period of several days or weeks. This is fundamentally different from other abdominal inflammatory disorders such as appendicitis, perforated ulcer or diverticulitis. Tissue damage, necrosis and infection evolve over time and may progress slowly. Thus a more prolonged (or repeated) surgical approach may be better suited for the disease process. We believe it is best to débride necrotic tissue gently. This way, bleeding is minimized but, more importantly, débridement is more complete and infection is better controlled. Repeated operations can be tailored according to the patient's physiological condition and complications such as colonic necrosis or intestinal fistula can be recognized as they occur. One disadvantage of the multiple laparotomy approach may be an increased risk of bowel injury associated with gauze packing. This is especially likely with open packing techniques or when gauze remains in contact with the intestine for longer than 48 hours. Our technique at the Medical College of Wisconsin involves repeated gentle débridement with temporary abdominal closure using either a Silastic sheet or a velcro device, the Wittmann Patch™ (Starsurgical, Burlington, WI). The latter is especially useful and well suited to the repeated laparotomy concept. Using either technique, it is possible to keep the abdominal contents enclosed and appropriately moist such that iatrogenic fistulas are avoided. We use gauze packing only at the initial débridement or as required for bleeding – but we try not to débride extensively such that bleeding occurs. All débridements are performed in the operating room. The numbers of débridements vary but have ranged from 5 to 26. Using the concepts of multiple, gentle débridements and temporary abdominal closure, we achieved excellent results in a series of renal transplant recipients who developed necrotizing pancreatitis [76].

The overall results for surgical management of infected pancreatic necrosis have improved significantly in recent years [70, 72, 75]. With adherence to the above mentioned concept, mortality rates have declined into the 10–20% range.

MANAGEMENT OF PANCREATIC ABSCESS AND INFECTED PANCREATIC PSEUDOCYSTS

Occasionally a pure pancreatic abscess (without necrosis) may present. As an isolated fluid collection this may respond to percutaneous catheter drainage. Infected pseudocysts may also be managed effectively with percutaneous drainage. In either case, a pancreatic fistula may ensue if the fluid collection (or pseudocyst) exhibits a connection to the pancreatic ductal system. This can be determined by performing an ERCP either before or after drainage. In the case of a suspected pancreatic abscess, it should be re-emphasized that the majority of these "fluid collections" are found in fact found to contain substantial amounts of necrotic tissue (as illustrated in Figure 1). Therefore surgical drainage remains the preferred treatment.

Summary

The overall risk of pancreatic infection in acute pancreatitis is approximately 5% but this may rise to 30–50% in cases of severe pancreatitis. Most infections arise from enteric bacteria. There is sufficient evidence for a beneficial effect of prophylactic antibiotics in severe pancreatitis such that patients who meet appropriate criteria should probably receive a course of antibiotic such as imipenem or a quinolone until clinical recovery occurs. The presence of pancreatic or peripancreatic necrosis itself does not mandate surgical intervention, but should prompt a diagnostic percutaneous aspirate to detect early infection, even in patients who are clinically stable. Patients with negative aspirates should undergo repeated aspirates as dictated by clinical progress or surgical intervention if deterioration occurs. Patients with positive aspirates should undergo prompt surgical intervention, as there is no role for medical or percutaneous management of infection in the presence of pancreatic or peripancreatic necrosis. Patients who are admitted to a medical service for management of acute pancreatitis should be seen in consultation by surgeons experienced in the management of pancreatic infection.

References

1. Lillemoe KD, Yeo CJ. Management of Complications of Pancreatitis. Current Problems in Surgery 1:1, 1998.
2. Farion AM, Ricci GL, Sianesi M, *et al.* Physiopathologic role of microlithiasis in gallstone pancreatitis. Surg Gynecol Obstet 164:252, 1987.
3. Klar E, Warshaw AL. Infections of the Pancreas. In Howard RJ, Simmons RL (eds). Surgical Infectious Diseases. Appleton & Lange 41:1059, 1995.
4. Ranson JHC, Rifkind DM, Roses DF, *et al.* Prognostic signs and the role of operative management in acute pancreatitis. Surg Gynecol Obstet 139:69, 1974.
5. Blamey SL, Imrie CW, O'Neill J, Gilmour WH, Carter DC. Prognostic factors in acute pancreatitis. Gut 25:1340, 1984.
6. Knaus WA, Draper EA, Wagner DP, *et al.* APACHE II: a severity of disease classification system. Crit Care Med 13:818, 1985.
7. Bradley EL. A clinically based classification system for acute pancreatitis. Summary of the International Symposium on Acute Pancreatitis, Atlanta, Ga., 1992. Arch Surg 128:586, 1993.
8. Kellum JM, Demeester TR, Elkins RC, *et al.* Respiratory insufficiency secondary to acute pancreatitis. Ann Surg 175:657, 1972.
9. Kimura T, Toung JK, Margolis S, *et al.* Respira-

tory failure in acute pancreatitis: a possible role for triglycerides. Ann Surg 189:509, 1979.

10. Maciver AG, Metcalfe IL, Possmayer F, *et al.* Altercation of surfactant chemistry in experimental acute pancreatitis. J Surg Res 23:311, 1977.
11. Ranson JHC, Turner JW, Roses DF. Respiratory complications in acute pancreatitis. Ann Surg 179:557, 1974.
12. Jacobs ML, Daggett WM, Cirett JM, *et al.* Acute pancreatitis: analysis of factors influencing survival. Ann Surg 186:43, 1977.
13. Powell JJ, Miles R, Siriwardena AK. Antibiotic prophylaxis in the initial management of severe acute pancreatitis. Br J Surg 85:582, 1998.
14. Ho HS, Frey CF. The role of antibiotic prophylaxis in severe acute pancreatitis. Arch Surg 132:487, 1997.
15. Widdison AL, Karanija ND, Reber HA. Routes of spread of pathogens into the pancreas in a feline model of acute pancreatitis. Gut 35:1306, 1994.
16. Lange JF, van Gool J, Tytgat GN. The protective effect of a reduction in intestinal flora on mortality of acute haemorrhagic pancreatitis in the rat. Hepatogastroenterology 34:28, 1987.
17. Webster MW, Pasculle AW, Myerowitz RL, *et al.* Postinduction bacteremia in experimental acute pancreatitis. Am J Surg 138:419, 1979.
18. Tarpila E, Nystrom PO, Franzen L, *et al.* Bacterial translocation during acute pancreatitis in rats. Eur J Surg 159:109, 1993.
19. Runkel NS, Moody FG, Smith GS, *et al.* The role of the gut in the development of sepsis in acute pancreatitis. J Surg Res 51:18, 1991.
20. Medich DS, Lee TK, Melhem MF, *et al.* Pathogenesis of pancreatic sepsis. Am J Surg 165:46, 1993.
21. Arendt T, Wendt M, Olszewski M, *et al.* Cerulein-induced acute pancreatitis in rats: does bacterial translocation occur via a transperitoneal pathway? Pancreas 15:291, 1997.
22. Luiten EJ, Hop WC, Endtz HP, *et al.* Prognostic importance of Gram-negative intestinal colonization preceding pancreatic infection in severe acute pancreatitis. Results of a controlled clinical trial of selective decontamination. Intensive Care Med 24:438, 1998.
23. Beger HG, Bittner R, Block S, *et al.* Bacterial contamination of pancreatic necrosis. A prospective clinical study. Gastroenterology 91:433, 1986.
24. Gerzof SG, Banks PA, Robbins AH, *et al.* Early diagnosis of pancreatic infection by computed tomography-guided aspiration. Gastroenterology 93:1315, 1987.
25. Bassi C, Falconi M, Girelli R, *et al.* Microbiological findings in severe acute pancreatitis. Surg Res Commun 5:1, 1989.
26. Banks PA. Infected necrosis: morbidity and therapeutic consequences. Hepatogastroenterology 38:116, 1991.
27. Uhl W, Buchler M, Malfertheiner P, *et al.* PMN-elastase in comparison with CRP, antiproteases, and LDH as indicators of necrosis in human acute pancreatitis. Pancreas 6:253, 1991.
28. Schmid SW, Uhl W, Steinle A, *et al.* Human pancreas-specific protein. A diagnostic and prognostic marker in acute pancreatitis and pancreas transplantation. Int J Pancreatol 19:165, 1996.
29. Klar E, Herfarth C, Messmer K. Therapeutic effect of isovolumic hemodilution with dextran 60 on the impairment of pancreatic microcirculation in acute biliary pancreatitis. Ann Surg 211:346, 1990.
30. Choi TK, Mok F, Zahn WH, *et al.* Somatostatin in the treatment of acute pancreatitis: a prospective randomized controlled trial. Gut 30:223, 1989.
31. D'Amico D, Favia G, Biasiato R, *et al.* The use of somatostatin in acute pancreatitis-results of a multicenter trial. Hepatogastroenterology 37:92, 1990.
32. Buchler M, Malfertheiner P, Uhl W, *et al.* Gabexate mesilate in human acute pancreatitis. Gastroenterology 104:1165, 1992.
33. Valderrama R, Perez-Mateo M, Navarro S. Multicenter double-blind trial of gabexate mesilate (FOY) in unselected patients with acute pancreatitis. Digestion 51:65, 1992.
34. Schmid SW, Uhl W, Friess H. The role of infection in acute pancreatitis. Gut 45:311, 1999.
35. Farkas G, Marton J, Mandi Y, Szederkenyi E. Surgical strategy and management of infected pancreatic necrosis. Br J Surg 83:930, 1996.
36. Foitzik T, Fernandez-del Castillo C, Ferraro MG, *et al.* Pathogenesis and prevention of early pancreatic infection in experimental acute necrotizing pancreatitis. Ann Surg 222:179, 1995.
37. Bradley EL III. A fifteen-year experience with open drainage for infected pancreatic necrosis. Surg Gynecol Obstet 177:215, 1993.
38. Luiten EJ, Hop WC, Lange JF, *et al.* Differential prognosis of Gram-negative versus Gram-positive infected and sterile pancreatic necrosis; results of a randomized trial in patients with

severe acute pancreatitis treated with adjuvant selective decontamination. Clin Infect Dis 25:811, 1997.

39. Finegold SM. Anaerobic bacteria. In Surgical Infectious Disease, Howard RJ, Simmons RL (eds). Appleton & Lange 6:81, 1995.
40. Foizik TF, Fernandez-del Castillo C, Ferraro MJ, Mithofer K, Rattner DW, Warshaw AL. Pathogenesis and prevention of early pancreatic infection in experimental acute necrotizing pancreatitis. Ann Surg 222:179, 1995.
41. Mithofer K, Fernandez-del Castillo C, Ferraro MG, Lewandrowski K, Rattner DW, Warshaw AL. Antibiotic treatment improves survival in experimental acute necrotizing pancreatitis. Gastroenterology 110:232, 1996.
42. Widdison A, Karanjia ND, Reber HA. Antimicrobial treatment of pancreatic infection in cats. Br J Surg 81:886, 1994.
43. Trudel JL, Wittnich C, Brown RA. Antibiotics bioavailability in acute experimental pancreatitis. J Am Coll Surg 178:475, 1994.
44. Roberts EA, Williams RJ. Ampicillin concentrations in pancreatic fluid bile obtained at endoscopic retrograde cholangiopancreatography (ECRP). Scand J Gastroenterol 14:669, 1979.
45. Buchler M, Malfertheiner P, Friess H, Isenmann R, Vanek E, Grimm H, *et al.* Human pancreatic tissue concentration of bactericidal antibiotics. Gastroenterology 103:1902, 1992.
46. Foitzik T, Hotz HG, Kinzig M, Sorgel F, Buhr HJ. Influence of changes in pancreatic tissue morphology and capillary blood flow on antibiotic tissue concentrations in the pancreas during the progression of acute pancreatitis. Gut 40:526, 1997.
47. Drewelow B, Koch K, Otto C, Franke A, Reithling AK. Penetration of ceftazidime into human pancreas. Infection 21:229, 1992.
48. Bassi C, Pederzoli P, Vesentini S, Falconi M, Bonora A, Abbas H, *et al.* Behavior of antibiotics during human necrotizing pancreatitis. Antimicrob Agents Chemother 38:830, 1994.
49. Pederzoli P, Bassi C, Vesentini S, Campedelli A. A randomized multicentre clinical trial of antibiotic prophylaxis of septic complications in acute pancreatitis with imipenem. Surg Gynecol Obstet 176:480, 1993.
50. Sainio V, Kemppainen E, Puolakkainen P, Taavitsainen M, Kivisaari L, Valtonen V, *et al.* Early antibiotic treatment in acute necrotizing pancreatitis. Lancet 346:663, 1995.
51. Schwartz M, Isenmann R, Meyer H, Beger HG. Antibiotic use in necrotizing pancreatitis. Results of a controlled study. Dtsch Med Wochenschr 122:356, 1997.
52. Golub R, Siddiqi F, Pohl D. Role of antibiotics in acute pancreatitis: A meta-analysis. J Gastrointestinal Surg 2:496, 1998.
53. Warshaw AL, Jin G. Improved survival in 45 patients with pancreatic abscess. Ann Surg 202:408, 1985.
54. Fedorak IJ, Ko TC, Kjuricin G, *et al.* Secondary pancreatic infections: are they distinct clinical entities? Surgery 112:824, 1992.
55. Wilson C, Heads A, Shenkin A, Imrie CW. C-reactive protein, antiproteases and complement factors as objective markers of severity in acute pancreatitis. Br J Surg 76:177, 1989.
56. Buchler M, Malfertheiner P, Schoetensack C, *et al.* Sensitivity of antiproteases, complement factors and C-reactive protein in detecting pancreatic necrosis. Results of a prospective clinical study. Int J Pancreatol 1:227, 1986.
57. McMahon MJ, Bowen M, Cooper EH, Mayer AD. C reactive protein: an aid to assessment and monitoring of acute pancreatitis. J Clin Pathol 37:207, 1984.
58. Puolakkainen P, Valtonen V, Paananen A, Schroder T. C-reactive protein (CRP) and serum phospholipase A2 in the assessment of the acute pancreatitis. Gut 28:764, 1987.
59. Schmidt J, Fernandez-del Castillo C, Rattner DW, *et al.* Trypsinogen activation peptides in experimental pancreatitis in the rat. Prognostic implications and histopathologic correlates. Gastroenterology 103:1009, 1992.
60. Gudgeon AM, Heath DI, Hurley P, *et al.* Trypsinogen activation peptides assay in the early prediction of severity of acute pancreatitis. Lancet 335:4, 1990.
61. Balthazar EJ, Robinson DL, Megibow AJ, Ranson JHC. Acute pancreatitis: value of CT in establishing prognosis. Radiology 174:331, 1990.
62. Balthazar EJ, Ranson JHC, Naidich DP, *et al.* Acute pancreatitis: prognostic value of CT. Radiology 156:767, 1985.
63. Fink AS, Hiatt JR, Pitt HA, *et al.* Indolent presentation of pancreatic abscess: experience with 100 cases. Arch Surg 123:1067, 1988.
64. Rattner DW, Legemate DA, Mueller PR, Warshaw AL. Early surgical debridement of pancreatic necrosis is beneficial irrespective of infection. Am J Surg 163:105, 1992.
65. Gerzof S, Banks P, Robbins AH, Johnson WC, Spechler SJ, Wetzner SM, Snider JM, Langevin RE, Jay ME. Early diagnosis of pancreatic infec-

tion by computed tomography-guided aspiration. Gastroenterology 93:1315, 1987.

66. Karlson KB, Martin EC, Fankuchen EI, Mattern RF, Schultz RW, Casarella WJ. Percutaneous drainage of pancreatic pseudocysts and abscesses. Radiology 142:619, 1982.
67. Gerzof SG, Johnson WC, Robbins AH, Spechler SJ, Nabseth DC. Percutaneous drainage of infected pancreatic pseudocysts. Arch Surg 119:888, 1984.
68. Barkin JS, Pereiras R, Hill M, Levi J, Isikoff M, Rogers AI. Diagnosis of pancreatic abscess via percutaneous aspiration. Dig Dis Sci 27:1011, 1982.
69. Hill MC, Dach JL, Barkin J, Isikoff MB, Morse B. The role of percutaneous aspiration in the diagnosis of pancreatic abscess. AJR 141:1035, 1983.
70. Warshaw AL, Gongliang J. Improved survival in 45 patients with pancreatic abscess. Ann Surg 202:408, 1985.
71. Stanten R, Frey CF. Comprehensive management of acute necrotizing pancreatitis and pancreatic abscess. Arch Surg 125:1269, 1990.
72. Bradley EL. A fifteen year experience with open drainage for infected pancreatic necrosis. Sur Gynecol Obstet 177:215, 1993.
73. Malangoni MA, Richardson D, Seiler JG, Polk HC. Factors contributing to fatal outcome after treatment of pancreatic abscess. Ann Surg 203:605, 1986.
74. Pemberton JH, Nagorney DM, Becker JM, Ilstrup D, Dozois RR, Remine WH. Controlled open lesser sac drainage for pancreatic abscess. Ann Surg 203:600, 1986.
75. Orlando R, Welch JP, Akbari CM, Bloom GB, Macaulay WP. Techniques and complications of open packing of infected pancreatic necrosis. Surg Gynecol Obstet 177:65, 1993.
76. Slakey DP, Johnson CP, Cziperle DJ, Roza AM, Wittman DH, Gray DWR, Roake JA, Britton J, Morris PJ, Adams MB. Management of severe pancreatitis in renal transplant recipients. Ann Surg 225:217, 1997.

47. BILIARY TRACT INFECTIONS

Josep M. Badia and Robin C.N. Williamson

Introduction

Biliary tract infections are a group of severe diseases that threaten thousands of people each year. The world-wide prevalence of gallstones and the increasing number of biliary operations and diagnostic interventions explain the high incidence of sepsis originating from the biliary tract. Gallstones affect about 10% of the population of the United States [1] and 17% of the population of Asian countries [2].

The incidence of bacteremia can be up to 0.8% in patients undergoing biliary operations [3]. Nonoperative interventions on the biliary tract, such as endoscopic retrograde cholangiography (ERCP) or percutaneous transhepatic cholangiography (PTC), are associated with a similar risk of sepsis [4]. Critically ill patients in ICUs are at increased risk of developing biliary complications unrelated to their original conditions, notably acute calculous or acalculous cholecystitis, which are frequently difficult to diagnose in the presence of severe intercurrent disease. New technologies for diagnosis and treatment are now available for managing these severe complications. This article addresses the main pathological features of biliary infection, emphasizes recent advances in diagnosis, and reviews operative and nonoperative treatment available for this condition.

Bacteriology of Biliary Infection

The presence of gallstones and its relationship to bacterbilia is the most single important factor for the development of biliary infection. The gallbladder and bile ducts in man are usually sterile. They may become colonized in the presence of stones or ductal obstruction or after construction of a biliary-enteric anastomosis. Specimens of the gallbladder bile taken at routine cholecystectomy for gallstones will yield positive cultures in 10–20% of patients [5]. Moreover, choledocholithiasis is associated with bile colonization in 70% of cases [6].

In the presence of gallstones, the incidence of positive gallbladder bile cultures increases progressively with advancing age from 10–20% below age 60 to 100% at and above 80 years of age. Other risk factors for bactibilia include acute cholecystitis, obstructive jaundice, biliary stricture, malignant obstruction, external cannulation and previous biliary bypass procedures [7–9]. Bacteria are isolated from the common duct in 36% of patients with common duct stones without cholangitis and in 84% of patients with acute cholangitis [10]. There is a direct correlation between the number of organisms present in choledochal bile and the severity of biliary tract disease.

The bacterial flora in biliary infection is mainly enteric organisms. The Gram-negative aerobes *Escherichia coli*, *Klebsiella spp* and *Enterobacter spp* account for approximately 50% of isolates. The enterococcus is third in frequency, accounting for an average of 13% of the isolates [5, 11]. In early reports, the anaerobes *Bacteroides fragilis* and *Clostridium perfringens*, accounted for approximately 5% each [5, 11]. However, this low rate of anaerobic isolation was probably due to the difficulty in isolating anaerobic organisms. The correct culture of infected bile allows isolation of anaerobic bacteria in 40% of patients with acute cholecystitis [12], 50% with acute cholangitis [8, 13] and 72% with gangrenous cholecystitis [8] (Table 1). Thus, agents effective against anaerobic bacteria should be given when treating severe biliary infection.

The route of colonization of the biliary tract has not been firmly established. Bacteria have three potential means of access: 1) ascending colonization from the duodenum, 2) lymphatic spread from the pancreas and duodenum, and 3) vascular dissemination from the portal vein or hepatic artery.

1) The ascending route of infection seems logical and has received most credit, because the organisms recovered from the gallbladder are enteric flora. No experimental or clinical evidence, however, has been found to demonstrate bacterial reflux in the presence of normal sphincteric function [14]. This is not the case in the absence of a functioning sphincter, when colonization of the biliary tree develops within a few weeks [15, 16].

2) In a series of experimental studies, the lymph was demonstrated to flown in a caudad manner from the liver to the periduodenal area [17]. Bacteria were not recovered from the bile after injection of organisms into the intestinal wall [18]. Thus, the evidence does not support the lymphatic pathway as a major route of access of bacteria into the biliary tract.

3) Bacteremia originating from the hepatic artery can be a cause of hepatic abscess, but this is an uncommon mechanism for bacteria to reach the biliary tree [14]. Conversely, Dineen experimentally demonstrated the spread of bacteria to the bile from portal vein bacteremia [17]. Portal vein bacteremia has been also shown in patients with ulcerative colitis and oriental cholangitis [19, 20], and this venous source seems to be the most important route by which bacteria gain access to the biliary tree. It is believed that bacteria are frequently removed from the blood by the reticuloendothelial system and are excreted into bile through the hepatocytes [21].

TABLE 1. Aerobic and anaerobic bacteria isolated from bile and blood in 125 patients with acute cholecystitis or acute cholangitis. (Taken from [8])

Microorganism	Number of isolates	
Aerobic	Bile	Blood
Escherichia coli	37	9
Klebsiella pneumoniae	12	
Klebsiella oxytoca	9	
Enterococcus faecalis	17	1
Streptococcus faecium	3	
Viridans streptococci	7	1
Enterobacter cloacae	5	1
Enterobacter aerogenes	2	1
Enterobacter agglomerans	2	
Proteus vulgaris	3	
Aeromonas hydrophila	3	
Pseudomonas putrefaciens	2	
Lactobacillus spp.	2	
Miscellaneous*	5	
Anaerobic		
Bacteroides fragilis	7	1
Bacteroides distasonis	1	1
Bacteroides ovatus	1	
Bacteroides melaninogenicus	1	
Fusobacterium sp.	1	
Clostridium perfringens	6	
Clostridium spp.	2	
Peptostreptococcus spp.	2	
Capnophilic streptococci	4	

* *Pseudomonas aeruginosa*, *Haemophilus influenzae*, *Serratia marcescens*, *Citrobacter freundii* and *Salmonella typhi*.

Antibiotics

Many papers address the relevance of antibiotic concentrations in bile. The most important factor for treatment success seems to be the antimicrobial activity of the drug against the organisms encountered in biliary infections [14, 22]. The initial antimicrobial therapy of biliary infections is usually empirical due to sampling limitations that hamper the establishment of a microbiological diagnosis. Thus, antibiotic treatment for biliary infection must cover enterobacteriaceae, enterococci and, in severe cases, anaerobes.

Despite the fact that biliary infections are frequent and severe, there is no standardized approach to antibiotic therapy, probably due to the limited number of randomized clinical trials addressing this issue. For years, the traditional combination of antibiotics has been an aminoglycoside and a penicillin with coverage for enterococci, with or without an anaerobicidal agent. Several studies have compared different single-agent regimens versus such a combination of antibiotics. New penicillins, such as mezlocillin, amoxicillin-clavulanic acid, ticarcillin-clavulanate, ampicillin-sulbactam, piperacillin-tazobactam and imipenem, and fluoroquinolones as ciprofloxacin and ofloxacin have good coverage for the organisms found in biliary infection; they avoid the potential risks of aminoglycosides in critically ill patients.

Ureidopenicillins have a broad spectrum of activity that includes Gram-positive cocci (including enterococci), Gram-negative bacilli (including *Pseudomonas aeruginosa*), and many anaerobes. Monotherapy with mezlocillin has been shown to be clinically more effective than the combination of ampicillin plus gentamicin for the treatment of acute cholecystitis and cholangitis [23, 24]. Piperacillin was equally efficacious when compared to ampicillin plus tobramycin in two randomized trials on biliary infection [25, 26]. However, over the last decade, the onset of a high level of resistance of *Escherichia coli* to piperacillin has been reported [27]. Current patterns of resistance now require the administration of piperacillin together with a beta-lactamase inhibitor, which makes piperacillin-tazobactam a good alternative. In acute cholangitis related to invasive endoscopic or percutaneous explorations of the biliary tree, the combination of an aminoglycoside with an ureidopenicillin covering *Pseudomonas aeruginosa* and *Enterobacter spp* is recommended [22]. In a randomized study analyzing severe biliary infections, cefoperazone was more effective than ampicillin plus tobramycin [28]. Ciprofloxacin showed comparable results to the combination of ceftazidime, ampicillin and metronidazole in acute cholangitis [29], whereas ofloxacin was as effective as ceftriaxone in patients with cholecystitis and cholangitis [30]. A combination with an aminoglycoside should also be recommended when ciprofloxacin is used in severe biliary sepsis if infection with *Pseudomonas aeruginosa* seems likely. When beta-lactam antibiotics or quinolones are chosen, adequate coverage for *Bacteroides fragilis* is needed in acute emphysematous cholecystitis and severe acute cholangitis.

The author's treatment of choice for acute cholecystitis, acute emphysematous cholecystitis and acute cholangitis (before bacteriologic results are available) is piperacillin-tazobactam. When serious *Pseudomonas aeruginosa* infection is present, an aminoglycoside such as gentamicin or tobramycin should be added.

Diagnosis of Biliary Infection

Biliary tract infection may present as localized upper abdominal sepsis or as systemic sepsis of unknown origin. In the approach to the patient with pain and signs of sepsis in the upper abdomen, the most common conditions to be considered are acute cholecystitis and acute cholangitis. Acute pancreatitis, although not a septic condition at an early stage, can sometimes also mimic upper abdominal sepsis. Typical clinical findings of biliary infection are abdominal pain and tenderness, fever, abdominal mass and jaundice. The routine screening tests include blood count, liver function tests, serum amylase, prothrombin and partial thromboplastin time, blood cultures, chest and abdominal x-rays and abdominal ultrasonography. These tests together usually allow differentiation between the three clinical entities mentioned above.

Ultrasonography is invaluable for determining the presence of gallstones. It has a sensitivity of 86% and a specificity of 99% in making the diagnosis of acute cholecystitis [31], but it is not as helpful in diagnosing acute cholangitis. A less common test is the radionuclide excretion scan using technetium-99m-labeled dimethyl acetanilide imino diacetic acid (HIDA). Tc-HIDA scan can differentiate acute cholecystitis from acute biliary colic, but it takes a long time to perform and is not widely available. Contrast-enhanced CT scan of the abdomen is helpful in differentiating difficult cases of acute pancreatitis and is good at diagnosing acute cholecystitis, acute cholangitis and their complications. Other useful investigations include ERCP and magnetic resonance cholangiopancreatography (MRCP). In most cases, the combination of these tests will lead promptly to the diagnosis of biliary infection.

At the other end of the clinical spectrum of biliary sepsis, infection can present as systemic toxicity with few clinical findings to direct the search. In this setting, a high level of clinical suspicion is needed to achieve the diagnosis. Moreover, in certain situations infection in the biliary tract can be more advanced than clinically suspected on the basis of clinical signs, especially for an elderly patient, in whom prompt decisions and early interventions are needed. Septic patients in the intensive care unit (ICU), who often have intercurrent disease, may develop occult biliary infection during their clinical course. However, biliary sepsis represents less than 5% of ICU nosocomial infections [32, 33] or bacteremias [34].

Acute Cholecystitis

ETIOLOGY

Acute cholecystitis with biliary colic is the third most common cause of acute abdominal pain, following nonspecific abdominal pain and appendicitis [35]. Between 85 and 95% of cases of cholecystitis are related to gallstones [36–38], the rest being acalculous. In calculous cholecystitis, a stone impacted in Hartmann's pouch producing total obstruction of the cystic duct appears to be the most important etiological factor. The trauma accompanying gallstone impaction triggers the formation of an abnormal bile, with more deoxycholic acid, less lecithin [39], increased lysolecithin: lecithin ratio [40], and release of arachidonic acid [41], which leads to mucosal damage with or without the assistance of enteric bacteria [42]. Bacterial invasion seems to be a secondary event, as the percentage of positive cultures increases with time from the onset of symptoms [43, 44]. In elective cholecystectomy for gallstones, 19% of bile cultures are positive [45]. This same prevalence of bacterbilia is found during the two first days after the onset of cholecystitis [43, 44], but it increases from the third day to reach 58% at the end of the first week [44]. This fact is important when considering the timing of surgical treatment, as the incidence of postoperative complications correlates with the presence of bacterbilia [44–47].

DIAGNOSIS

Acute cholecystitis usually develops between the fourth and eighth decades of life. Patients complain of upper abdominal pain, usually in the right upper quadrant or the epigastrium. Nausea, vomiting, fever and chills are common [36]. Mild jaundice is present in 20% of cases [48] and may reflect the presence of ductal calculi, cholangitis or partial obstruction of the bile duct by inflammatory edema caused by impaction of a stone in Hartmann's pouch [42]. The incidence of choledocholithiasis in patients with acute cholecystitis is around 3% [48], similar to the rate found during elective cholecystectomy. Therefore, jaundice is not a compelling reason for choledochotomy or preoperative ERCP. An intraoperative cholangiogram should suffice to exclude common bile duct stones. On physical examination, there is tenderness below the right costal margin, which may be associated with guarding or a palpable gallbladder. Blood studies, including liver function tests, are nonspecific. There is frequently leucocytosis plus elevated bilirubin and transaminase levels. Mild elevation in serum amylase can be seen in uncomplicated cholecystitis, but values over 1000 IU/L suggest acute pancreatitis [42].

Ultrasonographic signs, especially the thickness of the gallbladder wall, are the cornerstone of diagnosis. A positive US Murphy's sign (localized pain on pressure with the probe over the gallbladder), visualization of calculi and a thickened gallbladder wall have a sensitivity of 96%, 95% and 75% respectively [49]. Specificity is lower, being 38–83% for a thickened gallbladder wall [49, 50]. Color and power Doppler sonography of the gallbladder wall may be more accurate in diagnosing acute cholecystitis than conventional gray-scale sonography [31, 49, 51].

Radionuclide cholescintigraphy with technetium-99 (HIDA or PIPIDA) can also be diagnostic when acute cholecystitis is clinically suspected; the radionuclide is detected within the common bile duct and small intestine but not in the gallbladder. Morphine-augmented hepatobiliary scintigraphy uses intravenous morphine sulphate as an adjunct to promote gallbladder filling and diminish the investigation time of standard cholescintigraphy. In a metaanalysis, this test showed greater specificity (84%) for diagnosing acute cholecystitis than conventional scintigraphy (68%), while there were no differences in sensitivity (96% vs 97%) [52]. The main drawback of some of these studies is that they are not readily available in most hospitals.

TIMING OF OPERATION

Surgical operation is the treatment of choice for acute cholecystitis, but conflicting opinions concerning the optimal timing for surgical intervention have been expressed over the past few decades. This issue has been put to the test in several studies, both in the era of open operation and laparoscopy. When the results of the published controlled trials are analyzed, early operation is preferred [42, 53]. In a retrospective series in 1960, Wright and Holden found higher morbidity and mortality rates when cholecystectomy was performed beyond the fourth day after the onset of symptoms [54]. These findings triggered five clinical trials over the next decades, which demonstrated fewer deaths and complications when operation was performed within 72 hours of the onset of the acute process [55–59]. No particular risks were encountered in those receiving early operation, and sometimes an important missed diagnosis was corrected. These results have been reproduced with laparoscopic surgery [60, 61]. Laparoscopic cholecystectomy has been shown to be a safe and effective treatment for severe acute cholecystitis in several trials [62–65] and can be recommended when appropriate surgical skills are available [66]. Although, some biliary tract injuries have been reported in this situation when severe inflammation was present in the Calot's triangle [67], this increased risk has not been confirmed in one randomized prospective study [65]. A low threshold for conversion to open operation is recomended, nevertheless, to avoid major complications in laparoscopic cholecystectomy for acute cholecystitis. In cases of severe inflammation or fibrosis of the gallbladder, subtotal cholecystectomy, leaving *in situ* the back wall of the gallbladder or part of Hartmann's pouch, can be accomplished laparoscopically as in open operation [68].

A reasonable therapeutic approach to acute cholecystitis is a planned "early" cholecystectomy within 24 to 48 hours of admission to the hospital, once the disease has been diagnosed, operative risk has been assessed, antibiotics have been initiated, and the medical condition of the patient has stabilized [42]. Immediate cholecystectomy is only mandatory in a septic patient with a palpable tender gallbladder, especially when it is associated with diabetes, or in the case of emphysematous cholecystitis [35, 69, 70]. The presence of diabetes *per se* is not a reason for urgent operation [71]. In frail patients, at an especially high risk because of co-morbid disease (a frequent situation in the ICU setting), a percutaneous transhepatic drainage of the gallbladder under sonography or CT guidance can be an appropriate alternative strategy [72]. Once stable, the patients should undergo definitive treatment of cholelithiasis by open or laparoscopic cholecystectomy. In exceptional cases, the stones can be removed from the gallbladder by endoscopic means [72].

Emphysematous acute cholecystitis, characterized by the presence of gas within the gallbladder on a plain x-ray of the abdomen, is a severe condition caused by gas-forming bacilli (mainly *Escherichia coli* and *Clostridium perfringens*). It is associated with gallstones in 50% of patients, being more frequent in diabetic patients. Typical radiographic findings are a globular air shadow in the region of the gallbladder, intramural or submucosal gas and even pericholecystic gas (Figure 1). The incidence of free perforation is around 40–60%, and the mortality rate is higher than in non-emphysematous cholecystitis. Antibiotic treatment against Gram-negative and clostridial organisms should be administered [36], and an emergency operation is mandatory.

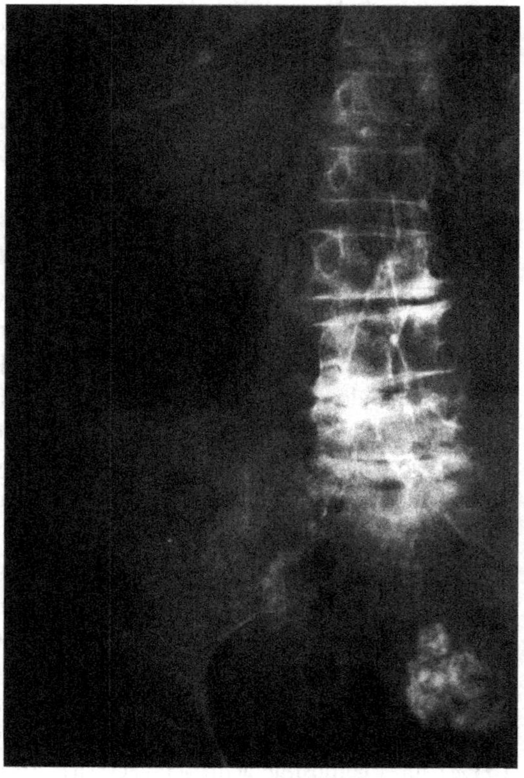

FIGURE 1. Detail of a plain abdominal film showing an emphysematous acute cholecystitis. Gas in the lumen of the gallbladder and within its wall can be seen. *Clostridium perfringens* was isolated from the bile culture.

Acute Acalculous Cholecystitis (AAC)

INCIDENCE

Kocher and Matti described the first operated case of acute acalculous cholecystitis in 1906 [73]. In 1947, Glenn defined the entity of "acute cholecystitis following the surgical treatment of unrelated disease" in a series in which only one case of acalculous postoperative cholecystitis was included [74]. However, in a cholecystectomy survey published in 1970, 7% of acute cholecystitis was acalculous [75]. In 1982, Glenn and Becker found a linear increment of incidence of AAC from 5.4% between 1932–1934 to 9.5% of all acute cholecystitis between 1975–1979 [37], confirming the perception of its increase over the years. Deaths associated with AAC were also significantly increased over this time. In a series of AAC in an American tertiary university hospital, 52% of cases of AAC occurred in critically ill patients and 63% in patients recovering from non-biliary tract operations. The condition was found in 0.19% of surgical ICU admissions and accounted for 14% of all cases of acute cholecystitis [76].

CLINICAL PATTERNS

Two different forms of clinical presentation in acute acalculous cholecystitis can be distinguished: the primary acalculous cholecystitis complicating other severe disease, and the secondary infection of an acalculous gallbladder during a systemic infection [77].

Early reports of primary acalculous cholecystitis described this condition as a complication of trauma, operations or burns. Signs and symptoms are similar to calculous cholecystitis: right upper quadrant abdominal pain, nausea, vomiting, fever, abdominal mass, and jaundice [78]. Currently, AAC is considered to be a complication of major surgery and critical illness, and a long list of other medical or surgical illnesses have been associated with this condition. AAC has been reported to complicate 0.7% of aortic reconstructions [79], 1.1% of aneurysms repairs [80] and 13.6% of ruptured abdominal aortic aneurysms [81]; it has also been described after trauma [82, 83], burns [84, 85], conventional cardiac surgery [86–88], and cardiac transplantation [89, 90]. Solid organ transplant recipients could be at increased risk of gallbladder perforation due to chronic immunosupression [91].

Several medical diseases have been associated with primary AAC: tuberculosis [92], diabetes mellitus [93], vasculitis [94], systemic lupus erythematosus [95], congestive heart failure [96], relapse of acute myeloid leukemia [97], bone marrow transplant [98], and in 1.65% of acute leukemias [99]. AAC can also complicate certain therapeutic interventions such as hepatic artery infusion chemotherapy [100], percutaneous transhepatic drainage of the biliary tree [101], or interleukin-2 treatment [102]. Similarly, AAC has been associated with total parenteral nutrition (TPN) [103], and, in this setting, its pathogenesis is probably related to the cholestasis observed during prolonged absence of oral feeding [104].

Recently, attention has been given to AAC appearing *de novo* in outpatients without evidence of acute illness or trauma. In one study, serious vascular disease was observed in 72% of such patients, who were mainly elderly and male [194]. However, the condition has also been described in young patients without such predisposing factors [106].

Secondary AAC appears during systemic bacterial, fungal or viral infections, such as *Salmonella typhi* [107], brucellosis [92], disseminated *Candida* infections [108, 109], systemic leptospirosis [110], and *Cytomegalovirus* (CMV) infection related to acquired immunodeficiency syndrome (AIDS), where CMV inclusions can be observed in gallbladder tissue sections [111–113]. It has also been described in relation to *Taenia saginata* infestation [114].

PROGNOSIS

AAC has a worse prognosis than its calculous counterpart. In several series, it has been associated with a high incidence of gangrene (52% to 63%), perforation (11% to 15%) and abscess (4%) [76, 83]. The mortality rate is between 33–71% [76, 115], being 33% after trauma [83], 45% after cardiac surgery [77], 50% after aortic aneurysm repair [80, 81], and 71% after aortic reconstruction [79].

PATHOGENESIS

The pathogenesis of AAC is different from that of acute calculous cholecystitis [37]. Its occurrence in patients with vasculitis or after hypotensive episodes has drawn attention to ischemia of the gallbladder wall as a likely cause. Barie and Fischer suggest that diminished left ventricular function is a pathogenic event in AAC complicating cardiac surgery [77]. In this setting, visceral hypoperfusion related to operation and hemodynamic shock secondary to ruptured aortic aneurysm, burns or trauma, could lead to ischemia of the gallbladder and initiate the inflammatory changes that end in acute cholecystitis. This sequence could explain the high percentage of mucosal necrosis, arteriolar thrombosis, gangrene and perforation observed in AAC [116]. Increased intraluminal gallbladder pressure [117], bile stasis secondary to fasting and gastrointestinal hypomotility [118], biliary sludge secondary to TPN [119], cystic duct obstruction [120], spasm of the sphincter of Oddi secondary to opioid analgesics [77], and increased common bile duct pressure by mechanical ventilation with positive end-respiratory pressure [121], are all factors that could interact with gallbladder ischemia to produce AAC.

DIAGNOSIS

The diagnosis of AAC can be extremely difficult in the critically ill patient with signs of nonspecific sepsis admitted to an ICU and often unable to express his symptoms. Biochemical markers are often equivocal and contribute to the delay in diagnosis and treatment. Confronted with a situation of sepsis with no obvious source, the clinician should suspice AAC and investigate the possibility, especially in the presence of biochemical cholestasis or jaundice. The definitive diagnosis is made by radiological tests, some of which can be performed at the bedside. Ultrasonography, one of the most available radiological explorations in the critically ill patient, is a reliable method for early detection and follow-up of AAC [122]. The diagnosis is based on a combination of hydrops of the gallbladder, increased wall thickness (>3.5 mm), and the demonstration of biliary sludge. Ultrasonography has proved valuable in many studies, with a diagnostic sensitivity of 82% [88].

Some authors advocate the use of radionuclide cholescintigraphy with technetium-99 (HIDA or PIPIDA) in ICU patients when acalculous disease is suspected [123] or as a part of a diagnostic work-up of occult sepsis. When delayed filling is present, morphine augmentation reduces the total examination time of cholescintigraphy to less than two hours and decreases the number of false-positive results [124]. Morphine cholescintigraphy has been extensively evaluated in critically ill patients; it has a diagnostic accuracy of 91%, sensitivity of 100%, specificity of 88%, positive predictive value of 75% and negative predictive value of 100% [125]. However, false-negative cholescintigraphy may occur in the absence of cystic duct obstruction in cholecystitis [126]. In a series of 27 patients with AAC in a tertiary surgical ICU, Kalliafas *et al.* found the highest diagnostic sensitivity for morphine cholescintigraphy (90%), followed by CT (67%) and ultrasonography (29%) [76].

Mirvis and colleagues published in 1986 a retrospective comparison of sonography, cholescintigraphy and CT [127]. Sonography and CT showed the highest sensitivity (92% and 100%, respectively) and specificity (96% and 100%). CT may have superior ability to assess pericholecystic inflammation, and it can show gallbladder wall abnormalities, perforation or fluid collections not demonstrated by ultrasonography [128]. Sonography is much less expensive, however, and is easier to perform in critically ill patients.

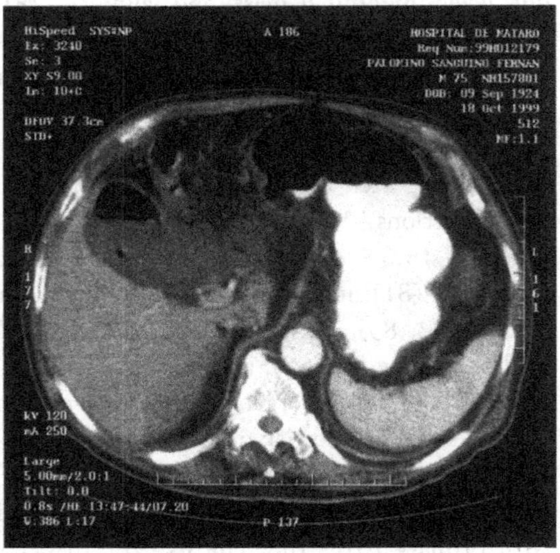

FIGURE 2. Abdominal CT scan showing emphysematous acute cholecystitis in a frail patient admitted to the ICU. An air-fluid level can be seen in the lumen of a wall-thickened gallbladder.

In summary, due to its low cost, high sensitivity and specificity and its availability at the bedside, ultrasonography is the radiological study of choice when AAC is suspected in the ICU setting. Morphine cholescintigraphy and CT can provide valuable additional information in doubtful cases in which a thorough ultrasonography of the gallbladder has not been diagnostic.

SURGICAL TREATMENT

Cholecystectomy, when feasible, affords the best overall results for AAC, providing early confirmation of diagnosis and surgical cure. It is thus the mainstay for decreasing morbidity and mortality rates in this condition [77]. However, some critically ill patients are too unstable to undergo general anesthesia. In this situation,

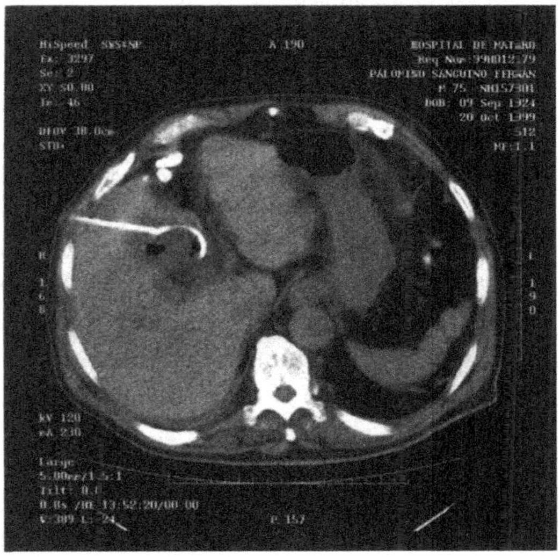

FIGURE 3. CT scan of the same patient from Figure 2. A percutaneous transhepatic catheter was inserted for gallbladder drainage. The patient recovered uneventfully and underwent an elective operation for cholelithiasis three months later.

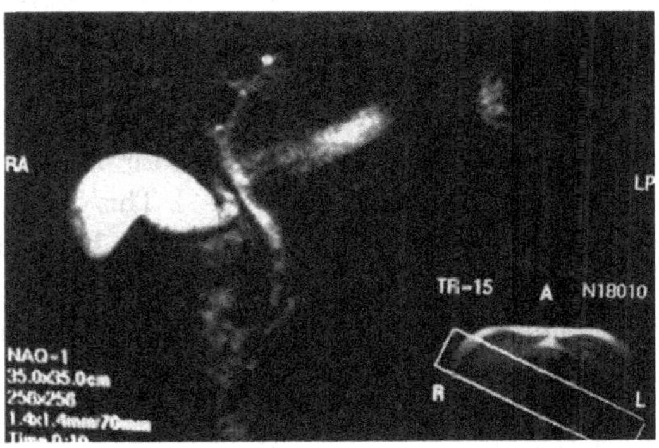

FIGURE 4. MRC image in a patient with gallbladder stones and choledocholithiasis. Two small stones are seen as a filling defect at the distal common bile duct. (Image courtesy of Dr A. Salvador).

open cholecystostomy under local anesthesia has been used for years with good results as an alternative to cholecystectomy [86], but its usefulness is limited in those who might have gangrene or perforation of the gallbladder. An open localized exploration allows the surgeon to determine whether the gallbladder wall is intact, necrotic or perforated, and to perform the appropriate surgical procedure. Laparoscopic cholecystostomy has recently been described as a minimally invasive approach to AAC in high-risk patients [129], with the same limitations as open cholecystostomy.

NON-OPERATIVE TREATMENT

Excellent results can be obtained in poor-risk patients with percutaneous transhepatic drainage of the gallbladder [130–132] (Figures 3 and 4). Radiologically controlled percutaneous cholecystostomy is a safe procedure that can be performed under local anesthesia at the bedside. A major complication rate of around 9% and a 30-day mortality rate of 3% have been reported [133]. The feasibility rate is near 100% and the success rate is 91% [134]. The technique can be curative, it has gained wide acceptance as an alternative to open operation, and for some authors it is now the treatment of choice for AAC [134, 135]. However, an erroneous diagnosis of cholecystitis, the presence of a pericholecystic abscess, perforation or gangrene of the gallbladder wall are drawbacks to consider.

During endoscopic retrograde cholangiography (ERC) it is also possible to cannulate the cystic duct and perform a naso-vesicular drainage of the gallbladder [136, 137], although this technique requires further evaluation.

Acute Cholangitis

Cholangitis is caused by the combination of biliary obstruction and bactibilia. This condition has a wide spectrum of severity, ranging from mild cases that will respond easily to antibiotic therapy to the most severe forms, which are termed suppurative cholangitis or toxic cholangitis. The presence of pus in the bile ducts does not correlate with the clinical severity of cholangitis, however.

In acute cholangitis, bacteria can reflux into the perihepatic lymphatics and hepatic veins, resulting in systemic bacteremia. The classical clinical presentation comprises Charcot's triad of fever, jaundice and right upper quadrant abdominal pain, although milder forms of the disease may not show all these features [14]. In fact, only 19% of patients develop the full triad [138]. Reynold's pentad is present in the most severe cases, in which hypotension and mental confusion are added to the three Charcot features. Non-operative treatment, either radiological or endoscopic (together with improved antibiotic management), can offer relief of biliary obstruction; it has replaced emergency surgical operation in the treatment of these often critically ill patients.

CHOLESTASIS AND CHOLANGIOVENOUS REFLUX

From the hepatocytes distally, the biliary tree is made up of the biliary canaliculi, ductules of Hering, bile ductules, bile ducts, extrahepatic bile ducts, gallbladder and cystic duct, and the ampulla of Vater [21]. The canaliculi are formed by spaces between adjacent hepatocytes, while Disse's space, situated between the hepatocyte and the sinusoid, is separated from the canaliculi by the tight junctions of the hepatocytes.

Bile flow into the duodenum is a passive event mostly controlled by the sphincter of Oddi, which shows phasic pressure changes that can be associated with a rhythmic ampullary emptying [139, 140]. The normal common bile duct pressure is below 5 cm H_2O [141], but in the presence of an obstruction this pressure can rise to 25 cm H_2O [141, 142], which sets off a series of changes at microscopic level. The ultrastructural hallmark of cholestasis is the presence of biliary material in dilated bile canaliculi [143]. In scanning electron micrographs, the canaliculi appear not only dilated but also tortuous, saccular and associated with diverticula [144]. No communications with the space of Disse have been found. The bile canaliculi do not rupture even in the face of prolonged biliary obstruction. The regurgitation of bile into the vascular stream appears to be transcellular and occurs by way of vesicles that transport biliary materials from the canalicular pole to the sinusoidal region of the liver cell, where the biliary material is released by reverse pinocytosis [143].

Raper and co-workers demonstrated experimentally that increased biliary pressure was the main determinant of bile reflux of bacteria into the bloodstream, and that the organisms gain access to the hepatic veins through the hepatocytes [145]. Flemma *et al.* showed that bacterbilia in concentrations greater than 10^5 could occur without bacteremia if there was no concomitant obstruction of the biliary tract [146].

BACTEREMIA

Operative bile cultures in acute cholangitis are positive in 82–100% of cases [10, 147, 148]. *Escherichia coli*, *Proteus* spp and *Klebsiella* spp are common isolates [149]. Bile cultures are polymicrobial in 60% of cases, and bacteraemia is detected in 25 to 75% of patients with cholangitis [143, 147, 150, 151]. Anaerobic bacteria can be isolated from the bile in 50% of patients with cholangitis [8, 13]. Some authors suggest a shift in the bacteriological profile of this condition during the last two decades. Lipsett and Pitt reviewed different time periods at John Hopkins and found a significant rise of *Enterobacter* and *Pseudomonas* species [14]. This change could be due to differences in the hospital population, with more complicated surgical and endoscopic operations performed in iller patients.

ETIOLOGY

The causes of biliary obstruction that predispose to bacterial cholangitis are multiple. The most common conditions include ductal calculi, benign or malignant biliary strictures, stenosis of a biliodigestive anastomosis, bile duct instrumentation and stent obstruction. The relative frequence of these causes of cholangitis probably depends on the area of the world analyzed, the type of institution (secondary or tertiary care), and the characteristics of the patients.

Early reports found that between 70% and 80% of cases of acute cholangitis were due to gallstones [14, 152]. However, at least in tertiary hospitals the etiology of cholangitis has changed, with increasing frequency of malignant strictures, sclerosing cholangitis, non-operative biliary manipulations of the biliary tree, the use of stents and endoprostheses [14], biliary anastomosis, and liver transplantation [153].

The biliary tree may also be the site of parasitic and mycotic infections leading to acute cholangitis. Candidal fungal balls have been described as a cause of obstructive jaundice and cholangitis [154]. In some parts of the world, parasites in the biliary tree play an important role in the pathogenesis of acute cholangitis. The parasites are the cause of inflammation, necrosis, fibrosis, strictures and cholangiectasis of the bile duct. In a 1998 review, Carpenter distinguished several mechanisms that lead to these changes: direct irritation from the chemical composition of the parasite, parasitic secretions or eggs, physical obstruction of the bile ducts, induction of formation of biliary calculi, and introduction of bacteria into the biliary system during migration from the duodenum [149]. Infestation by the nematode *Ascaris lumbricoides* [155], the cestodes *Echinococcus granulosus* and *multilocularis*, the trematodes *Opisthorchis viverrini* and *felineus*, *Clonorchis sinensis* and *Fasciola hepatica* [149] are other known causes of cholangitis.

Septic complications of non-operative biliary tract interventions, such as PTC, ERCP or endoscopic sphincterotomy, have been reported [4]. Bacteremia has been detected after 16% of ERCs [156], and cholangitis can develop in 7% of patients undergoing PTC [146] when these studies are performed without antibiotic prophylaxis. Lai and colleagues emphasized the necessity to drain an obstructed biliary tree after an ERCP exploration [157].

DIAGNOSIS

Acute cholangitis should be considered in any septic patient with abdominal pain who rapidly deteriorates with fever, signs of bacteremia and mental status changes, particularly if there is no obvious source of infection [158]. Fever and jaundice are the most common physical signs, followed by chills in two thirds of cases [159]. Most patients have an elevated white cell count, and nearly all of them have abnormalities in liver function tests [160]. One third of patients presents with a mild elevation of serum amylase, and 10% suffer concomitant clinical acute pancreatitis [161]. It is noteworthy that 28% of patients with acute cholangitis have an elevated serum CA 19-9 [162].

Ultrasonography is usually the first diagnostic test performed when cholangitis is suspected. It may reveal dilation of the bile ducts, stones, or a pancreatic tumor. In a comparative study in the evaluation of biliary obstruction, Baron and colleagues found that CT was more effective than sonography for demonstrating the cause (70% versus 38%) and the level of obstruction (88% versus 60%) [163]. Radionuclide cholescintigraphy is helpful at demonstrating the presence and degree of common bile duct or cystic duct obstruction, but it does not provide sufficient anatomic detail to be useful in acute cholangitis [14, 159]. Cholangiography, either endoscopic retrograde or transhepatic, gives an accurate anatomic definition of the biliary tree. These invasive procedures not only confirm the diagnosis of cholangitis, but can also offer palliation and definitive biliary decompression. However, when contrast is injected into an obstructed biliary tree, there is a high risk of cholangitis and bacteremia [4, 146, 156]. For this reason, antibiotic prophylaxis must be given and an adequate biliary drainage be secured after these procedures. Furthermore, ERCP has some important limitations: sedation is frequently required, cannulation of papilla is obtained only in 70–91% of patients, morbidity rates range from 1 to 7% [164], mortality rate is 0.2% [4], and opacification of the biliary tree proximal to a complete obstruction cannot be obtained.

Recently, magnetic resonance cholangiography (MRC) has been included in the medical armamentarium for the study of the biliary tract. MRC is a non-invasive imaging modality that produces high-resolution images of the biliary and pancreatic ducts in multiple planes of section. It could become the test of choice in certain situations in the near future. The technique has some potential advantages over invasive imaging of the biliary tree, avoiding the morbidity and mortality rates associated with ERCP and PTC. In the work-up of obstructive jaundice, MRC avoids contamination of the obstructed ducts by injection of contrast material and gives simultaneous visualization of the ducts proximal and distal to the site of obstruction. It can be useful in diagnosing ductal bile calculi, ampullary lesions, cholangiocarcinoma and inflammatory stenosis [165, 166] and sclerosing cholangitis [167] (Figures 4 and 5). Strictures appear as focal areas of ductal narrowing or as a signal void with proximal dilatation. The cause of such strictures may be difficult to determine on the basis of MRC alone, and the combination of clinical and radiographic data is needed for diagnosis. The sensitivity of MRC for the diagnosis of choledocholithiasis is over 90%, with one large study reporting a 100% diagnostic accuracy [168]. Lomanto and co-workers found a 92% sensitivity, 100% specificity, and an overall accuracy of 97% [166]. The sensitivity of MRC is superior to that of ultrasonography and computed tomography [169–171]. However, in a prospective comparative study of MRC and other imaging methods (ERC, endosonography, and intraoperative cholangiography), stones smaller than 6 mm were often missed by MRC when standard equipment was used [172]. In summary, although it is too early to predict its impact on the management of patients with cholangitis, MRC may play an increasingly important role in the selection of patients for endoscopic sphincterotomy. As the technique improves, it may come to replace ERC in the initial diagnosis of the obstructed biliary tract.

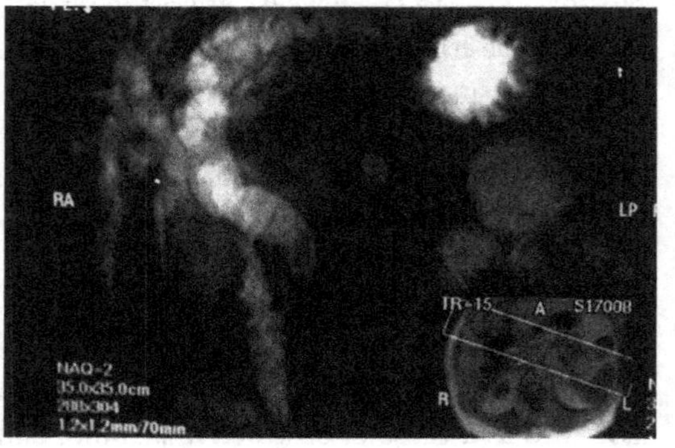

FIGURE 5. MRC image in a patient with obstructive jaundice. Several stones are depicted in the distal end of the main bile duct, which shows wide dilatation above the obstruction. (Image courtesy of Dr A. Salvador).

TREATMENT

General support. A policy of nil by mouth and intravenous fluids must be started at diagnosis. Depending on the severity of the illness, intensive care therapy may be required. Obstructive jaundice worsens the prognosis of acute cholangitis and is associated with a high rate of renal dysfunction. In the postoperative period in jaundiced patients, a 65% impairment of glomerular filtration can be found [173]. In a review of 15 series of patients with obstructive jaundice, an 8% incidence of acute renal failure was observed [174]. Furthermore, the overall mortality rate for jaundiced patients with acute renal failure was found to be 68 per cent. Acute renal failure is a particularly common complication of acute cholangitis *per se* [14], since in addition to the renal disturbances of biliary obstruction, hypotension, endotoxemia and aminoglycoside toxicity can further damage the kidney.

A key element in the treatment of cholangitis and in the prevention of its associated renal failure is adequate intravenous hydration. Jaundice produces an extracellular volume depletion, followed by a 15% isotonic reduction of the plasma volume due to a reduced water intake (hypodipsia) [175, 176], and an impaired ability to concentrate urine, mediated by release of atrial natriuretic peptide [177–181]. These findings have led to the recommendation of prophylactic volume expansion with approximately three liters of crystalloid every 24 hours in the man-

TABLE 2. Suggested antibiotic regimens for acute cholangitis [22,29,30,215,216]

Antibiotic regimen	Dosage
Ampicillin	Ampicillin 2 g/6 h
+ gentamicin	Gentamicin 5.1 mg/kg/d
+ metronidazole	Metronidazole 0.5 g/6 h
Imipenem	0.5 g/6 h
Ticarcillin-clavulanate	3.1 g/6 h
Ampicillin-sulbactam	3 g/6 h
Piperacillin-tazobactam	3.75 g/6 h
Ciprofloxacin	0.2 g/12 h
Ofloxacin	0.2 g/12 h
Aztreonam	Aztreonam 2.0 g/8 h
+ clindamicin	Clindamicin 450–900 mg/8 h

agement of jaundiced patients, and before any surgical, endoscopic or radiological intervention [174, 182].

Antibiotics. The mainstay of treatment is a regimen of broad spectrum intravenous antibiotics followed by prompt decompression of the obstructed biliary tract. Biliary concentration of antibiotics is less important than antibacterial spectrum and serum levels [14], as complete biliary obstruction prevents almost all biliary excretion of antibiotics and biliary bactericidal concentrations cannot be achieved [141, 183]. Adequate coverage for Gram-positive (including enterococci), Gram-negative bacilli, and anaerobes is needed in acute cholangitis. Suggested antibiotic regimens are summarized in Table 2.

General supporting measures and antibiotic treatment are initially effective in 74% to 85% of patients with acute cholangitis [147, 148, 184]. Failure to respond to antibiotic therapy is more likely to occur in biliary cancer and congenital lesions. Factors responsible for these therapeutic failures are a malignant cause of obstruction, positive blood culture, bilirubin level >2.2 mg/dl (40 μmol/l), more than two organisms per bile culture, and the isolation of *Candida spp* or any multiresistant organism from the bile [184]. In a multivariate analysis of risk factors in patients with acute cholangitis, Gigot and colleagues identified seven factors with significance in predicting death: acute renal failure, liver abscess, cirrhosis, high malignant biliary strictures, female gender, age over 50, and cholangitis secondary to percutaneous transhepatic cholangiography [185]. They developed a scale of 0–27 based on these factors. A score less than seven was associated with a 1.8% mortality rate, while a score greater or equal to seven carried a mortality rate of 49%. Furthermore, a mortality rate of 1.5% was observed among patients who responded immediately to antibiotics versus a 62% mortality rate in those who did not improve. These observations lead to the identification of a group of high-risk patients who need urgent biliary decompression.

Non-operative treatment. Biliary decompression can be achieved by operative or non-operative (endoscopic or transhepatic) means. Early studies demonstrated the efficacy and safety of transhepatic and endoscopic treatment of acute cholangitis [186–188]. Lois and co-workers in 1987 observed a 17% mortality rate and 30% morbidity rate after percutaneous transhepatic drainage in cholangitis [188], suggesting that the underlying disease process is more important than the presence of cholangitis in determining the outcome. In several studies, early ERCP with endoscopic sphincterotomy (ES) has been associated with a lower rate of complications and death than surgical or transhepatic decompression [186, 189]. In a British study, overall 30-day deaths after ES in acute cholangitis were associated with significantly lower serum albumin and higher serum urea levels. A randomized study by Lai and co-workers showed that endoscopic nasobiliary drainage for severe cholangitis caused by common bile duct stones was safer and more effective than emergency operation. The mortality rate was 32% in the operated group as opossed to 10% in the endoscopy group [190]. In critically ill patients with sepsis, urgent biliary decompression can be accomplished without sphincterotomy by placing a small-diameter nasobiliary drain or an internal stent across the sphincter. A 3.3% mortality rate was found in a recent report of 89 patients with acute cholangitis requiring drainage [191]. Endoscopic procedures performed were ES with stone extraction, ES with endoscopic nasobiliary drainage (ENBD), and ES with stent placement. Ninety per cent of patients responded to the endoscopic treatment within 48–72 h, and an overall complication rate of 4.4% was observed. Interestingly, all the complications were seen after ES and stone extraction. As an initial step, ENBD or stent placement appears safer than ES with stone extraction in acute cholangitis.

Surgical treatment. Emergency operation should be reserved for acute attacks of cholangitis that cannot be successfully treated by nonoperative means. However, when performed on these septic unstable patients, operation is associated with a high level of complications [148, 192]. In a multivariate analysis the risk predictors were concomitant medical illness, arterial blood pH < 7.4, total bilirubinemia >5.2 mg/dl (90 μmol/l), thrombocytopenia (<150.000 × 10^9/l) and serum albumin <30 g/l [192]. In the presence of three risk factors, postoperative morbidity and mortality rates were 91% and 55%, respectively. Elective operation is indicated to prevent recurrent disease in patients with benign strictures who initially respond to antibiotic treatment and who are then better treated surgically than by placement of endoscopic stents. Surgical options range from cholecystectomy with open choledochotomy, common duct exploration, surgical sphincteroplasty and T-tube placement, to biliary-enteric by-pass. In patients with gross suppurative cholangitis, any biliary anastomosis is at risk of leaking and it is safer just to insert a T-tube. The types of biliary-enteric drainage in common use today are basically the choledochoduodenostomy and the choledochojejunostomy. The choice will depend on the patient's condition, the etiology and site of the biliary stricture and the operating conditions. A choledochoduodenostomy is an easy procedure that can be performed when a dilated common duct is encountered in patients with low strictures, often associated with stones and/or chronic inflammatory changes in the head of the pancreas. Roux-en-Y choledochojejunostomy or hepaticojejunostomy would be the procedure of choice for many authors for definitive biliary drainage. Among its advantages are the feasibility of an eventual access to the biliary tract in case of anastomotic stenosis, the defunctioned isoperistaltic intestinal segment, and the possibility of performing either a side-to-side or a end-to-side anastomosis. Postoperative stricture of the biliary-enteric anastomosis is frequent. To provide an easy access to the hepaticojejunostomy, several types of access Roux-en-Y loop have been described. The subcutaneous placement of the afferent end of the loop near the umbilicus, or the efferent loop along the right abdominal wall marked with metallic clips, will allow percutaneous access to the jejunal limb. Thereafter, standard interventional catheter techniques and balloon dilatation can effectively resolve the stricture [193].

Oriental Cholangitis

Recurrent pyogenic cholangitis (oriental cholangitis, cholangiohepatitis) is a complex biliary tract disease, endemic to Southeast Asia, which is increasingly seen in Western countries. It is characterized by the presence of intrahepatic and extrahepatic pigment stones in the absence of gallbladder disease and is said to be the commonest cause of acute abdominal pain in Hong Kong [194].

Several factors have been implicated in the pathogenesis of hepatolithiasis. Differences in incidence among Chinese people living in different Asian countries, together with wide variations according to social status in Japan, suggest that environmental rather than ethnic factors are important in its etiology [195]. Parasitic infestation of the biliary tree with *Ascaris lumbricoides* and *Clonorchis sinensis* have a relationship with the pathogenesis of hepatic stones, although the evidence is inconclusive [196].

The condition presents with abdominal pain in almost all patients, fever in one half and jaundice in one third [197]. A history of biliary tract disease in a patient originating from an endemic area should raise the suspicion of recurrent pyogenic cholangitis. Diagnosis is confirmed by ultrasonography [198], CT scan [199], cholangiography [197], or MRC.

Surgical treatment consists of choledochotomy, exploration of the common duct and extensive cleansing of the intrahepatic biliary ducts. This maneuver frequently requires the use of the choledochoscope and operative cholangiography. New technologies such as laser and ultrasonic fragmentation are helpful in removing the intrahepatic stones. Attention must be given to the definitive treatment of the associated intrahepatic biliary strictures that sometimes require segmental hepatic resections. Roux-en-Y hepaticojejunostomy with an access loop (as described above) is sometimes necessary to permit further postoperative endoscopic or radiological dilatation of strictures [200].

Pyogenic Liver Abscess (PLA)

Pyogenic liver abscess is a life-threatening disorder that is relatively rare in the Western world but is more commonly encountered in tropical regions. Its incidence has remained constant despite improvements in diagnosis and antibiotic therapy. Historically, most PLAs arose by hematogenous spread from an infective intrabdominal focus, often involving pylephlebitis secondary to acute appendicitis. However, the etiology of PLA has altered during recent decades and is now mainly associated with hepatobiliary pathology. At present, the most common etiological cause of PLA is acute cholangitis [201]. The cholangitis is mainly secondary to hepatolithiasis in the Eastern world [202], whereas it is either cryptogenic or secondary to biliary tract malignancy in the Western world [203, 204]. In the experience of Seeto and colleagues, when pylephlebitis is responsible for PLA the common sites of primary sepsis are diverticulitis, appendicitis, perforated small intestine and inflammatory bowel disease [203].

The most frequent symptoms and signs of PLA are pain, fever, vomiting and right upper quadrant tenderness [202]. However, 60% of patients may present without symptoms suggestive of infection in the right upper quadrant [203]. Patients with hematogenous liver abscess have the shortest prodromal period (three days), while those with pylephlebitis have the longest (42 days) [203]. Abnormal laboratory findings include leukocytosis, low serum albumin, high alkaline phosphatase, gamma-glutamyl transpeptidase and C-reactive protein [204]; the fall in serum albumin can be particularly marked.

Blood cultures are frequently positive (70%). Abscess cultures are positive in 76% of cases and polymicrobial in 55%. Common organisms are *Escherichia Coli*, *Klebsiella* spp, *Streptococcus milleri*, anaerobes and enterococci [202, 204]. There are important differences in culture positivity rates among patients in different etiologic groups. Those with cryptogenic abscesses are most likely to have negative cultures, particularly from the blood. Those with biliary infection tend to have positive cultures both from the blood and the abscess cavity, and several organisms may be obtained [203].

The diagnosis of PLA is made by a combination of clinical findings, conventional X-ray films, ultrasonography, computed tomography, and, lately, magnetic resonance imaging. A yield of purulent material by percutaneous fine needle aspiration confirms the diagnosis. In patients with toxic cholangitis not responding to antibiotic therapy, the possibility of PLA should always be considered.

Treatment options are 1) antibiotics alone, 2) antibiotics plus percutaneous aspiration/drainage, and 3) antibiotics plus open surgical drainage. Patients with signs of sepsis or organ failure should be treated in an intensive care setting. Management should be directed to the treatment of underlying biliary obstruction (when present), combined with the treatment of the liver abscess itself. Antibiotic treatment must cover the organisms commonly encountered and should be combined with percutaneous aspiration of pus, with or without catheter drainage. Parenteral antibiotics can be changed to an oral form after two to three weeks [203]. A total course of six weeks of antibiotics is recommended [202], although a shorter treatment has also been suggested [205].

Early radiologically-guided drainage of the abscess is the mainstay for interventional management of PLA and may be life-saving in a frail patient. Percutaneous aspiration alone is used when small multiple abscesses are found [204]. Percutaneous catheter drainage of the collection is usually performed initially under ultrasonography or CT guidance, followed by fluoroscopy for the insertion and manipulation of appropriate drains. Catheters are left in place until symptoms and signs have settled, until drainage ceases or until the abscess is shown to have resolved on CT scan or tubography [204]. The reported success rate of percutaneous drainage in a 5-year experience was 90%, with no recurrences and a mortality rate of 5% [203].

Surgical drainage is reserved for patients with clinical signs of peritonitis (suggesting rupture of the abscess), ongoing deterioration of the condition despite percutaneous aspiration, or CT evidence of a persistent abscess [202]. Laparoscopic drainage of PLA has been suggested as an alternative to open operation [206], but the technique requires further evaluation.

The mortality rate of PLA ranges from 5% to 35% [202–204]. It is directly related to the number of abscesses, to the underlying hepatobiliary disease [201], and to the average time before definitive therapy is undertaken [203]. Malignancy, hyperbilirubinemia and elevated partial thromboplastin time have been found to be independent risk factors for death [202]. In association with hepatobiliary malignancy, PLA has a particularly high hospital mortality rate of 67% [204].

Prophylaxis of Biliary Infection

Antibiotic prophylaxis in biliary surgery. It is best to select the antibiotic prophylaxis to cover biliary procedures according to the presence of certain clinical factors related to the presence of bacterbilia [207]. Wound infection after biliary operation correlates with bacterbilia. Among the clinical factors associated with infection in bile are age over 60 years, choledocholithiasis, diabetes, jaundice and morbid obesity [208]. An antibiotic covering Gram-negative enteric bacteria will suffice in most cases. Routine coverage of anaerobic bacteria is of uncertain value. The only factor significantly associated with anaerobic biliary infection is a previous history of biliary tract surgery, particularly biliary-enteric anastomosis [7]. The conclusion of a meta-analysis conducted by Meijer and co-workers was to recommend a single preoperative dose of a first generation cephalosporin in the prophylaxis of biliary tract operations [209]. When cholangitis is suspected or when a previous biliary-enteric anastomosis is present, antibiotic coverage for clostridia and enterococci must be administered [207].

Antibiotic prophylaxis before endoscopic/radiological procedures. Several trials analyzing the usefulness of antibiotic prophylaxis before ERCP have given conflicting data. Although some prospective studies failed to demonstrate any benefit from prophylaxis [156, 210, 211], others observed a reduction in bacteremia and cholangitis, especially when obstructive jaundice was managed by interventional ERCP [212, 213]. Antibacterial prophylaxis with coverage for *P. aeruginosa* is thus indicated in patients with obstructive jaundice, a history of cholangitis or previous ERCP or with a malignant cause of the obstruction [214]. The most important factor in preventing infection after endoscopic or radiological procedures is succesful drainage of the biliary tree. Antibiotic prophylaxis should be continued after ERCP until complete drainage is obtained [22].

References

1. Motson RW, Way LW. Cholecystitis. In Blumgart LH (ed). The biliary tract. London: Churchill Livingstone, 1982:121.
2. Chen CY, Lu CL, Lee PC, Wang SS, Chang FY, Lee SD. The risk factors for gallstone disease among senior citizens: an Oriental study. Hepatogastroenterol 46:1607, 1999.
3. McLeish AR, Kerghley MR, Bishop HM, Burdon DW, Quoraishi AH, Dorricot NJ, Oates GD, Alexander Williams J. Selecting patients requiring antibiotics in biliary surgery by immediate Gram stains of bile at operation. Surgery 81:473, 1977.
4. Bilbao MK, Dotter CT, Lee TG, Katon RM. Complications of endoscopic retrograde cholangiopancreatography (ERCP): a study of 10,000 cases. Gastroenterology 70:314, 1976.
5. Keighley MRB. Preventing infections in bilary surgery. Infect Surg 2:711, 1983.
6. Smith JAR. Gastrointestinal tract infection. In Taylor EW (ed). Infection in surgical practice. Oxford: Oxford University Press, 1992:154.
7. Bourgault AM, England DM, Rosenblatt JE, Forgacs P, Bieger RC. Clinical characteristics of anaerobic bacteribilia. Arch Int Med 139:1346, 1979.
8. Marne C, Pallarés R, Martín R, Sitges-Serra A. Gangrenous cholecystitis and acute cholangitis associated with anaerobic bacteria in bile. Eur J Microbiol 5:35, 1986.
9. Ulualp K, Condon RE. Antibiotic prophylaxis for scheduled operative procedures. Infect Dis Clin North Am 6:613, 1992.
10. Csendes A, Mitru N, Maluenda F, Diaz JC, Burdiles P, Csendes P, Pinones E. Counts of bacteria and pyocites of choledochal bile in controls and in patients with gallstones or common bile duct stones with or without acute cholangitis. Hepatogastroenterol 43 800, 1996.
11. Morrow DJ, Thompson J, Wilson SE. Acute cholecystitis in the elderly. Arch Surg 113:1149, 1978.
12. England DM, Rosenblatt JE. Anaerobes in human biliary tracts. J Clin Microbiol 6:494, 1977.
13. Shimada K, Noro T, Inamatsu T, Urayama K, Adachi K. Bacteriology of acute obstructive suppurative cholangitis of the aged. J Clin Microbiol 14:522, 1981.
14. Lipsett PA, Pitt HA. Acute cholangitis. Surg Clin N Am 70:1297, 1990.
15. Rosseland AR, Midvedt T, Aasen AO. Gallbladder and duodenal bacterial flora after papillotomy in rabbits. Scan J Gastroenterol 17:785, 1982.
16. Gregg JA, De Girolami P, Carr-Locke DL. Effects of sphincteroplasty and endoscopic sphincterotomy on the bacteriologic characteristics of the common bile duct. Am J Surg 149:668, 1985.
17. Dineen P. The importance of the route of infection in experimental biliary obstruction. Surg Gynecol Obstet 119:1001, 1964.
18. Kune GA, Hibbard J, Morahan R. The development of biliary infection. Med J Aust 1:301, 1974.
19. Brooke BN, Slaney G. Portal bacteremia in ulcerative colitis. Lancet 1:1206, 1958.
20. Ong GB. A study of recurrent pyogenic cholangitis. Arch Surg 84:199, 1962.
21. Goldman LD, Silen WA, Steer ML. Biliary sepsis. In Davis JM, Shires GT (ed). Principles and management of surgical infections. Philadelphia: JB Lippincott, 1991:395.
22. Westphal JF, Brogard JM. Biliary tract infections: a guide to drug treatment. Drugs 57:81, 1991.
23. Brogarg JM, Kopferschmitt J, Arnaud JP, Dorner M, La Villaureix J. Biliary elimination of mezlocillin: an experimental and clinical study. Antimicrob Agents Chemother 18:69, 1980.
24. Gerecht WB, Henry NK, Hoffman WW, Muller SM, LaRusso NF, Rosenblatt JE, Wilson WR. Prospective randomized comparison of mezlocillin therapy alone with combined ampicillin and gentamicin therapy for patients with cholangitis. Arch Intern Med 149:1279, 1989.
25. Muller EL, Pitt HA, Thompson JE Jr, Doty JE, Mann LL, Manchester B. Antibiotics in infections of the biliary tract. Surg Gynecol Obstet 165:285, 1987.
26. Thompson JE Jr, Pitt HA, Doty JE, Coleman J, Irving C. Broad spectrum penicillin as an adequate therapy for acute cholangitis. Surg Gynecol Obstet 171:275, 1990.
27. Chamberland S, Lécuyer J, Lessard C, Bernier M, Provencher P, Bergeron MG. Antibiotic susceptibility profiles of 941 gram-negative bacteria isolated from septicemic patients throught Canada. Clin Infect Dis 15:615, 1992.
28. Bergeron MG, Mendelson J, Harding GK, Mandell L, Fong IW, Rachlis A, Chan R, Biron S, Feld R, Segal NB. Cefoperazone compared

with ampicillin plus tobramycin for severe biliary tract infections. Antimicrob Agents Chemother 32:1231, 1988.

29. Sung JJ, Lyon DJ, Suen R, Chung SC, Co AL, Cheng AF, Leung JW, Li AK. Intravenous ciprofloxacin as treatment for patients with acute suppurative cholangitis: a randomized, controlled clinical trial. J Antimicrob Chemother 35:855, 1995.
30. Karachalios GN, Nasiopoulou DD, Bourlinou PK, Reppa A. Treatment of acute biliary tract infections with ofloxacin: a randomized, controlled clinical trial. Int J Clin Pharmacol Ther 34:555, 1996.
31. Soyer P, Brouland JP, Boudiaf M, Kardache M, Pelage JP, Panis Y, Valleur P, Rymer R. Color velocity imaging and power Doppler sonography of the gallbladder wall: a new look at sonographic diagnosis of acute cholecystitis. Am J Roentgenol 171:183, 1998.
32. Vincent JL, Bihari DJ, Suter PM, Bruining HA, White J, Nicolas-Chanoin MH, Wolff M, Spencer RC, Hemmer M. The prevalence of nosocomial infection in intensive care units in Europe. JAMA 274:639, 1995.
33. Richards MJ, Edwards JR, Culver DH, Gaynes RP. Nosocomial infections in medical intensive care units in the United States. Crit Care Med 27:887, 1999.
34. Edgeworth JD, Treacher DF, Eykyn SJ. A 25-year study of nosocomial bacteremia in an adult intensive care unit. Crit Care Med 27:1421, 1999.
35. de Dombal FT. The O.M.G.E. acute abdominal pain survey. Progress report, 1982. Scandinavian J Gastroenterol 95:28, 1984.
36. Schwartz SI. Gallbladder and extrahepatic biliary system. In Schwartz SI, Shines GT, Spencer FC, Stores EH (eds). Principles of surgery. New York: McGraw-Hill, 1984: 1326.
37. Glenn F, Becker CG. Acute acalculous cholecystitis: an increasing entity. Ann Surg 195:131, 1982.
38. Williamson RCN. Acalculous disease of the gallbladder. Gut 29:860, 1988.
39. Heuman R, Norrby S, Sjödahl R, Tiselius HG, Tagesson C. Altered gallbladder bile composition in gallstone disease. Relation to gallbladder wall permeability. Scand J Gastroenterol 15:581, 1980.
40. Sjödahl R, Wetterfords J. Lysolecithin and lecithin in the gallbladder wall and bile; their possible roles in the pathogenesis of acute cholecystitis. Scand J Gastroenterol 9:519, 1974.
41. Pellegrini CA, Way LW. Acute cholecystitis. In Way LW, Pellegrini CA (eds). Surgery of the gallbladder and bile ducts. Saunders: Philadelphia, 1987.
42. Williamson RCN. Acute cholecystitis, calculous and acalculous. In Williamson RCN, Cooper MJ (eds). Emergency Abdominal Surgery. Edinburgh: Churchil Livingstone, 1990.
43. Way LW, Sleisenger MH. Acute cholecystitis. In Sleisenger MH, Fordtran JS (eds). Gastrointestinal disease. Phyladelphia: WB Saunders, 1983:1374.
44. Sianesi M, Ghirarduzzi A, Percudani M, Dell'Anna B. Cholecystectomy for acute cholecystitis: timing of operation, bacteriologic aspects and postoperative course. Am J Surg 148:609, 1984.
45. Reiss R, Eliashiv A, Detusch AA. Septic complications and bile cultures in 800 consecutive cholecystectomies. World J Surg 6:195, 1982.
46. Chetlin SH, Elliott DW. Biliary bacteremia. Arch Surg 102:303, 1971.
47. Van Leeuwen PAM, Keeman JN, Butzelaar RMJM, van den Bogaard AEJM. Correlation between a positive gallbladder culture and subsequent wound infection after biliary surgery. A retrospective study of 480 patients. Neth J Surg 37:179, 1985.
48. Cheung LY, Maxwell JG. Jaundice in patients with acute cholecystitis. Am J Surg 130:746, 1975.
49. Uggowitzer M, Kugler C, Schramayer G, Kammerhuber F, Grôll R, Hausegger KA, Ratschek M, Quehenberger F. Sonography of acute cholecystitis: comparison of color and power Doppler sonography in detecting a hypervascularized gallbladder wall. Am J Roentgenol 168:707, 1997.
50. Park MS, Yu JS, Kim YH, Kim MJ, Kim JH, Lee S, Cho N, Kim DG, Kim KW. Acute cholecystitis: comparison of MR cholangiography and US. Radiology 209:781, 1998.
51. Schiller VL, Turner RR, Sarti DA. Color doppler imaging of the gallbladder wall in acute cholecystitis: sonographic-pathologic correlation. Abdom Imaging 21:233, 1996.
52. Cabana MD, Alavi A, Berlin JA, Shea JA, Kim CK, Williams SV. Morphine-augmented hepatobiliary scintigraphy: a meta-analysis. Nucl Med Commun 16:1068, 1995.

53. Badia JM, Sitges-Serra A. Tratamiento actual de la colecistitis aguda. Enf Infec y Microbiol Clin 6:159, 1988.
54. Wright HK, Holden WD. The risks of emergency surgery for acute cholecystitis. Arch Surg 81:341, 1960.
55. Van der Linden W, Suzel H. Early versus delayed operation for acute cholecystitis. A controlled clinical trial. Am J Surg 120:7, 1970.
56. McArthur P, Cuschieri A, Sells RA, Shields R. Controlled clinical trial comparing early with interval cholecystectomy for acute cholecystitis. Br J Surg 62:850, 1975.
57. Lahtinen J, Alhava EM, Aukee S. Acute cholecystitis treated by early versus delayed surgery. A controlled clinical trial. Scand J Gastroenterol 13:673, 1978.
58. Van der Linden W, Edlun G. Early versus delayed cholecystectomy: the effect of a change in management. Br J Surg 68:753, 1981.
59. Norrby S, Herlin P, Holmin T, Sjödahl R, Tagesson C. Early or delayed cholecystectomy in acute cholecystitis? A clinical trial. Br J Surg 70:163, 1983.
60. Lo CM, Liu CL, Fan ST, Lai EC, Wong J. Prospective randomized study of early versus delayed laparoscopic cholecystectomy for acute cholecystitis. Ann Surg 227:461, 1998.
61. Lai PB, Kwong KH, Leung KL, Kwok SP, Chan AC, Chung SC, Lau WY. Randomized trial of early versus delayed laparoscopic cholecystectomy for acute cholecystitis. Br J Surg 85:764, 1998.
62. Wilson RG, Macintyre IM, Nixon SJ, Saunders JH, Varma JS, King PM. Laparoscopic cholecystectomy as a safe and effective treatment for severe acute cholecystitis. Br Med J 15:394, 1992.
63. Estes NC, Mc Elhinney C, Estes MA, Opie H, Johnson M. Acute cholecystitis treated urgently by nonselective laparoscopic cholecystectomy. Am Surg 62:598, 1996.
64. Eldar S, Sabo E, Nash E, Abrahamson J, Matter I. Laparoscopic versus open cholecystectomy in acute cholecystitis. Surg Laparosc Endosc 7:407, 1997.
65. Kiliiluoto T, Siren J, Luukkonen P, Kivilaakso E. Randomised trial of laparoscopic versus open cholecystectomy for acute and gangrenous cholecystitis. Lancet 351:321, 1998.
66. Schwesinger WH, Sirinek KR, Strodel WE III. Laparoscopic cholecystectomy for biliary tract emergencies: state of the art. World J Surg 23:334, 1999.
67. Richardson MC, Bell G, Fullarton GM, and The West of Scotland Laparoscopic Cholecystectomy Audit Group. Incidence and nature of bile duct injuries following laparoscopic cholecystectomy: an audit of 5913 cases. Br J Surg 83:1356, 1996.
68. Michalowski K, Bornman PC, Krige JE, Gallagher PJ, Terblanche J. Laparoscopic subtotal cholecystectomy in patients with complicated acute cholecystitis or fibrosis. Br J Surg 85:904, 1998.
69. Mentzer RM, Golden GT, Horsley JS III. A comparative appraisal of emphysematous cholecystitis. Am J Surg 129:10, 1975.
70. Hermann RE. Surgery for acute and chronic cholecystitis. Surg Clin N Am 70:1263, 1990.
71. Lewis RT, Barkun J. Infection in the upper abdomen: biliary tract, pancreas, liver and spleen. In Meakins JL (ed). Surgical Infections. Diagnosis and treatment. New York: Scientific American, 25:311, 1994.
72. Lee KT, Wong SR, Cheng JS, Ker CG, Sheen PC, Liu YE. Ultrasound-guided percutaneous cholecystostomy as an initial treatment for acute cholecystitis in elderly patients. Dig Surg 15:328, 1998.
73. Kocher T, Matti H. Under 100 operationen an den gallenwegen mit berucksichtigung der daurerfolge. Arch Clin Chir 81:655, 1906.
74. Glenn F. Acute cholecystitis following the surgical treatment of unrelated disease. Ann Surg 126:411, 1947.
75. Gallbladder Survey Committee. Ohio Chapter, American College of Surgeons. 28,621 cholecystectomies in Ohio. Am J Surg 119:714, 1970.
76. Kalliafas S, Ziegler DW, Flancbaum L, Choban PS. Acute acalculous cholecystitis: incidence, risk factors, diagnosis, and outcome. Am Surg 64:471, 1998.
77. Barie PS, Fischer E. Acute acalculous cholecystitis. J Am Coll Surg 180:232, 1995.
78. Coelho JC, Campos AC, Moreira M, Moss AA Jr, Artigas GV. Acute acalculous cholecystitis. Int Surg 76:146, 1991.
79. Hagino RT, Valentine RJ, Clagett GP. Acalculous cholecystitis after aortic reconstruction. J Am Coll Surg 184:245, 1997.
80. Ouriel K, Green RM, Ricotta JJ, DeWeese JA, Adams JT. Acute acalculous cholecystitis complicating abdominal aortic aneurism resection. J Vasc Surg 1:646, 1984.
81. Scher KS, Sarap D, Jaggers RL. Acute acalculous cholecystitis complicating aortic

aneurism repair. Surg Gynecol Obstet 163:475, 1986.
82. Lindberg EF, Grinnan GLB, Smith L. Acalculous cholecystitis in Vietnam casualties. Ann Surg 171:152, 1970.
83. DuPriest RW, Khaneja SC, Cowley RA. Acute cholecystitis complicating trauma. Ann Surg 189:84, 1979.
84. Munster AM, Goodwin MN, Pruitt BA Jr. Acalculous cholecystitis in burned patients. Am J Surg 122:591, 1971.
85. Slater H, Goldfarb IW. Acute septic cholecystitis in patients with burn injuries. J Burn Care Rehabil 10:445, 1989.
86. Savino JA, Scalea TM, del Guercio LRM. Factors encouraging laparotomy in acalculous cholecystitis. Crit Care Med 13:377, 1985.
87. Leitman IM, Paull DE, Barie PS, Isom OW, Shires GT. Intraabdominal complications of cardiopulmonary by-pass surgery. Surg Gynecol Osbtet 165:251, 1987.
88. Sessions SC, Scoma RS, Sheikh FA, McGeehin WH, Smink RD Jr. Acute acalculous cholecystitis following open heart surgery. Am Surg 59:74, 1993.
89. Steed DL, Brown B, Reilly JJ, Peitzman AB, Griffith BP, Hardesty RL, Webster MW. General surgical complications in heart and heart-lung transplantation. Surgery 98:739, 1985.
90. Merrell SW, Ames SA, Nelson EW, Rendlund DG, Karwande SV, Burton NA, Sullivan JJ, Jones KW, Gay WA Jr. Major abdominal complications following cardiac transplantation. Arch Surg 124:889, 1989.
91. Feltis BA, Lee DA, Gruessner RW. Acute acalculous cholecystitis (AAC) resulting in gallbladder perforation in a solid organ transplant recipient: a case report. Clin Transplant 12:278, 1998.
92. Cabrero F, Liaño JL. Colecistitis aguda alitiásica: a propósito de 5 casos. Rev Esp Enferm Ap Dig 53:277, 1978.
93. Barie PS, Jacobson IM. Gallbladder disease. In Zakim D, Boyer TD (eds). Hepatology. Philadelphia: WB Saunders Co., 1990.
94. Papaioannou CC, Hunder GG, Lie JT. Vasculitis of the gallbladder in a 70 year old man with giant cell arteritis. J Rheumatol 6:71, 1979.
95. Kamimura T, Mimori A, Takeda A, Masuyama J, Yoshio T, Okazaki H, Kano S, Minota S. Acute acalculous cholecystitis in systemic lupus erythematosus: a case report and review of the literature. Lupus 7:361, 1998.
96. Smith JP, Bodai BI. Empyema of the gallbladder-potential consequence of medical intensive care. Crit Care Med 10:451, 1982.
97. Hurley R, Weisdorf DJ, Jessurun J, Vercellotti GM, Miller WJ. Relapse of acute leukemia presenting as acute cholecystitis following bone marrow transplantation. Bone Marrow Transplant 10:387, 1992.
98. Jardines LA, O'Donnell MR, Johnson DL, Terz JS, Forman SJ. Acalculous cholecystitis in bone marrow transplant patients. Cancer 71:354, 1993.
99. Buyukasik Y, Kosar A, Demiroglu H, Altinok G, Ozcebe OI, Dundar S. Acalculous acute cholecystitis in leukemia. J Clin Gastroenterol 27:146, 1998.
100. Lafon PC, Reed K, Rosenthal D. Acute cholecystitis associated with hepatic arterial infusion of floxuridine. Am J Surg 150:687, 1985.
101. Lillemoe KD, Pitt HA, Kaufman SL, Cameron JL. Acute cholecystitis occurring as a complication of percutaneous transhepatic drainage. Surg Gynecol Obstet 168:348, 1989.
102. Chung-Park M, Kim B, Marmolya G, Karlins S, Wojcik E. Acalculous lymphoeosinophylic cholecystitis associated with interleukin-2 and lymphokin-activated killer cell therapy. Arch Pathol Lab Med 114:1073, 1990.
103. Petersen SR, Sheldon GF. Acute acalculous cholecystitis: a complication of hyperalimentation. Am J Surg 138:814, 1979.
104. Sitges-Serra A. Complications of parenteral nutrition. In Sitges-Serra A (ed). Parenteral nutrition and the surgical patient. Bruxelles: Institut Danone, 1999.
105. Savoca PE, Longo WE, Zucker KA, McMillen MM, Modlin IM. The increasing prevalence of acalculous cholecystitis in outpatients. Results of a 7-year study. Ann Surg 211:433, 1990.
106. Parithivel VS, Gerst PH, Banerjee S, Parikh V, Albu E. Acute acalculous cholecystitis in young patients without predisposing factors. Am Surg 65:366, 1999.
107. Yulevich A, Cohen Z, Maor E, Bryk T, Mares AJ. Acute acalculous cholecystitis caused by *Salmonella typhi* in a 6-year-old child. Eur J Pediatr Surg 2:301, 1992.
108. Miller DD. Postoperative acalculous cholecystitis due to *Torulopsis glabrata*. Arch Surg 111: 1404, 1976.
109. Hiatt JR, Kobayashi MR, Doty JE, Ramming KP. Acalculous *Candida* cholecystitis: a complications of critical surgical illness. Am Surg 57:825, 1991.

110. Monno S, Mizushima Y. Leptospirosis with acute acalculous cholecystitis and pancreatitis. J Clin Gastroenterol 16:52, 1993.
111. Kavin H, Jonas RB, Chowdorhu L, Kabins S. Acalculous cholecystitis and cytomegalovirus infection in the acquired immunodeficiency syndrome. Ann Intern Med 104:53, 1986.
112. Keshavjee SH, Magee LA, Mullen BJ. Acalculous cholecystitis associated with cytomegalovirus and sclerosing cholangitis in a patient with acquired immunodeficiency syndrome. Can J Surg 36:321, 1993.
113. Ramos-Ruiz JL, Elosegui-Martínez F. Colecistitis alitiásica por citomegalovirus en paciente con SIDA. An Med Interna 15:155, 1998.
114. Daou R, Achram M, Abousalb M, Dannaoui M. Cholecystite aigue alithiasique due a Taenia saginata. Chirurgie 123:195, 1998.
115. Frazee RC, Nagorney DM, Mucha P Jr. Acute acalculous cholecystitis. Mayo Clin Proc 64: 163, 1989.
116. Thompson JW, Ferris DO, Beggenstoss AH. Acute cholecystitis complicating operation for other disease. Ann Surg 155:489, 1962.
117. Orlando R, Gleason E, Drezner AD. Acute acalculous cholecystitis in the critically ill patient. Am J Surg 145:472, 1983.
118. Niderheiser DH. Acute acalculous cholecystitis induced by lysophosphatidyl choline. Am J Pathol 124:559, 1986.
119. Messing B, Bories C, Kunstlinger F, Bernier JJ. Does total parenteral nutrition induce gallbladder sludge formation and lithiasis? Gastroenterology 84:1012, 1983.
120. Andry G, Turnbull AD, Botet J, Kurtz RC. Cholesonographic characteristics of cystic duct metastases causing acute acalculous cholecystitis: case report. J Surg Oncol 31:178, 1986.
121. Johnson EE, Hedley-White J. Continous positive-pressure ventilation and portal flow in dogs with pulmonary edema. J Appl Physiol 33:385, 1972.
122. Imhof M, Raunest J, Ohmann C, Roher HD. Acute acalculous cholecystitis complicating trauma: a prospective sonographic study. World J Surg 16:1160, 1992.
123. Grossman SJ, Joyce JM. Hepatobiliary imaging. Emerg Med Clin North Am 9:853, 1991.
124. Kim EE, Pjura G, Lowry P, Nguyen M, Pollack M. Morphine-augmented cholescintigraphy in the diagnosis of acute cholecystitis. Am J Roentgenol 147:1177, 1986.
125. Flancbaum L, Choban PS. Use of morphine cholescintigraphy in the diagnosis of acute cholecystitis in critically ill patients. Intensive Care Med 21:120, 1995.
126. Ohrt HJ, Posalaky IP, Shafer RB. Normal gallbladder cholescintigraphy in acute cholecystitis. Clin Nucl Med 8:97, 1983.
127. Mirvis SE, Vainright JR, Nelson AW, Johnston GS, Shorr R, Rodriguez A, Whitley NO. The diagnosis of acute acalculous cholecystitis: a comparison of sonography, scintigraphy, and CT. Am J Roentgenol 147:1171, 1986.
128. Blankenberg F, Wirth R, Jeffrey RB Jr, Mindelzun R, Francis I. Computed tomography as an adjunct to ultrasound in the diagnosis of acute acalculous cholecystitis. Gastrointest Radiol 16:149, 1991.
129. Yang HK, Hodgson WJ. Laparoscopic cholecystostomy for acute acalculous cholecystitis. Surg Endosc 10:673, 1996.
130. Eggermont AM, Laméris JS, Jeekel J. Ultrasound-guided percutaneous transhepatic cholecystostomy for acute acalculous cholecystitis. Arch Surg 120:1354, 1985.
131. Klimberg S, Hawkins I, Vogel SB. Percutaneous cholecystectomy for acute cholecystitis in high-risk patients. Am J Surg 153:125, 1987.
132. Vauthey JN, Lerut J, Martini M, Becker C, Gertsch P, Blumgart LH. Indications and limitations of percutaneous cholecystostomy for acute cholecystitis. Surg Gynecol Obstet 176:49, 1993.
133. VanSonnenberg E, D'Agostino HB, Goodacre BW, Sanchez RB, Casola G. Percutaneous gallbladder puncture and cholecystostomy: results, complications, and caveats for safety. Radiology 183:167, 1992.
134. Boggi U, Di Candio G, Campatelli A, Oleggini M, Pietrabissa A, Filipponi F, Bellini R, Mazzotta D, Mosca F. Percutaneous cholecystostomy for acute cholecystitis in critically ill patients. Hepatogastroenterology 46:121, 1999.
135. Taylor S, Rawlinson J, Malone DE. Technical report: Percutaneous cholecystostomy in acute acalculous cholecystitis. Clin Radiol 45:273, 1992.
136. Johlin FC Jr, Neil GA. Drainage of the gallbladder in patients with acute acalculous cholecystitis by transpapillary endoscopic cholecystostomy. Gastrointest Endosc 93:645, 1993.
137. Dumas R, Caroli-Bosc FX, Demarquay JF, Zanaldi H, Hastier P, Conio M, Maes B,

Delmont JP. Cholecystite aigue inoperable traitee par drainage nosavesiculaire endoscopique. Etude chez 15 malades. Gastroenterol Clin Biol 21:854, 1997.
138. Pitt HA, Couse NF. Biliary sepsis and toxic cholangitis. In Moody FG, Carey LC, Jones RS (eds). Surgical treatment of digestive disease, 2nd edn. Chicago: Year Book, 1990.
139. Toouli J. Sphincter of Oddi motility. Br J Surg 71:251, 1984.
140. Hauge CW, Mark JBD. Common bile duct motility and sphincter mechanism. Ann Surg 162:1028, 1965.
141. Leung JW, Chan RC, Cheung SW, Sung JY, Chung SC, French GL. The effect of obstruction on the biliary excretion of cefoperazone and ceftazidime. J Antimicrob Chemother 25:399, 1990.
142. Jacobsson K, Ellander J, Rosengren B. Cholangiovenous reflux. Acta Chir Scand 123:316, 1962.
143. Phillips MJ, Latham PS, Poucell-Hatton S. Electron microscopy of human liver diseases. In Schiff L, Schiff ER (eds). Disease of the liver, 7th edn. Philadelphia: JB Lippincott Co., 1993.
144. Compagno J, Grisham JM. Scanning electron microscopy of extrahepatic biliary obstruction. Arch Pathol 97:348, 1974.
145. Raper SE, Baker ME, Jones AL, Way LW. Anatomic correlates of bacterial cholangiovenous reflux. Surgery 105:352, 1989.
146. Flemma RJ, Flint LM, Osterhout S, Shingleton WW. Bacteriologic studies of biliary infection. Ann Surg 166:563, 1967.
147. Saharia PC, Cameron JL. Clinical management of acute cholangitis. Surg Gynecol Obstet 142: 369, 1976.
148. Boey JH, Way LW. Acute cholangitis. Ann Surg 191:264, 1980.
149. Carpenter HA. Bacterial and parasitic cholangitis. Mayo Clin Proc 73:473, 1998.
150. Thompson JE, Tomkins RK, Longmire WP. Factors in management of acute cholangitis. Ann Surg 195:137, 1982.
151. Lau WY, Chu KW, Yuen WK, Poon GP, Hwang JS, Li AK. Operative choledochoscopy in patients with acute cholangitis: a prospective, randomized study. Br J Surg 78:1226, 1991.
152. Saik RP, Greenburg AG, Farris JM, Peskin GW. Spectrum of cholangitis. Am J Surg 130:143, 1975.
153. Mazariegos GV, Molmenti EP, Kramer DJ. Early complications after orthotopic liver transplantation. Surg Clin North Am 79:109, 1999.
154. Wig JD, Singh K, Chawla YK, Vaiphei K. Cholangitis due to candidiasis of the extra-hepatic biliary tract. HPB Surg 11:51, 1998.
155. De Andrade DR Jr, Karam JA, Warth M do P, de Marca AF, Jukemura J, Machado MC, Rocha AD. Massive infectation by Ascaris lumbricoides of the biliary tract: report of a succesfully treated case. Rev Inst Med Trop Sao Paulo 34:71, 1992.
156. Sauter G, Grabein B, Huber G, Mannes GA, Ruckdeschel G, Sauerbruch T. Antibiotic prophylaxis of infectious complications with endoscopic retrograde cholangiopancreatography. A randomized controlled study. Endoscopy 22: 164, 1990.
157. Lai EC, Lo CM, Choi TK, Cheng WK, Fan ST, Wong J. Urgent biliary decompression after endoscopic retrograde cholangiopancreatography. Am J Surg 157:121, 1989.
158. Glenn F, Moody FC. Acute obstructive suppurative cholangitis. Surg Gynecol Obstet 113:265, 1961.
159. Sinanan MN. Acute cholangitis. Infect Dis Clin North Am 6:3, 571, 1992.
160. Raraty MGT, Finch M, Neoptolemos JP. Acute cholangitis and pancreatitis secondary to common duct stones: management update. World J Surg 22:1155, 1998.
161. Neoptolemos JP, Carr-Locke DL, Leese T, James D. Acute cholangitis in association with acute pancreatitis: incidence, clinical features, outcome and the role of ERCP and endoscopic sphincterotomy. Br J Surg 74:1103, 1987.
162. Ker CG, Chen JS, Lee KT, Sheen PC, Wu CC. Assessment of serum and bile levels of CA 19-9 and CA 125 in cholangitis and bile duct carcinoma. J Gastroenterol Hepatol 6:505, 1991.
163. Baron RL, Stanley RJ, Lee JKT, Koehler RE, Melson GL, Balfe DM, Weyman PJ. A prospective comparison of the evaluation of biliary obstruction using computed tomography and ultrasonography. Radiology 145:91, 1982.
164. Teplick SK, Flick P, Brandon JC. Transhepatic cholangiography in patients with suspected biliary disease and non-dilated intrahepatic bile ducts. Gastrointest Radiol 16:193, 1991.
165. Reinhold C, Bret PM, Guibaud L, Barkun ANG, Genin G, Atri M. MR cholangiopancreatography: potential clinical applications. Radiographics 16:309, 1996.

166. Lomanto D, Pavone P, Laghi A, Panebianco V, Mazzocchi P, Fiocca F, Lezoche E, Passariello R, Speranza V. Am J Surg 174:33, 1997.
167. Ernst O, Asselah T, Sergent G, Calvo M, Talbodec N, Paris JC, Lherminé C. MR cholangiography in primary sclerosing cholangitis. Am J Roentgenol 171:1027, 1998.
168. Fulcher AS, Turner MA, Capps GW, Zfass AM, Baker KM. Half-Fourier RARE MR cholangiopancreatography: experience in 300 subjects. Radiology 207:21, 1998.
169. Cronan JJ, Mueller PR, Simeone JF, Oconnell RS, vanSonnenberg E, Wittenberg J, Ferrucci JT Jr. Prospective diagnosis of choledocholithiasis. Radiology 146:467, 1983.
170. Jeffrey RB, Federle MP, Laing FC, Wall S, Rego J, Moss AA. Computed tomographic features of biliary obstruction. Am J Roentgenol 140: 1179, 1983.
171. Baron RL, Stanley RJ, Lee JKT, Koehler RE, Levitt RG. Computed tomographic features of biliary obstruction. Am J Roentgenol 140: 1173, 1983.
172. Zidi SH, Prat F, Le Guen O, Rondeau Y, Rocher L, Frtsch J, Choury AD, Pelletier G. Use of magnetic resonance cholangiography in the diagnosis of choledocholithiasis: prospective comparison with a reference imaging method. Gut 44:118, 1999.
173. Gubern JM, Sancho JJ, Simó J. Sitges-Serra A. A randomized trial on the effect of mannitol on postoperative renal function in patients with obstructive jaundice. Surgery 103:39, 1988.
174. Fogarty BJ, Parks RW, Rowlands BJ, Diamond T. Renal dysfunction in obstructive jaundice. Br J Surg 82:877, 1995.
175. Martínez-Ródenas F, Oms LM, Carulla X, Segura M, Sancho JJ, Piera C, Fernández-Espina MR, Sitges-Serra A. Measurements of body water compartments after ligation of the common bile duct in the rabbit. Br J Surg 76: 461, 1989.
176. Sitges-Serra A, Carulla X, Piera C, Martínez-Ródenas F, Franch G, Pereira J, Gubern JM. Body water compartments in patients with obstructive jaundice. Br J Surg 79:553. 1992.
177. Oms LM, Martínez-Ródenas F, Valverde J, Jiménez W, Sitges-Serra A. Reduced water and sodium intakes associated with high levels of natriuretic factor following common bile duct ligation in the rabbit. Br J Surg 77:752, 1990.
178. Valverde J, Martínez-Ródenas F, Pereira JA, Carulla X, Jiménez W, Gubern JM, Sitges-Serra A. Rapid increase in plasma levels of atrial natriuretic peptide after common bile duct ligation in the ribbit. Ann Surg 216:554, 1992.
179. Pereira JA, Torregrosa MA, Martínez-Ródenas F, Clària J, Pallarés L, Gubern JM, Ruano-Gil D, Sitges-Serra A. Increased cardiac exocrine activity after common bile duct ligation in the rabbit. Ann Surg 219:73, 1994.
180. Martínez-Ródenas F, Pereira JA, Jiménez W, Gubern JM, Sitges-Serra A. Circulating bile is the main factor responsible for atrial natriuretic peptide release in experimental obstructive jaundice. Br J Surg 85:480, 1998.
181. Gallardo JM, Padillo J, Martín-Malo A, Miño G, Pera C, Sitges-Serra A. Increased plasma levels of atral natriuretic peptide and endocrine markers of volume depletion in patients with obstructive jaundice. Br J Surg 85:28, 1998.
182. Diamond T, Parks RW. Perioperative management of obstructive jaundice. Br J Surg 84:147, 1997.
183. Van den Hazel SJ, De Vries XH, Speelman P, Dankert J, Tytgat GN, Huibregtse K, van Leewen DJ. Biliary excretion of ciprofloxacin and piperacillin in the obstructed biliary tract. Antimicrob Agents Chemother 40:2658, 1996.
184. Thompson J, Bennion RS, Pitt HA. An analysis of infectious failures in acute cholangitis. HPB Surgery 8:139, 1994.
185. Gigot JF, Leese T, Dereme T, Coutinho J, Castaing D, Bismuth H. Acute cholangitis. Multivariate analysis of risk factors. Ann Surg 209:435, 1989.
186. Leese T, Neoptolemos JP, Baker AR, Carr Locke DL. Management of acute cholangitis and the impact of endoscopic sphincterotomy. Br J Surg 73:988, 1986.
187. Gogel HK, Runyon BA, Volpicelli NA, Palmer RC. Acute suppurative obstructive cholangitis due to stones: treatment by urgent endoscopic sphincterotomy. Gastrointest Endosc 33:210, 1987.
188. Lois JF, Gomes AS, Grace PA, Deutsch LS, Pitt HA. Risks of percutaneous transhepatic drainage in patients with cholangitis. Am J Roentgenol 148:367, 1987.
189. Siegel JH, Rodriguez R, Cohen SA Kasmin FE, Cooperman AM. Endoscopic management of cholangitis: a critical review of an alternative technique and report of a large series. Am J Gastroenterol 89:1142, 1994.
190. Lai EC, Mok FPT, Tan ESY, Lo CM, Fan ST, You KT, Wong J. Endoscopic biliary drainage for acute severe cholangitis. N Engl J Med 326:1582, 1992.

191. Sharma BC, Agarwal DK, Baijal SS, Saraswat VA, Choudhuri G, Naik SR. Endoscopic management of acute calculous cholangitis. J Gastroenterol Hepatol 12:874, 1997.
192. Lai EC, Tam PC, Paterson IA, Ng MM, Fan ST, Choi TK, Wong J. Emergency surgery for severe acute cholangitis: the high risk patients. Ann Surg 211:55, 1990.
193. Hutson DG, Russell E, Yrizarry J, Levi JU, Livingstone AS, Guerra J, Reddy R, Jeffers L, Schiff ER, Scagnelli T, Mendez K. Percutaneous dilatation of biliary strictures through the afferent limb of a modified Roux-en-Y cholecochojejunostomy of hepaticojejunostomy. Am J Surg 175:108, 1998.
194. Carmona R, Crass R, Lim RJ, Trunkley D. Oriental cholangitis. Am J Surg 148:117, 1984.
195. Saunders KD, Cates JA, Roslyn JJ. Pathogenesis of gallstones. Surg Clin North Am 70:1197, 1990.
196. Nakayama F, Koga A. Hepatolithiasis: present status. World J Surg 8:9, 1984.
197. Harris HW, Kumwenda ZL, Sheen-Chen S, Shah A, Schecter WP. Recurrent pyogenic cholangitis. Am J Surg 176:34, 1998.
198. Lim J. Oriental cholangiohepatitis: pathologic, clinical and radiologic features. Am J Roentgenol 157:1, 1991.
199. Fan ST, Choi TK, Chan FL, Lai EC, Wong J. Role of computed tomography in the management of recurrent pyogenic cholangitis. Aust N Z Surg 60:599, 1990.
200. Tompkins RK. Surgical management of bile duct stones. Surg Clin North Am 70:1329, 1990.
201. Pitt HA, Zuidema GD. Factors influencing mortality in the treatment of pyogenic hepatic abscess. Surg Gynecol Obstet 140:228, 1997.
202. Chu KM, Fan ST, Lai ECS, Lo CM, Wong J. Pyogenic liver abscess: an audit of experience over the past decade. Arch Surg 131:148, 1996.
203. Seeto RK, Rockey DC. Pyogenic liver abscess: changes in etiology, management, and outcome. Medicine (Baltimore) 75:99, 1996.
204. Rintoul R, O'Riordain MG, Laurenson IF, Crosbie JL, Allan PL, Garden OJ. Changing management of pyogenic liver abscess. Br J Surg 83:1215, 1996.
205. Bowers ED, Robison DJ, Doberneck RC. Pyogenic liver abscess. World J Surg 14:128, 1990.
206. Tay KH, Ravintharan T, Hoe MNY, See ACH, Chng HC. Laparoscopic drainage or liver abscesses. Br J Surg 85:330, 1998.
207. Condon RE. Antibiotic prophylaxis in gastrointestinal surgery. In Davis JM, Shires GT (eds). Principles and management of surgical infections. Philadelphia: JB Lippincott Co, 1991:131148.
208. Keighley MR, Flinn R, Alexander-Williams J. Multivariate analysis of clinical and operative findings associated with biliary sepsis. Br J Surg 63:528, 1976.
209. Meijer WS, Schmitz PI, Jeekel J. Meta-analysis of randomized controlled clinical trials of antibiotic prophylaxis in biliary tract surgery. Br J Surg 77:283, 1990.
210. Brandes JW, Scheffer B, Lorenz-Meyer H, Körst HA, Littmann KP. ERCP: complications and prophylaxis. A controlled study. Endoscopy 13: 27, 1981.
211. Finkelstein R, Yassin K, Suissa A, Lavy A, Eidelman S. Failure of cefonicid prophylaxis for infectious complications related to endoscopic retrograde cholangiopancreatography. Clin Infect Dis 23:378, 1996.
212. Niuderau C, Pohlman U, Lübke H, Thomas L. Prophylactic antibiotic treatment in therapeutic or complicated diagnostic ERCP: results of a randomized controlled clinical study. Gastrointest Endosc 40:533, 1994.
213. Byl B, Devière J, Struelens MJ, Roucloux I, De Coninck A, Thys JP, Cremer M. Antibiotic prophylaxis for infectious complications after therapeutic endoscopic retrograde cholangiopancreatography: a randomized double-blind, placebo-controlled study. Clin Infect Dis 20:1236, 1995.
214. Motte S, Deviere J, Dumonceau JM, Serruys E, Thys JP, Cremer M. Risk factors for septicemia following endoscopic biliary stenting. Gastroenterology 101:1374, 1991.
215. Polk HC Jr, Fink MP, Laverdiere M, Wilson SE, Garber GE, Barie PS, Hebert JC, Cheadle WG. Prospective randomized study of piperacillin/tazobactam therapy of surgically treated intra-abdominal infection. The Piperacillin/Tazobactam Intra-Abdominal Infection Study Group. Am Surg 59:598, 1993.
216. Gilbert DN, Moellering RC Jr, Sande MA. The Sanford guide to antimicrobial therapy. Antimicrobial Therapy, Inc. 1999.

48. SEPSIS IN OBSTETRICS

Humberto Correa

Severe infections originated in the gravid or recently evacuated uterus nearly always lead to fetal death in the former case and always place the mother's life at risk. They present some important features among which we highlight the following:

- They are related with human reproduction
- The protagonist is a woman with reproductive capacity who may have other small children
- They undoubtedly present social and economical implications
- The main site of the infection is in an organ which may be totally excised
- It is frequently accompanied by an infected thrombosis of the pelvic large veins and septic embolism.

The risk of maternal death due to obstetric infection is present when the chorioamnionitis, endomyometritis, pelvic thrombophlebitis or peritonitis, which may be simultaneously present, are the starting point of multiple organ failure (MOF) and transform the condition into a Severe Sepsis or Septic Shock.

Our Western tradition's interest and knowledge in obstetric sepsis began, or have as one of their most important landmarks in Ignaz Philipp Semmelweiss, a Viennese physician (1818–1865), who recognized and stressed the severity of postpartum infection in women undergoing delivery at medical centres during the nineteenth century. He wrote about the mortality of this clinical condition, the means of transmission of the infection (the contaminated hands of the physicians examining the pregnant women in labor) and implemented an effective form of prevention.

The medical and academic interest in obstetric sepsis-OS-(sepsis following delivery, cesarean section or abortion) has varied during the last third of the twentieth century. A great concern regarding this problem was observed at the beginning of this period, in the type and number of publications. But this interested faded rapidly in later years. This temporal variation has been clear in the developed Western countries. Although this trend has been maintained elsewhere in the rest of the world, an important variability is observed in the different continents in relation with the different technological and economic development throughout the globe.

In a search carried out in the MEDLINE duringe October 1999 including publicaciones since 1970 it was possible to obtain 705 references. We observed that 65% had been produced during the 1970s, 24% during the 1980s and 11% during the 1990s. In the first of these decades, the most publications originated in the USA and Western Europe, followed by scientific papers from Eastern Europe (the former socialist block). Most of the Western European publications come from Germany and France In Eastern Europe, most publications came from Russia. Production in the other continents was much smaller. During the second decade the production in Eastern Europe was maintained, increasing Africa, and decreasing in all other places, more abruptly in developed countries. During the third decade it decreased in all the sectors mentioned.

	1970-79	1980-89	1990-99
USA	75	30	15
West.Eur.	72	31	17
East.Eur.	49	44	6
Latin Amer	31	8	5
Asia	23	13	10
Africa	8	17	10
Oceania	8	5	1

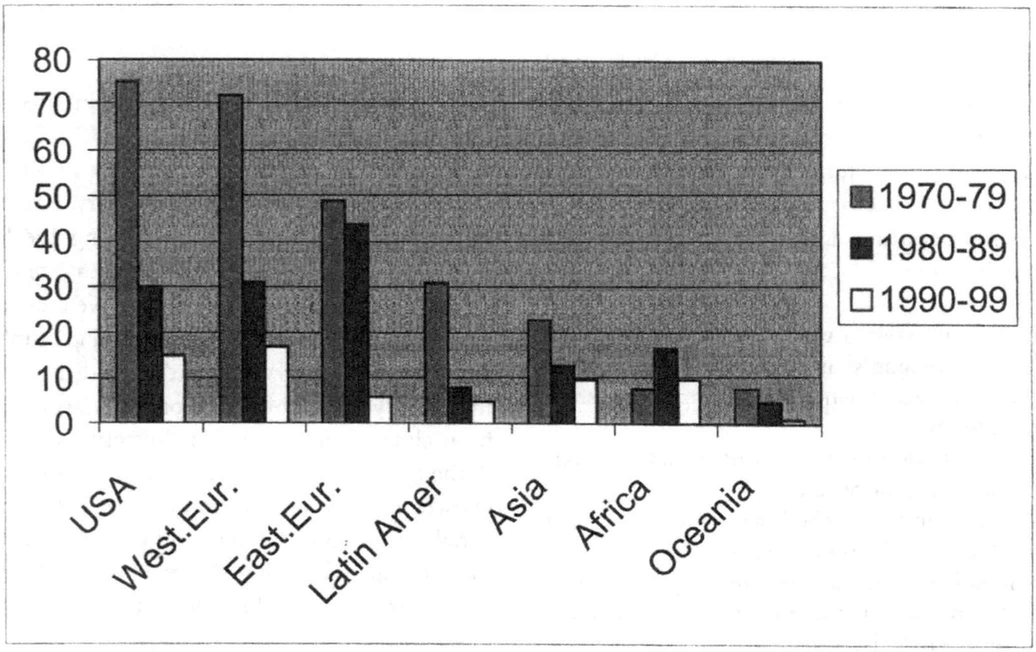

FIGURE 1. Distribution of publications in puerperal sepsis and septic abortion in differents continents during the last 30 years. Source: MEDLINE, search in November 1999.

It is worthwhile noting that most of the Asian work has been carried out India, and that most of the Latin American papers are mainly from Chile and Mexico, while the Africans are mainly from South Africa and Kenya. There are few references from Oceania and Japan, and none from China (see Figure 1).

The OS is more commonly related with emotional, moral, legal, social and sanitary organization factors than other severe infections. These are, in turn, dependent on economical and technical development, community patterns and traditions.

Some of the specific factors impinging with greater or lesser frequency on obstetric sepsis are: 1) existence or absence of early sexual education plans; 2) existence or absence of family planning programs; 3) dissemination and extensive knowledge of contraceptive methods; 4) national medical surveillance plans for pregnant women (mother-child health plans); 5) health care provisions for complicated pregnancies and delivery, which depend on the sanitary development (good enough, accessible and efficient hospitals or sanitary, networks); 6) legal framework for carrying out abortions (banned, partially permitted, or free and facilitated abortion). Practically all these factors are especially influenced by the degree of economic development. There are authors in many countries who in their publications request an increase in sexual education, the knowledge and use of contraceptive methods, together with radical changes in the laws that penalize abortion [1–4].

The results obtained in the MEDLINE search may partly reflect the status of the problem in different parts of the world.

Definition and Classification

The present study does not include all infections that may occur in obstetrics, but only obstetric sepsis. When we say obstetric sepsis we refer to the severe infectious conditions that pose a risk for the mother's life. This is why we will restrict ourselves to Severe Sepsis or Septic Shock of obstetric origen. We therefore exclude all obstetric infections that only present the Systemic Inflamatory Response Syndrome (SIRS), but do not present organ failure. Since our first studies on the subject we have defined sepsis as the severe clinical alteration of several vital systems due to an infectious site [5–7]. When the site of infection is in the uterus, gravid or recently evacuated, we speak of obstetric sepsis [8] The Chicago Consensus on Sepsis [9] spoke of severe sepsis in the presence of multiple organ dysfunction (MOD) or multiple organ failure associated to a site of infection and caused by it. A further step occurs in Septic Shock, a sepsis associated with hemodynamic failure. The hemodynamic failure called septic shock is produced by an infection and is characterized by a generalized hypoperfusion of tissues associated with hypotension that needs to be corrected through intravenous infusion of inotropic medication. When we use the acronym OS we refer to severe sepsis or sepsis with shock.

The OS may originate in: a) Infections secondary to the evacuation of an early pregnancy: provoked abortion – generally clandestine – or, very rarely, miscarriage. b) Endometritis following the evacuation of pregnancy at term spontaneously through the vagina or by cesarean section. c) Infections of the amniotic fluid during pregnancy: chorioamnionitis following amniocentesis or related with cerclage complications. d) In many cases peritonitis or septic pelvic thrombophlebitis may be associated as additional sites of infection.

Frequency

The occurrence of OS has decreased in Western developed countries and other parts of the world when compared to the situation 30 years ago [10, 11]. The exact frequency of pregnancies ending in OS is not well known. The available epidemiological data of infections following delivery allows us to suppose, after studying limited series of patients, the number of focalized infections produced, but not how many develop MOD. Maternal mortality data in different countries leads us to think about the frequency of maternal death due to OS following delivery, although it is not possible to know its frequency of development. Exact total birth figures are known in most countries, but the total number of illegal abortions is naturally unknown.

Feim and Duvivier [10] comment that puerperal endometritis occurs in 1 to 4 out of every 100 deliveries, and that it is much more frequent if there are predisposing factors or a cesarean section has been carried out. Dare *et al.* [12] communicate that, in a university centre in Nigeria, a total 146 episodes of puerperal endometritis occurred in 8428 deliveries assisted during a 10 year period (1.7%). In his study, puerperal infection was particularly associated with certain factors: anemia, protracted labor lasting more than 12 hours, more than 5 vaginal examinations during labor, premature rupture of membranes and lack of asepsis. We might conclude that 1 to 2% of deliveries are complicated with puerperal infection, but that very few of these cases develop into OS.

In the case of abortion, the infection apears more frequently when is it provoked compared to miscarriages, and more frequently in those provoked with dilatation and curetage than in those using the vacuum extraction [1]. Most authors agree that clandestine or illegal abortions, in patients admitted after it, cause three times more septic abortions than legal abortions [2, 3, 13]. Canas *et al.* [14] in Barcelona carried out a 5 year trial (1971–1975) and found that 20.2% of admittances to a hospital gynecology service were due to abortion. Of this group, 7.8% presented endometrial infections and, in turn, 15.2 of the infected patients presented OS. We could conclude that the frequency of OS in patients with abortion (clandestine or spontaneous) admitted to hospital during the 1970s, in a European country was approximately 1%.

Chorioamnionitis is the infection of the amniotic fluid, and may occur following the puncture of the intact egg or cerclage complications. Golstein *et al.* [15] carried out bacteriological cultures in amniotic fluid obtained through puncture, for karyotype studies, in 157 pregnant women. They found that in 8 cases presented pathogenic bacteria in the fluid in the absence of visual signs of infection and leucocytes in the cytological smear (5.8%). One of the 8 patients ended with a septic abortion (12% of those who presented bacterial growth and 0.6% of the pregnant women undergoing puncture). The hypothesis was that there had been a previous infection with intact membranes, although the germ might have been introduced through the puncture procedure. Siekman *et al.* [16] communicate that 13 out of 3122 amniocentesis were complications of chorioamnionitis and abortion (0.4%), although they do not state if any of them ended with OS.

In Uruguay we have carried out several studies between 1971 and 1999 [5, 17–20]. Between 1971 and 1974, 1 of every 4 admittances due to severe sepsis in the Intensive Care Unit of the University Hospital were due to OS [5]. This figure decreased after 1980. In our experience, 66% of obstetric sepsis are due to abortion, most frequent cause, 24% occur following vaginal delivery (most with previous foetal death and late evacuation) and 10% following cesarean section [8, 18].

In the ICU of the Italian Hospital of Montevideo, a private medical centre, 51 out of a total 6500 pacientes admitted during the 1975–1995 period were due to OS (0.78% of all admittances). Fifty of these cases presented an etiology similar to that indicated for the University Hospital, although there were less abortions. One case was due to chorioamnionitis following amniocentesis (2%). The frequency of OS in Uruguay tends to decrease, but, even in the present decade, remains between 0.5 and 0.6% of the total ICU admittances. On the other hand, Brun-Buisson *et al.* [21], analyzing an extensive number of sepsis in 30 French ICUs in 1995, do not communicate the existence of OS in their series.

Mortality

Mortality due to OS impinges in general maternal mortality (MM). The MM varies greatly from one country to another and has likewise varied in time. Its trend, as occurs with OS mortality, tends to descend although with varying rhythm according to the development of the regions considered. The MM in Sweden is currently of 6.6 per 100,000 born alive [22]. Between 1952 and 1986 15% of female deaths in the USA following delivery of a live baby were due to infection. The MM decreased 90% [10] throughout this period. During the 1990s MM in USA was 9.8/1,000,000 live births, and of those who died, only 8% were due to infection. In Uruguay in 1980 MM was 51/100,000 live births. It later descended more than 50%. During the 1988–1998 period it varied between 14 and 26/100,000 live births [23]. We do not know how many of these deaths were due to infection. Ayhan *et al.* [11] communicated the outcome of a trial encompassing 25 years at a hospital centre which shows that 108 women died due to pregnancy and delivery complications out of a total number of 59,993 pregnant women assisted. Of those who died, 59.8% were due to infection, 3/4 following abortion and 1/4 following delivery. Between the beginning and the end of the period studied mortality decreased 5 times and mortality due to infection among the mothers who died decreased from 74% to 9%.

Mortality in women with OS of all etiologies was greater than 50% during 1974 at the University Hospital of Montevideo [5, 17]. After 1980 these mortality figures decreased suddenly at the same centre to 10%, after the adoption of aggressive early surgery associated with other measures [19]. Aguilar and Estebam [23] indicated that in 1995, 38 (22%) out of a total 169 patients admitted due to septic abortion and MOD to the Argerich Hospital in Buenos Aires died. In 1999, Bagnulo and Barbato [20] communicated a series including 30 patients with OS following clandestine abortion, studied at the Maciel Hospital in Montevideo, 6 of which died (20%).

In summary, we might say that: 1) mortality in mothers who deliver live babies has varied during the present decade between 10 and 25 per 100,000 deliveries in the countries of the American continent mentioned, and is even lower in Sweden; 2) possibly 1 of every 10, or 1 out of every 7 of these deaths or more are due to infection; 3) the MM has descended in some countries in several continents during the last 40 years in proportions that have varied between 90 and 50%; 4) OS mortality was high 30 years ago, and has decreased to 10 to 20% at present in the places already mentioned.

Pathology

ENDOMETRITIS, MYOMETRITIS, PANMETRITIS

In OS following abortion, delivery or cesarean section, uterine infection occurs in the endometrium, and practically always in the myometrium. Histological lesions include inflamation, hemorrhage, supuration and necrosis. In many circumstances all the uterine wall is involved, and this may be observed from outside the uterus. In cases where manouevres to abort have been carried out there may be perforations of the fundus, and occasionally traumatic lesions of neighboring organs (intestinal perforation). These macroscopic lesions sysematically produce peritonitis. But peritonitis may be present without perforation when all the uterine wall is invaded. Peritonitis may be present in 6 out of 10 endomyometritis requiring surgery [8]. Uterine lesions may be visible macroscopically in the majority cases during exploratory surgery or resection. Nevertheless, on occasions this organ does not seem to be infected during external inspection and when it is sectioned and studied histologically always shows microabcesses and necrosis.

VENOUS THROMBOSIS: SEPTIC PELVIC THROMBOPHLEBITIS (SPTP)

The venous vessels of the uterine wall are systematically thrombosed, and nearly always infected. The histology enables the individualization of thrombi with bacterial colonies inside. In a study of 40 uterine specimens obtained from surgery or post-mortem examination, intramural septic thrombophlebitis was present in 36 (90%) [8]. These intramural thrombi continue in the extramural veins. They invade the utero-ovarian veins in 40% of cases, the illiac veins in 12–20% and even the inferior vena cava in 4% of patients. Collins carried out pathological studies of these phenomena many years ago [25, 26]. The SPTP is very frequently observed in pathological examinations, although it may be clinically invisible in the vaginal examination. In a total of 36 cases of SPTP confirmed in the anatomical and histological studies, only one was detected by an expert gynecologist in the genital examination [8]. Septic pelvic thrombophlebitis is a typical epiphenomenon of OS, and may cause protracted febrile conditions and septic lung thromboembolism (SLTE) in spite of treatment. Occasionally the SPTP is only manifest later, when the OS condition seems to have been cured, or appears alone, without previous clinical manifestations. It then causes protracted febrile conditions and abdominal pain. Rumhlan *et al.* [27] found SPTP in 1 out of every 600 deliveries, always associated with puerperal endometritis; he stresses the difficulty in confirming it through the vaginal examination. Janky *et al.* recommend the diagnosis using CT-scan or MRI [28].

The SPTP is the source and origin of *septic lung thromboembolism*. The SLTE is present in up 40% of the cases with OS. The clinical manifestations of SLTE are: episodes of dyspnea of sudden onset accompanied by cough, tachicardia and, occasionally bloody sputum. The chest X-ray shows them as irregular dense images, more frequently observed in the lower lobes and sometimes accompanied by pleural fluid. It is impossible to distinguish them from a non-infectious clott embolism, unless they later progress to cavitation or empyema. The irrefutable demostration of their existence may only be carried out through an anatomical examination. These episodes cannot therefore be confirmed during the patient's life. In spite of this, post-mortem studies frequently show them. When these episodes occur during OS we must first consider them as septic. They may cause an acute cor pulmonale [29, 30].

Right heart endocarditis (RHE) is another complication of OS. This phenomenon has been especially studied by Vic Dupont *et al.* since 1969 [31], and later by other authors such as Pimentel *et al.* [32] and Grover *et al.* [33]. Grover *et al.* [33] have communicated the results of a trial carried out in central India during the 80s where they found that 7.3% of a total 109 acute endocarditis only affected the righ heart (RHE) without previous congenital disorders, and that 60% of them occurred following obstetric sepsis. In that series, and during that time, none of the cases of RHE occurred in drug addicts. OS shares, together with the venous lesions of drug addicts and phlebitis secondary to venous catheterisms, the doubtful privilege of being one of the three common causes of tricuspid endocarditis. The repeated septic microembolism could be a common etiopathogenical cause in the three conditions. In our experience, the frequency of RHE in OS is 2% [8]. Left heart endocarditis may be present, together with RHE or isolated, although it is less frequent. When RHE occurs, it is another factor contributing to septic lung embolism.

Bacteriology

Beta hemolytic Streptococcus A and *Clostridium perfringens* were the classical agents of puerperal sepsis. These pathogens now represent a minimum fraction of the total group of bacterial agents proven responsible for OS during the past 30 years. It is currently known that infections and obstetric sepsis are of mixed etiology in 90% of cases, and that strict anaerobes are most frequently found. The microrganisms causing OS most often than not come from the cervico-vaginal environment, and therefore in the majority of cases correspond to the usual flora found in the female genital tract. Anaerobes are present in at least half of the cases of OS and in most of the series studied reach figures of 70% and more [34–36].

In healthy conditions the vagina has an abundant bacterial flora, the cervix is only occasionally colonized, and the endometrium is normally sterile. The vaginal flora is varied [37] and includes more strict anaerobes: *lactobacillus* (70% of the cases studied), several classes of *bacteroides* with a predominance of *bacteroides fragilis* (30%), *clostridium perfringens* (10–30%), *peptococcus and peptostreptococcus*. Facultative anaerobes and aerobes include: *Staph epidermidis* (30–80%); several enterobacteria (18–40%), the most important of which are *E coli*, *Klebsiella* and *Enterobacter; group D Streptococcus* (36%), *Streptococcus A* (5–20%), *Staph aureus* (5–15%); *group B Streptococcus-Agalactiae* (3–5%), and yeasts. During normal pregnancy there is a progressive increase of *lactobacilli* and yeasts and a reduction in the number of facultative anaerobes (Gram-negative enteric bacilli) and pathogenic strict anaerobes. Furthermore, these two last groups suddenly increase their presence during the three days following normal delivery [37].

The more frequent agents of OS are *bactercides fragilis* and other anaerobes together with enterobacteria. Among them, *E coli* is the most frequent, and is found in up to 39% of cases [8]. *Streptococcus, types A* or *B*, *Clostridium*, *Enterococcus*, *Candida* and *Pseudomonas* are rare. *Clostridium* species were only found to be responsible in 3% of the cases of OS in Montevideo [8]. *Streptococcus type A*, although currently infrequent, may provoke OS following abortion or labor, and may also cause the toxic shock syndrome with a mortality of 30 to 60% [38]. *Streptococcus type B* (Agalactiae) colonizes the vagina in some patients, particularly in the black race. It has been communicated that it causes OS in 2 out of every 1000 deliveries, and that it occurs in previously colonized patients [39]. *Candida*, which has never caused OS in our experience [8, 18], has been proven responsible in 8 cases following abortion or pregancy, especially in patients who previously underwent antibiotic treatment. Mortality has reached 37% [40]. *Staph aureus* is an infrequent agent of puerperal OS, but is very frequent as an agent of OS due to clandestine abortion in the countries where it is practised. We have found it in 35% of cases Its empirical treatment with antibiotics should be systematic in OS following illegal abortion [18].

Clinical Condition

The OS of different origins (abortion, delivery, cesarean section) present the same systemic symptoms and have a different manifestation in the genital-obstetric sector. All of them share a similar toxic infectious syndrome (fever, frequently elevated leukocytosis, postration and shivers), and the multiple organ dysfunction syndrome that makes them a severe sepsis. This syndrome is already classical [9, 41] and is due to the association of varying degrees of pulmonary edema, renal failure, low platelets and hemorrhage, hemodynamic instability or clear shock, jaundice and consciousness disorders.

As to the local aspect, the clinical signs and symptoms very.

In OS following delivery (puerperal sepsis) there is a history of childbirth, and in most cases purulent and foetid secretions may be demonstrated in the vaginal canal, the uterus is enlarged and tender. This lack of uterine involution is in some cases accompanied by evidences of a cavity occupied with non-evacuated residues (sectors of the placenta). Ultrasound is a useful aid for diagnosis. Nevertheless, local signs may be absent. In our experience all this local uterine and vaginal symptomatology is absent in 1 of 5 episodes of puerperal sepsis, in spite of the presence of endomyometritis [8, 18].

In sepsis following cesarean section the local elements are manifest at abdominal level: there is abdominal distension, absence of intestinal movements (frequently) and intense or moderate pain. We should recall that during the manual examination of the abdomen pain or contractures of the abdominal wall may be absent due to the poor reactivity during the peurperal period, although peritonitis is very frequently present in this type of OS. The genital examination in OS following cesarean section is inexpressive in 2 out of every 3 cases of OS. It is important to make a differential diagnosis with the spontaneous rupture of the ceacum. The latter may occur during the pueperal period following cesarean section, and the signs and symptoms may be similar.

In sepsis following provoked abortion the local symtomatology at the level of the genital tract includes genital bleeding, foetid secretions, pain during genital examination and the palpation of the hypogastrium. In our experience, all or some of these symptoms are present in 92% of cases, while in 8% they are all absent. In approximately half of the cases there is abdominal pain of varying intensity, indicating the possible presence of peritonitis. There are some interesting problems related to legal and social factors and their influence on the clinical situation. If the abortion has been carried out in countries where it is banned (and is therefore a crime) or carries a heavy moral social sanction, the person affected, generally of poor economic status, or some family member who knows about the fact, may deny or hide its existence to the physician, even when there is a risk of death. This has occurred in 7% of cases in our experience [8, 18].

In all the cases of severe sepsis in a woman who is pregnant, during the course of the pregnancy or at term, it is necessary to discard a urinary infection as a cause of sepsis. Pyelonephritis during pregnancy or the peripartum period is a severe clinical entity that may confuse the clinician, manifesting a symptomatology that may be interpreted as caused by endometrial infection [10].

Treatment

The treatment of OS requires four main steps:

1) Support of the organs and systems with dysfuntion or failure
2) Prescription of appropriate antibiotic therapy
3) Elimination of the site of infection
4) Prevention of septic embolism.

Support of the altered functions may include oxygen therapy, assisted ventilation, intravenous infusions, the use of inotropic adrenergic agents, hemodialysis, and other measures.

Antibiotic therapy: should be initiated immediately, always intravenous, following blood extractions for bacteriological tests. The antibiotics prescribed initially in an empirical manner aim to eliminate the potentially infectious agents. As mentioned before, they are most frequently Gram-negative enteric bacilli and different sorts of anaerobes. Third generation cephalosporins, fluorquinolones or aminoglucosides may be used in order to combat the Gram-negatives. It is always necessary to associate an anaerobicide. OS mortality decreased since more anaerobicides have been employed to treat it [42]. First choice anaerobicides are Metronidazol or *Clindamycin* [43]. The association of an effective anaerobicide together with an agent against Gram-negative is considered an "essential plan" for OS. There are 4 variables that motivate changes or additions to this "essential plan". In our milieu, and in the case of illegal abortion, it is mandatory to choose *clindamycin* instead of metronidazol, due to its proven effect in the presence of *Methycillin Susceptible Staph aureus* (*MSSA*), very frequent in this disorder. Given that abortions are practiced outside hospitals we rarely find *Methycillin Resistant Staph aureus* (*MRSA*). Due to the severity of this condition, when the presence of clostridium type (infrequent) agents is suspected or demonstrated, it is necessary to associate high doses of penicillin and maintain the metronidazol. When it is a nosocomial infection, as is the case of OS following cesarean section, it is prudent to employ Vancomycin empirically at the beginning in association with the basic plan due to the risk of *MRSA*. When the presence of *Pseudomonas aeruginosa* (rare) is confirmed, specific treatment should be initiated. People have recommended associating Ampicillin to the "basic plan" in order to treat a possible *Streptococcus A* or *Enterococcus*. These agents may be present in puerperal sepsis, but only in few cases.

Eliminate the site of infection: the site of infection is in the uterine wall (endo or panmetritis) and inside (egg parts). It also may occur in the peritoneum (peritonitis) or inside the pelvic veins (SPTP). When peritonitis is suspected, exploratory and cleansing surgery should be indicated. If perforation of the uterus, disseminated infection or necrosis are confirmed during the laparotomy, hysterectomy should be performed, generally accompanied by bilateral annexectomy. In cases where there is no suspicion of peritonitis actions on the infected uterus may be of two types:

a) in cases with OS, with organic dysfunction of moderate intensity requiring little replacement treatment (which do not require assisted ventilation, hypotension is not severe, conciousness is preserved and there is no bleeding due DIC or low platelets) the uterus may be treated in a conservative manner. It is necessary to evacuate the uterine cavity (residues of the product of conception in abortions or in puerperal sepsis) after initiating the antibiotics, and later continue with support measures, strict surveillance and prevention of pulmonary embolism with heparin (*Minor therapeutic plan*).

b) On the other hand, if the organic dysfunction is severe, it is mandatory to consider early on installing an aggressive excision policy: complete early hysterectomy with annexectomy. One of the first authors to propose and practice this form of treatment was an intensivist, Professor V. Vic Dupont [44]. This tactic is applied in Uruguay and elsewhere, and in the same procedure the inferior vena cava is nearly always ligated below the renal veins (*Major therapeutic plan*). This ligation has few immediate consequences, it does not affect the hemodynamic situation, and the post-ligation femoro-illiac thrombosis appears in less than 5% of cases and less frequently if heparin has been prescribed. We have observed that a supplementary paravertebral return circulation develops during a period 8 to 12 weeks.

It is worthwhile indicating some facts regarding hysterectomy. There are some authors with experience in OS caused by provoked abortion [24] who only indicate hysterectomy taking into account the local condition of the uterus: uterine gangrene, uterine perforation and myometritis which does not respond to medical treatment. This group (an Argentinean team [24]) treated 169 patients with severe sepsis caused by illegal abortion, and performed hysterectomy in 54 patients (32% of cases) obtaining a general survival figure of 78%. Our experience in Montevideo was different: until 1975 mortality due to OS of obstetric cause was greater than 50% [5]. In a study [17] we found that treatment defects included a late recognition of the sepsis, the non-realization of the hysterectomy in spite of a poor response to the initial treatment or its late implementation, and the absence of prevention of septic embolism. Taking into account the poor outcomes, a consensus and evaluation meeting was called gathering intensivists and obstetricians. The meeting produced a plan for systematic management. Only conservative treatment or the "minor" therapeutic plan (evacuate the uterus without excision) were allowed in patients with moderate organic dysfunctions during OS which generally did not require function replacement. But in all the other cases, or when the "minor plan" did not show a tendency towards improvement after 24 hours, the proposal was total hysterectomy and ligation of the inferior vena cava, or "major plan". In our case, we included the Argentine team indications for hysterectomy and added severe organ dysfunction, without taking into account the uterine status. The outcome of the application of this tactic, carried out by the same medical teams in the same hospital in Montevideo, reduced OS mortality to less 10%, and definitely changed the course of this type of sepsis [19]. Table 1 shows a comparison between two groups of patients: the first included 65 women and assisted between 1971 and 1979 at the University Hospital ICU in Montevideo. This group was treated without the existence of a systematic and concertated plan. Hysterectomies were performed in 60%, but nearly all were late, and venous ligations in 22%. Mortality was 54%. The other group, including 34 patients, was assisted at the same place during the 1980–84 period. These patients were treated according to a previously agreed systematic plan. Surgery was more frequent and earlier. Hysterectomy was performed in 91%, and venous ligations in 71%. Mortality was 6% ($p < 0.001$). We think that this "major" therapeutic tactic should be implemented early on in all OS with severe MOD [18]. Regarding the possibility of oophorectomy in the cases of hysterectomy, it is interesting to indicate that de Jonge and Venter [45] in South Africa found that only 28% of the ovaries excised during hysterectomy due to OS following abortion presented infection. They likwsie observed that none of the ovaries described as normal during laparatomy presented infection. This finding

TABLE 1. Comparison between two series of obstetric severe sepsis treated in the University Hospital ICU in Montevideo

SERIES	1971–79	1980–84	
Number of patients	65	34	
Abortions	39 (60%)	22 (65%)	
Deliveries	20 (31%)	9 (26%)	
Cesarean sections	6 (9%)	3 (9%)	
Peritonitis (operated)	26/44 (59%)	17/31 (55%)	
Average age	28.5 years	28.4 years	
Hysterectomy	39 (60%)	31 (91%)	
Annexectomy	15 (23%)	28 (85%)	
Ligation of veins	14 (22%)	24 (71%)	
Septic PTE	24 (37%)	3 (10%)	P < 0.01
Period between the initiation of the sepsis and admittance to a specialized environment	7.8 dias	2.9 dias	P < 0.01
Surgery before 74 hours following admittance/total number operated	25/44 (56.8%)	28/31 (90.3%)	
Survival	46%	94%	P < 0.001

could lead us to respect the ovaries in case of hysterectomy in sepsis when they seem normal in the gross examination.

Summary

- The OS occurs following abortion, delivery or cesarean section and its mortality affected half the patients several decades ago.
- The main agents are Gram-negative bacilli and associated anaerobes.
- The main site is the endometritis, frequently associated with peritonitis.
- The genital (vaginal) examination may not show abnormal elements in 7% of abortions, 20% of deliveries and 60% of cesarean sections.
- It nearly always associates infected thrombosis of the pelvic veins and may be complicated with septic PTE and tricuspid endocarditis.
- The imaging studies (ultrasound, CT-scan or MRI) may serve as important aids.
- The early recognition of sepsis has been partly thanks to the existence of intensive care medicine, while more aggressive therapeutic measures have collaborated towards a drastic reduction in mortality.
- The frequency of OS, which seems to decrease in some parts of the world, should decrease further. This requires a more intense and broader sexual education, and training in the use of contraceptive methods. It is necessary to consider legalization of abortion; it is likewise essential to optimize and generalize the mother health care systems during pregnancy and delivery.

References

1. Chi IC, Miller ER, Fortney J, Bernard RP. A study of abortion in countries where abortions are legally restricted. J Reprod Med 18:15, 1977.
2. Figueroa Damian R, Arredondo García JL. Conceptos actuales en la patogenia y tratamiento

de aborto y shock septico. I Epidemiología, patogenia y manejo del aborto septico. Ginecol Obstet Mex 61:305, 1993.

3. Lassey AT. Complications of induced abortions and their preventions in Ghana. East Afr Med J 72:774, 1995.
4. Ladipo OA. Preventing and managing complications of induced abortion in Third World countries. Suppl Int J Gynecol Obstet 3:21, 1989.
5. Correa Rivero H, Bagnulo H, Hiriart JC, Bagattini JC. Sepsis. Análisis de 80 casos en un CTI. El Tórax (Montevideo) 24:168, 1975.
6. Correa Rivero H, Bagnulo H, Hiriart JC. Sepsis repercusiones sistémicas. El Tórax (Montevideo) 24:182, 1975.
7. Correa Rivero H, Bagnulo H. Conceptos actuales en sepsis. Arch Med Int 2:2, 1980.
8. Correa Rivero H, Bagnulo H, Olazábal M. Sepsis en obstetricia. In Bagnulo H, Bagattini JC (eds). Seminarios en medicina interna. Montevideo: Prensa Médica Latinoamericana, 1982:97.
9. ACCP/SCCM Consensus Conference Commitee. Definition for sepsis and organ failure and guidelines for the use of innovative therapies in sepsis. Chest 101:1644, 1992.
10. Feim AM, Duvivier R. Sepsis in pregnancy. Clin Chest Dis 13:709, 1992.
11. Ayhan A, Bilgin F, Tuncer ZS, Yanik A, Kisnisci HA. Trends in maternal mortality at a university hospital in Turkey. Int J Gynaecol Obstet 44: 223, 1994.
12. Dare FO, Bako AU, Ezechi OC. Puerperal sepsis: a preventable post-partum complication. Trop Doct 28:92, 1998.
13. Macebo TG, Tsadic T. A six month prospective study on different aspects of abortion. Ethiop Med J 31:165, 1993.
14. Canas E, Cararach V, Fortuny A. Septic abortion. Complications and therapeutic considerations. Med Clin (Barc) 74:43, 1980.
15. Goldstein I, Zimmer EZ, Merzbach D, Peretz BA, Paldi E. Intraamniotic infection in the very early phase of the second trimester. Am J Obstetric Gynecol 163:1261, 1990.
16. Siekmann U, Daschner F, Heilmann L. Chorioamniotic infections following diagnostic amniocentesis in the 2d. trimester. Z Geburtshilfe Perinatol 3:119, 1985.
17. Correa Rivero H, Di Giovanni J, Nin Ferrari J. Sepsis de orígen genital en la mujer. Parte II. Arch Ginecol Obstet 28:81, 1978.
18. Correa Rivero H, Bagnulo H. Sepsis: concepto, clasificación, diagnóstico, tratamiento. In Artucio H, Correa H, Mazza N, Recarte M (eds). Medicina intensiva. Montevideo: Librería Médica, 1987:301.
19. Belloso A, Correa Rivero H, Bagnulo H. Elaboración de un plan terapéutico para Sepsis origen obstétrico. In Congreso Panamericano de Infectología, 2nd. Buenos Aires. 1984: 64.
20. Bagnulo H, Barbato M. Sepsis postaborto una problemática persistente en Latinoamérica. In Raad J (ed). Congreso Panamericano Ibérico de medicina intensiva y terapia intensiva. 1999:185.
21. Brun-Buisson C, Doyon F, Carlet J, *et al.* Bacteremia and severe sepsis in adults. A multicenter prospective survey in ICUs and wards of 24 hospitals. Am J Respir Crit Care Med 154:617, 1996.
22. Hogberg U. Maternal death in Sweden, 1971–1980. Acta Obstet Gynecol Scand 65:161, 1986.
23. Estadística de Mortalidad Materna 1980–1998. República Oriental del Uruguay. Ministerio de Salud Pública. División Estadística 1999.
24. Aguilar L, Esteban M. Aborto séptico. In Pacin J, Dubin A, Gallesio A, Laffaire E, Maskin B, San Roman E (eds). Terapia intensiva, 2nd edn. Buenos Aires: Panamericana, 1995:501.
25. Collins C, Mac Callum E. Suppurative pelvic thrombophlebitis. 1. Incidence pathology and etiology. Surgery 30:311, 1951.
26. Collins CG. Suppurative pelvic thrombophlebitis. Am J Obstet Gynecol 105:681, 1975.
27. Ruhmlan B, Reiher H, Randow H. A case of septic ovarian vein thrombosis. Zentralbl Gynakol 112:383, 1990.
28. Janky E, Cambon D, Leng JJ, Cormier P, Baste JC. Thrombophlebitis of the ovarian veins. A case report. Review of the literature. Rev Fr Gynecol Obstet 85:615, 1990.
29. Griffite G, Maull I, Sachatello R. Septic pulmonary embolization. Surg Gynecol Obstet 144:105, 1977.
30. Bagnulo H, Correa Rivero H, Bianchi A, Olazábal M. Tromboembolismo pulmonar séptico en obstetricia. Arch Med Int (Montevideo) 4:1, 1982.
31. Vic-Dupont V, Binet JP, Cachera JP Witchtz S, Amstutz P, Bazin C, *et al.* Post-abortum staphylococcal tricuspid endocarditis cured by surgical excision and Starr's prosthesis. Presse Med 77:661, 1969.
32. Pimentel M, Barbas CS, de Carvalho CR, Takagaki TY, Mansur AJ, Grinberg M, *et al.*

Septic pulmonary embolism and endocarditis caused by staphylococcus aureus in the tricuspid valve after infectious abortion. Report of 2 cases. Arq Bras Cardiol 52:337, 1989.
33. Grover A, Anand IS, Varma J, Choudhury R, Khattri HN, Sapru Rp, *et al.* Profile of right-sided endocarditis: an Indian experience. Int J Cardiol 33:83, 1991.
34. Finegold SM. Anaerobic bacteria in human disease. New York: Academic Press, 1977.
35. Tally FP, Gorbach SL. Antibiotics in surgery. Adv Surg 9:41, 1975.
36. Ledger WJ. Antibiotics in obstetric and gynecologic patients. In Kagan BM (ed). Antimicrobial therapy, 3rd edn. Philadelphia: Saunders, 1980:200.
37. Pedreira W. Antibioticoterapia profiláctica en ginecología y obstetricia. Bacteriología. In Bagnulo H, Bagattini JC (eds). Seminarios en medicina interna. Montevideo: Prensa Académica Latinoamericana, 1982:63.
38. Dotters DJ, Katz VL. Streptococcal toxic shock associated with septic abortion. Obstet Gynecol 78:549, 1991.
39. Pass MA, Gray BM, Dillon HC. Puerperal and perinatal infections with group B streptococci. Am J Obstet Gynecol 143:147, 1982.
40. Potasman I, Leibovitz Z, Sharf M. Candida sepsis in pregnancy and the postpartum period. Rev Infect Dis 13:146, 1991.
41. Marshall JC. Criteria for the description of organ dysfunction in sepsis and SIRS. In Fein AM, Abraham EM, Balk RA, Bernard GR, Bone RC, Dantzker DR, Fink MP (eds). Sepsis and multiorgan failure. Baltimore: Williams & Wilkins, 1997:286.
42. Rivlin Me, Hung JA. Surgical management of diffuse peritonitis complicating obstetrics/gynecologic infections. Obstet Gynecol 67:652, 1986.
43. Zambrano D. Clindamycin in the treatment of obstetric and gynecolonic infections: a review. Clin Ther 13:58, 1991.
44. Vic-Dupont V, Vachon F, Witchtz S, Gibert C, Bruniaux J. Post-abortion and post-partum septico-pyemia. Apropos of 27 cases. Ann Med Interne (Paris) 124:291, 1973.
45. de Jonge ET, Venter PF. Hysterectoy for septic abortion – is bilateral salpingo-oophorectomy necessary? S Afr Med J 74:291, 1988.

49. PERITONITIS

Gina Quaid and Joseph S. Solomkin

Introduction

Diffuse peritonitis remains a surgical disease where history and physical diagnosis are sufficient for the critical decision of whether to proceed with laparotomy. For patients with peritonitis due to a perforated viscus, intra-operative decisions regarding such items as extent of resection, anastamosis vs ostomy, and fascial closure or open management determine morbidity and mortality.

Patients with peritonitis also represent difficult management problems in critical care. Ongoing soiling of the peritoneal cavity and the dynamics of the local peritoneal response to contamination often produce dilemmas in timing of operation and resuscitation and support strategies. The organism(s) responsible for infection, adjuvant factors such as mucin, blood, or feces, and the integrity of host defenses are key variables determining the clinical presentation and treatment. In fact, most of the technological advances in radiographic diagnosis and intervention and in hemodynamic and respiratory support benefit these patients only after a major operative intervention.

This chapter is intended to provide an overview of the physiology of peritoneal response to contamination and to then review the disease processes and management falling under the heading of peritonitis.

Host Defenses

The peritoneal cavity is lined with mesothelium and several potential spaces are present. In normals, this space contains only a small amount of serous, sterile fluid. This fluid also contains a population of free floating cells that include large numbers of lymphocytes, monocytes/macrophages and a small percentage of eosinophils and mast cells [1]. Under normal conditions, homeostasis is regulated via a constant entry of cells into the peritoneal cavity and their exit via lymphatics of the diaphragm [2]. Fluid, particulate matter, and many microorganisms can be cleared by translymphatic absorption that occurs through specialized structures found only on the peritoneal mesothelium on the underside of the diaphragm. Stomata (10 to 16 μm) are formed between mesothelial cells that lead into lymphatic structures (lacunae) that subsequently drain into larger mediastinal lymphatic vessels. Material is then passed to the thoracic duct and the venous system sequentially. Particulates of all types, including bacteria, are rapidly removed from the peritoneal cavity into the systemic circulation. Inoculation of bacteria into the peritoneum leads to bacteremia within minutes.

Introduction of microorganisms into the normally sterile peritoneal environment invokes several potent specialized host antimicrobial defense mechanisms-clearance, phagocytosis and killing, and sequestration.

Resident and recruited phagocytic cells rapidly engulf those microbes that are not cleared by lymphatic channels. Resident macrophages constitute a minor mechanism of bacterial uptake and killing. Their primary function is as signaling sources. Signaling from these cells involves the production of various cytokines. Most important for recruitment of neutrophil (professional) phagocytes is Interleukin-8. The accumulation of neutrophils into the peritoneal cavity is delayed several hours, first by time needed to induce cytokine synthesis (69–90 minutes), the time needed to alter the endothelium in a manner allowing neutrophil attachment, and then the time needed for recruitment of sufficient numbers of cells to have a biological effect.

This delay may be viewed as a window during which more primitive host defense mechanisms, including exudation of plasma proteins, is central. During peritoneal contamination, a fibrinogen-rich inflammatory exudate containing plasma opsonins develops rapidly, and fibrin polymerization occurs. Fibrin complexes provide a variety of attachment sites for bacterial adhesins, and this affords a mechanism of sequestering microorganisms and thereby preventing bacterial entry into the vascular space [3, 4]. This mechanism has the capacity to trap large numbers of bacteria. Sequestration is a process that appears to be relatively nonspecific, trapping particulates as well as bacteria, regardless of external charge or structure characteristics.

These host defenses are also contributory to the development of pathology. For example, bacteremia occurs when lymphatic clearance mechanisms act to transport microbes into the thoracic duct. Intraabdominal abscess formation is promoted both by the fluid influx into the peritoneal cavity inhibiting opsonization and phagocytosis and by fibrin clots that isolate the bacteria from the phagocytes.

In the setting of bowel perforations, the drainage is halted by either resolution of the inflammatory process and repair of the damage and/or abscess formation. Acting in conjunction with the omentum and other mobile viscera, perforations are sealed; as ileus develops, contaminated enteric contents are walled off, thereby preventing continued soilage of the peritoneal cavity. The omentum is a pivotal element of host defense, and it has been characterized as, "the policeman of the abdomen" [5]. Containment of infection is one of its major functions. Currently, the omentum is thought to move to sites of infection by random movement and gravitational forces. With technical advances and a greater understanding of cellular molecular biology, the future may elucidate signaling and adhesion molecules working in concert to direct the omentum to areas of infection or injury.

Another important role the omentum plays in infection is deposition of phagocytes and acquisition of foreign particles or bacteria. The portal and regulation of these functions is thought to occur at sites known as "Milky spots". These are opaque patches in the greater omentum. They were first described by von Recklinghausen [6] as white spots in the omentum of rabbits and were named "taches laiteuses" by Ranvier [7, 8]. Milky spots are present in most mammals, and were described by Seifert on the greater omentum 70 years ago [9]. In humans, the number of milky spots per unit area is the greatest in infancy, and gradually decreases with age.

Milky spots are composed of cellular aggregations of mesenchymal cells, mainly macrophages and lymphocytes, surrounding capillary convolutions termed omental glomeruli [10]. The cellular composition of the milky spots include macrophages (40%), b lymphocytes (30%) and tlymphocytes (12%) [10]. Mast cells are rare (6%). Macrophages covering the milky spots, which face the peritoneal cavity, trap and digest the circulating antigens and foreign bodies which are introduced into the peritoneal cavity. The macrophages transfer information to lymphocytes in the central part of the milky spots. Thus, functional cellular zonation of omental milky spots corresponds to the structural relation between macrophages lining the lymph sinus wall and lymphocytes in the germinal center of the lymph node. From a clinical standpoint, the omental milky spots may function to absorb antigenic proteins or bacteria which are introduced into the peritoneal cavity during gut inflammation, perforation or at operation. Milky spots also serve as a major site of entry for recruited neutrophils during inflammatory processes.

During inflammation, the number and size of omental milky spots dramatically increase, and some develop germinal centers within the lymphatic follicles and produce antibodies. During intraperitoneal immunotherapy, the omental milky spots and their cellular elements may be activated by intraperitoneal administration of biological response modifiers, and thereby represent an important immunoregulatory system for the peritoneal cavity.

Major Types of Peritonitis

PRIMARY PERITONITIS

Primary peritonitis refers to infection of the peritoneal cavity without a documented source of contamination from the gastrointestinal tract. There are four major variants of primary peritonitis, which are based on pathophysiology and microbiology. Primary peritonitis has declined in frequency, but still accounts for approximately two per cent of all pediatric abdominal emergencies. Primary peritonitis follows a bimodal age distribution [11]. In infants, it occurs within the first two months of life, and females are predominately affected. The second peak is from 5 to 9 years of age (mean 8.5), and a more equal distribution of males and females is seen Children with nephrotic syndrome or cirrhosis are at particularly high risk [12–14]. *Streptococcus pneumoniae* and group A streptococci are the most common isolates in primary peritonitis of childhood.

A second type of primary peritonitis is from the urogential tract. It is often linked to sexually transmitted diseases, with *Chlamydia trachomatis* as the major etiologic agent. The likely mechanism is retrograde flow through the fallopian tubes reaching the peritoneal cavity continuing cephalad along the paracolic gutters. This type of peritonitis is characterized by a localized inflammatory process involving Glisson's capsule and adjacent peritoneum, referred to as perihepatitis, or Fitz-Hugh-Curtis syndrome. Other variants are rare and include periappendicitis and perisplenitis. Primary peritonitis can also occur in women with intrauterine devices, supporting a transfallopian route.

Primary peritonitis can develop in immunocompromised patients. In these patients, spontaneous bacterial peritonitis develops secondary to either translocation from the intestines or hematogenous spread that cannot be cleared by resident macrophages. Patient may have systemic syndromes such as systemic lupus erythematosus on steroids, immunosuppressed following transplantation or chemotherapy for neoplasia, or can have some type of severe viral illness like the acquired immunodeficiency syndrome. These types of patients can be a diagnostic problem, as 10 to 37 per cent of patients will manifest abdominal pain as a part of their symptomatology-the majority of which represent other peritoneal inflammatory syndromes, such as serositis, vasculitis, or pancreatitis.

The most common form of primary peritonitis is termed spontaneous bacterial peritonitis (SBP) which occurs in cirrhotic patients with ascites. It has also been reported in patients with normal livers and ascites due to congestive heart failure, metastatic malignant disease, and, rarely, adults with no obvious disease. Hematogenous seeding of the ascitic fluid is the most likely mechanism by which the peritoneal fluid becomes infected, although bacterial translocation through the intact gut or lymphogenous spread is also believed possible. Bacterial translocation from the gut to mesenteric lymph nodes, depressed activity of the reticuloendothelial phagocytic system and decreased antimicrobial capacity of ascitic fluid seem to be the main steps in the pathogenesis of ascitic fluid infection. Patients at highest risk are those with ascitic fluid protein concentrations of less than 1 g/dl.

The infection is monomicrobial in 90 per cent of cases. The most common isolates are *E. coli*, *Streptococcus* species, and *Klebsiella* species. Characteristic of SBP is the low concentrations of organisms encountered in the peritoneal fluid. Routine admission paracentesis documented an incidence of 27 per cent in this patient population and it accounts for 30 per cent of all infections in cirrhotic patients [15, 16].

Diagnosis of ascitic fluid infection is based on clinical suspicion and analysis of ascitic fluid, especially white cell count and culture in blood culture bottles. A low threshold for performing an abdominal paracentesis is the key for an early diagnosis and treatment. The leukocyte count is usually $>300/mm^3$, with most having $>1000/mm^3$. A leukocyte count $>500/mm^3$ is considered diagnostic. Lactate concentrations and pH are also of help in diagnosing primary bacterial peritonitis [17].

A third-generation cephalosporin is the treatment of choice, achieving a cure rate higher than 80%. Nonazotemic patients with uncomplicated SBP may be treated with oral quinolones. Prophylactic selective intestinal decontamination with oral norfloxacin or trimethoprim-sulfamethoxazole may be useful in preventing SBP in patients that are at high risk for developing SBP, such as hospitalized cirrhotic patients with gastrointestinal hemorrhage or low ascitic fluid total protein [18, 19].

Both tuberculous peritonitis and peritonitis due to *Coccidiodes immitis* also rarely occur. The presentation is of a subacute disease and is diagnosed by appropriate cultures and histology.

SECONDARY PERITONITIS

Secondary peritonitis occurs as a result of contamination of the peritoneal cavity following perforation of a hollow viscus or transmural necrosis of the gastrointestinal tract. The most common causes of secondary peritonitis are perforated gastric or duodenal ulcer, perforated appendicitis, perforation of the colon due to either diverticulitis, carcinoma or volvulus, and postoperative peritonitis occurring as a result of anastomotic disruption or failed treatment for intraabdominal infection.

The delay in diagnosing and treating gastric or duodenal perforation determines the anticipated microbiology. If operation is undertaken within 24 hours of perforation, either a sterile chemical peritonitis or contamination with low levels of acid-resistant microorganisms, including *Candida* and lactobacilli, may be encountered. This situation warrants only brief prophylactic antimicrobial therapy, typically with an agent such as cefazolin. In the event that *Candida* is isolated in this setting of acute perforation in otherwise healthy hosts, no treatment is indicated.

Infections arising from perforations in the distal ileum or colon present far more complex microbiology. Most commonly, the resultant infection is polymicrobial, containing a mixture of aerobic and anaerobic bacteria. In a recent study of 339 peritoneal culture specimens in patients with peritonitis, 76 per cent contained mixed aerobic and anaerobic bacteria with the most frequent combination being *Escherichia coli* and *Bacteroides fragilis* [20]. Table 1 is a composite of the most common peritoneal isolates at laparotomy.

Synergism between various microorganisms present at the site of contamination favors the progression of infection. The best studies example of this is the interaction between *Bacteroides fragilis* and lipopolysaccharide-expressing Gram-negative organisms. The presence of *Bacteroides fragilis* in relatively low numbers greatly

TABLE 1. Common community acquired peritoneal isolates at laparotomy

Gram-Negative aerobic and facultative anaerobes	Escherichia coli Pseudomonas aeruginosa Klebsiella species Enterobacter species Proteus mirabilis Morganella morganii
Gram-Positive aerobic and facultative anaerobes	Nonenterococcal streptococci Enterococci Staphylococcus aureus S. epidermidis
Anaerobic Organisms	Bacteroides fragilis Other Bacteroides Clostridium species Peptococci/streptococci
Yeast	Candida species

reduces the number of *E. coli* needed to establish infection [21]. *Bacteroides fragilis* expresses a complex capsular polysaccharide that inhibits phagocytosis and suppresses NK cell functioning [22, 23]. Conversely, lipopolysaccharide, which is easily shed from the bacterial surface, causes an intense local reaction by inducing cytokines from resident macrophages. These cytokines, most notably TNFα, have profound effects on local perfusion. By inducing local coagulation, enhanced vascular permeability, and constriction of arterioles, TNFα effectively devascularizes the local area, greatly limiting the influx of blood-borne host defense mechanisms.

Bacterial peritonitis is associated with an immense intraperitoneally compartmentalized cytokine response, with plasma levels of cytokines representing only the tip of the iceberg. Although small amounts of cytokines appear beneficial to peritoneal defense, higher levels correlate with adverse outcome [24].

PRESENTATION

Peritonitis has variable presentations dependent on the specific disease causing perforation, location of the perforation in relation to other viscera and serosal surfaces, and host factors such as immunocompetence or recent operation. Secondary peritonitis causes a rapid contamination of the peritoneum which usually produces the classic acute abdomen: pain is of recent onset and may be sudden or appear over several hours, onset could be localized, but generalized pain develops rapidly and movement, coughing, or jarring the bed aggravates the symptoms. For diffuse peritonitis, tenderness is found over the entire abdomen. The patient lies still, with shallow respirations and voluntary muscular guarding of the abdomen and as the parietal peritoneum becomes inflamed, rigidity ensues due to reflex muscular spasm. Anorexia, nausea, and vomiting are present from the onset, but the patient is thirsty, and urine output is low. Ileus results in abdominal distention and hyperresonance, and bowel sounds are usually diminished or absent.

LABORATORY/IMAGING STUDIES

A leukocytosis greater than 11,000/mm^3 with bandemia is a common finding in peritonitis. Leukopenia is likely a consequence of C5a generation and indicates greater mediator production. Elevated blood urea nitrogen level and a metabolic acidosis may be present reflecting dehydration. Microscopic hematuria and pyuria occur with inflammation adjacent to the urinary tract, but the presence of bacteria, white blood cell casts, and large numbers of erythrocytes in the urine should suggest a urinary tract source of the pain. Amylase levels are usually normal unless pancreatitis, a proximal gastrointestinal tract perforation, or bowel infarction are responsible for the peritoneal inflammation. Blood cultures are positive 30 to 40% of the time [4, 25]. However, it is important to note that bacteremia itself does not worsen the outcome from intraabdominal infection. Bacteremic organisms from intraabdominal foci typically have low invasiveness (as compared to *Staphylococcus aureus*) and thus the presence of bacteremia does not mandate prolonged or otherwise altered anti-infective therapy. Anti-infective therapy is begun empirically, before the results of cultures and susceptibility data are know. Generally, such therapy is designed in anticipation of a mixed flora infection. Particularly in the setting of community acquired infection, regimens commonly utilized will cover the bacteremia organism. It is worth obtaining such cultures, however, primarily to provide a database of identities and susceptibilities of organisms seen in the particular hospital.

Plain film evaluation of the abdomen in an ICU patient include a supine and left lateral decubitus provide evidence of mechanical intestinal obstruction, volvulus (Figure 1), intussusception, and uncommonly mass effects due to abscesses or neoplastic processes. They may also reveal mild distention of the small and large intestine with air-fluid levels. A chest x-ray may reveal a non-gastrointestinal etiology of upper abdominal pain, such as pneumonia. Gas found within the biliary tree or gallbladder suggests a fistulous communication, emphysematous cholecystitis, or cholangitis. Gas within the mesenteric and portal venous systems suggests an advanced gastrointestinal inflammatory or ischemic process (Figure 2). Rarely, pneumatosis intestinalis or retroperitoneal air may be seen following endoscopy. Extraluminal gas with a fluid level or gas bubbles is suggestive of an abscess in which the infecting organism are undergoing anaerobic metabolism.

Computed tomography (CT) scanning of the abdomen may be useful in some cases of peritonitis were the diagnosis is not obvious. It should be done with intravenous, oral, and rectal contrast. If there is a question of perforation, especially in the sigmoid and rectal region, rectal contrast is not recommended. Intravenous contrast is very important in the evaluation of solid organs such as the liver, spleen, pancreas, and kidneys. In the setting of renal failure, intravenous contrast is contraindicated. CT is very accurate in demonstrating small-bowel obstruction with the use of oral contrast. It has proven very helpful in the elucidation of closed-loop intestinal obstruction. Arteriography or digital subtraction venography may be required in cases of suspected intestinal ischemia.

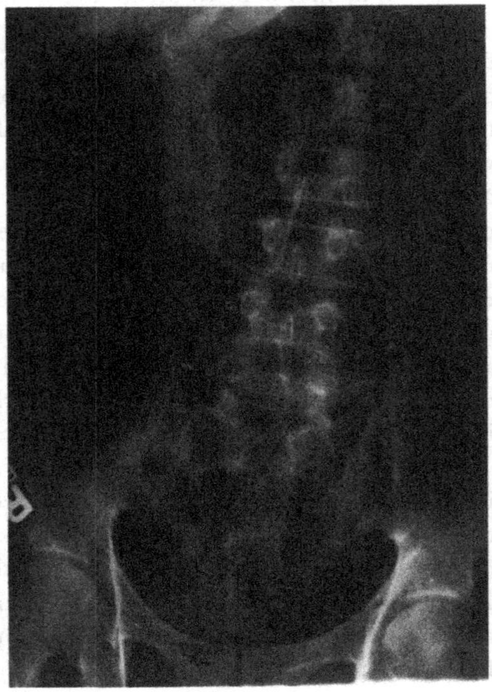

FIGURE 1. Plane film of the abdomen. The patient presented with abdominal pain and distention for two hours. The plane film reveals a sigmoid volvulus.

TERTIARY PERITONITIS

Tertiary peritonitis is a well known but poorly understood phenomenon. It is characterized by fever, leukocytosis, hyperdynamic cardiovascular parameters, a general hypermetabolic state, and progression to multisystem organ failure, similar to that seen in overtly infected patients. Usually these patients have been aggressively treated for a secondary peritonitis via surgical intervention and antimicrobial therapy.

The microbial flora of patients with tertiary peritonitis is very different from patients with secondary peritonitis. Potentially pathogenic organisms traditionally thought to be of low virulence such as *Enterococcus*, *Candida*, *Staphylococcus epidermidis*, *Pseudomonas* and *Enterobacter* spp. are the predominate microbes [26]. These organisms are also resistant to most first-line antibiotics used in the surgical ICU and may reflect a shift secondary to antibiotic pressures.

An additional component of this syndrome is dysfunctional immune system with diminished capability of clearing these organisms. Early studies of multiple organ failure in patients with peritonitis demonstrated a strong association between organ failure and the presence of uncontrolled residual infection in the peritoneal cavity [27–29]. This resulted in a trend toward exploratory or "blind" laparotomy in patients with organ dysfunction and was extended to patients without recent gastrointestinal tract manipulations and negative imaging studies. The concern was for poorly loculated infection and varying degrees of a thick fibrinous peel of

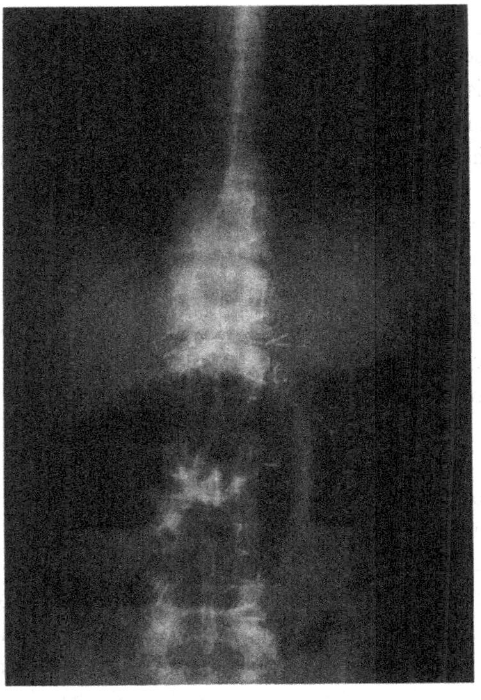

FIGURE 2. Plane film of the abdomen. This is a 37 year old male with a history of previous abdominal surgery who presented to an ER in septic shock and a distended abdomen. The plane film shows a small bowel obstruction and portal venous air.

the peritoneal and serosal surfaces [26]. Subsequent studies documented that it is rare to find intra-abdominal infection in the majority of cases diagnosed with tertiary peritonitis [26, 30] and reoperation in this case is associated with an exaggerated host inflammatory response without obvious benefit to the clinical course [31].

In a multitude of studies, alteration of treatment does not alter the morbidity and mortality of this disease [26, 30, 32, 33]. This would suggest that in the setting of immunologic and therapeutic intervention fail this syndrome will appear. This entity may be viewed as an ICU-acquired infections, such as pneumonia, in which the role for antimicrobial (or surgical) therapy in improving outcome is modest and the specific impact of infection on mortality is uncertain [26, 34–36].

Treatment

ANTIMICROBIAL THERAPY

The goals of antibiotic therapy for intraabdominal infection are as with any other infectious process, to quickly eliminate the microorganisms, decrease the possibility of recurrence and shorten or eliminate further clinical manifestations. Surgical wounds can be heavily contaminated by infecting microogranisms, and it is important that effective antimicrobial therapy be begun prior to operation. Necrotizing fascitis and other forms of extension of infection to the surgical wound represent catastrophic failures of antimicrobial treatment.

Once the diagnosis of intraabdominal infection is suspected antimicrobial therapy is begun, prior to the establishment of an exact diagnosis and before results of appropriate cultures are available. The adequacy of initial empiric regimen dose affects outcome. Inappropriate treatment (antibiotics that do not cover all possible bacteria in the infection) results in an increase in treatment failures and mortality rates [37, 38]. Empiric therapy must be chosen based on historical information identifying organisms at specific sites and guided further by local resistance patterns. Antibiotics used for intraabdominal infections should be active against enteric Gram-negative aerobic, facultative and obligate anaerobic bacilli. The microbiology of community acquired intraabdominal infection has been well defined (Table 1). Depending on the site of the gastrointestinal tract perforation, the identity and density of microorganisms can be predicted. In general, a small number of Gram-positive aerobic and Gram-negative anaerobic organisms are found in gastric, duodenal, and proximal jejunal perforations. Defense mechanisms in intact hosts and first or second generation cephalosporins eradicate these organisms.

Distal small bowel perforations into the peritoneum usually contain Gram-negative facultative organisms with variable density. Colonic anaerobes such as *Bacteroides fragilis* are variably present. Colon-derived intraabdominal infections contaminate the peritoneal cavity with large numbers of facultative and obligate anaerobic Gram-negative organisms.

In 20 per cent of patients with acute perforations of the gastrointestinal tract, *Candida albicans* or other fungi are cultured. Treatment in these cases with antifungal agents is unnecessary unless the patient has recently received immunosuppressive therapy for neoplasm, transplantation, or inflammatory disease, or has recurrent intraabdominal infection.

Intraoperative cultures should guide decisions regarding antimicrobial therapy. Fluid collections, particularly if purulent, should be sampled for Gram stain and culture. Infected intraabdominal fluid specimens should either be sent to the laboratory in a capped airless syringe with no needle or collected in appropriate (separate) aerobic and anaerobic transport media. If the Gram-stained smear reveals predominance of Gram-positive cocci, which may indicate that enterococci or other fecal streptococci are significant copathogens at the site of infection, the clinician should consider alterations in the antibiotic regimen to include agents specifically active against enterococci.

Although the appropriate role of anti-enterococcal therapy is controversial, most authorities believe that specific anti-enterococcal therapy should be given only when enterococci are the only organisms isolated or are isolated from blood. Isolation of enterococci as part of a mixed Gram-positive and Gram-negative flora should not prompt addition of ampicillian or vancomycin to the antibiotic regimen. The incidence of treatment failure for patients harboring enterococci and not treated for it is the same as for patients treated with imipenem or other agents effective against enterococci. Enterococci are low-level pathogens, meaning that they incite little host response and do not cause invasive infection in intact hosts. However, patients who have had one major episode of sepsis are sufficiently immunosuppressed so that isolation of enterococci from a second infectious site (including recurrent infection within the abdomen) should mandate specific anti-enterococcal therapy. If the smear reveals Gram-negative bacilli, failure to isolate either facultative or obligate anaerobes on culture does not obviate the need to continue providing antimicrobial agents against both. Antimicrobial susceptibility patterns within each hospital should be heeded in selecting initial empiric therapy.

In vitro data, especially antimicrobial susceptibility test, are predictive of the *in vivo* response of infecting bacteria to particular antibacterial agents. While a variety of susceptibility testing techniques are available, disk or automated testing is appropriate for bacteria isolated from intraabdominal infections except in extraordinary circumstances. Evidence from *in vitro* data, animal studies, and clinical trials has led to widespread acceptance of the need to provide empiric antimicrobial therapy directed against Eschericia coli and other common members of the family Enterobacteriaceae and B. fragilis. B fragilis and E. coli are the most common isolates from intraabdominal infections and are the organisms most likely to cause bacteremia in abdominal sepsis, further attesting to their pathogenicity.

The evidence in support of broadening therapy to cover organisms other than common facultative and obligate anaerobes such as E. coli and B fragilis is more controversial. In a study by Yellin *et al.*, initial empiric coverage of Pseudomonas aeruginosa was associated with a decreased likelihood of persistent or recurrent abdominal infection when these organisms were isolated from the site of infection [39]. In patients with recurrent (nosocomial) peritonitis, resistant organisms are routinely found and primary therapy covers both Pseudomonas and Enterococci [40].

A large number of agents are broadly active against the bacteria found in intraabdominal infection. These are best discussed as classes of drugs and include aminoglycosides, carbapenems, cephalosporins, penicillins plus beta-lactamase inhibitors and quinolones. Aztreonam is considered as a cephalosporin-class agent. Table 2 summarizes anti-infective agents commonly used for treating intraabdominal infections.

Aminoglycosides have been the mainstay of therapy for serious Gram-negative infections for the past 30 years. Due to their potential for nephrotoxicity and ototoxicity, there has been considerable movement away from aminoglycosides as first-choice agents for community-acquired intraabdominal infections. The use of beta-lactams combined with beta-lactamase inhibitors, or single-agent imipenem/cilastatin in mixed flora infections has given clinical results equivalent to or better than those seen with aminoglycoside-based combinations. Aminogylcosides no longer represent the "gold standard" for therapy of intraabdominal infections and need not be used for community-acquired intraabdominal infections. Some data, however, suggest that hypotensive patients with Gram-negative bacteremias have higher survival rates if treated at least initially with aminoglycoside-based combination therapy [41]. Aminoglycoside-contining regimens may result in more rapid clearance of organisms and abbreviate host deterioration. When aminoglycosides are prescribed, it is usually for nosocomial infections due to multiply resistant organisms

If β-lactam resistant isolates are suspected because of poor antibiotic treatment, intermittent dosing of gentamicin or tobramycin given once every 24 hours (7–10 mg/kg) is now the gold standard of therapy. The rationale for this form of treatment is based on two key antimicrobial properties of aminoglycosides: dose-dependent killing and a post-antibiotic effect. If cultures reveal organisms sensitive to a non-aminoglycoside use, single agent anti-Gram-negative therapy may be continued after 48 hours.

"First-generation" cephalosporins, including cefazolin, cephapirin and cephalothin, have excellent Gram-positive activity, moderate Gram-negative activity, and no anaerobic activity. Cefonocid, cefamandole, and cefuoxime may be grouped with these agents because none have anaerobic activity. Other second generation agents, including cefotxitin, cefotetan, and cefmetazole, all have some anaerobic activity, improved facultative Gram-negative activity, and less Gram-positive coverage. The anaerobic activity of these agents against B. fragilis is unimpressive; in general surveys, about a third to a half of tested isolates are resistant. Because of the high incidence of B. fragilis and relatively large inoculum loads encountered in colon-derived infections, these agents are best used for prophylaxis and for treatment of low-inoculum infections such as appendicitis.

The "third-generation" agents, cefotaxime, ceftizoxime, cefoperazone, ceftriaxone, and ceftazidime, have considerable facultative Gram-negative activity but no anaerobic and limited Gram-positive coverage. Aztreonam, termed a monobactam, has activity against facultative Gram-negative organsims equivalent to third-generation cephalosporins. It has no Gram-positive or anaerobic activity. Metronidazole has remained highly effective against Bacteroides species, in contradistinction to clindamycin, and is now the preferred agent for combination therapy.

The specific choice of one third-generation cephalosporin or aztreonam over another is not a major issue. As clinical experience with these agents has widened, it has become apparent that the differences between agents do not affect outcome. Many hospitals have therefore taken the position that cephalosporins can be grouped into classes and that within each class the agents are therapeutically interchangeable. Commonly, acquisition costs now determine which cephalosporin is used within each class. Ceftazidime is not recommended for general empiric therapy because broad usage of the agent is associated with decreasing susceptibility of P. aeruginosa, and this agent is the only cephalosporin reliably effective against this

TABLE 2. Antimicrobial reagents

Agents	Dosage	Comments
Aminoglycosides		All aminoglycosides can cause ATN, deafness due to cochlear toxicity, vertigo due to damage to vestibular organs and rarely neuromuscular blockade
Gentamicin	5–7 mg/kg q24 hrs	
Tobramycin	5–7 mg/kg q24 hrs	
Amikacin	15 mg/kg q24 hrs	
Monobactam		Can be used in Pen allergic patients
Aztreonam	2 g q8–12 hrs	
Fluoroquinolones		Concerns are drug-drug interactions, CNS toxicity, phototoxicity, nausea/vomiting, and potential adverse effect on joint cartilage
Ciprofloxacin	750 mg q12 hrs	
Levofloxacin	250–500 mg q24 hrs	
Oflaoxacin	200–400 mg q12	
Anaerobic Antibiotics		
Clindamycin	600–900 mg q8 hrs	Frequent cause of C. difficile toxin-mediated diarrhea.
Metronidazole	500 mg q6 hrs	Can be given rectally or vaginally (gel form). Neuro side effects include peripheral paresthesias or neuropathy, ataxia, seizures, and aseptic menigitis
Cephlosporins		Prospective data has demonstrated a correlation with the use of cephlosporins and increased risk of C. difficile toxin-mediated diarrhea. Increased risk of vancomyocin resistant enterococci
Cefoxitin	1–2 g q4–6 hrs	
Cefotetan	1–2 g q12 hrs	
Ceftizoxime	2 g q8 hrs	
Ceftazidime	1–2 g q8–12 hrs	
Ceftriaxone	2 g q24 hrs	
Cefepime	1–2 g q12 hrs	
Cefpirome	1–2 g q12 hrs	
Penicillin + B-Lactamase inhibitors		Hypersensitivity reactions, diarrhea, hypokalemic alkalosis, elevation of serum aminotransferases and inhibition of platelet aggregation especially at high doses
Ampicillin/sulbactam	3 g q6 hrs	
Ticarcillin/clavulanate	3.1 g q4–6	
Piperacillin/tazobactam	3.375 g q6 hrs	
Carbapenems		
Imipenem/cilastatin	0.5 g q6 hrs	Seizures with higher doses
Meropenem	1 g q8 hrs	

pathogen. Additionally, ceftazidime therapy is associated with an increased incidence of enterococcal superinfections.

An alternative strategy to the use of beta-lactamase-resistant cephalosporins is to utilize currently available beta-lactams in combination with beta-lactamase inhibitors, such as sulbactam, clavulanic acid, and tazobactam. These agents are potent inhibitors of beta-lactamases from Gram-positive and anaerobic organisms.

They have little activity against the chromosomal beta-lactamases seen in many strains of Enterobacteriaceae and do not compensate for the marginal Gram-negative activity of the penicillin derivative. The primary concern has to do with organisms that constitively express Beta-lactamases. Organisms that typically do this include Enterobacter species, P. aeruginosa, Citrobacter, Serratia and Actinetobacter species. These organisms are most commonly encountered in nosocomial infections but are also present in about 15 per cent of community-acquired infections. Clinical trials with these agents for intraabdominal infections have been generally confined to patients with acutely perforated gastroduodenal ulcers and acute appendicitis.

Imipenem, a carbapenem derivative, has broad activity against facultative and obligate Gram-negative anaerobes and excellent Gram-positive activity (excepting methicillin-resistant staphylococci). This agent is formulated with cilastatin, a renal dehydropeptidase inhibitor that prevents renal tubal epithelial metabolism of the drug. In situations where plasma accumulation of the drug occurs (high dose levels or renal failure), the drug can cause seizures. With lower dose levels (500 mg every six hours) and appropriate adjustments for renal failure, seizures have not been a problem. Meropenem is now available, with an equivalent antimicrobial spectrum to imipenem/cilastatin without equivalent neurotoxicity. This agent has been used in doses up to 6 gm/day in treatment of severe infections.

As clinical experience has accumulated, quinolone antibiotics appear to be quite useful for intraabdominal infections. These agents act by inhibiting DNA replication and have shown similar if not improved activity to imipenem in clinical trials for pneumonia and intraabdominal infection. Available quinolones have little anti-B. fragilis activity and should be combined with metronidazole. Quinolones are attractive because serum levels following oral absorption parallel those seen with intravenous infusion. In patients with anatomically extensive infections, such as diffuse peritonitis, prolonged therapy with oral quinolones may be an attractive strategy.

The pharmacokinetics of antimicrobials is an important area, since prediction of treatment outcome correlates with whether or not very specific dosing parameters are met (peaks for aminoglycosides, AUC/MIC for others).

Dosing of cephalosporins, penicillin, carbapenem, and quinolone antibiotics should be optimized based on the known pharmacodynamics of these agents. Cell-wall-active agents are effective at the minimum inhibitory concentration (MIC) of the drug for the organisms being treated. Increasing the drug concentration substantially above about two to four times the MIC does not increase the rate of killing. Once the drug level falls below the MIC, the organisms begin regrowth immediately. Dosage regimens for cell-wall-active agents in critically ill patients should involve dosing intervals sufficiently short to maintain serum levels about the MIC. Therefore, the general rule with these agents should be to give relatively small doses frequently to maintain the trough levels above the MIC and avoid the costs and toxicities seen with high doses. This is best accomplished by administering these drugs every four half-lives, with adjustments as needed for renal compromise.

SURGICAL INTERVENTION

Intraoperative management of diffuse peritonitis involves immediate evacuation of all purulent collections, with particular attention to subphrenic, subhepatic, interloop, and pelvic collections. Radical peritoneal debridement, developed by Hudspeth in the 1970s, employs a xiphoid to pubis midline incision and the meticulous dissection of all fibrin from the peritoneal surface and from the serosal surface of the intestine [42]. Radical surgical debridement increases operative time and is associated with increased blood loss and fistula formation. Theoretically the idea of removing all bacteria-laden fibrinous debris from within the peritoneal cavity seems to be a logical choice, but the technical consequences do not appear to justify the method. A prospective randomized trial also did not show any benefit over conventional means of handling peritonitis [43].

Perforated bowel should be resected and an end colostomy with Hartman's pouch is recommended. A primary anastomosis in the setting of septic shock has been accompanied by a high complication and mortality rate, therefore should be avoided. In less severe cases, primary anastomosis has a high success rate and obviates the need for a second (major) procedure [44].

Peritoneal lavage is useful for removing debris and bacteria from the abdominal cavity. Antibiotics in the irrigation solution have not proven to be of benefit in patients who are receiving systemic antibiotics [45, 46]. There appears to be no benefit to postoperative peritoneal irrigation.

Abdominal wound closure in operations for peritonitis can be challenging. Patients with diffuse peritonitis, especially secondary to colonic perforation or anastomotic leakage, develop significant bowel and abdominal wall edema making closure difficult. If closure can be accomplished without tension, a single fascial layer of either interrupted or running monofilament suture may be used to close the abdominal wall. In the malnourished or immunocompromised patient, retention sutures may be required in addition to the fascial closure. We do not favor retention sutures secondary to ischemia generated from sutures being tied too tightly or abdominal wall edema development.

ABDOMINAL COMPARTMENT SYNDROME

If the abdomen is closed in the face of severe bowel and abdominal wall edema, there will then be a significant increase in intraabdominal pressure, this in turn may lead to multisystem organ dysfunction. Specifically, acute pulmonary failure secondary to compressive atelectesis, associated with high peak inspiratory pressures and impaired gas exchange, acute renal failure with marked oliguria without hypernaturia, intestinal and hepatic ischemia possibly leading to bacterial translocation or necrosis with peritonitis, increased intracranial pressures which may cause brain dysfunction or aggravate head injury edema, venous thrombosis and thromboembolism, and abdominal wall ischemia or necrosis. The diagnosis is made clinically in a patient with high peak inspiratory pressures, oliguria and an apparently tight abdomen. A bladder pressure is an indirect measurement of the abdominal pressure. Twenty centimeters of mercury is suggestive, but greater than 30 is definitive. However, chronically increased intraabdominal pressure as is seen in the morbidly obese, pregnancy and cirrhosis may be misleading.

Treatment includes leaving the fascia open and closing the skin with return to the operating room once the patient has stabilized and has mobilized enough fluid to close the fascia. Another option is to leave the skin open, attach IV bag or a Gore-Tex mesh of some type to the fascia, and place an impermeable dressing atop the entire wound. This will allow for continued sterility of the wound and decrease fluid loss from the abdomen. As the patient is mobilizing fluid, the IV bag or Gore-Tex may be cinched to help re-approximate the fascia, which can then be closed at a later date. Abdominal compartment syndrome is a deadly entity that must be recognized early and treated rapidly.

There are two surgical approaches to prevention of recurrent intra-abdominal infection: scheduled relaparotomy and open management. In general, the planned relaparotmy at 24 to 48 hours has been shown not to improve mortality nor decrease the incidence of late abscess formation [47]. It is not indicated for episodes of peritonitis in which peritoneal soiling is minimal or when inflammatory exudates are readily debrided at initial operation. Relaporotomy still may be useful in cases where significant quantities of necrotic material and foreign debris can not be adequately debrided (e.g., colonic perforation with massive fecal spillage and infected pancreatic necrosis). Current surgical therapy of infected lesser sac collections associated with pancreatic necrosis includes repetitive scheduled debridement at 48 hour intervals. Usually three or four such debridements are sufficient.

The difficulties arising from frequent exploration, with its forceful, repeated closure of the abdominal wall, have resulted in the development of the open abdomen approach, or laparostomy. Reported benefits include the conceptual advantage of treating the entire peritoneal cavity as ones large collection, with its exposure allowing for drainage. Other possible advantages include improved ventilation and renal perfusion [48, 49]. The open abdomen technique classically leaves the fascia opened with saline gauze packing. Complications of this technique include evisceration, massive fluid losses, spontaneous fistulas, and contamination of the open wound. It has also become apparent that an open abdomen does not obviate the need for repeat abdominal exploration.

The use of Marlex or Dexon mesh with or without an in sewn zipper provides ready access to the peritoneal cavity. In addition, the mesh prevents evisceration in the early postoperative period, allows for drainage of fluid and pus through its interstices, and may function as an exit site for a stoma or drain. The use of the zipper in this technique allows for entire abdominal exploration, fractionation of abdominal adhesions, removal of fibrous exudates, debris and fluid. Repeated laparotomies may be performed daily to ensure prompt treatment of new septic foci and early recognition of enteric fistulas. Once clinical evidence of sepsis subsides and the peritoneal cavity appears clean exploration are discontinued. Definitive repair can include skin graft or secondary intention healing over the mesh or removal of the mesh and definitive closure performed.

Some reports evaluating this technique have been quite favorable. Objective interpretation is difficult due to the heterogeneity of the patient populations with regard to severity of illness and underlying disease processes. Two studies used the APACHE II stratification system to define the severity of illness, thereby permitting comparison of outcome to an accepted standard [50, 51]. In one, the technique was applied to patients with diffuse, nonlocalizing peritonitis [51]. The mortality in patients receiving a mesh at the time of reoperation for postoperative peritonitis was one-third the rate predicted on the basis of APACHE II scores. Evaluation of the subgroups of APACHE II scores indicated that critically ill patients with scores higher than 25 had a mortality of 100 per cent, whereas those with low scores already had a low mortality that was independent of treatment. These data suggest that patients with midrange APACHE II scores are the ones who may derive the greatest benefit from this approach, a finding confirmed by Garcia-Sabrido *et al.* [50].

However, based on a compilation of 642 patients from 22 series, Schein *et al.* concluded that there was insufficient evidence to recommend that either open management or planned relaparotomy improves outcome in postoperative peritonitis [52]. Enteric fistulas are a significant complication associated with the open abdomen approach despite the use of mesh. Mastboom *et al.* demonstrated a fistula rate of 13 per cent in patients treated with such an approach with 14 patients developing 53 small bowel perforations attributable to the use of mesh [53]. Another study done by van Goor *et al.* concluded that planned relaparotomy seems to be associated with appreciable morbidity and does not reverse organ dysfunction [54]. The Peritonitis Study Group of the Surgical Infection Society-Europe determined that infectious complications due to suture leaks, recurrent intraabdominal sepsis and septicemia were more common in patients who had undergone planned relaparotomy compared to relaparotomy on demand [55].

Conclusion

Early diagnosis and treatment is paramount in decreasing the morbidity and mortality of peritonitis. This complex disease process can be effectively treated with microorganism directed antimicrobial therapy and excellent surgical debridement at the primary operation. Tertiary peritonitis is most likely a nosocomial infection secondary to multiple insults endured during the ICU stay resulting in a declining immune status. Planned relaparotomies are controversial, but may be very useful in specific patient populations.

References

1. Meltzer MS. Peritoneal mononuclear phagocytes from small animals. Methods for studying mononuclear phagocytes. Academic Press, New York, 1981.
2. Leak LV, Rahil K. Permeability of the diaphragmatic mesothelium: the ultrastructural basis for stomata. Am J Anat 151:557, 1978.
3. Dunn DL, Barke RA, Knight NB, Humphrey EW, Simmons RL. Role of resident macrophages, peripheral neutrophils, and translymphatic absorption in bacterial clearance from the peritoneal cavity. Infect Immun 49:257, 1985.
4. Hau T, Ahrenholz DH, Simmons RL. Secondary bacterial peritonitis: the biologic basis of treatment. Curr Probl Surg 16:1, 1979.
5. Morison R. Function of the omentum. Br Med J 1:76, 1906.
6. von Recklinghausen FT. Uber Eiter- und Bindeqewebskorperchen. Virchow's Arch 28:157, 1863.
7. Ranvier L. Du developmentet de l"accrossment des vaisseux sanguins. Arch De Physiol 1:429, 1874.
8. Ranvier L. Recherches sur la formation des mailes du grand epiploon. Arch De Physiol 1:421, 1874.
9. Seifert E. Zur Biologie des menschlichen groben. Netezes 116:510, 1921.
10. Shimotsuma M, Shields JW, Simpson-Morgan MW, Sakuyama A, Shirasu M, Hagiwara A, Takahashi T. Morpho-physiological function and role of omental milky spots as omentum-associated lymphoid tissue (OALT) in the peritoneal cavity. Lymphology 26:90, 1993.
11. Fowler R. Primary peritonitis: changing aspects 1956–1970. Aust Paediatr J 7:73, 1971.
12. McDougal WS, Izant RJ, Jr, Zollinger RM, Jr. Primary peritonitis in infancy and childhood. Ann Surg 181:310, 1975.
13. Speck WT, Dresdale SS, McMillan RW. Primary peritonitis and the nephrotic syndrome. Am J Surg 127:267, 1974.
14. Wilfert CM, Katz SL. Etiology of bacterial sepsis in nephrotic children 1963–1967. Pediatrics 42:840, 1968.
15. Hoefs JC, Runyon BA. Spontaneous bacterial peritonitis. Dis Mon 31:1, 1985.
16. Wyke RJ. Problems of bacterial infection in patients with liver disease. Gut 28:623, 1987.
17. Elsakr R, Johnson DA, Younes Z, Oldfield EC. Antimicrobial treatment of intra-abdominal infections. Dig Dis 16:47, 1998.
18. Grange JD, Roulot D, Pelletier G, Pariente EA, Denis J, Ink O, Blanc P, Richardet JP, Vinel JP, Delisle F, Fischer D, Flahault A, Amiot X. Norfloxacin primary prophylaxis of bacterial infections in cirrhotic patients with ascites: a double-blind randomized trial [see comments]. J Hepatol 29:430, 1998.
19. Singh N, Gayowski T, Yu VL, Wagener MM. Trimethoprim-sulfamethoxazole for the prevention of spontaneous bacterial peritonitis in cirrhosis: a randomized trial [see comments]. Ann Intern Med 122:595, 1995.
20. Brook I. A 12 year study of aerobic and anaerobic bacteria in intra-abdominal and postsurgical abdominal wound infections. Surg Gynecol Obstet 169:387, 1989.
21. Onderdonk AB, Bartlett JG, Louie T, Sullivan Seigler N, Gorbach SL. Microbial synergy in experimental intra-abdominal abscess. Infect Immun 13:22, 1976.
22. Simon GL, Klempner MS, Kasper DL, Gorbach SL. Alterations in opsonophagocytic killing by neutrophils of Bacteroides fragilis associated with animal and laboratory passage: effect of capsular polysaccharide. J Infect Dis 145:72, 1982.
23. Tzianabos AO, Kasper DL, Onderdonk AB. Structure and function of Bacteroides fragilis capsular polysaccharides: relationship to induction and prevention of abscesses. Clin Infect Dis 20 (Suppl 2):S132, 1995.
24. Schein M, Wittmann DH, Holzheimer R, Condon RE. Hypothesis: compartmentalization of cytokines in intraabdominal infection. Surgery 119:694, 1996.
25. Solomkin JS, Dellinger EP, Christou NV, Busuttil RW. Results of a multicenter trial comparing imipenem/cilastatin to tobramycin/clindamycin for intra-abdominal infections. Ann Surg 212:581, 1990.
26. Nathens AB, Rotstein OD, Marshall JC. Tertiary peritonitis: clinical features of a complex

nosocomial infection. World J Surg 22:158, 1998.
27. Bose SM, Kalra M, Sandhu NP. Open management of septic abdomen by Marlex mesh zipper. Aust N Z J Surg 61:385, 1991.
28. Junor BJ, McMillan MA. Immunosuppression in sclerosing peritonitis. Adv Perit Dial 9:187, 1993.
29. Melnicoff MJ, Horan PK, Morahan PS. Kinetics of changes in peritoneal cell populations following acute inflammation. Cell Immunol 118:178, 1989.
30. Chung YF, Eu KW, Nyam DC, Leong AF, Ho YH, Seow-Choen F. Minimizing recurrence after sigmoid volvulus [In Process Citation]. Br J Surg 86:231, 1999.
31. Ferrer TJ, Webb JW, Wallace BH, Bridges CD, Palmer HE, Robertson RD, Cone JB. Interleukin-10 reduces morbidity and mortality in murine multiple organ dysfunction syndrome (MODS). J Surg Res 77:157, 1998.
32. Sawyer RG, Rosenlof LK, Adams RB, May AK, Spengler MD, Pruett TL. Peritonitis into the 1990s: changing pathogens and changing strategies in the critically ill. Am Surg 58:82, 1992.
33. Watson CJ, Finlay-Jones JJ, McDonald PJ, Hart PH. IL-4 mRNA expression by peritoneal cells during episodes of peritonitis in patients on continuous ambulatory peritoneal dialysis. Clin Exp Immunol 100:253, 1995.
34. Cheadle WG. Current perspectives on antibiotic use in the treatment of surgical infections. Am J Surg 164:44S, 1992.
35. Chou CK, Chen LT, Sheu RS, Wang ML, Jaw TS, Liu GC. MRI manifestations of gastrointestinal wall thickening [see comments]. Abdom Imaging 19:389, 1994.
36. Hammoudeh M, Siam AR. Recurrent peritonitis with ascites as the predominant manifestation of systemic lupus erythematosus. Clin Rheumatol 14:352, 1995.
37. Montravers P, Gauzit R, Muller C, Marmuse JP, Fichelle A, Desmonts JM. Emergence of antibiotic-resistant bacteria in cases of peritonitis after intraabdominal surgery affects the efficacy of empirical antimicrobial therapy. Clin Infect Dis 23:486, 1996.
38. Mosdell DM, Morris DM, Voltura A, Pitcher DE, Twiest MW, Milne RL, Miscall BG, Fry DE. Antibiotic treatment for surgical peritonitis [see comments]. Ann Surg 214:543, 1991.
39. Yellin AE, Heseltine PN, Berne TV, Appleman MD, Gill MA, Riggio CE, Chenella FC. The role of Pseudomonas species in patients treated with ampicillin and Sulbactam for gangrenous and perforated appendicitis. Surg Gynecol Obstet 161:303, 1985.
40. Montravers P. Antibiotic therapy of secondary nosocomial peritonitis. Presse Med 28:948, 1999.
41. Calandra T, Cometta A. Antibiotic therapy for gram-negative bacteremia. Infect Dis Clin North Am 5:817, 1991.
42. Hudspeth AS. Radical surgical debridement in the treatment of advanced generalized bacterial peritonitis. Arch Surg 110:1233, 1975.
43. Polk HC Jr, Fry DE. Radical peritoneal debridement for established peritonitis. The results of a prospective randomized clinical trial. Ann Surg 192:350, 1980.
44. Belmonte C, Klas JV, Perez JJ, Wong WD, Rothenberger DA, Goldberg SM, Madoff RD. The Hartmann procedure. First choice or last resort in diverticular disease? Arch Surg 131:612, 1996.
45. Hau T, Nishikawa R, Phuangsab A. Irrigation of the peritoneal cavity and local antibiotics in the treatment of peritonitis. Surg Gynecol Obstet 156:25, 1983.
46. Moesgaard F, Nielsen ML, Hjortrup A, Kjersgaard P, Sorensen C, Larsen PN, Hoffmann S. Intraincisional antibiotic in addition to systemic antibiotic treatment fails to reduce wound infection rates in contaminated abdominal surgery. A controlled clinical trial. Dis Colon Rectum 32:36, 1989.
47. Farthmann EH, Schoffel U. Principles and limitations of operative management of intraabdominal infections. World J Surg 14:210, 1990.
48. Caldwell CB, Ricotta JJ. Evaluation of intra-abdominal pressure and renal hemodynamics. Curr Surg 43:495, 1986.
49. Richardson JD, Trinkle JK. Hemodynamic and respiratory alterations with increased intra-abdominal pressure. J Surg Res 20:401, 1976.
50. Garcia-Sabrido JL, Tallado JM, Christou NV, Polo JR, Valdecantos E. Treatment of severe intra-abdominal sepsis and/or necrotic foci by an "open-abdomen" approach. Zipper and zipper-mesh techniques. Arch Surg 123:152, 1988.
51. Walsh GL, Chiasson P, Hedderich G, Wexler MJ, Meakins JL. The open abdomen The Marlex mesh and zipper technique: a method of managing intraperitoneal infection. Surg Clin North Am 68:25, 1988.

52. Schein M, Hirshberg A, Hashmonai M. Current surgical management of severe intraabdominal infection. Surgery 112:489, 1992.
53. Mastboom WJ, Kuypers HH, Schoots FJ, Wobbes T. Small-bowel perforation complicating the open treatment of generalized peritonitis [see comments]. Arch Surg 124:689, 1989.
54. van Goor H, Hulsebos RG, Bleichrodt RP. Complications of planned relaparotomy in patients with severe general peritonitis. Eur J Surg 163:61, 1997.
55. Hau T, Ohmann C, Wolmershauser A, Wacha H, Yang Q. Planned relaparotomy vs relaparotomy on demand in the treatment of intra-abdominal infections. The Peritonitis Study Group of the Surgical Infection Society-Europe. Arch Surg 130:1193, 1995.

SECTION 8: INFECTIONS WITH SURGICAL IMPLICATIONS

J. Valles

50. SURGICAL SITE INFECTION CONTROL IN THE CRITICAL CARE ENVIRONMENT

Charles E. Edmiston, Jr

Introduction

Over the past 20 years there has been a significant change in the demographics of hospitalized patients, reflected in patients being admitted with more severe disease process resulting in a higher risk for infection. This is especially true for surgical patients, many of whom require admission to the ICU and are recipient of various lines, catheters and other intravascular devices. The number of surgical procedures performed annually in the United States approaches 30 million and based upon data derived from the CDC's National Nosocomial Infection Surveillance (NNIS) program, surgical site infections (SSIs) are the third most frequently reported nosocomial infection [1, 2]. Several studies suggest that surgical site infections are associated with both an increased length of stay (up to 7.3 days) and increased total hospital charges amounting to approximately $3000 dollars [3, 4]. In addition, the acquisition of SSI has been suggested to be associated with increased mortality when compared to closely matched hospitalized patients without SSI.

The NNIS program developed through cooperation with the Centers for Disease Control and Prevention is an operation specific index with a fairly high discriminatory power compared to previous risk stratified index systems. Currently, within most institutions in the United States the infection control team monitors those surgical procedures, which by virtue of historical experience, possesses the greatest risk for postoperative infection. At Froedtert Memorial Lutheran Hospital, the major teaching affiliate institution associated with the Medical College of Wisconsin, decisions as to which procedures are to be monitored are made by an interdisciplinary committee, the *Surgical Wound Taskforce*. The efforts of this group to reduce/prevent postoperative surgical site infections may, however, be impacted by external risk factors such as nosocomial resistance. In addition, ignorance or disregard for appropriate infection control practices is often equally to blame for failure to prevent nosocomial infections in both the medical and surgical ICU.

Strategies for preventing postoperative surgical site infections require attention to infection control practices and appropriate patient care management. Three factors have been identified as influencing the development of a postoperative surgical site infection: (a) the patient's intrinsic risk factor, (b) extrinsic factors associated with the operation itself, and finally (c) microbial virulence. The following discussion will focus upon these three factors and also emphasize the recent Guidelines for the Prevention of Surgical Site Infections that have been developed by the Hospital Infection Program of the Centers for Disease Control and Prevention.

Microbiology and Pathogenesis of Surgical Site Infections

Surgical site infections may be caused by endogenous or exogenous microbial contamination. Table 1 demonstrates the distribution of pathogens associated with surgical site infections in the United States. This data from the NNIS program encompasses two study intervals, 1986–1989 and 1990–1996 [5]. In addition to understanding the etiology and pathogenesis of the predominant pathogens associated with SSIs, it is also important to recognize that the emergence of antimicrobial resistance among both Gram-positive and Gram-negative microorganisms has a profound impact on the care of surgical patient in the ICU, limiting therapeutic options and emphasizing reinforcement of stringent infection control practices.

Gram-Positive Microorganisms

Staphylococcus aureus is the most common surgical site pathogen at 20%, followed by *Staphylococcus epidermidis* (14%) and *Enterococcus* species at 12%. Overall, Gram-positive pathogens are responsible for 53% of surgical site infections. *Staphylococcus aureus* has been recognized to be a significant nosocomial pathogens since the late 19th century. According to data derived from the NNIS program the incidence of methicillin-resistant *Staphylococcus aureus* (MRSA) has increased from less than 2.5% in the mid 1970s to almost 30% in the 1990s [6]. While early reports placed the greatest incidence of MRSA in tertiary medical centers, it is now obvious that this organism is ubiquitous within the healthcare environment, with even small hospitals (less than 200 beds) reporting rates approaching 20%. It is important to note that quite often these organisms will express resistance to antibiotics other than the beta-lactam group such as the fluoroquinolones. For example, it has been pointed out in one study that resistance to methicillin is often accompanied by resistance to both the 2nd and 3rd generation quinolone, such as ciprofloxacin and levofloxacin [7]. At present, vancomycin remains the drug of choice for the treatment of MRSA. However, a growing number of institutions are reporting intermediate level resistance to vancomycin, due to the presence of a thick exopolysaccharide capsular material surrounding the bacterial cell [8]. This nontraditional mechanism of resistance is rather problematic, especially since routine susceptibility testing often suggests that these organisms are fully sensitive to vancomycin.

TABLE 1. Predominant microbial pathogens associated with surgical site infections (NNIS 1986–1996)

	Percentage of Isolates	
Organism	1986–1989	1990–1996
Staphylococcus aureus	17	20
Coagulase negative staphylococci	12	14
Enterococcus spp	13	12
Escherichia coli	10	8
Pseudomonas aeruginosa	8	8
Enterobacter spp	8	7
Proteus mirabilis	4	3
Klebsiella pneumoniae	3	3
Streptococcus spp	3	3
Candida albicans	2	3
Miscellaneous Gram-positives	–	4
Bacteroides fragilis	–	2

It is important to note that the development of antimicrobial resistance among the staphylococci may involve a myriad of genetic mechanisms including transposon, plasmid or chromosomal mediated resistance. While, *Staphylococcus aureus* is recognized as the most virulent member of this genus, *Staphylococcus epidermidis* is presently the most common pathogen recovered from intravascular device infections [9]. In addition, 60% of the *Staphylococcus epidermidis* strains at our institution express resistance to the 1st generation cephalosporins. This has significant implications for the selection of a surgical prophylactic agent for high-risk patients undergoing clean surgical procedure and has prompted the substitution of a 2nd generation agent for patients undergoing surgery. The presence of MRSA in the surgical ICU and other units of the hospital has necessitated the adoption of strict isolation guidelines that while controversial, these policies have been successful in limiting or preventing nosocomial dissemination to other patients or units of the healthcare environment.

The enterococci have been traditionally viewed as a second class pathogen in surgery, often found as a component of normal flora and recovered in mixed infections. However, many enterococci express multidrug resistance and drug susceptibility is highly variable, dependent upon the microbial species. In most institutions, *Enterococcus faecalis* is still highly sensitive to ampicillin (>90%), while greater than 80% of *Enterococcus faecium* strains will express resistance to ampicillin. Prior to 1994, the vast majority of hospital microbiology laboratories in the United States did not speciate the enterococci, but rather reported their results to genus level. It is obvious that with the emergence of these multi-resistance strains greater efforts are needed to document the epidemiology of these organisms within the hospital environment. Susceptibility to other beta-lactam agents may also demonstrate significant variation. While in some surveys sensitivities to piperacillin may exceed 90%, high rates or resistance (>95%) are demonstrated against many of the 3rd generation cephalsporins [7]. In the last 10 years, the appearance of high level aminoglycoside resistance has reduced the therapeutic efficacy of the synergistic combination of penicillin and gentamicin for the treatment of enterococcal bacteremias. In the face of high level beta-lactam and aminoglycoside resistance, vancomycin has emerged as the therapy of choice for many enterococcal infections.

However, in 1989 reports suggested that selected strains of enterococci were developing resistance to the glycopeptides, in particular among strains of *Enterococcus faecium*. Over the past 10 years there have been numerous studies demonstrating nosocomial outbreaks associated with vancomycin-resistant enteroccal (VRE) strains expressing high level (Van A) vancomycin resistance [10, 11]. This high level type of resistance is carried on a single transposable element that is incorporated into a bacterial plasmid. A moderate and low level resistance to vancomycin has also been identified but the precise genetic mechanisms are presently unclear. In an effort to reduce the risk of vancomycin resistance among the enterococci and to prevent the spread of this resistance to the more virulent staphylococci, the CDC has developed criteria for the appropriate use of vancomycin through the Hospital Infection Control Practice Advisory Committee [12]. This important document encompasses four separate areas: (a) development of microbiologic criteria for the identification, susceptibility testing to detect vancomycin resistance and screening for VRE in hospitalized patients, (b) development of educational program that enhance health care worker understanding of the epidemiology and pathogenesis of VRE, (c) development of prevention and control strategies to reduce the incidence of VRE in the health care environment, and finally (d) criteria for the prudent use of vancomycin.

Gram-Negative Microorganisms

Data from the NNIS hospitals suggest that Gram-negative microorganisms continue to be a significant source of morbidity and mortality for surgical patients. *Pseudomonas aeruginosa* is currently responsible for approximately 9% of surgical site infections, while *Enterobacter, Escherichia coli* and *Klebsiella pneumoniae* occur as nosocomial SSIs pathogens approximately 8.8%, 7.1%, and 3.5% of the time, respectively. Anaerobic bacteria on the other hand such as the Gram-negative *Bacteroides fragilis* occur as a surgical site pathogens less than 3% of the time [5]. Members of the Enterobacteriaceae and *Pseudomonas aeruginosa* have all been associated with selected mechanisms of resistance, some of which have occurred quite rapidly over the past 10 years. Strains of *Klebsiella pneumoniae* that express resistance to the 3rd generation cephalosporins including ceftriaxone, cefotaxime or ceftazidime are increasing at a rate or 1–2% a year [7]. This resistance is due to an extended spectrum beta-lactamase (ESBLs) enzyme that is capable of hydrolyzing not only the 3rd generation cephalosporin antibiotics but also aztreonam. Unfortunately, under laboratory conditions these organisms will often appear to be sensitive to these agents, therefore rendering false-positive antibiogram data [13]. This type of resistance is occurring at a much faster pace among ICU patients than the general hospital population. It has been proposed that increased duration of stay in the ICU is associated with acquisition of this type of resistance in strains of *Klebsiella pneumonae* [7]. Quinolone resistance in *Pseudomonas aeruginosa* has increased more dramatically over the past 10 years with resistance rates ranging from 20% to 35%. However, it is important to note that it does not appear that the increase in quinolone resistance among strains of *Pseudomonas aeruginosa* is solely an ICU phenomenon, but rather occurs throughout the hospital. At present, in our institution we are seeing an 18% rate of resistance among *Pseudomonas aeruginosa* to the carbapenems which is due to an altered bacterial membrane porin, preventing the entry of the antimicrobial into the bacterial cell. It is obvious that the increase in resistance that is currently being seen in the SICU is related to several important variables. First the high-risk status of the patient population coupled with their severity of illness contributes to the overall problem of host susceptibility to nosocomial infection. Second, the failure to ascribe to basic infection control practices exacerbates the problem of acquisition and dissemination. Finally, a less than prudent pattern of antimicrobial use has intensified the pressure placed upon patients in the critical care environment.

Endogenous versus Exogenous Sources of Contamination

Historically most SSIs have been viewed as derived from the patient's own endogenous flora, whether from the skin, oropharyngeal or gastrointestinal tract. For instance, vascular, orthopaedic or plastic surgical procedures often involve the skin or skin structures and therefore tend to involve a Gram-positive flora if infection occurs, while general surgical procedures involving the gastrointestinal tract have a more Gram-negative focus [14, 15]. Alternatively, exogenous contamination may occur within the intraoperative environment as a result of contaminated instruments, breaks in aseptic technique or from members of the surgical team. Studies conducted in our institution have shown that potential nosocomial pathogens, both Gram-positive and Gram-negative are present in the air of the operating room environment [16]. As a result of these findings a special effort is undertaken to ensure that implantable biomedical devices are immediately covered upon removal from sterile packaging so as to reduce the potential for intra-operative contamination.

The infecting inoculum required to produce a postoperative surgical site infection has been determined to be in the order of magnitude of $5.0 \log_{10}$ colony forming units or greater per gram of tissue [17]. This value was from studies conducted in experimental animal models of infection. The inoculum size however, required to produce an infection is diminished when an inert foreign body is present in the wound. It has been suggested that 100 microorganisms or less per gram of tissue may be sufficient to produce an biomedical-associated infection [18]. Unfortunately, patients presenting for surgery in the year 2000 are often high-risk, exhibiting multi-organ disease states and demonstrating varying levels of anergy. Therefore, it is likely that patients with diminished phagocytic cell function and poor wound healing characteristics, such as in the diabetic patient are at higher risk for infection and that the microbial threshold dose for producing a postoperative infection is less well defined in this patient population.

Problematic Risk Factors Associated with Surgical Site Infections

Multivariant analysis has been used to analyze the association of two or more risk factors upon development of surgical site infection. Table 2 identifies several intrinsic (patient) and extrinsic (operation) factors that may influence the risk of developing a surgical site infection. While it is reasonable to assume that diminished nutritional status (severe-protein calorie malnutrition) may predispose one to development of a surgical site infection, it has been very difficult to assess the benefit of nutritional supplementation on decreasing the risk of SSI [19–21]. The diabetic patient offers another case in point. Previous scientific studies have demonstrated that diminished leucocytic cell function and poor wound healing occurs in patients with hyperglycemia [22, 23]. A recent study has demonstrated that glucose levels above 200 mg/dl increase the risk for surgical site infections [24]. There are however, no controlled studies which document the benefit of maintaining tight control of glucose as a preventative strategy for reducing surgical site infections in diabetic patients. It would stand to reason that preoperative use of immunosuppressive agents would appear to place surgical patients at risk for infection, since these compounds diminish the host's ability to respond to an infectious challenge. However, scientific studies validating this universal assumption are presently lacking. Another area of continued controversy is the role that *Staphylococcus aureus* nares colonization plays in the development of a postoperative surgical site infection. Studies have documented the impact or preoperative nares colonization of *S. aureus* on the subsequent development of surgical site infections [25]. Mupirocin, a topical antibiotic, has been shown to be effective for eliminating *S. aureus* from the anterior nares of both patients and health care professionals. The response to this phenomenon has been the implementation of decolonization protocol for selected patients. A study utilizing cardiothoracic patients has suggested that mupirocin when applied preoperatively to the nares resulted in reduced risk of SSIs [26]. However, a recent report from a Veterans Administration Hospital quite clearly demonstrated that the use of mupirocin to control endemic MRSA resulted in the recovery of MRSA *S. aureus* isolates exhibiting high level resistance to mupirocin [27]. In addition, recent reports have documented that mupirocin is only marginally effective in reducing MRSA nasal colonization and infections within an endemic environment. The precise role for this compound in the surgical patient population is yet to be determined. Clearly, *S. aureus* carriage appears to be a significant independent risk factor for sugical site infection following selected surgical procedures, however further studies are needed to assess the most effective and judicious use of mupirocin in surgical patients. While it may be difficult to assess the relative importance of these

TABLE 2. Intrinsic (patient) and extrinsic (operation) risk factors that may influence the development of a surgical site infection

Intrinsic Factors	Extrinsic Factors
Patient gender	Site of surgery
Patient age	Surgical scrub
Nutritional status	Surgical skin prep
Diabetes	Hair removal
Smoking	Duration of surgery
Severity of disease	Perioperative prophylaxis
Immunocompetence	OR ventilation
Weight	Drains & packs
Presence of other infections	Surgical attire & drapes
Microbial colonization	Surgical technique
Duration of preoperative stay	Poor hemostasis
	Dead space
	Tissue trauma

intrinsic factors in the development of a postoperative surgical site infections, it is prudent to view each of these characteristics such as obesity, smoking and even age, as factors that may potentially engender the risk of infection for our patients.

Several extrinsic factors have also been suggested as contributing to the risk of surgical site infections. The surgical site is an obvious factor since procedures involving the gastrointestinal tract will expose the wound to potential contamination involving a myriad of microbial population, while a breast biopsy will have a much lower risk for contamination. Skin asepsis and perioperative prophylaxis will be discussed in a separate section since both of these issues merit careful consideration when determining sentinel events that result in increased surgical site infection rates. Ongoing efforts to reduce the microbial burden in the operating room are viewed as a priority among health care professions. Current standards that direct a minimum of 15 air changes per hour in the operating room indicate the relative importance placed upon operating room ventilation as a potential risk factor for infection [28]. The standards that address room ventilation as well as policies and procedures for the disinfection and sterilization of surgical equipment and devices have reduced the iatrogenic sources of intraoperative contamination [29]. The importance of surgical attire as a risk factor for infection is a topic of some debate. The use of gowns, gloves and masks actually play a two-fold role in the operation room: (a) protects the health care worker from contamination by blood and body fluids, and (b) reduces the potential for microbial shedding, which may contaminate operative field or devices inserted at the time of surgery [5]. Unlike the intrinsic or patient risk factors, many of the extrinsic risk factors influence the intraoperative level of microbial contamination. Efforts to reduce the level of microbial contamination in the OR have been universally viewed as appropriate and beneficial to reducing the overall risk of postoperative infection. Finally, the cornerstone for good surgical care resides with exquisite surgical technique and when coupled with judicious infection control practices results in reduced wound morbidity and favorable patient outcomes.

Strategies for the Prevention of Surgical Site Infections

PREOPERATIVE SKIN PREPARATIONS

For over 100 years surgeons, infectious disease experts and other health professionals have recognized that infections may be transmitted to patients within the operating room environment. Because of the luxurious nature of the microbial flora colonizing the surface of the skin, great attention has been paid to the surgical site and several antiseptic agents are available for preoperative disinfection of the incisional site. In general, preoperative skin preps should provide a broad spectrum of activity against both Gram-positive and Gram-negative bacteria. This is also true for agents that are use as hand and forearm scrubs. Table 3 lists the three agents currently used as surgical site preparations. Alcohol, chlorhexidine and iodine/iodophors all demonstrate excellent activity against Gram-positive bacteria such as the staphylococci or enterococci. Alcohol demonstrates the best antiseptic activity against Gram-negative bacteria compared to chlorhexidine and iodine/iodophor. At our institution we require our patients to bath the night before surgery with an antiseptic agent, which in most cases involves using a chlorhexidine gluconate soap. This is done to reduce the microbial burden on the surface of the body. While, this may appear prudent, there are, however, no scientific studies validating this practice as efficacious in reducing the incidence of surgical site infections. Of all the various compounds that are used as antiseptics agents in the OR, chlorhexidine gluconate has the greatest residual activity and is not inactivated by blood or other body fluids [5]. Studies conducted in our laboratory using an FDA endorsed protocol demonstrate that a 3-minute surgical prep with chlorhexidine

TABLE 3. Antiseptic agents currently available for preoperative surgical skin prep (SSP) and surgical scrub (SS)

Agent	Spectrum of Activity[a]				Rapidity	Residual	Uses
	GP	GN	FN	VR			
Alcohol	E	E	G	G	Fast	None	SSP/SS
Chlorhexidine	E	G	F	G	Moderate	E	SSP/SS
Iodine/Iodophors	E	G	G	G	"	Minimal	SSP/SS
PCMX[b]	G	F	F	F	"	G	SS
Triclosan	G	G	F	U	"	E	SS

[a]GP, Gram-positive bacteria; GN, Gram-negative bacteria; FN, fungi; VR, virus; E, excellent; G, good; F, fair; P, poor; U, unknown.
[b]PCMX, para-chloro-meta-xylenol.

results in at least 8-hours of suppressed growth on the surface of unexposed skin (unpublished data). Concentration is an important variable and chlorhexidine is most effective as a surgical scrub when used at 4%. Likewise, aqueous alcohol at a concentration of 70%–90% is germicidal against bacteria, fungi and viruses [30]. However, a distinct problem associated with using alcohol solutions in the operating room is the issue of flammability. Alcohol fires are dramatic when they occur and can be catastrophic within the operating room [31]. Alcohol, chlorhexidine and iodine/iodophors have also been formulated into surgical hand scrub solutions, 0.5% chlorhexidine in 70% isopropanol has been found to have the greatest residual activity as a surgical hand scrub [23, 33].

ANTIMICROBIAL PROPHYLAXIS IN SURGERY

The perioperative use of antibiotic has become an essential standard of care for all operations or classes in which it has been shown to reduce the rate of SSI [34, 35]. The rules or principles governing the appropriate use of antimicrobial prophylaxis include the following [36]:

1. There is a probably risk of infection in the absence of a prophylactic agent.
2. There is a knowledge of the probable contaminating flora associated with operative wound or organ/space site.
3. The activity of the chosen prophylactic agent should encompass the majority of pathogens likely to contaminate the wound or organ/space site.
4. The prophylactic agent must be administered as a dose which provides an effective tissue concentration prior to intraoperative bacterial contamination, Administration must occur 30–60 minutes prior to incision (usually with the induction of anesthesia).
5. The effective dose must be governed by the weight of the patients. For example with the cephalosporins, patients weighing >70 kg, dosage should be doubled.
6. If the surgical procedure last ≤ 3-hours, a single prophylactic dose is usually sufficient. However, procedures lasting > 3-hours require an additional effective dose. Procedures in which there is rapid blood loss and/or fluid administration will dictate more frequent dosing. Postoperative prophylaxis is strongly discouraged, there is no evidence to suggest that multiple doses are more efficacious at preventing postoperative surgical site infections than a single effective dose.

The first generation cephalosporin, cefazolin or the 2nd generation agent cefuroxime are frequently used as prophylactic agents for many clean-contaminated operations. In general, antimicrobial prophylaxis is discouraged for elective clean surgical cases. However, patients with comorbid risk factors such as diabetes, obesity or who are receiving concommitant immunosuppressive therapy may receive a single prophylactic dose when undergoing an elective surgical procedure. Patients undergoing an elective operation involving the distal gastrointestinal tract will usually receive 1–2 doses of either cefoxitin or cefotetan (2nd generation agents) which provides broad-spectrum coverage for any anticipated contaminants. The use of antibiotic prophylaxis for the insertion of a biomedical device is in general an exception to the clean surgery rule. Biomedical device-associated infections are often seen as catastrophic and recalcitrant to traditional antibiotic therapy, therefore administration of 1–2 perioperative antimicrobial doses is viewed as prudent in light of the perceived risk. Patients unable to receive a cephalosporin because of previous hypersensitivity reactions can be given either clindamycin or vancomycin for Gram-positive coverage or aztreonam as an alternative for effective Gram-negative coverage. Finally, vancomycin should never be used as a routine agent for prophylaxis unless there is evident of MRSA clustering on the selected surgical service.

PERIOPERATIVE ADMINISTRATION OF BLOOD AND OXYGEN

It has been widely reported that the administration of blood perioperatively is associated with a two-fold increase in the surgical wound infection rate in patients undergoing elective colon resection for cancer [37]. However, a closer examination of the data suggests that the rationale for withholding whole blood or blood products are fundamentally flawed since multivariant analysis was not perfomed on a myriad of confounding variables that may have influenced the studies outcome. Therefore, it is generally viewed as safe and appropriate to administer whole blood or blood products to patients during the intraoperative period. A recent report from a multicentered trial has suggested that use of 80% supplemental oxygen results in a reduction in the surgical site infection rate in colorectal surgery [38]. Elevating the percentage of inspired oxygen was viewed as beneficial for tissue perfusion and neutrophil function. This is a provocative hypothesis, which deserves further consideration. Unfortunately, a major flaw of the study was the failure of the investigators to adopt a standardized perioperative antibiotic prophylaxis regimen. It is also important to note that the antibiotic prophylaxis that was used in the course of the investigation involved parenteral agents alone. It would have been interesting to see if the addition of an oral regimen, as used in the United States for colorectal procedures, would have altered the wound infection rate. In addition, the authors failed to provide an adequate criteria for defining a surgical site infection. Microbial recovery from cultured pus was the sole criteria for determining the presence or absence of an infection and no postdischarge surveillance was performed, which significantly limited the period of surveillance, if not the outcome. Therefore, until additional studies are performed which address the shortcomings of this recent publication, the use of supplemental oxygen to reduce surgical site infection in elective colon procedures is unwarranted, if not unfounded.

Classification of Surgical Site Infections

Surgical wounds are classified into four groups based upon selected criteria. developed by the National Academy of Science/National Research Council (NAS/NRC) [39]. **Class I** or "Clean" wounds represent an uninfected operative wound in which there is no inflammation and the hollow viscus sites such as the GI, urinary, respiratory or genital tract have not been breeched. Clean wounds are primarily closed with closed drainage. **Class II** or "Clean-Contaminated" wounds may involve controlled entry into the GI, urinary, respiratory or genital tract in a mannner where there is little or no contamination. Elective procedures involving the oropharynx, appendix or biliary tract are typical of Class II procedures providing no break in aseptic technique is encountered. **Class III** or "Contaminated" wounds involve procedures in which there has been a major break in sterile technique or there has been gross spillage of gastrointestinal contents. This classification includes, open, fresh, accidental wounds in which there may be evident of acute inflammation. Finally, **Class IV** or "Dirty-Infected" wounds involves perforated viscera, tissues in which there is an existing infection, or traumatized, devitalized tissues. In most cases, patients with Class IV wounds are already received antimicrobial therapy.

While, the NAS/NRC classification has been helpful in defining which patients would benefit from antimicrobial prophylaxis, it does not provide us with a standarized criteria for defining the site of infection. The Centers for Disease Control and Prevention has developed with the National Nosocomial Infection Surveillance program a standarized surveillance criteria for defining surgical site infections. Surgical site infections are now classified as either superficial incisional, deep incisional or organ space infection. Designation to one of three sites is defined as follows:

SUPERFICIAL INCISIONAL SURGICAL INFECTIONS

Any infection that occurs within 30 days post surgical procedure and involves only the skin or subcutaneous tissue of the incision. In addition, at least one of the following must occur:

1. Purulent drainage from the superficial incisional site with or without laboratory confirmation.
2. Microorganisms are recovered from culture of tissue or fluid from the incisional site.
3. The wound is deliberately opened by the surgeon because of one of the following signs or symptoms of infection: pain or tenderness, swelling, redness or heat.
4. Surgeon or attending physician renders a diagnosis of infection.

Simple stitch abscesses, episiotomy wounds, infection burn wounds or SSI that involve the fascia and muscle layers are not defined as superficial SSIs.

DEEP INCISIONAL SURGICAL SITE INFECTION

Any infection involving the deep soft tissues (fascia and muscle layers) that occurs within: (a) 30 days post surgical procedure provided no biomedical device has been inserted, or up to (b) one year if a biomedical device has been inserted and the infection appears related to that device. In addition, at least one of the following must occur:

1. Purulent drainage originating from the deep incision.
2. Wound spontaneous dehisces or is deliberately opened in response to fever, localized pain or tenderness.
3. There is an abscess of other clinical evidence of an infection of the deep incisional site.
4. A diagnosis of infection is made by the attending physician.

When the infection involves both the superficial and deep incision sites, the infection is reported as a deep incisional. Any organ/space surgical site infection that drains through the incision is reported as deep incisional.

ORGAN SPACE SURGICAL SITE INFECTION

Any infection involving any part of the anatomy (organ or cavity space) other than the incision that occurs within: (a) 30 days post surgical procedure provided no biomedical device has been inserted, or up to (b) one year if a biomedical device has been inserted and the infection appears related to that device. In addition, at least one of the following must occur:

1. Evidence of purulent drainage from a drain position through a stab wound into the organ/space.
2. Recovery of bacterial from organ/space culture.
3. Evidence of abscess of infection of organ/space.
4. A diagnosis of organ/space infection is made by attending physician.

TABLE 4. Classification of site-specific organ/spaces for surveillance of surgical site infections

Arterial/venous infection	Eye (orbit)	Meningitis
Breast abscess	GI tract	Myocarditis
Ear, mastoid	Intracranial	Oral cavity
Endocarditis	Osteomyelitis	Sinusitis
Endometritis	Joint/bursa	Spinal Abscess
Upper respiratory tract	Vaginal cuff	

Examples of the classification of site-specific organ/spaces are presented in Table 4.

Surveillance of Surgical Site Infections

Surveillance of surgical site infections is a sentinel component of an overall infection control strategy that involves collection, management, analysis and reporting of wound infection data in an effort to determine baseline nosocomial infection rates, which are reported to surgeons in an effort to reduce the surgical site infection risk. In the development of a surgical site surveillance program the overall goals must be clearly focused, addressing the priorities and objectives of the health care institution's infection control program. The National Nosocomial Infection Surveillance program has been an important resource for: (a) identifying the role of sentinel patient risk factors through stratification strategies, (b) establishing benchmark rates for specific surgical procedures, and (c) providing primary reference for precise definitions of selected surgical site infections.

Predictors of Surgical Site Infections

Three categories have been established which are recognized as accurate predictors of surgical site infections. First, the level of potential microbial contamination of the surgical site during the intraoperative period is an important variable when assessing the relative risk of a SSI. This was briefly discussed in an earlier section and essentially involves classifying the surgical procedures based upon the NAS/NRC definitions of clean, clean-contaminated, contaminated and dirty. The second predictor is the duration of the operative procedure and the final predictor is the physiologic status of the host as measured by the ASA (American Society of Anesthesiology) score [40].

These three predictors in essence provide a risk index that is operation specific. The index ranges from 0 to 3 and is derived through assigning points based upon the following:

1. One point is assigned when the ASA score is ≥3; the ASA score ranges from 1 to 5 with a score of defining a normally healthy patient, while a score of 5 is reflective of a patient who is not expected to survive for 24 hours.
2. One point is assigned whenever the operation is classified as either a "contaminated" or "dirty" based upon the NAS/NRC classification scheme.
3. One point is assigned if the surgical procedure lasts greater than a defined time interval, reflective of the 75th percentile durational period of the specific operation being performed.

Therefore, a patient with a risk index score of 0 would by definition have the lowest risk of infection for the specific surgical procedure. On the other hand, a score of 3 would place the patient within the highest risk category for that specific operation.

Surveillance Strategies

One of the weaknesses of the current surveillance program in US hospitals is that our data collection strategies are based upon reviewing in-patient surgical procedures. In our own institution, over 40% of surgical procedures are performed in the outpatient or ambulatory environment. This percentage is growing daily and presently in many communities there are free-standing facilities both pubic and private that exclusively perform out-patient surgeries. This has created a dilemma in the infection control communities; how do we best target our surveillance efforts in the current health care environment? In addition, most of the operations upon which the NNIS benchmark data is based involve data derived from traditional surgical (open) procedures. Rapid advances in the field of laprascopic surgery within all of the surgical professions are not reflected whithin the NNIS data pool. Therefore, few if any benchmark rates are currently available for minimally invasive surgical procedures. This deficiency is currently under study however, it will be several years before our surveillance teams have stratification rates reflective of these new minimally invasive technologies.

INPATIENT SURVEILLANCE

Few, if any health care facilities have the luxury of time, personnel and monetary resources to indulge in global surgical site surveillance. Many institutions practice a "targeted" type of surveillance of selected surgical procedures which may in part be based upon: (a) knowledge of surgical procedures performed upon high-risk patient population, (b) concerns associated with selected surgical techniques (biomedical implantation), (c) recognition of increased incidence of infection in selected patient or procedure specific populations [41]. Table 5 reports the surgical procedures currently selected for surveillance with our institution. Selected surgical procedures are added or deleted from surveillance based upon volume, intrinsic risk of patient population, and prior history of surgical site infections. While "targeted" surveillance may address the historical or current infection trends, care must be taken so that no clusters or outbreaks are overlooked within those non-selected surgical procedures. It is also prudent to design your surveillance strategies so that a broad band of surgical disciplines are included in the census. Finally, flexibility is an inherent characteristic of a successful program since resources may have to be rapidly shifted in response to a dynamic change in surgical site infection rates, albeit service or procedure selected.

TABLE 5. Surgical procedures selected for surveillance at Froedtert Memorial Lutheran Hospital, 1999 and 2000

Procedures	Operation Cutpoint (hrs)	1999	2000
Abdominal hysterectomy	2	yes	yes
Hernia repair with mesh	2	no	yes
Gastric bypass	4	no	yes
Coronary bypass (chest)	5	yes	yes
Coronary bypass/valves	5	yes	no
Valve replacement	5	yes	no
Cesarean section	1	yes	yes
Colon surgery	3	yes	yes
Craniotomy/ Craniectomy	4	yes	yes
Vascular surgery	3	yes	yes
Fusion-cervical with implant	4	yes	no
Fusion-lumbar with implant	4	yes	yes
Fusion-thoracic with implant	4	yes	no
Hip replacement	2	yes	yes
Knee replacement	2	yes	no
Kidney/pancreas transplant	7	yes	yes
Liver transplant	7	yes	yes

The preferred method as documented in the surgical literature for identifying a surgical site infection is direct observation of the surgical site by a trained practitioner. Infection control personnel (ICP) should be regular visitors to the clinical wards or units since visibility is essential for promoting trust and collegiality. It is also possible at this time for the ICP to interact with the attending physician and nursing staff or answer questions relative to specific policy or procedures. Also a visible presence in the patient care areas allows the infection control staff to observe sentinel infection control practice such as hand washing or adherence to isolation policies. Often the ICP is viewed as the harbinger of bad news rather than a colleague who is available as a clinical resource. Surgical site infections represent an adverse outcome that may upon reflection have been prevented. Direct observation is also beneficial since it allows the ICP to observe whether appropriate wound care pratices are being used.

While direct observation represents the "best" of infection control practices, much of the data reported within the infection control literature is actually derived from indirect case-finding studies. Indirect measurement are represented by chart reviews, daily review of laboratory reports, pharmacy reports and "curbside" discussions with health care professions. Essentially any clinical resource is available for indirect audit however, many of these strategies are stagenant in time since infections detected retrospectively after the patient has been discharged often leave a "cold trail" especially if the infection falls outside of a traditional cluster. Sorting out all of the potential intrinsic and extrinsic variables that may contribute to a surgical site infection after the patient has been discharged often leads to more questions that answers, if not inconclusive findings. Regardless of the surveillance strategy, institutions that utilize NNIS benchmarks tend to collect similar data such as, date of operation, NNIS operative procedure category, surgeon and patient indentifier, usual patent demographics, duration of operation, wound class, ASA score, discharge date, etc.

POSTDISCHARGE AND OUTPATIENT SURVEILLANCE

Several studies have suggested that between 12% and 84% of SSIs can be detected after the patient has been discharged from the hospital [42, 43]. This creates a problem for most hospital-based infection control programs, especially if post discharge follow-up occurs at a site remote to where the original operation was performed. It would not be heretical to suggest that even the most diligent of infection control programs likely fails to capture anywhere from 25% to 40% of their surgical site infections, the majority of which are probably superficial incisional site infecitons. It is interesting to note that institutions which emphasize the use of clinical pathways to manage the routine "clinical continuum" are experiencing shorter hospital stays for selected procedures than hospitals relying upon traditional order and patient care directives. It is ironic that in an effort to improve the efficiency and quality of patient care, we are omitting significant outcome data for surgical patients. Several strategies have been proposed for capturing postdischarge data that include remote review of clinic charts, and physician and/or patient surveys utilizing the mail or direct telephone contact. It is unsettling to contemplate that the credibility of an institution's surgical site surveillance program could possibly rest squarely upon the shoulders of a patient population that is requied to assess their own wounds for infection [44].

A recent study has proposed that "electronic surveillance" of pharmacy records within an integrated health infromation system may offer the best possibilities for tracking surgical site infections after the patient has left the hospital [45]. At present, even under the best of scenarios, surveillance strategies that rely upon questionaires or telephone surveys are probably failing to capture anywhere from 15% to 60% of infections post discharge [46, 47]. It is evident that leadership is needed in this arena since at this time the CDC and other professional bodies can offer no clear guidance regarding which detection method should be used for postdischarge or outpatient surveillance. It is possible that future efforts may focus on selecting a few "targeted" surgical procedures which are then intensely monitored with the result of this surveillance used to interpolate (indicator) the overall quality of the combined surgical services within the institution. While this approach may have several potential minefields, it may come to pass that selecting a few key surgical procedures with sufficient statistical power coupled to electronic surveillance may in fact, be a plausible way to assess surgical site infection rates in the postdischarge and outpatient environments.

Some Final Thoughts on Wound Management and Infection Control

The basic principles of effective surgical wound management are also grounded in appropriate infection control practices. The presence of necrotic debris in the wound is recognized to facilitate the growth of microorganisms [48]. Abscesses should be drained and any sinus tract excised. The principle that wounds that are kept moist, heal better than wound left open has been a source of constant debate. When caring for the wound the clinical practitioner must avoid at all cost any contamination between themselves, other patients or multiple wound on the same patient. All disposable or contaminated material must be placed in an appropriate labeled (biohazard) container [49].

Infection control practices vary widely between institutions. The use of sterile gloves and aseptic technique is well documented for the prevention of wound sepsis during the peioperative period. The Centers for Disease Control and Prevention has suggested that sterile gloves be used for the first 24 hours of incisional care. However, no specific glove recommendations are offered for the management of postoperative wounds beyond this period. A recent survey found that nurses in acute care facilities were more likely to wear sterile gloves when managing postoperative surgical wounds beyond the 24-hour postoperative window [50]. The use of chemically clean versus sterile gloves for managing wounds has emerged as a major discussion point primarily because of the issue of cost. The use of chemically clean but nonsterile gloves has been shown within our institution to be a major cost savings over sterile, individually wrapped surgical gloves. The impact of this strategy on infection control practices within an institution is debatable and subject to individual interpreation. Whether or not sterile or chemically clean gloves are used when caring for an open wound is likely dependent upon the type of wound or clinical setting. Sterile technique is indicated when managing wounds in immunosuppressed patients or open surgical wounds involving exposed organ/space sites.

There are at present several emerging technologies which may impact upon infection control practices by reducing the potential for wound colonization/contamination in acute wounds. This includes the use of dressings that attempt to manipulate the biology of the wound and thereby accelerate normal wound which will have measureable infection control benefits. Another strategy has been the incorporation of antimicrobial or antiseptic substances into the matrix of the wound dressing. The incorporation of selected metals with antiseptic activity such as silver has potential intrinsic value in reducing wound contamination postoperative wounds such as sternal incisions. The use of such dressings may have an initial benefit in selected high-risk surgical patient populations including the morbidly obese and poorly controlled diabetic. Finally, the ideal strategy would involve application of an active dressing that exhibits antiseptic properties while stimulating the activation of various cell types such as neutrophils or macrophages within the wound itself. The morbidity and mortality associated with surgical site infections has an impact not only on patient care but also on those infection control practices that attempt to limit or reduce the acquisition/dissemination of nosocomial pathogens within the hospital environment.

References

1. Centers for Disease Control and Prevention, National Center for Health Statistics. Vital and Health Statistics, Detailed Diagnoses and Procedures, National Hospital Discharge Survey, 1994. Vol 127, Hyattsville, Maryland: DHHS Publication; 1997.
2. Emori TG, Gaynes RP. An overview of nosocomial infections, including the role of the microbiology laboratory. Clin Microbiol Rev 6:428, 1993.

3. Cruse PJ, Foord R. The epidemiology of wound infection: a 10-year prospective study of 62,939 wounds. Surg Clin North Am 60:27, 1980.
4. Boyce JM, Potter-Bynoe G, Dziobek L. Hospital reimbursement patterns among patients with surgical wound infections following open heart surgery. Infec Control Hosp Epidemiol 11:89, 1990.
5. Hospital Infection Program, National Center for Infectious Diseases, Center for Disease Control and Prevention. Guidelines for Prevention of Surgical Site Infection. Infect Control Hosp Epidemiol 20:247, 1999.
6. Gaynes RP. Surveillance of nosocomial infections: a fundamental ingredient for quality. Infect Control Hosp Epidemiol 18:475, 1997.
7. Fridkins SK, Gaynes RP. Antimicrobial resistance in intensive care units. Clin Chest Med 20:303, 1999.
8. Turco TF, Meldo GP, Williams R. Vancomycin intermediate-resistant *Staphylococcus aureus*. Ann Pharmacother 32:758, 1998.
9. Schaberg DR. Resistant Gram-positive organisms. Ann Emerg Med 24:462, 1994.
10. Centers for Disese Control and Prevention. Nosocomial enterococci resistant to vancomycin-United States, 1989–1993. MMWR 42:597, 1993.
11. Gin AS, Zhanel GG. Vancomycin-resistant enterococci. Ann Pharmacother 30:615, 1996.
12. Hospital Infection Program, Hospital Infection Control Advisory Committee. Recommendations for preventing the spread of vancomycin-resistance. Infect Control Hosp Epidemioal 16:105, 1995.
13. Tenover FC, McGowan JE. Reasons for the emergence of antibiotic resistance. Am J Med Sci 311:9, 1996.
14. Altemeier WA, Culbertson WR, Hummel RP. Surgical consideration of endogenous infections-sources, types, and methods of control. Surg Clin North Am 48:227, 1968.
15. Wiley AM, Ha'eri GB. Routes of infection: a study of using "tracer particles" in the operating room. Clin Orthop 139:150, 1979.
16. Edmiston CE, Sinski S, Seabrook G, Simons D, Goheen M. Airborne particulates in the OR environment, AORNJ 69:1169, 1999.
17. Krizek TJ, Robson MC. Evolution of quantitative bacteriology in wound management. Am J Surg 130:579, 1975.
18. James RC, MacLeod CJ. Induction of staphylococcal infections in mice with small inocula introduced on sutures. Br J Exp Pathol 42:266, 1961.
19. Mullens JL, Gertner MH, Buzby GP, Goodhart GL, Rosato EF. Implications of malnutrition in the surgical patient. Arch Surg 114:121, 1979.
20. Campos AC, Mequid MM. A critical appraisal of the usefulness of perioperative nutrition support. Am J Clin Nutr 55:117, 1992.
21. Winsor JA, Hill GL. Protein depletion and surgical risk. Aust NZJ Surg 58:711, 1988.
22. Lilienfeld DE, Vlahov D, Tenney JH, McLaughlin JS. Obesity and diabetes as risk factors for postoperative wound infections after cardiac surgery. Am J Infect Control 16:3, 1988.
23. Terranova A. The effect of diabetes mellitus on wound healing. Plast Surg Nurs 11:20, 1991.
24. Zerr KJ, Furnay AP, Grunkemeier GL, Bookin S, Kanhere V, Starr A. Glucose control lowers the risk of wound infection in diabetics after open heart operations. Ann Thorac Surg 63:356, 1997.
25. Kluytmans JA, Mouton JW, Ijzerman EP, Vandenbroucke-Grauls CM, Maat AW, Wagenvoot JH, *et al*. Nasal carriage of *Staphylococcus aureus* as a major risk factor for wound infections after cardiac surgery. J Infect Dis 171:216, 1995.
26. Kluytmans JA, Mouton JW, VandeBergh MF, Manders MJ, Maat AP. Reduction of surgical site infections in cardiothoracic surgery by elimination of nasal carriage of *Staphylococcus aureus*. Infect Control Hosp Epidemiol 17:780, 1996.
27. Vasquez JE, Walker ES, Franzus BW, Overbay BK, Reagan DR, Sarubbi FA. The epidemiology of mupirocin resistance among methicillin-resistant *Staphylococcus aureus* at a Veterns' Affairs Hospital. Infect Control Hosp Epoidemiol 21:459, 2000.
28. American Institute of Architects. Guidelines for design and construction of hospitals and health care facilities. Washington (DC): American Institute of Architects Press: 1999.
29. Centers for Disease Control and Prevention. Postsurgical infections associated with nonsterile implantatble devices. MMWR 41:263, 1992.
30. Larson E. Guidelines for use of topical antimicrobial agents. Am J Infect Control 16:253, 1988.
31. Hardin WD, Nichol RL. Handwashing and patient skin preparation. In Malangoni MA, (ed). Critical Issues in Operating Room Management. Philadelphia: Lippincott-Ravens, 1997:133.
32. Larson EL. APIC guidelines for handwashing and hand antisepsis in health care settings. Am J Infect Control 23:251, 1995.

33. Wade JJ, Casewell MW. The evaluation of residual antimicrobial activity on hands and its clinical relevance. J Hosp Infect 18 (Suppl B):23, 1991.
34. Wittman DH, Condon RE. Prophylaxis of post-operative infections. *Infection* 19:S337, 1991.
35. Nichols, RL. Postoperative wound infections. *N Engl J Med* 307:1701, 1982.
36. FMLH Suggested Recommendations and Guidelines for Surgical Prophylaxis, Froedtert, Memorial Lutheran Hospital Antibiotic Utilization Guideline. 2000.
37. Vamvakas EC, Carven JH, Hibberd PL. Blood transfusion and infection after colorectal surgery. Transfusion 36:1000, 1996.
38. Grief R, Akca O, Horn EP, Kurz A, Sessler DL. Supplemental perioperative oxygen to reduce the incidence of surgical-wound infections. Outcomes Research Group. N Eng J Surg 342:161, 2000.
39. B'erard F, Gandon J. Postoperative wound infections: the influence of ultraviolet irradiation of the operating room and various other factors. Ann Surg 160 (Suppl 1):1, 1964.
40. SHEA, APIC, CDC < SIS. Consensus paper on the surveillance of surgical wound infections. Infect Control Hosp Epidemiol 13:599, 1992.
41. Pottinger JM, Herwaldt LA, Perl TM. Basics of surveillance-an overview. Infect Control Hosp Epidemiol 18:513, 1997.
42. Law DJ, Mishriki SF, Jeffery PJ. The importance of surveillance after discharge from the hospital in the diagnosis of postoperative wound infection. Ann R Coll Surg Eng 72:207, 1990.
43. Weigelt JA, Dryer D, Haley RW. The necessity and efficiency of wound surveillance after discharge. Arch Surg 127:77, 1992.
44. Seaman M, Lammers R. Inability of patients to self-diagnose wound infections. J Emerg Med 9:215, 1991.
45. Sands K, Vineyard G, Platt R. Surgical site infections occurring after hospital discharge. J Infect Dis 173:963, 1996.
46. Fanning C, Johnston BL, MacDonald S, LeFort-Jost S, Dockerty E. Postdischarge surgical site surveillance. Can J Infect Control 10: 75.
47. Zoutman D, Pearce P, McKenzie M, Taylor G. Surgical wound infections occurring in day surgery patients. Am J Infect Control 18:277, 1990.
48. Robson MC. A failure of wound healing caused by an imbalance of bacteria. Surg Clin N Am 77:637, 1997.
49. Witte MB, Barbul A. Gerneral principles of wound healing. Surg Clin N Am 77:509, 1997.
50. Wise LC, Hoffman J, Grant L, Bostrum J. J Wound Ost Cont Nurs 24:144, 1997.

51. SEVERE SOFT TISSUE INFECTIONS: A SYNDROME-BASED APPROACH

Antonio Sitges-Serra

Introduction

Severe soft tissue infections (SSTI) rank among the most common and potentially dangerous infections that can be acquired either in the community setting or in hospital. Community-acquired SSTI may occur in previously healthy people but most often are diagnosed in immunocompromised patients, in patients with advanced cancer, with diabetes, receiving steroids or with AIDS. Diabetic patients are particularly susceptible to SSTI acquired at home probably as a result of tissue ischemia secondary to micro or macroangiopathy. Healthy individuals may develop SSTI either spontaneously, after trauma or after insect or animal bites. SSTI developing in hospitalized patients often represent a post-operative complication, particularly of emergency operations, in patients with severe trauma, intrabdominal infections or vascular disease. Patients undergoing solid organ transplantation may also develop insidious and severe infections of the soft tissues as, for example, mucormycosis. Finally, bed-ridden patients may develop SSTI complicating decubitus ulcers.

Depth of Infection and Time Evolution

There are several well-characterized clinical syndromes revealing the presence of a SSTI. These should be familiar to all practitioners dealing with ill patients since appropriate recognition and early treatment may be live saving or, at least, may prevent the development of severe systemic complications. For this reason, SSTI will be presented in this chapter as separate clinical syndromes characterized by four fundamental parameters: the presence of systemic symptoms, the macroscopic appearance, the depth of microbial invasion (as assessed from physical examination and/or surgical exploration) and the time from onset to overt disease. These are the most useful clinical guides available to the clinician to help him in making a good differential diagnosis and to appropriately treat SSTI. In particular, clinicians should be able to recognize the layer or layers of soft tissue involved: the skin, the fatty subcutaneous tissue, the muscular fascia and the muscle itself. In addition, an appropriate assessment of the tempo (a musical term used to designate the speed and brio that should be employed to interpret a score) of the infection is also of paramount importance. Many SSTI progress quite rapidly and may cause serious systemic complications if therapy is not instituted early enough.

When Should a Severe Soft Tissue Infection be Suspected?

Mild dermal and subdermal infections are rather common in primary care and are usually the result of minor trauma (superficial wound infections, puerperal mastitis, paronychia) or may develop into abnormal anatomical structures (pilonidal sinus, omphalitis, perianal abscess). These are well-circumscribed suppurative lesions that respond to standard therapy with oral antibiotics and/or surgical drainage. These minor common infections are to be distinguished from the most severe forms that may either complicate an apparently innocent superficial infection in an immunocompromised host or start *de novo* with an aggressive clinical picture. When examining a patient with a soft tissue infection, there are several hints that should lead the clinician to suspect that he or she is dealing with a SSTI rather than a mild one. These can be summarized as follows:

1. **Systemic symptoms.** High fever, tachycardia and prostration are often found in patients with SSTI such as streptococcal gangrene, necrotizing fasciitis or gas gangrene. In addition, these patients may progress rapidly to septic/toxic shock and die within a few hours no matter the treatment they receive.

2. **Skin lesions: necrosis or bullas.** The presence of skin lesions, particularly of bullas or necrosis, is typical of some syndromes of SSTI such as necrotizing cellulitis or severe *Str. pyogenes* infections. Necrotic tissues are often gray to black colored, do not bleed and are not painful when incised with a scalpel. Bullas are also found in some SSTI and in these cases the skin lesion usually reveals a more deep involvement.

3. **Crepitation.** Crepitus is a typical sign of SSTI due to gas-producing microorganisms. Once mechanical causes of crepitation are ruled out (lung lesion, magnesium salts, accidental subdermal air injection) infection is the most probable cause of this ominous sign. Crepitation is not a pathognomonic sign of *Clostridium* spp. infections since it can also be observed in infections due to gas-forming enterobacteriaceae such as *E. coli* (i.e. crepitant cellulitis). A mixed flora producing necrotizing fasciitis causes subcutaneous crepitation in roughly 25% of cases.

4. **Progressing disease.** Skin lesions that do not heal after an "appropriate" initial treatment characterize some SSTI. A non-healing perineal incision after debridement of a seemingly banal perianal abscess may signal the presence of a necrotizing fasciitis due to a mixed enteric flora, particularly in a diabetic or immunocompromised patients. In other circumstances, as happens in cases of Meleney's synergistic gangrene, necrosis progresses and the lesion tends to expand centrifugally despite a seemingly appropriate antibiotic therapy.

5. **Absence of pus.** From the Hippocratic empiric days to the days of Ambroise Paré in the XVI century, suppuration of a wound was considered an essential phase of the normal healing process and regarded as a good prognostic sign (*pus bonum et laudabile*). Time has proved that surgeons of the classical period were essentially right since most SSTI are not associated with the production of pus. Instead, they are characterized by the presence of a gray or brown fluid discharge that in the case of *Clostridium* spp. infections or mixed infections with anaerobic Gram-negative bacilli is typically foul smelling.

Physical Exploration

Adequate assessment of the extension and depth of a SSTI cannot be achieved if the lesions are not thoroughly explored. If there is no a preexistent surgical wound and surgical drainage is not indicated, soft tissue infections are explored superficially. Tenderness, edema and dermal necrosis should be looked for. If present, crepitation is a revealing sign of the severity of a soft tissue infection. If SSTI arise in a preexistent surgical wound or, if surgical drainage is indicated, thorough exploration is mandatory. Inspecting a wound should be carried out with sterile gloves. Stitches, if present, must be removed. The wound margins should be opened wide and the color and consistency of the fatty tissue noted. Necrotizing cellulitis is characterized by a grayish to black discoloration of the subcutaneous fat. The index finger should be used to look for separation of the subcutaneous fat from the muscular fascia, an ominous sign typical of necrotizing fasciitis. Gentle lateral pressure with the fingertip is exerted deep in the wound. If the tissues do not offer resistance, the gloved finger dissects easily the plane existing between the subcutaneous fat and the muscle. Muscle state should be assessed by opening the fascia. There may be massive muscular edema with a compartmental syndrome and then the muscle herniates through the fascial incision. This happens preferentially in whole-thickness Group A streptococcal infections (often called streptococcal "gangrene"). In cases of muscle necrosis (clostridial myonecrosis), the muscle appears gray instead of pink red and does not bleed when cut.

In all circumstances, physical exploration of a SSTI should reach the limits of the lesion until healthy tissues are found. This is an essential part of the surgical treatment of SSTI. Failure to identify the limits of the infection means also failure to actually debride and excise all the infected or necrotic tissue, a common cause of treatment failure.

Microbiology and Pathogenesis

Many microorganisms may cause SSTI. The Gram-positive cocci *S. aureus* and *Str. pyogenes* rank among the most commonly involved bacteria. *S. aureus* is usually implicated in less severe forms of tissue infections above the diaphragm such as puerperal mastitis, anthrax or paronychia. In some immunocompromised hosts, however, it may give rise to pyomyositis or extensive soft tissue infections as a result of surgical wound or catheter site infections ("tunnelitis"). *Str. pyogenes* is responsible for relatively minor superficial infections (impetigo, erysipela) but is also responsible for whole-thickness extremely SSTI in previously healthy individuals, in surgical wounds and in neutropenic patients. Other Gram-positive cocci involved, mostly in infections developing after animal or human bites, are the anaerobic streptococci (Peptostreptococci) and *Str. viridans*. The particularly virulent association of anaerobic or microaerophilic streptococci with *S. aureus* was originally reported by Meleney [1] as the cause of one of the most representative SSTI: progressive synergistic gangrene.

A mixed flora involving enteric bacteria (*B. fragilis*, enterobacteriaceae, *E. faecalis*) is often found in necrotizing infections arising in the perineal area due to anal or urogenital disease. Other Gram-negative non-fermenting bacilli may be recovered from SSTI. Dog bites may be occasionally complicated by *Capnocytophaga canimorsus* infection. *P. aeruginosa* may be recovered from mixed necrotizing infections.

Anaerobic Gram-positive bacilli of the genus *Clostridium* (*C. perfringens, C. septicum, C. novyi*) are involved in severe suppurative infections or as part of a mixed enteric flora causing necrotizing fascitis and in gas gangrene, a fulminant, predominantly muscular, highly lethal necrotizing infection.

Finally, fungus of the order *Mucorales* are involved in whole thickness infections in severely immunocompromised hosts, usually receptors of solid organ transplantation. The pathogenesis of SSTI is multifactorial The three most important determinant factors influencing the clinical manifestations and the time evolution are now described.

INTRINSIC VIRULENCE OF THE MICROORGANISM – TOXIC SHOCK

Some of the bacteria involved in SSTI are extremely virulent due to their having exotoxins that can trigger both a systemic inflammatory reaction and a local devastating disease due to extensive and rapidly spreading necrosis and superimposed ischemia due to vascular compression or thrombosis. Apparently superficial or even occult skin infections (up to 20% of cases) due to *Str. pyogenes* or *S. aureus* may lead to a severe systemic response characterized as the toxic shock syndrome. Patients are profoundly ill and may develop sudden shock and rash associated with multiorgan failure, particularly acute renal failure. Other clinical findings include high temperature, diffuse macular erythroderma and desquamation.

Some group A *Str. pyogenes* secrete potent pyrogenic exotoxins (spe) that play a major role in the pathogenesis of toxic shock. The production of these exotoxins is enhanced by the M protein, also an inhibitor of phagocytosis. The spe exotoxins exert their effects in two ways: they stimulate mononuclear cells and they interact with T lymphocytes as "superantigens", namely, antigens that do not require preprocessing by monocytes and bind directly to the major histocompatibility complex class II molecules on the surface of T-cells. This occurs in a much higher proportion of T-cells (5–20%) than would happen in a regular pre-processed antigen presentation. Clonal proliferation of this large T-cell subset results in the massive release of lymphokines. As a consequence of mononuclear and T-cell activation, production of TNF-a and b, IL-1, IL-2 and IL-6 is triggered resulting in multiple organ dysfunction and shock [2, 3].

TISSULAR OR ENVIRONMENTAL FACTORS

Good tissue perfusion is an essential component of the local mechanisms preventing bacterial proliferation and invasion by providing the necessary elements to support the local antibacterial response: leukocytes, macrophages, complement, nutrients and oxygen. Tissue ischemia is a determinant factor for invasive *Clostridium* spp. infections and infections complicating ischemic limbs, particularly in the diabetic patient. Gas gangrene almost always develops on necrotic and devitalized tissues resulting from severe trauma, vascular disease, inappropriate surgery or unresected gangrenous bowel. More rarely, clostridial myonecrosis may develop spontaneously due to *C. septicum* bacteremia arising from an unsuspected colonic cancer [4] or minor injuries such as intramuscular injections. Once *Clostridium* spp. proliferate in the ischemic tissues, they release many potent exotoxins such as lecithinase, which destroys cell membranes and caues hemolysis and diffuse tissue damage, or θ-toxin which seems to be the main responsible for muscle tissue necrosis.

Foreign bodies facilitate the proliferation of bacteria by protecting the microorganisms from local host defenses. Prosthetic materials in close contact with the bowel may induce bacterial translocation through local inflammation of the bowel wall [5]. Thus, in some circumstances foreign materials may be the essential trigger of a deeply initiated SSTI.

Defective lymphatic drainage is a well-known tissular factor increasing the susceptibility to infections. *Str. pyogenes*, in particular, shows a marked preference for edematous limbs (arm edema after mastectomy, lower limb edema and ulcer due to venous insufficiency).

Obesity may also play a major role in favoring bacterial proliferation in the relatively hypovascularized fatty tissue. In addition, SSTI may be more difficult to eradicate in obese individuals for clear anatomical reasons.

THE HOST FACTOR

Patients with a blunted inflammatory response (Table 1) are at high risk of developing a SSTI even after a minor injury or as complication of a superficial infection (i.e., perirectal abscess, appendectomy wound). Absence of a cellular and humoral immune and inflammatory response at the site of a primary infection results in failure of the host to circumscribe the septic focus, rapid spreading of bacteria and impressive skin lesions. Patients with neutropenia or on high-dose steroids may harbor a spontaneous or postopera-

TABLE 1. Associated conditions which may impair the inflammatory response and facilitate the origin and spreading of soft tissue infections

Treatment with steroids
Treatment with immunosuppressors
Disseminated cancer
AIDS
Organ transplantation
Neutropenia
Chemotherapy
Polytrauma
Multiorgan failure
Diabetes mellitus
Old age

tive SSTI with few, if any, local inflammatory changes.

Initiating Factors

SPONTANEOUS INFECTIONS

Absence of a definite, clinically obvious, portal of entry is not uncommon for necrotizing fasciitis, pyomyositis or severe streptococcal infections. In some of these cases minor breaches allowing bacterial to penetrate the tissues can be indentified such as perianal fistula, prostatitis or minimal dermal abrasions on the upper or lower extremities. In necrotizing perineal infections, anal, urological or genital disease is the usual responsible of the infection. A perirectal abscess, as the initial septic focus, is involved in about 50% of cases [6]. Necrotizing fasciitis of the neck region, potentially extending to the mediastinum, is usually secondary to a protracted dental infection involving the second or third mandibular molars or to an progression of a retropharyngeal abscess secondary to trauma [7]. Exceptionally, even gas gangrene may occur without an apparent focus in patients with colonic malignancies (see below).

POSTOPERATIVE INFECTIONS

Almost all syndromes of SSTI can develop in surgical wounds. Severe streptococcal infections may complicate minor surgical interventions such as meniscectomy or herniorraphy. Gas gangrene may occur after surgery of the appendix, small bowel or colon. Left-*in situ* necrotic bowel and conservative limb amputation for ischemic vascular disease are two of the procedures that carry a higher risk of postoperative gas gangrene. Necrotizing fasciitis can follow abdominal surgery, often of the septic type, mostly in debilitated and diabetic patients.

POSTRAUMATIC INFECTIONS

SSTI often follow complex trauma of the extremities or trauma involving the abdominal viscera. Clostridial myonecrosis was once the paradigm of this syndrome and was responsible for many deaths, particularly following war injuries. Modern trauma management, including early excision of all devitalized tissues, has almost eliminated this dreaded infection. In the late 1970s, however, it was still the first cause of gas gangrene in a referral unit [6]. Insect or dog bites may cause Meleney's gangrene in healthy individuals. Dog and human bites are also a well known antecessor of SSTI due to the very high bacterial colonization of the oral cavity in which angerobes outnomber aerobes by $1/10^3–10^6$.

ILLICIT DRUG INJECTION

An increasing number of cases of SSTI, usually of the upper extremities, are observed in parenteral drug abusers with or without AIDS. These may present initially as a local subcutaneous abscess that may lead the clinician to ignore a deeper infection involving the fascia and muscle. Mortality in this type of patients can be as high as 20% [8].

FISTULA ARISING FROM THE GASTROINTESTINAL TRACT

Colonic cancer, acute appendicitis and sigmoid diverticulitis may give rise to a necrotizing infection as a first clinical manifestation. This is preceded by inflammatory adhesion to the abdominal wall and fistulization of the bowel lumen to the muscles and subcutaneous fat of the lower abdomen, the groin or even the upper third of the thigh if the infection follows the plane of the psoas muscle [9].

Classification, Diagnosis and Treatment of the Main Syndromes

There have been numerous attempts to classify SSTI to help clinicians to better diagnose and treat these disorders. Some authors have used a microorganism-based approach but this is not entirely satisfactory since some SSTI syndromes are due to a specific bacterium (i.e. streptococcal severe infections or clostridial myonecrosis) while others are not (Meleney's gangrene, necro-

TABLE 2. A cassification of severe soft tissue infections based on the depth of infection and the time course

	Rapid (<72 h)	Subacute (<7 days)
Skin and dermis	Erysipela Necrotizing cellulitis Crepitant cellulitis	Meleney's gangrene (Progressive synergistic gangrene)
Fascia	Necrotizing fasciitis	Necrotizing fasciitis
Muscle	Gas gangrene Postraumatic Postoperative Spontaneous	Pyomyositis
All layers	Gas gangrene Streptococcal gangrene	Diabetic foot/leg Mucormycosis

tizing fasciitis). In Table 2 we put forward a classification that combines depth of infection (layer or layers predominantly affected) with the time course. Some bacteria-specific syndromes such as *pyoderma gangrenosum* due to *P. aeruginosa*, carbuncle due to *B. anthracis* or erysipeloid will not be discussed.

CELLULITIS (DERMAL AND SUBDERMAL INFECTIONS)

Group A *Streptococcus pyogenes* is a relatively common cause of less severe cellulitis (erysipela) which is easily diagnosed on the basis of a typical clinical picture (high fever, erythema and pain) and responds to penicillin therapy (4 million units/4 h.). Streptococcal cellulitis should be differentiated from *S. aureus* purulent infection. Presence of a regional enlarged node and systemic symptoms (high fever and malaise) with a short incubation period are most often found in streptococcal infections. Blisters or bullas can also be found although, in our experience, these are more characteristic of whole-thickness streptococcal infections (Figure 1).

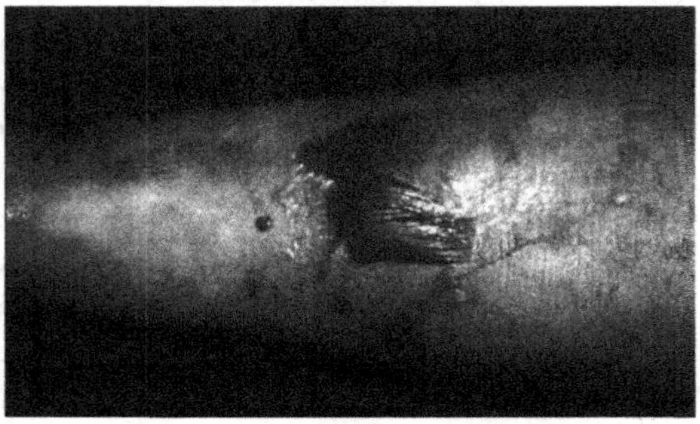

FIGURE 1. Extensive bullae and erythroderma of the leg in a leucopenic female patient with disseminated breast cancer with a lethal *Streptococcus pyogenes* infection.

Suprafascial SSTI are represented mainly by three major syndromes: necrotizing cellulitis, crepitant cellulitis and Meleney's gangrene.

Necrotizing cellulitis is a rare rapidly progressing skin and subcutaneous fat necrosis usually due to a mixed flora involving entrobacteriaceae, Gram-positive cocci. *Bacteroides* spp. and even *Clostridium* spp. It is characterized by necrosis of the deep fatty subcutaneous tissue layer progressing centrifugally and to the skin. Dermal involvement is seen with patchy areas of necrosis and erythema (Figure 2). There is no necrosis of the underlying fascia or muscle. Severe toxicity is the rule and the disease usually runs a rapid and fatal course. It has been reported as a postoperative complication of different surgical procedures often involving the abdominal wall (cholecystectomy, colectomy, hysterectomy). It can also involve the extremities as a result of trauma. Wide spectrum antibiotic therapy (i.e. piperacillin-tazobactam 12 g/day) needs to be instituted immediately and appropriate samples for culture obtained as soon as

FIGURE 2. Patchy areas of skin necrosis in a patient with lethal *necrotizing cellulitis* due to *E. coli* and *B. fragilis* after in intramuscular injection.

possible. Extensive excision of the skin and subcutaneous tissue needs to be carried out leaving exposed wide fascial surfaces requiring a local treatment similar to that of infected burn wounds after scar excision.

Crepitant cellulitis is usually due to gas-forming *E. coli, Streptococcus spp., Bacteroides fragilis* or *Clostridium spp.* The hallmark of this syndrome is absence of skin lesions in a febrile patient with local tenderness and crepitation. These are most commonly found in:1) surgical wounds of the abdomen, and 2) in lower limbs of diabetic patients [10]. Deeper microbial invasion should be ruled out and a Gram stain of the exudate may help to establish the diagnosis between clostridial and non-clostridial crepitant cellulitis. Treatment consists of antibiotics, debridement and, eventually, limb revascularization or amputation.

Meleney's synergistic gangrene is a form of progressive subacute necrotizing cellulitis characterized by an enlarging wound which demarcates in three zones: a wide peripheral zone of erythema surrounding a tender purple zone, the center of which becomes black and necrotic with subsequent ulceration (Meleney's "ulcer"). There may be no or little systemic toxicity. In healthy people, SSTI may be caused by insect or dog bites. Meleney's gangrene may also complicate a surgical or a venipuncture wound. From the bacteriological point of view, Meleney's ulcer usually results from the synergistic action of an anaerobic or microaerophilic microorganism with an aerobic one. A characteristic combination is that of *Peptostreptococcus* with *S. aureus*, but enterobacteriaceae and other anaerobes may also be involved. Meleney's ulcer enlarges in a period of days and may not respond to antibiotic therapy if the central necrosis is not excised. The muscle fascia is usually preserved. Decubitus ulcers typically evolve to Meleney's gangrene when they get infected. They enlarge progressively uncovering large surfaces of the affected body areas. Debridement of the necrotic and "purple" zones is essential to stop the progression of the skin and subcutaneous fat necrosis.

NECROTIZING FASCIITIS

In some studies, deep streptococcal infections are often included under this heading. For example, Bisno and Stevens [3] term as necrotizing fasciitis 2, the group A streptococcal whole-thickness infections, whereas they refer as necrotizing fasciitis 1 those mixed infections with predominance of anaerobes and enteric bacteria. In a historical paper, Rea and Wyrick [11] described as necrotizing fasciitis, infections caused mostly by hemolytic streptococci and *S. aureus*. In more recent studies, however, the term necrotizing fasciitis is reserved for preferentially mixed infections in connection with trauma, or originating spontaneously around the oral or perineal areas [6, 7, 12, 13]. We also prefer to reserve the term "necrotizing fasciitis" for non-streptococcal fascial necrosis with extensive subdermal undermining.

Necrotizing fasciitis is often seen in patients with associated conditions such as diabetes, cancer or receiving steroids. In a recent series of necrotizing fasciitis involving the male genitalia (Fournier's gangrene) two thirds of the patients were diabetic, alcoholic or both [14].

In about 25% of the cases skin lesions (echymosis, bullas) and/or crepitation may be present. In general, however, superficial lesions are not prominent and this may erroneously lead to underestimate the severity of the disease. The hallmark of necrotizing fasciitis is extensive skin undermining of the deep subcutaneous tissue. This is easily diagnosed by physical exploration with a gloved finger or with a surgical instrument. Underlying muscle is usually spared. The lesion content is usually dark-brown, liquid and devoid of frank pus.

The incubation period of necrotizing fasciitis is usually less than a week and by the time the diagnosis is made, fasciitis usually extends more than 10 cm around the initiating focus and severe systemic symptoms are present. Renal failure, jaundice, metabolic acidosis and hypoalbuminemia are very often found. About 20% of the patients are in septic shock and almost all of them will die of the disease despite aggressive treatment.

The most common origins of necrotizing fasciitis are surgical wounds (usually after abdominal surgery for a septic condition), spontaneous perineal due to anorectal or genitourinary disease, spontaneous cervical (secondary to an odontogenic infection) and posttraumatic, after accidental trauma or illicit drug injection.

Treatment of necrotizing fasciitis includes three major chapters: wide surgical debridement and drainage, antibiotic therapy and metabolic support. Surgical debridement usually implies extensive fascia resection through wide skin "windows". Aggressive skin resection is seldom required. Drains should be placed in all the skin incisions and these should follow as far from the initiating focus as indicated by the presence of undermining. Frozen-section biopsies have been proposed to better identify the margins of the infection [15] but they are probably unnecessary if debridement is appropriately guided by the presence of skin undermining.

Cultures should be taken from the deepest infected areas and empiric antibiotic therapy of wide spectrum initiated. The microorganisms most often involved are *E. coli*, *K. pneumoniae*, *Proteus* spp., *P. melaninogenica*, *Fusobacterium* spp., *B. fragilis*, *Streptococcus* spp., *P. aeruginosa* and *E. faecalis*. About 30% of necrotizing fasciitis are monomicrobial and a case due to *S. enteritidis* was reported by our group [16]. Because these patients are often in renal failure, piperacillin-tazobactam (12 g/day) is administered as the antibiotic of choice. It has the additional advantage of being very active against *Enterococcus* spp. and *P. aeruginosa*, two bacterial species commonly found in patients with necrotizing fasciitis of the perineal region.

Metabolic and nutrition support is essential in these debilitated often-malnourished patients [17]. Hydroelectrolitic balance should be reestablished, diabetes should be controlled with insulin and artificial nutrition considered in all cases, if possible, by the enteral route.

Mortality ranges from 10 to 30% and is negatively influenced by the delay to undertake a prompt and radical surgical debridement [18].

MUSCLE INFECTIONS: PYOMYOSITIS AND CLOSTRIDIAL MYONECROSIS

Pyomyositis is the presence of an abscess involving skeletal muscle. It may be a secondary metastatic infection due to *S. aureus* bacteremia of any origin, or present as a primary muscular abscess developing spontaneously or after trauma. Pyomyositis has been extensively reported in tropical countries but is rare in Europe and the USA [19]. Clinically, pyomyositis presents with pain and swelling over a muscle group, typically in the proximal regions of the upper extremities (thighs, buttocks and shoulder). Fever is usually present. Limitation of motion and local inflammatory signs may precede the development of systemic symptoms. Differential diagnosis should be made with thrombophlebitis, bone trauma, septic arthritis, fibrillar rupture and soft tissue sarcoma. Nuclear magnetic resonance or computed tomography have proved extremely useful for the diagnosis of all musculoskeletal mass lesions and usually gives the correct diagnosis). Although very frequently pyomyositis is due to *S. aureus*, many different bacteria have been associated with this syndrome such as the enterobacteriaceae. Thus, initial empiric antibiotic therapy should cover both Gram-positive cocci and Gram-negative rods. A Gram stain and appropriate cultures of a pus sample should be taken as soon as possible either by puncture or at the time of surgical intervention. In addition, wide surgical debridement is often required when an abscess cavity can be delineated. The skin and the muscle fascia should be treated conservatively. Drainage of the purulent cavity and excision of necrotic muscle is usually limited to the muscle compartment. *Clostridial myonecrosis* or "gas gangrene" is the most dramatic SSTI. Strictly speaking, gas gangrene should be described under the heading of "whole-thickness infections" since it usually involves also the skin and subcutaneous tissue, causing extensive necrosis and bullas of the most superficial layers of the soft tissues. However, because the hallmark of gas gangrene is myonecrosis, it is better included in the group of infections affecting primarily the skeletal muscle.

Gas gangrene is due to *Clostridium* spp. a strictly anaerobic Gram-positive sporulated rod easily identifiable on a Gram stain. Most of the postraumatic and postoperative clostridial myonecrosis are due to *C. perfringens* while the sponatenous or bacteremic form is caused by *C. septicum*. As mentioned earlier, clostridial myonecrosis is fundamentally an "exotoxin disease" caused by the proliferation of *Clostridium* spp. under anaerobic conditions favored by the presence of ischemic and necrotic tissues either as a result of trauma or surgery. The organism is characterized by its ability to produce numerous extracellular toxins including alpha-toxin or phospholipase C, theta-toxin or perfringolysin O, kappa-toxin or collagenase, as well as a sporulation-associated enterotoxin. Alpha-toxin is the key virulent determinant exotoxin. It is a 370-residue, zinc metalloenzyme that has phospholipase C activity, and can bind to membranes in the presence of calcium [20, 21].

Clostridial myonecrosis presents under three major syndromes: post-traumatic, post-operative and spontaneous. Post-traumatic gas gangrene has become and uncommon complication of trauma and has the lowest mortality (15–20%). In the recent Bosnian war (1991–1992), no amputation for gas gangrene was carried out on over 1200 lower extremity war wounds [22]. Clostridial myonecrosis may also follow apparently minor trauma such as in inappropriately given intramuscular injections. Post-operative gas gangrene is usually secondary to abdominal septic operations, often involving the small bowel or the colon, or to inappropriate vascular procedures leaving behind devascularized muscle. It has a mortality of 50%. Spontaneous gas gangrene is due to a *C. septicum* bacteremia arising from a malignancy in the gastrointestinal tract, usually a colonic carcinoma, or observed in patients with leukemia or severe enteritis due to chemotherapy induced mucosal damage, and is a fatal disease [23, 24]. It has a mortality close to 100% and patients usually die within 24 hours of onset.

Gas gangrene is a fulminant disease. It has a very short time of incubation and may cause death within the first 48 hours. Thus, the only chance for survival is early recognition and appropriate treatment. Clinical signs that may help in the diagnosis of gas gangrene is severe general deterioration (hypotension, oliguria, disorientation, jaundice and local pain) beginning early after trauma or surgery, extensive crepitation and an ominous purple discoloration of the skin with bullas containing a blackish exudate. The necrotic skin is not painful. Hemoglobinuria secondary to massive intravascular hemolysis can also be found. Multisystem organ failure may develop rapidly and the patient dies of uncontrollable hypotension and hemolysis.

Treatment is based in wide tissue excision and debridement, high dose penicillin and intensive care support. The addition of hyperbaric oxygen has been shown to have a synergistic effect in reducing morbidity and mortality in both canine and murine models. Although no prospective human data are available, retrospective data indicate that concomitant hyperbaric oxygen therapy has resulted in a twofold reduction in mortality. It has also been shown that production of alpha-toxin stops at high pO_2 (240 mmHg). Where feasible, hyperbaric oxygen therapy should be incorporated into the treatment plan for gas gangrene.

WHOLE-THICKNESS INFECTIONS: STREPTOCOCCAL "GANGRENE" AND MUCORMYCOSIS

Str. pyogenes may be the cause of severe, invasive and rapidly evolving whole-thickness soft tissue infections. In a recent epidemiological study in Ontario, Canada, about 1.5 cases of severe streptococcal infections were observed per 100,000 inhabitants/year, 50% of them being of invasive Group A streptococcal soft tissue infections [26]. Most of these affect the children and the elderly. The most extreme clinical manifestation of SSTI due to *Str. pyogenes* is the toxic shock syndrome. In a recent report, Wood *et al.* [27] have reviewed the main clinical manifestations in 59 patients (Table 3).

Initially described by McLennan [28], deep streptococcal infections cause diffuse swelling of the involved muscle (usually in the extremities), often associated with a compartmental syndrome and inflammatory changes in the overlying fascia, subcutaneous fat and skin. Superficial signs suggestive of streptococcal infection (erythema, edema and bullas) are the rule, but deeper invasion should be suspected if there is limited motion, limb swelling and severe systemic symptoms suggestive of toxic shock. Immediate recognition and differential diagnosis with streptococcal cellulitis is important since delay in surgical debridement carries a poor prognosis. In situations where superficial signs are scarce, measurement of muscle compartment pressure may be helpful, and, if pressures are above 40 mmHg, fasciotomy is indicated [3]. Surgical intervention is indicated if patients do not respond to penicillin, present already with established acute renal failure or there is vascular compromise due to massive muscle edema. It also helps in making a definitive diagnosis by obtaining deep sample for bacteriological culture and Gram's staining. Debridement may be conservative (sparing the overlying skin) with excision of necrotic tissues and wide fasciotomy to relieve compartmental hypertension [27].

TABLE 3. Streptococcal toxic shock syndrome: Summary of clinical manifestations of 59 patients (from reference 27)

	No. of patients (%)
Major criteria	
Shock	52 (88%)
Fever	50 (85%)
Rash	48 (81%)
Desquamation	24 (41%)
Associated systemic dysfunction criteria	
Renal	51 (86%)
Gastrointestinal	35 (59%)
CNS	31 (52%)
Myalgia or elevated CPK	27 (46%)
Mucous membrane	27 (46%)
Hepatic	26 (44%)
Hematologic	25 (42%)
Operation required	41 (69%)
Death	14 (24%)

Str. pyogenes is exquisitely sensitive to penicillin, which is the agent of choice for most streptococcal infections. In deep-seated infections, however, doubts have been expressed on the usefulness of this antibiotic used as single therapy [3]. This may be related to the presence of massive bacterial inoculum or the lack of expression of penicillin-binding proteins. A potent effect against *Str. pyogenes* has been ascribed to clindamycin because it appears to facilitate *Str. pyogenes* phagocytosis and to inhibit the synthesis of bacterial toxins. Thus, in view of the severeity of the disease it seems advisable to add clindamycin to penicillin when treating whole-thickness streptococcal infections.

Mucormycosis (zygomycosis) is an uncommon, subacute, frequently fatal, fungal infection which rarely arises in otherwise healthy people.

Different species of the order *Mucorales* are responsible for this disease such as *Mucor* spp., *Rizhopus* spp., *Apophysomyces* spp., *Saksenaea* spp. [29–31]. An underlying disease, frequently diabetes mellitus or immunesuppression after solid organ transplantation, is almost always present. It appears in different anatomic sites: paranasal, cerebral, pulmonary, and gastrointestinal areas; and in the soft tissue of the extremities. It can also progress to disseminated disease by aggressive vascular invasion. Tissue invasion by the hyphae of mucormycosis must be seen microscopically to establish the diagnosis, but culture is required to identify the fungal species involved. A study of 33 cases seen in one hospital over five decades [32] suggests that the incidence of this infection is increasing. There has been an improvement in outcome, which has been paralleled by a major shift from postmortem to premortem diagnosis. Premortem diagnosis gives the opportunity for metabolic stabilization, surgical excision, and liposomal amphotericin-B therapy appropriate to this disease. Successful use of hyperbaric oxygen has been reported in rhinocerebral mucormycosis, and it may be of benefit in high-risk patients with soft tissue infections by preventing local and systemic spreading of the fungus.

References

1. Sandusky WR. Frank L. Meleney, pioneer surgeon-bacteriologist. Arch Surg 118:151, 1983.
2. Lewis RT. Soft tissue infections. World J Surg 22:146, 1998.
3. Bisno AL, Stevens DL. Streptococcal infections of skin and soft tissues. N Engl J Med 334:240, 1996.
4. Case 49-1979. Fulminant illness with subcutaneous crepitance. N Engl J Med 301:1276, 1979.
5. Mora EM, Cardona MA, Simmons RL. Enteric bacteria and ingested inert particles translocate to intraperitoneal prosthetic materials. Arch Surg 126:157, 1991.
6. Bubrick MP, Hitchcock CR. Necrotizing anorectal and perineal infections. Surgery 86:655, 1979.
7. Estrera AS, Landay MJ, Grisham JM, Sinn DP, Platt MR. Descending necrotizing mediastinitis. Surg Gynecol Obstet 157:545, 1983.
8. Callahan TE, Schecter WP, Horn JK. Necrotizing soft tissue infection masquerading as cutaneous abscess following illicit drug injection. Arch Surg 133:812, 1998.
9. Nicell P, Tabrisky J, Lindstrom R, Peter M. Thigh emphysema and hip pain secondary to gastrointestinal perforation. Surgery 78:555, 1975.
10. Bessman AN, Wagner W. Nonclostridial gas gangrene. Report of 48 cases and review of the literature. JAMA 233:958, 1975.
11. Rea WJ, Wyrick WJ. Necrotizing fasciitis. Ann Surg 172:957, 1970.
12. Changyul OH, Chongwook L, Jacobson JH. Necrotizing fasciitis of perineum. Surgery 91:49, 1982.
13. Rouse ThM, Malangoni MA, Schulte WJ. Necrotizing fasciitis: A preventable disaster. Surgery 92:765, 1982.
14. Clayton MD, Fowler JE, Sharifi R. Causes, presentation and survival of fifty seven patients with necrotizing fasciitis of the male genitalia. Surg Gynecol Obstet 170:49, 1990.
15. Stamenkovic I, Lew PD. Early recognition of potentially fatal necrotizing fasciitis. The use of frozen section-biopsy. N Engl J Med 310:1689, 1984.
16. Sánchez C, Capell S, Casanovas A, Admetlla M, Sitges-Serra A. Necrotizing fasciitis caused by *Salmonella enteritidis*. Scand J Infect Dis 16:321, 1984.
17. Majeski JA, Wesley Alexander J. Early diagnosis, nutritional support and immediate extensive debridement improve survival in necrotizing fasciitis. Am J Surg 145:784, 1983.
18. McHenry CR, Piotrowski JJ, Petrinic D, Malangoni MA. Determinants of mortality for necrotizing soft-tissue infections. Ann Surg 221:558, 1995.
19. Schlech WF, Moulton P, Kaiser AB Pyomyositis: Tropical disease in a temperate climate. Am J Med 71:900, 1981.
20. Rood JI. Virulence genes of *Clostridium perfringens*. Annu Rev Microbiol 52:333, 1998.
21. Naylor CE, Eaton JT, Howells A, Justin N, Moss DS, Titball RW, Basak AK. Structure of the key toxin in gas gangrene. Nat Struct Biol 5:738, 1998.
22. Jovanovic S, Wertheimer B, Zelic Z, Getos Z. Wartime amputations. Mil Med 164:44, 1999.
23. Kudsk KA. Occult gastrointestinal malignancies

producing metastatic *Clostridium septicum* infections in diabetic patients. Surgery 112:765, 1992.

24. Bodey GP, Rodríguez S, Fainstein V, Elting LS. Clostridial bacteremia in cancer patients. A 12-year experience. Cancer 67:1928, 1991.
25. Stephens MB. Gas gangrene: potential for hyperbaric oxygen therapy. Postgrad Med 99:217, 1996.
26. Davies HD, McGeer A, Schwartz B, Green K, Cann D, Simor AE, Low DE. Invasive Group A streptococcal infections in Ontario, Canada. N Engl J Med 335:547, 1996.
27. Wood ThF, Potter MA, Jonasson O. Streptococcal toxic shock-like syndrome. The importance of surgical intervention. Ann Surg 217:109, 1993.
28. MacLennan JD. Streptococcal infections of muscle. Lancet 1:582, 1943.
29. Bearer EA, Nelson PR, Chowers MY, Davis CE. Cutaneous zygomycosis caused by *Saksenaea vasiformis* in a diabetic patient. J Clin Microbiol 32:1823, 1941.
30. Chakrabarti A, Kumar P, Padhye AA, Chatha L, Singh SK, Das A, Wig JD, Kataria RN. Primary cutaneous zygomycosis due to Saksenaea vasiformis and *Apophysomyces elegans*. Clin Infect Dis 24:580, 1997.
31. Holland J. Emerging zygomycoses of humans: *Saksenaea vasiformis* and *Apophysomyces elegans*. Curr Top Med Mycol 8:27, 1997.
32. Parfrey NA. Improved diagnosis and prognosis of mucormycosis. A clinicopathologic study of 33 cases. Medicine (Baltimore) 65:113, 1986.

52. INFECTIONS IN BURN PATIENTS

Enrique Cerdá, Miguel A. de la Cal and P. García-Hierro

Introduction

Experts agree that improvements in the management of burn patients have reduced their morbidity and mortality in the last few decades [1]. The most significant of these enhancements are: i) better resuscitation which has reduced the incidence of shock, acute renal failure and severe digestive haemorrhage; ii) the early excision of the burn followed by immediately covering the burn area, which has reduced colonization and infection of the burn and severe sepsis associated with this type of infection. This new situation has increased the relative importance of other infections such as pneumonia, in the morbidity and mortality of severe burn patients.

Nonetheless, in spite of the importance of the infections in burn patients, to our knowledge, there are no prospective studies specifically designed to shed light on the incidence of each one of these infections, the risk factors associated with their presence or the clinical relevance of each one in terms of mortality.

The general aim of this chapter is to describe the more relevant clinical aspects of infections in severe burn patients as well as to present out experience in diagnosis, prevention and treatment.

General Incidence

In a search of the literature covering the period 1990 to 1999 we have only found five prospective studies aimed at the analysis of infection rates in severe burn patients [2–6]. It can be deduced from these studies (Table 1) that: i) the total incidence of nosocomial infections in severe burn patients is high; ii) the burn wound infections (BWI) rate is low, possibly explained by the early excision surgical of the burn wound and the topical use of antimicrobial agents; iii) mechanical ventilation-associated pneumonia (VAP) is the most common infection.

The variations found in the infection rates from study to study depend on the definitions given of the infections in each study, the type of rates used to express the incidence and the severity of the patients as well as how often invasive devices are used [7], such as mechanical ventilation, central venous lines and bladder catheters. Although for the most part the studies have followed the definitions proposed by the Centres for Disease Control (CDC) [8] there is evidence of the low specificity of the definition of pneumonia [4] and it has been suggested that new definitions of BWI [9] and secondary bloodstream infection (BSI) are needed to give a more appropriate definition of the complete spectrum of infections in severe burn patients [5].

In a medical or surgical ward the rate of in-hospital acquired infections is 6%, in a general intensive care unit (ICU) the rate is 18% and in the ICU the overall rate is between 34 and 50% [10]. In the ICU of the Hospital Universitario de Getafe (HUG) [6] we followed 56 patients consecutively admitted to hospital out of which 66% had some kind of infection. This high rate was possibly linked to the percentage of body surface burned which in our series was higher, 41%, than those in the previously referred to studies, 29% [4] and 30% [5], and the high proportion, 46%, of patients suffering inhalation

TABLE 1. Infection rates in burn patients

	Taylor [2] n = 116	Wurtz [3] n = 52	Cremer [4] n = 140	Weber [5] n = 40	Cerdá [6] n = 56
Age (years) (mean)	32	–	36	Children	43
Total body surface burn (%) (mean)	–	–	29	>30	41
Inhalation injury (%)	28	–	33	–	46
Mechanically ventilated (%)	–	52	43	60	73
Mortality (%)	–	–	8	–	25
Infected patients (%)	34	50	40	–	66
Infections per 1000 patient-days	–	32	25	30	59
Infections per 100 infected patient	2.3	1.4	2.4	–	2.5
BWI per 100 patients	18	4	28	52	14
BWI per 1000 patient-days	7.6	–	7.4	8.0	5
BSI per 100 patients	12	4[a]	21	57	54
BSI per 1000 iv line days	–	–	–	>15.4	–
UTI per 100 patients	16	19	17	–	32
UTI per 1000 patient-days	6.6	–	7	4.2	9.7
UTI per 1000 bladder catheter-days	–	–	7	10.5	9.7
Pneumonia per 100 patients	19	42	5	23	66
Pneumonia per 100 patient-days	8.0	–	1.3	–	23.0
Pneumonia per 1000 mechanical ventilation-days	–	–	–	12.3	48

BWI = Burn wound infection. BSI = Bloodstream infection. UTI = Urinary tract infection. [a]Only primary BSI.

injury. This higher infection rate in burns, compared to other critically ill patients admitted to the polyvalent ICU wards, invariably holds for the infections when considered on an individual basis, both for urinary tract infections (UTI), BSI and VAP, just as the National Nosocomial Infection Surveillance System (NNISS) has shown in its figures comparing the different types of ICU (Table 2).

TABLE 2. National nosocomial infections surveillance system by type of ICU [11]

Type of ICU	UTI[a]	Central-line-associated BSI[b]	VAP[c]
Coronary	6.8	4.9	9.4
Medical	7.6	6.1	8.2
Medical/Surgical			
Major teaching	6.8	6.0	12.4
All others	4.5	4.1	10.3
Surgical	5.6	5.6	14.6
Neurosurgical	8.4	5.6	17.1
Trauma	7.7	7.3	16.9
Burns	10.1	12.2	19.9

[a] $\frac{\text{Number of urinary tract infections} \times 1000}{\text{Number of urinary catheter-days}}$

[b] $\frac{\text{Number of central-line-associated bloodstream infections} \times 1000}{\text{Number of central-line-days}}$

[c] $\frac{\text{Number of ventilator-associated pneumonias} \times 1000}{\text{Number of ventilator-days}}$

Pneumonia

INCIDENCE

The cumulative incidence ranges between 5 and 66 per 100 patients and the density incidence ranges between 12 and 48 episodes per 1000 days of mechanical ventilation (Table 1). According with the NNISS [11], based on the data from 14 burn ICUs, the average rate is 19.9 VAP per 1000 days of mechanical ventilation. This wide range is due to the different degrees of severity of the patients and the diagnostic criteria applied and the inclusion or exclusion of those pneumonia which may present in the first two or three days of admittance to burn ICU.

The study conducted at the HUG [6] included patients more severely ill than in other studies. Half the patients had inhalation injury, 73% required mechanical ventilation, the average percentage of body surface burned was 41% and mortality was 25%. The severity of the patient condition may explain the cumulative incidence of VAP observed in 66 out of 100 patients. On the contrary, the lowest rate of pneumonia published, 8%, in other studies corresponds to patients with an 8% death rate [4].

The VAP rates also vary according with the diagnostic method applied. The diagnosis based on clinical signs and symptoms only, with high sensitivity and low specificity, usually increases the rates [2, 3, 5], comparing these with the rates calculated on the basis of clinical signs plus quantitative cultures taken from the tracheobronchial samples obtained using invasive techniques such as protected bronchoscopic specimen brush or bronchoalveolar lavage [4].

Quite often studies into the incidence of nocosomial pneumonia take into consideration only those infections whose symptoms present 48 to 72 hours after admittance to the ICU, without taking into account those infections whose symptoms present in the first two or three days following admittance. The fact that these early pneumonia are excluded has no pathogenetical rationale, given that the burn patient is usually a subject free of previous infection who following a thermal lesion and admittance to the hospital, develops an infection, which in our opinion should be included among the nocosomial pneumonia. In the study undertaken by the ICU unit at the HUG, 28 out of 56 patients developed 37 episodes of VAP, six of which (21%) were diagnosed in the first 72 hours following their admittance to the ICU.

MORTALITY

Pneumonia's contribution to the mortality among burn patients has not been demonstrated in any prospective study. However, it is widely accepted that infections in general and particularly pneumonia make a significant contribution to increasing these figures. The risk factors generally included in the models used to predict mortality amongst burn patients are: age, body surface burned and inhalation injury [12–14]. The inclusion of the diagnosis of pneumonia in the predictive models does not increase their accuracy. Very often pneumonia must be considered as a marker of the severity of the patients instead of as a risk factor of mortality as it has been described in other groups of critically ill patients [15]. On the other hand, the effect of pneumonia on mortality may be partially or totally confunded by the effect of inhalation injury, which not only increase the death rates, but also the likelihood of developing VAP.

Shirani *et al.* [16] studied the independent contributions of pneumonia and inhalation injury to mortality in a retrospective study on 1058 burn patients, consecutively admitted to the hospital over a five year period (1980 to 1984). The relative risk of death related to inhalation injury in this population was 1.8. The relative risk or death of patients with pneumonia was 2.5 times higher than in those patients without pneumonia, after adjusting for age, percentage of body surface burned and inhalation injury. The expected death rate increased by 20% in the presence of only inhalation injury, 40% when there is only pneumonia, and 60% when inhalation injury and pneumonia are both present. These findings suggest that the effects of inhalation injury and pneumonia on mortality are not only independent but also additive. These data support the hypothesis that a significant proportion of deaths attributed to inhalation injury is really attributable to pneumonia. However, the main weak point of this study, its retrospective timing, implies an important problem in defining the presence of inhalation injury and/or pneumonia, which significantly limits the study validity. In the study conducted in the HUG [6] the risk of death related to pneumonia and inhalation injury are 2.25 and 1.6 respectively, similar to those cited by Shirani *et al.* [16].

PATHOGENESIS AND RISK FACTORS

The risk factors associated with the development of pneumonia give an idea of the pathogenesis of respiratory infections in burn patients (Table 3). These factors are the severity of the burns (estimated by according with age and the percentage of body surface burned), inhalation injury and the need to intubate the patient.

Immediately after the burn injury, a process of inflammation begins, and progresses, peaking at around seven days after the burn injury [17]. The physiological response is a systemic inflammatory response syndrome, without other signs of infection in more than half the cases. This syndrome is produced by the release of mediators, oxidants and arachidonic acid metabolites in the burn areas. The cascade of systemic mediators is activated, i.e., cytokines and the complement, and arachidonic acid is released. The ensuing syndrome is inmunosupression and organic damage, including pulmonary lesions. The colonization of the burn wound triggers of absorption of endotoxins which in turn triggers the release of more local and systemic anti-inflammatory mediators and thus amplify the whole process. The increased permeability of the gastrointestinal mucosa and the suppression of the immune function of the intestinal mucosa and the intestinal ischemia foster the absorption of endotoxins and possibly bacterial translocation, which has been demonstrated in animal models. Both inmunosupression and pulmonary injury are considered to be risk factors for the development of pneumonia, given that these factors weaken the defence mechanisms against adhesion of potential pathogen microorganisms to the respiratory mucosa enabling ensuing colonization and infection [18]. Inhalation injury is closely associated with mortality and pneumonia [17, 19]. Inhalation of smoke damages the airways, above all when this is sufficiently severe that is causes inflammatory changes visible on the bronchoscope. In animal models inhalation injury causes necrosis of the endobronchial mucosa and release of local mediators thus blocking the terminal bronchioles and interfering with the defence mechanisms against bacterial colonization and infection.

TABLE 3. Risk factors of ventilator associated pneumonia

	RR (95% CI)	p
Mechanical ventilation (yes/not)	10.46 (1.54 a 71.19)	0.003
Inhalation injury (yes/not)	3.65 (1.72 a 7.76)	0.0002
Percentage of body-surface area burned (per 1%)	1.07 (1.03 a 1.12)	0.002
Percentage of body-surface area full-thickness burned (per 1%)	1.06 (1.02 a 1.11)	0.005
Age (per year)	1.01 (0.99 a 1.04)	0.31

RR = Relative Risk. CI = Confidence Intervals.

A very high proportion of patients, 40%–80%, with severe inhalation injury requires intubation and mechanical ventilation, either due to stenosis of the upper respiratory tract or oedema, because of respiratory failure secondary to the smoke induced injury or pulmonary oedema caused by the infusion of liquids during resuscitation, or pulmonary lesion induced by systemic inflammation. Intubation and mechanical ventilation are the most important risk factors for the development of pneumonia in critical patients and that therefore encompasses burn patients.

Rue *et al.* [20] carried out a retrospective study of 370 patients who had required mechanical ventilation, in order to evaluate the impact of tracheal intubation and inhalation injury on pneumonia development. Over a 6-year period (1985–1991) they looked at all those patients who developed pneumonia more than three days after intubation. The cumulative incidence of pneumonia during intubation was 32% in 105 patients with no inhalation injury and 36% in 265 patients with inhalation injury. Pre-intubation pneumonia was diagnosed most frequently in those patients without inhalation injury (19% compared with 5%). The authors concluded that the risk of pneumonia associated with mechanical ventilation was not related to inhalation injury. However, due to their retrospective nature one must be very cautious with these conclusions in as far as the reliability of the diagnosis of pneumonia and inhalation injury. What is more, the diagnostic criteria used for pneumonia might underestimate the true infection rates because the early VAP may develop within the first three days.

DIAGNOSIS

The problem with diagnosing pneumonia in burn patients is similar to that of other types of critically ill patients who require mechanical ventilation or who suffer adult respiratory distress syndrome [21]. Nonetheless, there are some clinical aspects which are specific to the burn patients. Fever or hypothermia and leucocitosis are symptoms of the inflammatory response syndrome caused by burns, which are always present in burn patients in the first week. Radiological pulmonary infiltrates often show up when there is lung injury and pulmonary oedema post-resuscitation as a result of the high hydrostatic pressure in the lung capillaries and increased vascular permeability. Post-inhalation inflammation of the airways often causes purulent sputum. Therefore, the clinical and radiological signs included in the diagnosis of pneumonia are often of a very low specificity. However, most prospective studies into the incidence of pneumonia in burn patients [2, 3, 5] use the criteria of clinical suspicion to establish the diagnosis. Although quantitative cultures obtained by using invasive techniques have recently been proposed for the diagnosis of pneumonia in these patients [4] the efficacy of this technique has not as yet been sufficiently proven neither in critical patients nor in burn patients [22, 23].

In our opinion, the diagnostic criteria of pneumonia in burn patients for the purpose of monitoring and research should be similar to those proposed for other patients on mechanical ventilation [21].

POTENTIAL PATHOGEN MICROORGANISMS

The most useful classification is that which distinguishes between community flora and hospital flora as it comes enables one to come closer to empirical treatment. The relative frequency of community or hospital flora in the different studies hinges mainly on two factors: the percentage of early onset VAP, i.e., ≤5 days after admission in ICU, in relation to late onset VAP, >5 days, and the patient origin, whether they come from the community or from another hospital. Both factors condition the likelihood that the infective flora be predominantly community or hospital flora. The pathogens which caused pneumonia in burn patients in the HUG can be seen in Table 4. The early VAP were caused by community microorganisms, except for two cases, one caused by *Acinetobacter sp.* and another

TABLE 4. Potential pathogen microorganisms according with the onset of pneumonia[a]

Number of VAP	Early onset (≤5 days)	Late onset (>5 días)
Community acquired flora		
Staphylococcus aureus	12	0
Haemophilus influenzae	6	0
Streptococcus pneumoniae	6	0
ICU acquired flora		
Pseudomonas aeruginosa	0	3
Enterobacteriaceae	0	1
Acinetobacter sp.	1	0
Methicillin-resistant *Staphylococcus aureus*	1	11

[a]Twenty eight patients developed 37 VAP.

by methicillin-resistant *Staphylococcus aureus*. Both patients had been referred from other hospitals. The microorganisms responsible for the late onset VAP portray the flora endemic to the ICU, including the potential outbreaks of multiresistant microorganisms.

PREVENTION OF PNEUMONIA

Just like in other types of critical patients, in burn patients is important to recognize the relation between digestive, oropharyngeal and/or rectal colonization, and the development of infections [24]. Surveillance studies of oropharyngeal and rectal flora reveal that between 80% and 95% of pneumonia are caused by microorganisms which have previously colonized the patient digestive tract.

According with the results of the oropharyngeal and rectal sample cultures pneumonia can be classified as: i) primary endogenous, when the infections are caused by microorganisms which were present in the patient's oropharynx when admitted to the ICU; ii) secondary endogenous, when the infections are caused by microorganisms which the patient was not carrying when admitted to the ICU, but which colonized the digestive tract later, before causing the infection; iii) exogenous, when the microorganisms causing the infections are not previously found in the surveillance samples taken from the oropharynx and the rectum. The distribution of pneumonia in burn patients according with this classification can be seen in Table 5.

This classification enables clinicians to chose appropriate preventive measures according with the pathogenetical mechanism. The primary endogenous infections can never be prevented using the traditional methods of hygiene, as normally the infective microorganisms, generally acquired in the community, are passed directly, from the oropharynx, where they are already lodged when the patient is admitted to the ICU, to the tracheobronchial system upon intubation. In this case a short cycle of antibiotics (two to four days administering 2nd or 3rd cephalosporine) eradicates community flora of the oropharynx and the respiratory tract, preventing the development of pneumonia [25]. Secondary endogenous infections could be controlled by traditional methods of hygiene, to prevent cross-colonization, and using topical digestive antibiotics (tobramycin, amphotericin B and polymixin) to prevent and/or eradicate the abnormal carrier state ensuing from the acquisition of potential pathogen microorganisms following patient admittance to the ICU [26,

TABLE 5. Potential pathogen microorganisms according with the pathogenesis[a]

Number of VAP	Primary endogenous	Secondary endogenous	Exogenous
Community acquired flora			
Staphylococcus aureus	11	0	1
Haemophilus influenzae	6	0	0
Streptococcus pneumoniae	6	0	0
ICU acquired flora			
Pseudomonas aeruginosa	0	2	1
Enterobacteriaceae	0	1	0
Acinetobacter sp.	1	0	0
Methicillin-resistant *Staphylococcus aureus*	1	10	0

[a]Twenty eight patients developed 37 VAP.

27]. Exogenous infections can only be prevented by identifying where the barrier methods have been broken and by tightening hygiene. The majority of burn patients who develop pneumonia are normally intubated as a result of respiratory failure or obstruction of the airways secondary to direct lesions of the mucosa or edema. It would therefore be logical to think that those methods which have proven effective in the prevention of pneumonia in mechanically ventilated critically ill patients, would be efficacious in burn patients. These measures also include hygiene [28], proper management of the airways [29] and selective digestive decontamination [27].

Selective digestive decontamination using non-absorbable, topical antimicrobials (tobramycin, polymixin and amphotericin B) applied in paste form in the oropharynx and in solution form in the digestive tract, plus a short course of systemic antibiotics, have proven to reduce the incidence of pneumonia by 64% and mortality by 20% in critically ill patients, without any significant side effects for the patient and without increase in antimicrobial resistance, in the absence of endemia of methicillin-resistant *Staphylococcus aureus* [27]. Mackie *et al.* [30], have made a retrospective analysis of two historical series. The first included 33 consecutive patients with burns of more than 30% of the body surface who required mechanical ventilation support. The second group was of 31 similar patients admitted two years later who received selective digestive decontamination plus iv cephotaxime over a four day period. The incidence of pneumonia was 27% in the first group and 6.5% in the second one. The level of evidence provided by this study is low. So, the data regarding the effect of selective digestive decontamination on the general hospital population in ICUs require the confirmation of the effects on the burn patients.

Recently Kimura *et al.* [31], in a prospective, randomized placebo controlled study, looked at the effect on the prophylaxis of methicillin-resistant *Staphylococcus aureus* pneumonia with trimethoprim-sulfamethoxazole, commencing four to six days after admittance to the burn ICU and maintaining the treatment over a 10 period. The study population was 40 intubated patients, 57.5% had inhalation injury, with more than 20% body surface burned. The incidence of methicillin-resistant *Staphylococcus aureus* pneumonia was 4.8% in the trimethoprimsulfamethoxazole and 36.8% in the placebo group which implies a significant decrease in VAP incidence of 32% ($p = 0.017$).

TREATMENT

The treatment of pneumonia in burn patients follows the same principles as those applied to other critical patients. The empirical treatment should commence early, with the onset of the first symptoms. The choice of antibiotics should be based on epidemiological criteria. If the patient is a healthy subject prior to the burn injury, comes form the community and develops pneumonia in the first five days, a second generation cephalosporine would be the right choice against *Staphylococcus aureus*, *Streptococcus pneumoniae* and *Haemophilus influenzae*, which are the microorganisms responsible for causing the more prevalent forms of pneumonia in the community.

When the likelihood of the ICU endemic flora being the cause of infection is high (late onset pneumonia, transfer from other hospital, or previously ill patient), the antibiotic regimen should include an antipseudomonal beta-lactam as well as aminoglycosides in keeping with the antibiotic resistance patterns existing in the ICU. When outbreaks of methicillin-resistant *Staphylococcus aureus* occur, glycopeptides can be prescribed. The treatment can be adjusted according with the results of the sample cultures.

The dose of systemic antibiotics to be administered to the severe burn patients is a subject of discussion as the pharmacokinetics of the antimicrobials administered to burn patients shows huge individual variations [32]. In general terms, one should take into account that: i) aminoglycosides have a shorter half-life in burn patients than in healthy volunteers; ii) the beta-lactams have an augmented distribution volume; iii) vancomycin, aztreonam and carbapenems clearance is closely linked to creatinine clearance. The administration regimens for antibiotics in burn patients based on serum levels has not been evaluated from the point of view of the effects on relevant clinical objectives such as the cure rate of infections, clinical relapse or mortality. On the basis of the experimental data, the burn patients should be receiving higher doses of antimicrobials than other patients, at least for the first weeks during which the extracellular volume tends to be expanded. The usefulness of monitoring the serum levels of aminoglycosides and glycopeptides to enhance clinical efficacy and to reduce side effects has not as yet been assessed.

Bloodstream Infections

INCIDENCE

The cumulative incidence varies from 4 per 100 patients [3] to 57 per 100 patients [5] according to whether it refers to primary BSI alone or all types of BSI. This variability depends on the same factors commented upon in relation to the VAP. Weber *et al.* [5] observed in the paediatric population an overall incidence of primary BSI in patients with central venous catheters, of 12.5 per 100 patients, with a rate of 4.9 per 1000 central catheter-days. When the authors stratified the patients according with the body surface burned they found that in the subgroup of patients with less than 30% involvement there was no BSI. However, in the subgroup of patients with 30% to 60% burns the rate of primary BSI was 8.5 per 1000 central catheter-days and the rate of secondary BSI 11.3 per central catheter-days. In more severe subgroup with more than 60% burns the rates were 3.5 primary BSI per 1000 central catheter-days 15.0 secondary BSI per 1000 central catheter-days. According with these data the risk of having primary and secondary BSI increases as the involvement of body surface area augments. The mean rate found in the NNISS [11] is 12.2 central venous catheter associated BSI per 1000 central catheter-days, on the basis of the data from 17 burns ICUs and 25,660 patients. In the HUG study we observed 54 BSI per 100 patients, there was some difficulty in defining the type of BSI as being intravascular catheter associated or whether it was associated with burn wound colonization or infection because in 90% of the cases the microorganism isolated in blood culture was isolated in the intravascular catheters and in the burn exudate at the same time.

MORTALITY

Mason *et al.* [33] and Boucher *et al.* [34] in a retrospective study compared a population of 1605 burn patients admitted the ICU between 1974 and 1983 at a time when there were no individual rooms, whose average age was 31 years, and on average 47.5% of body surface burned and an average death rate of 42%, and a population of 914 other patients who had been through the unit between 1984 and 1993 when there was a new ICU with individual rooms, whose average age was 32, 43% of body surface burned and a death rate of 23.4%. The first group's BSI incidence was 31.2 per 100 patient caused by Gram-positive microorganisms and 31.8 per 100 patients caused by Gram-negative microorganisms. The patients who developed BSI showed a 32% excess of mortality compared with the expected mortality according with age and extent of burns. In the second time span the incidence was of 20 BSI per 100 patients caused by Gram-positive microorganisms and 12 BSI per 100 patients caused by Gram-negative microorganisms. In this second period no significant increase in mortality was observed in the patients with BSI in regard to age and extent of burns. The design of both studies prevents from deriving firm conclusions regarding death rates attributable to BSI in severe burn patients. Nonetheless, at the present time there is no evidence to support the idea that there is an excess of mortality which could be attributed to BSI.

In the population studied by the HUG group the presence of BSI was not significantly related to the death rate: mortality in patients with BSI was 22%; mortality in patients without BSI 27% ($p = 0.63$). The lack of association between BSI and death rates is possibly linked to: i) BSI in burn patients is often transitory, related to the way the burns are handled, cleaning and surgical excision [35]; ii) BSI are often related to intravascular catheters and deaths attributable to intravascular catheter BSI are nil in some population of critically ill patients [36].

PATHOGENESIS AND RISK FACTORS

The significance of a positive blood culture in a burn patient will depend on the relation between sample extraction and manipulation of the wounds, the presence of other foci of infection and the patients overall condition [1].

Sasaki *et al.* [35] showed that the procedures followed in treating the wound caused BSI in 20% of cases, and that this frequency increased the larger the area involved and the more intense the manipulation.

Franceshi *et al.* [37] made a prospective study of risk factors associated with colonization of 101 intravascular catheters in 89 burn patients. The main conclusions were: i) the frequency of colonization of the catheters depends on the extent of the burn and the distance between the point where the catheter is inserted and the burn wound; ii) the frequency of intra-arterial catheter colonization is similar to that of the central vein catheters; iii) skin colonization is more frequent than colonization of the hub, which suggests that the main pathway of catheter colonization is peri-catheter; iv) change of tubing every 48 or every 24 hours does not have any influence on the frequency of colonization of the intravascular catheters.

In keeping with the pathogenetical classification of infections mentioned above, based on the relation between colonization and infection, in the HUG 15 (50%) BSI were primary endogenous, i.e., they were caused by microorganisms already carried by the patient before admittance to the ICU, mainly *Escherichia coli*; 14 (47%). BSI were secondary endogenous, that is to say they were caused by microorganisms not carried by the patient prior to admittance to the burn ICU, but rather these were acquired during hospitalization in the ICU; 1 (3%) BSI was caused by a microorganism which the patient had not been carrying but was introduced during manipulation of the patient.

The origin of the BSI in the prospective studies on incidence of infection in burn patients is shown in Table 5, where one can see the predominance of the BSI associated with burn wound colonization and the colonization of the intravascular catheters. When interpreting these data it is worth considering that some authors have proposed [5] modifying the definition of BSI in these patients, considering that these BSI, which are caused by the same microorganisms which colonize burns, should considered secondary as opposed to primary BSI.

This confirms just how difficult it is to assign a primary foci of BSI in burn patients as often times more than one positive clinical sample, i.e. intravascular catheter, burn wound exudate and tracheal aspirate, with the same microorganism are found simultaneously.

POTENTIAL PATHOGEN MICROORGANISMS

In the 1970s and beginning of the 1980s reference is made to the predominance of Gram-negative microorganisms as being the cause of BSI. Later on, coinciding with changes in surgical approaches to burns, the topical treatment with anti-microbials and an improvement in isolation methods have all brought about a reduction in BSI, and now it is the Gram-positive which are most frequently isolated in some burn ICU. The causal flora of BSI are seen on Table 7.

PREVENTION AND TREATMENT

The high frequency of intravascular catheter and burn manipulation associated BSI suggest that the prophylaxis should be centred on both foci.

TABLE 6. Bloodstream infections

Type of infection	Taylor [2] n = 116	Wurtz [3] n = 52	Creme [4] n = 140	Weber [5] n = 345	Cerdá [6] n = 56
Number of bloodstream infections	14	12	29	42	28
Primary and central-line associated bloodstream infections	10	2	23	11	18
Secondary bloodstream infections:	5	0	6	35[a]	–
Primary focus					
Burn wound	1	0	NS	28[b]	20[c]
VAP	3	0	NS	3	4[d]
UTI	1	0	NS	3	1

NS = not specified.
[a] In 20 BSI cases the same micro-organism has been isolated in blood and in one or more sites.
[b] In fifteen cases the same micro-organism has been isolated in blood and in colonized burn wound (not infected according with CDC criteria).
[c] In 13 cases the same micro-organism has been isolated in blood and in burn wound exudate and in intravascular catheters.
[d] In one case the same micro-organism has been isolated in blood and in burn wound exudate and in intravascular catheters and tracheal aspirate.

TABLE 7. Bloodstream infections: Pathogen micro-organisms

	Taylor [2] n = 116	Wurtz[a] [3] n = 52	Weber [4] n = 345	Cerdá [6] n = 56
Number of bloodstream-infections	14	2	42	28
Gram-positive	11	2	26	23
Staphyloccoccus aureus	6	1	10	5
Methicillin-resistant *S. aureus*		1	0	7
Enterococcus sp.			7	5
Coagulase-negative *Staphylocccus*	5		7	4
Other Gram-positive micro-organisms			2	2
Gram-negative	3		13	6
Pseudomonas aeruginosa			6	3
Enterobacter cloacae			1	0
Escherichia coli	1		1	3
Proteus mirabilis			1	0
Other Gram-negative bacilli	2		4	0
Yeasts				
Candida sp	1	1	6	1

[a] Only primary bloodstream infections.

Although there are no clinical trials specifically designed to evaluate the effects of the different measures to prevent the colonization of catheters in burn patients, it is advised that the care taken with intravascular catheters be the same as for other critical patients. It has also been suggested that the vascular catheter be changed every five or six days, and that the access be as far away from the burn as possible [37].

In treating burns it is essential that BSI be prevented as frequent manipulation is associated with BSI and what is more the colonization of burns is often associated with the colonization of the catheters. Early excision and early grafting of the burned surface, as well as topical treatment with antimicrobials have been proposed to prevent colonization and over-growth of microorganisms in the burn wound. The prophylactic use of antibiotics prior to surgical manipulation of the burn is the subject of debate. However, the most accepted opinion is not in favor of the use of prophylactic antibiotics [35].

Burn Wound Infection

INCIDENCE

The cumulative incidence of BWI (Table 1) varies in different series between 4 per 100 patients and 52 per 100 patients. The numbers referred to in these studies range between 7.4 and 8.0 BWI per 1000 patient-days.

MORTALITY

Traditionally BWI have been considered crucial in determining the burn patients prognosis [1]. It is considered that in part today s survival rate of burn patients which is higher than in the 1980s rates is due to the prevention of colonization and burn wound infection by excising and early grafting.

DIAGNOSIS

The CDC diagnostic criteria published in 1988 [8] are: "a change in burn wound appearance or character such as rapid eschar separation, or dark brown, black or violaceous discolcration of the eschar, or edema at the wound margin and histologic examination of the burn biopsy showing invasion of microorganisms into the adjacent visible tissue or organisms cultured from blood in the absence of other identifiable infection".

Recently attention has been drawn to the limitations of these definitions: i) they do not sufficiently describe the present spectrum of burn wound infection. The macroscopic changes described are present before the excision of the eschar. Currently, with the early excision of the eschar, these macroscopic changes are rarely seen; ii) histological examination of the burn wound biopsy is highly specific, but is not usually done in burns units.

The American Burn Association has recently proposed new criteria for the diagnosis of BWI, aimed at encompassing the whole BWI clinical spectrum, without the need to biopsy the burns in the majority of cases [38]. Four types of infection are included in these definitions: burn wound impetigo, open burn-related surgical wound infection, burn wound cellulitis and invasive infection in unexcised burn wound. The last type of infection corresponds to the definition proposed by the CDC in 1988. The acceptance and the usefulness of this approach deserves further evaluation.

The quantitative eschar cultures are of limited value in handling burn patients. A value of $\geq 10^5$ cfu per gram of burn eschar is associated with high probability of graft failure. However, this is of little value for the diagnosis of burn wound infection. McManus *et al.* [39] studied the relationship between the quantitative cultures of biopsies and their histologic findings in 200 patients. In general, agreement was found between the biopsies with negative cultures and lack of histologic invasion by microorganisms. Of the positive culture biopsies, $\geq 10^5$ cfu per gram, only 36% presented histologic signs of microorganism invasion in viable tissue. These authors concluded that the quantitative cultures of the biopsies had a high negative predictive value and it is a useful tool to describe the predominant flora which colonizes the burn wound, which is helpful when choosing the most appropriate antimicrobial treatment.

PATHOGENESIS AND RISK FACTORS

The direct effect of heat on skin and adjacent tissue means that the burned area is susceptible to infection. It is accepted that the greater the extent of the burn the greater the risk of infection [1]. The burned tissue is a growth medium for microorganisms which are present on the skin surface. Moreover, thrombosis of local vessels caused by heat limit the delivery of blood borne antibiotics to the eschar. The microorganisms penetrate through the hair follicles and the sweat glands getting to the boundary limits between the viable tissue and nonviable tissue. In this sub-eschar area there is a proliferation of microorganisms which, if not counteracted by the local defence mechanisms, will invade the viable tissue. The environment surrounding burn patients, that usually is a reservoir of hospital flora in high concentrations, and the need for successive changes of dressing and cleaning, that causes some disruptions to the isolation measures and hygiene in these patients, constitute significant risks factors of BWI.

The cultures of the oropharyngeal and rectal samples show that the colonization and infection of burns is very often endogenous, i.e., produced by microorganisms previously isolated in the patient's digestive system, whose intestine is the main reservoir of the ICU endemic flora [40]. In the HUG series the eight BWI suffered by the 56 patients studied were endogenous in origin, seven were secondary endogenous and one was primary endogenous.

POTENTIAL PATHOGEN MICROORGANISMS

In an untreated burn first the community microorganisms would appear, coagulase-negative *Staphylococcus* and *Staphylococcus aureus* and *Streptococcus sp*. In the course of the next few days they are replaced by the ICU acquired microorganisms [1]. Table 8 shows that the existing predominance flora is community acquired in some series whilst in others the infective flora is predominantly acquired in the ICU.

TREATMENT

The prevention of burn wound infection is a priority objective in the treatment of burn patients. This is achieved by the appropriate surgical treatment, aseptic management of the burn wounds and topical antimicrobial treatment. The efficacy of the wound infection preventative measures is estimated through inspection of the burn wound and the graft, and by taking quantitative serial burn wound cultures, once or twice a week. The presence of overgrowth of microorganisms, i.e., 10^5 cfu/ml of exudate, increases the probability of there being BWI and graft loss [39].

TABLE 8. Burn wound infection: Potential pathogen micro-organisms

	Taylor [2] n = 116	Wurtz [3] n = 52	Weber [4] n = 345	Cerdá [6] n = 56
Number of burn wound infections	21	1	37	8
Gram-positive	15	1	30	7
Staphyloccoccus aureus	15		21	
Methicillin-resistant *S aureus*		1	1	6
Enterococcus sp.			2	1
Coagulase-negative *Staphylocccus*				
Other Gram-positive micro-organisms			6	
Gram-negative			23	1
Pseudomonas aeruginosa	1		8	1
Enterobacter cloacae			5	
Escherichia coli	2		2	
Proteus mirabilis			1	
Other Gram-negative bacilli	2			
			7	
Yeasts				
Candida sp	1		1	

The universally accepted treatment for burns is early excision and wound closure with grafts. In patients with less than 50% burn body surface the patients own skin can be used for the grafts (autologous grafts). In patients with greater percentages there is less likelihood that there will be sufficient healthy donor skin for grafting. In these cases recourse is taken to cadaver skin grafts (allografts) and synthetic skin, or culture grown epidermic queratinocytes, combining all the alternative treatments to cover all the affected areas.

The burns must be handled in an aseptic environment just like any other severe surgical lesion, in ICUs where the patient can be isolated and there are sufficient staff to keep preventive measures, such as handwashing, gloving and gowning, properly in order to prevent the transmission of flora from patient to patient or from inanimate environment to patient.

Topical antimicrobial agents can be used to limit the proliferation of bacteria and fungal colonization. The most commonly used are silver sulfadiazine, mafenide acetate and povidone-iodine. The advantages and disadvantages of each antimicrobial agent are beyond the scope of this chapter [41].

Given that the colonization of the burn is often brought about by enteric flora, there are physiopathological justifications for the use of selective digestive decontamination in burn patients. Nonetheless, the effect of this approach has not as yet been sufficiently assessed. Mackie *et al.* [30] presented a retrospective study comparing two consecutive series of 31 and 33 patients in which the administration of tobramycin and polymixin reduced the incidence of burn colonization by *Pseudomonas aeruginosa* in 61% and 29% and *Enterobacteriaceae* by 73% and 10%, respectively.

The treatment of BWI calls for a review of the evaluation of surgical approaches and systemic treatment with antimicrobial agents in accordance with the results obtained from the cultures.

References

1. Pruitt BA, McManus AT. The changing epidemiology of infections in burn patients. World J Surg 16:57, 1992.
2. Taylor GB, Kibsey P, Kiriland T, Burroughs E, Tredget E. Predominance of staphylococcal organisms in infections occurring in a burn intensive care unit. Burns 18:332, 1992.
3. Wurtz R, Karajovic M, Dacumos E, Jovanovic B, Hanumadass M. Nosomial infections in a burn intensive care unit. Burns 21:181, 1995.
4. Cremer R, Ainaud P, Le Bever H, Fabre M, Carsin H. Infections nosocomiales dans un service de brulés. Resultats d'une enquete prospective d'un an. Ann Fr Anesth Reanim 15:599, 1996.
5. Weber JM, Sheridan RL, Pasternack MS, Tompkins RG. Nosocomial infections in pediatric patients with burns. Am J Infect Control 25:195, 1997.
6. Cerdá E, de la Cal MA, Garcia-Hierro P. Pneumonia in severe burn patients. Clin Pulm Med 6:1, 1999.
7. Jarvis WR, Edwards JR, Culver DH, Hughes JM, Horan T, Emori TG, Banerjee S, Tolson J, Henderson T, Gaynes RP, Martone WJ, and the National Nosocomial Infections Surveillance System. Nosocomial infection rates in adult and pediatric intensive care unit in the United States. Am J Med 91(Suppl 3B):185S, 1991.
8. Garner JS, Jarvis WR, Emori TG, Horan TC, Hughes JM. CDC definitions for nosocomial infections, 1988. Am J Infect Control 16:128, 1988.
9. Peck MD, Weber J, McManus A, Sheridan R, Heimbach D. Surveillance of burn wound infections: A proposal for definitions. J Burn Care Rehabil 19:386, 1998.
10. Donowitz LG, Wenzel RP, Hoyt JW. High risk of hospital acquired infection in the ICU patient. 10:355, 1982.
11. National Nosocomial Infections Surveillance (NNISS) report: Data summary from January 1990–May 1999, issued June 1999. Am J Infect Control 27:520, 1999.
12. Tredget EE, Shankosky HA, Taerum TV Moysa GL, Alton JDM. The role of inhalation injury in burn trauma. A Canadian experience. Ann Surg 212:720, 1990.
13. Smith DL, Cairns BA, Ramadan F, *et al.* Effect of inhalation injury, burn size, and age on mortality: a study of 1447 consecutive burn patients. J Trauma 37:655, 1994.

14. Ryan CM, Schoenfeld DA, Thorpe WP, Sheridan RL, Cassem EH, Tompkins RG. Objetive estimates of the probability of death from burn injuries. N Engl J Med 338:362, 1998.
15. Heyland DK, Cook DJ, Griffith L, Keenan SP. Brun-Buisson C for the Canadian Critical Care Trials Group. The attributable morbidity and mortality of ventilator-associated pneumonia in the critically ill patient. Am J Respir Crit Care Med 159:1249, 1999.
16. Shirani KZ, Pruitt BA, Mason AD. The influence of inhalation injury and pneumonia on burn mortality. Ann Surg 205:83, 1987.
17. Youn YK, LaLonde C, Demling R. The role of mediators in the response to thermal injury. World J Surg 16:30, 1992.
18. Estes RJ, Meduri GU. The pathogenesis of ventilator-associated pneumonia: I. Mechanisms of bacterial transcolonization and airway inoculation. Intensive Care Med 21:365, 1995.
19. Clark WR, Bonaventura M, Myers RN. Smoke inhalation and airway management at a regional burn unit: 1974–1983. Part I. Diagnosis and consequences of smoke inhalation. J Burn Care Rehabil 10:52, 1989.
20. Rue LW, Cioffi WG, Mason AD, McManus WF, Pruitt BA. The risk of pneumonia in thermally injured patients requiring ventilatory support. J Burn Care Rehabil 16:262, 1995.
21. Niederman MS, Torres A, Summer W. Invasive diagnostic testing is not needed routinely to manage suspected ventilator-associated pneumonia. Am J Respir Crit Care Med 150:565, 1994.
22. Sanchez-Nieto JM, Torres A, Garcia-Cordoba F, *et al*. Impact of invasive and noninvasive quantitative culture sampling on outcome of ventilator-associated pneumonia. Am J Respir Crit Care Med 157:371, 1998.
23. Fagon JY, Chastre J, Wolff M, *et al*. Invasive and noninvasive strategies for management of suspected ventilator-associated pneumonia. A randomized trial. Ann Intern Med 132:621, 2000.
24. Van Saene HKF, Damjanovic V, Murray AE, de la Cal MA. How to classify infections in intensive care units: the carrier state, a criterion whose time has come. J Hosp Infect 33:1, 1996.
25. Sirvent JM, Torres A, El Biary M, Castro P, Batlle J, Bonet A. Protective effect of intravenously administered cefuroxime against nosocomial pneumonia in patients with structural coma. Am J Respir Crit Care Med 155:1729, 1997.
26. Baxby D, van Saene HFK, Stoutenbeek CP, Zandstra DF. Selective decontamination of the digestive tract: 13 years on, what it is and what it is not. Intensive Care Med 22:1, 1996.
27. Liberati A, D'amico R, Pifferi S. Effectiveness of antibiotic prophylaxis based on selective decontamination of the digestive tract (SDD) on respiratory tract infections and mortality in an intensive care unit population. In Douglas R, Bridges-Web C, Glaziou P (eds). Acute respiratory infections module of the Cochrane Database of Systemic Review. Updated December, 1997.
28. Tablan OC, Anderson LJ, Arden NH, Breiman RF, Butler JC, McNeil MM and the Hospital Infection Control Practices Advisory Committee. Guideline for Prevention on nosocomial pneumonia. Am J Infect Control 22:247, 1994.
29. Cook D, De Jonghe B, Brochard L, Brun-Buisson C. Influence of airway management on ventilator-associated pneumonia. Evidence from randomized trials. JAMA 279:781, 1998.
30. Mackie DP, van Hertum WAJ, Schumburg T, Kuipjer EC, Knape P. Prevention of infection in burns: Preliminary experience with selective decontamination of the digestive tract in patients with extensive injuries. J Trauma 32:570, 1992.
31. Kimura A, Mochizuki T, Nishizawa K, Mashiko K, Yamamoto Y, Otsuka T. trimethoprim-sulfamethoxazole for the prevention of methicillin-resistant *Staphylococcus aureus* pneumonia in severely burned patients. J Trauma 45:383, 1998.
32. Boucher BA, Kuhl DA, Hickerson WL. Pharmacokinetics of systemically administered antibiotics in patients with thermal injury. Clin Infect Dis 14:458, 1992.
33. Mason AD Jr, McManus AT, Pruitt BA Jr. Association of burn mortality and bacteremia: a 25 year review. Arch Surg 121:1027, 1986.
34. Boucher BA, Kuhl DA, Hickerson WL. Pharmacokinetics of systemically administered antibiotics in patients with thermal injury. Clin Infect Dis 14:458, 1992.
35. Sasaki TM, Welch GW, Herndon DN, Kaplan JZ, Lindberg RB, Pruitt BA, Jr. Burn wound manipulation-induced bacteremia. J Trauma 19:46, 1979.
36. DiGiovine B, Chenoweth C, Watts C, Higgins M. The attributable mortality and costs of primary nosocomial bloodstream infections in the intensive care unit. Am J Respir Crit Care Med 160:976, 1999.
37. Franceschi D, Gerding RL, Phillips G, Fratianne RB. Risk factors associated with intravascular catheter infections in burned patients: A

prospective randomized study. J Trauma 29:811, 1989.

38. Peck MD, Weber J, McManus A, Sheridan R, Heimbach D. Surveillance of burn wound infections: A proposal for definitions. J Burn Care Rehabil 19:386, 1998.
39. McManus AL, Kim SH, McManus WF, Mason AD, Pruitt BA. Comparison of quantitative microbiology and histopathology in divided burn-wound biopsy speciments. Arch Surg 122:74, 1997.
40. Van Saene HKF, Nicolai JPA. The prevention of wound infections in burn patients. Scand J Plastic Reconst Surg 13:63, 1979.
41. Mozingo DW, McManus AT, Pruitt BA. Infections in Burn Wounds. In Bennettt JV, Brachman PS (eds). Hospital Infections. 4th Edn. New York: Lippincott-Raven, 1998:587.

53. INFECTIOUS DISEASES IN TOXIC EPIDERMAL NECROLYSIS

José M. Arévalo, José A. Lorente, Carlos González-Herrada, José Jiménez-Reyes, Carlos Santonja and Paloma Garcia-Hierro

Summary

Lyell's syndrome or toxic epidermal necrolysis (TEN) is a diffuse exfoliative cutaneous disease with systemic involvement. The initial pathogenic mechanism involves T-cell mediated immunological skin damage triggered by the ingestion of drugs. The key subsequent event is an extensive epidermal detachment from the underlying dermis and exposure of extensive areas of denuded skin, inducing pathophysiological changes similar to those observed in superficial dermal burns. The disease is also characterized by loss of mucosal membranes, fever, systemic toxicity and an increased risk of infection and respiratory failure. Complications of TEN are similar to those observed in burned patients, including repeated episodes of sepsis and bacteremia, shock and sequential organ dysfunction.

The risk of infection is increased due to (i) the loss of the skin barrier function; (ii) a state of immunocompromise associated with TEN by itself; (iii) immunosuppressive therapy; (iv) mucositis that predisposes to bacterial colonization; (v) wound care promoting bacterial translocation; and (vi) techniques for cardiovascular monitoring or organ function support (i.e., intravascular access, endotracheal intubation) that violate the normal defense mechanisms. The incidence rate of infectious complications in patients with TEN, including bacteremia and pneumonia, is high. Mortality is primarily due to sepsis.

These concepts (immunological etiology, extensive dermal loss, sepsis-related mortality) provide the basis for what is considered by many specialists to be the modern treatment of this condition, which is based on: (i) the realization of the clinical and pathophysiological similarities between TEN and superficial burns; (ii) early transfer to an Intensive Care Burn Unit (ICBU), where expertise in the management of extensive skin loss can be provided by a multidisciplinary team; (iii) general supportive care, with emphasis on fluid therapy; (iv) adequate immunosuppressive treatment; (v) prevention and early treatment of infection; (vi) dermal coverage with skin substitutes; and (vii) nursing care and prevention of sequelae, with particular attention to corneal damage.

In this clinical scenario, it is clear that diagnosis and early treatment of infection is of utmost importance. The diagnosis of infection may be delayed since signs of infection are nonspecific and can be attributed to the systemic inflammatory response syndrome rather than to the presence of infection. Treatment of infection in patients with TEN must consider the high incidence of infectious complications, the immunocompromise state and the relationship between sepsis and mortality in these patients. The risk of infection, as in burns, remains high as long as the wound has not healed. Therefore, attempts to achieve an early epithelialization (by nutritional support, adequate immunosuppressive therapy and surgical wound care) have to be considered part of the measures for infection prevention and treatment.

Definition and Demographics

Toxic epidermal necrolysis was first described by Lyell in 1956 [1] as an exfoliative skin disease of sudden onset that may involve a large body surface area (BSA) as well as mucosal surfaces. Considerable confusion exists in the differential diagnosis of exfoliative cutaneous diseases, such as erythema exudativum multiforme (EEM), Stevens-Johnson syndrome (SJS) and TEN. It is sustained by some authors that all belong to the spectrum of the same disease with different degrees of skin involvement. EEM is associated with the recurrent typical target lesions occurring after infections (i.e., Herpes simplex, Mycoplasma pneumoniae), and has no associated mortality. SJS is characterized by exfoliative skin lesions, purpuric maculae and diffuse blistering, involving less than 30% of BSA and may be associated with considerable mortality (ranging between 0% and 38%). Finally, TEN involves more than 30% of BSA, and more than 1 mucosal surface [2–4].

Incidence of TEN is between one and three cases per million population per year [5, 6]. It is more frequent in adult women. Mortality varies widely in the different reported series, ranging from 25% to 80% [7, 8], and is probably strongly influenced by therapy. Extremes of age, the presence of comorbidity, previous use of corticosteroids, and delay in the ICBU referral, are factors that have been identified in different studies as indicators of a worse prognosis [8–10].

Etiology and Pathogenesis

TEN is characterized by an immunologically-mediated skin necrosis induced by the ingestion of drugs. An antecedent of drug ingestion is, however, not always obtained. A history of a potentially offending drug is obtained in 77%–94% of cases of TEN (less often in SJS). Drugs more commonly involved include antibiotics, antiinflammatory and anticonvulsant agents [5, 11, 12]. An infectious etiology (Mycoplasma pneumoniae and Herpes simplex infections) common in EEM, has been invoked in certain cases of SJS but not in TEN [5, 11–14].

Certain diseases have been associated with the development of TEN, such as Crohn's disease, ulcerative colitis, systemic lupus erythematosus, leukemia, graft versus host disease (GVHD), and infections caused by Epstein-Barr, influenza and human immune deficiency virus (HIV). In one series, 22% of cases with TEN had HIV infection [15].

The pathogenesis of TEN is not completely understood [13, 16, 17]. Clinical, histological and immunological similarities between TEN and graft versus host disease (GVHD) suggest an abnormality in the T cell-mediated immunity [18]. Both TEN and GVHD are characterized by lymphopenia, depletion of CD4 lymphocytes, and dermoepidermal junction necrosis with a minimal dermal lymphohistiocytic infiltrate.

Clinical Manifestations

The appearance of skin rash is usually preceded by a flu-like syndrome, with fever and general malaise [19]. The patient may have been taking the potentially offending drug for some time before for another indication (i.e., arthritis, gout, epilepsy), or may have started taking it coinciding with the flu episode. Usually one to three weeks after taking the medication, a skin rash appears. The development of the skin disorder after drug ingestion is idiosyncratic, dose-independent, and may progress even after drug discontinuation. The skin rash, initially noted as purpuric macules or papules, involves in a symmetric fashion the face, neck and upper thorax, and is painful and burning. The rash rapidly progresses over the first 2–3 days, sometimes over a few hours. The presence of the Nikolski's sign (epidermal detachment upon a slight digital abrasion) is useful to support the diagnosis of TEN (Figure 1). Skin lesions coalesce and form

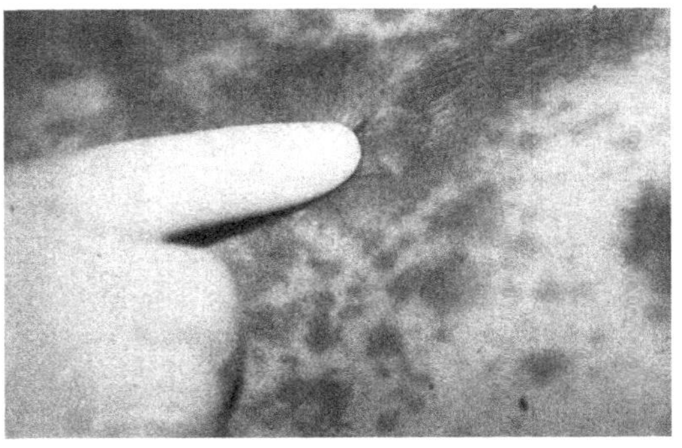

FIGURE 1. Nikolski's sign in a patient with toxic epidermal necrolysis. It is appreciated that apparently normal skin is easily removed upon slight digital abrassion.

A

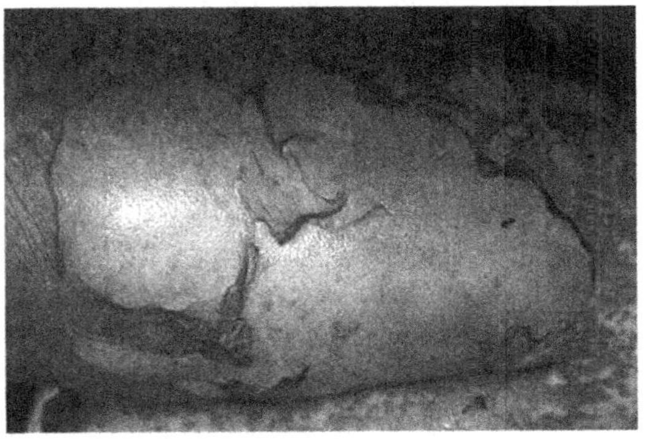

B

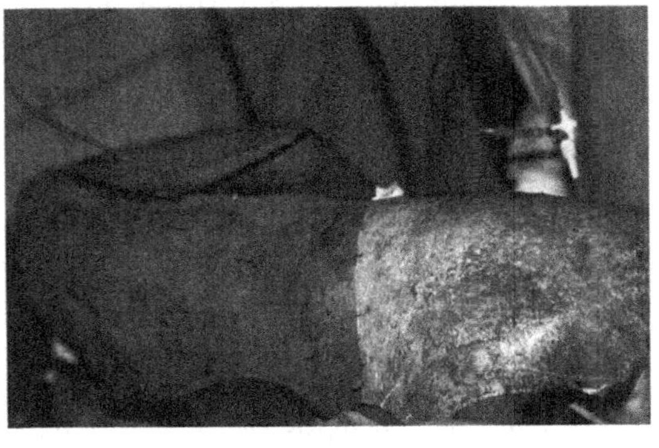

FIGURE 2. *Panel A*. Large skin areas showing epidermal detachment on the back of a patient with toxic epidermal necrolysis. Blisters easily break leaving large areas of exposed dermis. *Panel B*. After skin debridement of all necrotic and sloughed skin, a skin substitute (Biobrane) is applied to decrease fluid losses and pain.

diffuse bullae of different sizes. Large blisters break spontaneously or after minor trauma, leaving large areas of exposed dermis and detached and wrinkled epidermal remnants (Figure 2). Loss of a large skin surface area is associated with intense pain, fluid and electrolyte losses, heat losses, and increased risk of infection. Patients are usually prostrated, febrile, and appear "toxic". The appearance of TEN in this phase resembles that of superficial burns [8, 11].

More than 90% of patients with TEN present three or more mucosal sites involved. Mucosal damage (i) facilitates dermal colonization, due to the loss of the skin barrier, the normal presence of bacteria in septic sites (i.e., mouth, oropharynx), and the persistence of necrotic epidermal tissue; and (ii) may result in the formation of synechiae in the oral, otic, vaginal or conjunctival mucosae (further decreasing the ability to clear microorganisms). Particularly serious are eye complications, which include conjunctivitis, symblepharon, ectropion, entropion and corneal scarring with loss of vision [4, 20].

Oral and gastroesophagical mucosal involvement causes severe dysphagia, epiglottal swelling, diffuse bleeding, esophagitis, and gastrointestinal lesions resembling ulcerative or pseudomembranous colitis macroscopically [10, 21].

Bronchial mucosal detachment gives rise to inflammation of the upper airway, formation of fibrin casts, and alveolar cell desquamation, resulting in atelectasis, pulmonary edema, and infectious complications [10, 22, 23].

Involvement of external genitalia may originate phymosis in men and vaginal synechiae in women.

Diagnosis

The diagnosis should be suspected on the bases of a history of drug ingestion and a flu-like syndrome, and the appearance of the typical skin lesions with positive Nikoslki's sign (Figure 1). The diagnosis is confirmed by a skin biopsy.

The histopathological diagnosis of TEN is based on the finding of extensive keratinocyte necrosis associated with basal hydropic degeneration, leading to dermoepidermal detachment and bullae formation, and a mild dermal inflammatory infiltrate (Figure 3). Cellular components of the infiltrate are T cells with helper phenotype [24] or macrophages and dermal dendrocytes [25].

Different histological phases can be observed in the same biopsy, corresponding to different clinical stages of evolving lesions. The borders of the clinical lesions are characterized by isolated necrotic keratinocytes accompanied by moderate dermal inflammation. The central dark red areas correspond to areas of extensive necrosis of keratinocytes, subepidermal bullae and dermoepidermal detachment (Figure 3). Erythematosus peripheral areas correspond to intense papillary dermal edema, capillary plexus dilatation, vasodilatation, endothelial cell edema and mononuclear perivascular infiltrate. The reticullary dermis is normal [26].

Laboratory tests are consistent with the pathophysiological changes alluded to above, and are therefore nonspecific. There may be slight liver enzymes elevation, increase in BUN and serum creatinine concentration, thrombocytopenia, leukopenia and albuminuria. These laboratory changes may also appear in sepsis, and do not confirm or rule out the presence of infection [27].

Differential diagnosis includes EEM and staphylococcal scalded skin syndrome (SSSS). EEM is characterized by target lesions, is usually accompanied by signs of Mycoplasmal or herpetic infection, and has a benign and recurrent course. SSSS is due to a staphylococcal toxin. A skin biopsy shows intraepidermal blistering, with separation occurring in the midgranular layer (therefore, more superficial than in TEN). SSSS is associated with a mortality rate of 4% in children and 40% in adults [26]. The differential diagnosis should also include chemical burns, septic shock and various bullous skin diseases [2, 28].

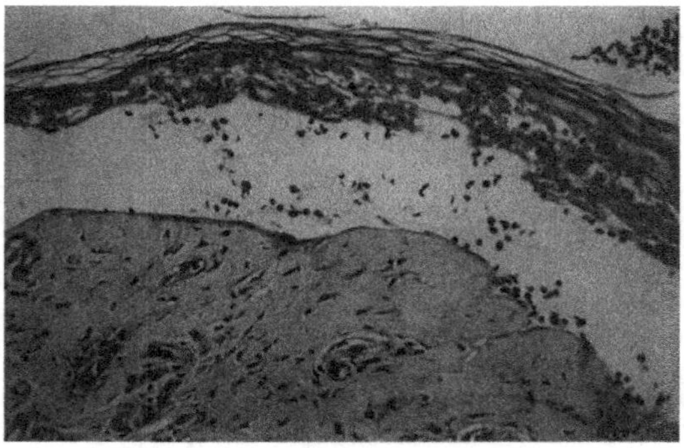

FIGURE 3. Skin biopsy from a patient with toxic epidermal necrolysis (Hematoxylin-Eosin, ×200), showing necrosis of the epidermis, detachment at the dermoepidermal junction and mild dermal mononuclear infiltrate.

Infectious Complications in TEN

The risk of infection in patients with TEN is increased because of a variety of mechanisms: (i) the loss of the skin barrier function and the exposure of extensive areas of denuded skin makes it more likely the passage of bacteria from the skin surface to the circulation; (ii) TEN by itself is associated with a state of immunocompromise; (iii) immunosuppressive therapy is usually administered to control the disease progression; (iv) mucosal damage (particularly airway mucositis), resulting in necrotic tissue and abundant exudate formation, predisposes to bacterial colonization and overgrowth; (v) wound care and aggressive debridement of necrotic tissue promotes bacterial translocation; (vi) techniques for monitoring or organ function support (i.e., intravascular access, endotracheal intubation) violate the normal defense mechanisms, as it occurs in other critically ill patients.

Mortality in these patients is most frequently due to infection and sepsis. Sepsis is very often manifested by subtle signs such as hypothermia, leukopenia or decreased mental status [29, 30]. These signs are nonspecific, and can be due to the underlying disease and the subsequent inflammatory response syndrome. Thus a high index of clinical suspicion for the diagnosis of infection is required. Failure to recognize signs of infection because they are attributed to the underlying inflammatory process rather than to infection, may result in a fatal delay in antimicrobial therapy. Management in the ICBU is most appropriate for early detection of signs of sepsis and timely antimicrobial treatment.

All published clinical series of patients with TEN report a high incidence of infections. Halebian *et al.* [9, 31] reported that 20 of 30 patients with TEN (BSA involved 71% ± 6%) had infections. Mortality was due in all cases to infection. Although sepsis was equally frequent in patients treated and not treated with corticosteroids, survival after sepsis was higher in the group not treated with corticosteroids. Kelemen *et al.* [8] revised a series of 37 patients (14 of them treated with corticosteroids), with a mean BSA involved of 54% ± 4%. Significant infections occurred in 26 patients (70%) with bacteremia (14/37, 38% of all patients), pneumonia (11/37, 30%) and urinary tract infection (9/37, 24%) being the most common. Infection was more frequent in those patients treated with corticosteroids for more than 48 hr (30% vs 74%). Khoo and Foo [32] studied 23 patients with TEN involving a mean BSA of 52%, and reported that sepsis was present in 14 of 23 patients (61%), respiratory tract infection in 8/23 (35%), urinary tract infection in 4/23 (17%) and skin infection in 2/23 (8%). Causative organisms included MRSA, Pseudomonas, Acinetobacter, Klebsiella, Enterobacter, S. aureus, Proteus and Candida spp. In another series of 19 patients (mean BSA involved 75% ± [SD] 20%), Heimbach *et al.* [33] reported bacteremia in 12/19 (63%), pneumonia in 9/19 (47%). Three died, all of infectious complications.

Thus previous reported series report a high infection rate in patients with TEN, as well as a possible relationship between treatment with corticosteroids and the incidence of infection.

In our series of patients with TEN, most patients (17/24, 71% of cases) suffered at least one episode of infection. Bacteremia, diagnosed in 14 of 24 patients (58%), was the most frequent infectious complication (Table 1).

These 14 patients had 17 episodes of bacteremia (18 bacteria were isolated because one episode was due to two different microorganisms), 12 of which occurred during the first week of ICBU admission (mean 2.9 + [SE] 0.6 days, range 1–6 days), and five were detected after the first week (Table 2). Among cases with early bacteremia (12 cases, 13 bacteria), five were due to Gram-negative bacilli and eight were due to Gram-positive cocci. Among all cases with bacteremia (early or late), in six cases a digestive origin of the bacteremia could be invoked, in five cases the wound, and in four the intravascular catheter (in several cases both the wound and the catheter could be the source of the bacteremia).

Based on these findings of cases with bacteremia, occurring sometimes very early after ICBU admission, and caused in some cases by enteric microorganisms, and in some others

TABLE 1. Infectious complications in patients with toxic epidermal necrolysis (n = 24)

	N (%)
Infection	17 (71)
Bacteremia (*)	
Patients with bacteremia	14 (58)
Episodes of bacteremia	17
Number of bacteria isolated	18
Episodes of early bacteremia (*)	12
Episodes of late bacteremia	5
Pneumonia (†)	
Patients with pneumonia	5 (21)
Episodes of pneumonia	5
Urinary tract infection	
Patients with urinary tract infection	8 (33)
Episodes of urinary tract infection	8

The number of patients in the group of 24 presenting each item is represented.

(*) early and late refer to whether blood cultures were positive within or after the first week of ICBU admission.

(†) Pneumonia was diagnosed by the following criteria: fever (>38.0 C or <35.5 C central temperature), presence of a purulent tracheal aspirate; new and persistent for more than 48 hr x-ray infiltrate; growth of more than 10^5 CFU of a pathogen in the tracheal aspirate; and leukocytosis or leukopenia (>12,000 or <4500 cells/μl).

TABLE 2. Bacteria causing bacteremia, pneumonia and urinary tract infection, and relationship with colonization of other sites and day of diagnosis of infection

	Colonization of other sites (*)	Day of diagnosis
Bacteria causing early bacteremia (12 cases)		
K. pneumonia	Gi	6
E. coli	W	6
E. cloacae	none	2
E. cloacae	W	1
Proteus	Cath/W	1
S. epidermidis	none	2
S. epidermidis	none	1
S. epidermidis	none	4
S. aureus	Cath/W	6
S. aureus	Tr	5
MRSA	Gi	3
MRSA	Tr	2
Enterococcus spp.	Cath/W	3
Bacteria causing late bacteremia (5 cases)		
Hafnia alvei	*Gi*	*47*
A. anitratus	*Cath*	*9*
E. faecalis	*Gi*	*39*
S. epidermidis	*Gi*	*30*
MRSA	*Gi*	*59*
Bacteria causing pneumonia (5 cases)		
S. aureus	Gi, Ph, W	2
S. aureus	none	1
MRSA	none	2
MRSA	W	11
E. faecalis	Gi, Ph	14
Bacteria causing UTI (8 cases)		
Enterococcus spp.	Gi	7
Candida spp.	Gi/W	26
Candida spp.	none	9
Candida spp.	none	22
E coli	Gi	1
P. mirabilis	Tr/W/Gi	59
P. mirabilis	Cath	27
MRSA	Gi	3

Definitions as in Table 1.
(*) Colonization of other sites indicates that the microorganism causing the infection also grew in the catheter tip culture (Cath), in the tracheal aspirate (Tr) culture, or in the rectal (Gi), pharyngeal (Ph) or wound (W) exudate cultures, in the same day or within the preceeding three days of the diagnosis of infection.

by skin microorganisms, we speculate that: mechanical abrasion and debridement of large areas of necrotic and detached skin may facilitate episodes of early bacteremia [34], possibly without having to cause infection *stricto sensu* (invasion of viable dermal tissue). Also, episodes of intestinal hypoperfusion, as has been shown in other critically ill patients, including burn patients, may give rise to intestinal hyperpermeability and subsequent bacterial translocation, which could explain cases of bacteremia due to enteric microorganisms [27, 35, 36].

Pneumonia was diagnosed in five cases, and all were due to Gram-positive cocci, possibly reflecting the primary endogenous origin of the pulmonary infection. The diagnosis of pneumonia was made between day one and day 14 of ICBU admission. Urinary tract infection was diagnosed in eight patients (Table 2).

Our results indicate that (i) infectious complications occur very frequently in patients with TEN; (ii) bacteria causing bacteremia may originate in the wound or in the digestive tract; and (iii) bacteremia may occur very early after ICBU admission. These observations have important therapeutic implications (vide infra).

In summary, patients with TEN, like burn patients, are immunocompromised, have an increased risk of infection, and sepsis is the most important cause of death. Although signs of sepsis are nonspecific, they must prompt an aggressive diagnostic search for infection and the appropriate antimicrobial therapy. Sometimes, leukopenia or hypothermia are the only signs anticipating the isolation of Gram-negative rods or MRSA in the blood. The condition of these patients does not allow for an expectant approach until the results of the different cultures are obtained, and antimicrobial therapy has to be started as soon as the infection is suspected.

Treatment: General Concepts and Resuscitation

Recent advances in treatment strategies for TEN have been accompanied by a reduction in the mortality rate of this condition from about 70% to about 20% [33]. We believe that morbidity and mortality in TEN can be minimized by: (i) realization of the clinical and pathophysiological similarities between TEN and superficial burns; (ii) early transfer to an ICBU; (iii) general supportive care, with emphasis on fluid therapy; (iv) adequate immunosuppressive treatment, (v) prevention and early treatment of infection; (vi) dermal coverage with skin substitutes; (vii) nursing care and prevention of sequelae, with particular attention to corneal damage.

Patients with TEN suffer extensive epidermal loss, which is associated with fluid loss, hypermetabolism, increased risk of sepsis, pain, and hypothermia. These complications are similar to those presented by burn patients. Therapy of TEN is therefore based on the same principles as those of burn patients [19, 37].

There are studies indicating that *early transfer to an ICBU* may improve the prognosis of these patients [8, 9, 31]. A recently published series of patients treated in burn centers report a mortality rate of 10% [32]. Appropriate multidisciplinary team management and expertise in the treatment of the pathophysiological changes and complications associated with extensive skin loss can be provided most adequately in the ICBU.

General supportive care includes monitoring, fluid resuscitation, and cardiovascular, respiratory and nuritional support. *Monitoring* requires an intravenous line, preferably peripheral and inserted through noninvolved skin [38]. An arterial line and a Foley catheter are also required for hemodynamic monitoring. Insertion of a nasogastric tube is very often indicated to warrant sufficient protein and calorie intake in the presence of gastroesophageal lesions and dysphagia that preclude spontaneous oral intake [38–40].

Fluid resuscitation is the first concern upon ICBU admission, once basic hemodynamic monitoring (insertion of venous and arterial lines) has been performed, and pulmonary function has be warranted (i.e., by endotracheal intubation if indicated). Fluid requirements of patients with TEN are not as high as in patients with burns of similar BSA involved, because the exfoliated areas in TEN do not exudate as much fluid as in thermal burns. However, insensible fluid losses may be considerably high, and patients may develop hypovolemia and severe hypernatremia over a few hours. Therefore, fluid losses should not be underestimated, and the patient's intravascular volume status should be adequately assessed [16, 41, 42].

Particular attention has to be paid to *respiratory function*. Respiratory failure may ensue in patients with TEN due to a variety of mechanisms. Bronchial mucosal involvement may cause airway obstruction, respiratory difficulty, hypoxemia due to atelectasis and ventilation/perfusion mismatch, and accumulation of bronchial secretions due to pain and difficulty in coughing. These patients are also at risk of presenting noncardiogenic pulmonary edema, cardiogenic pulmonary edema (due to overzealous fluid resuscitation in patients with compromised cardiac function), or pneumonia [23, 41]. As in burns, a large BSA exposed and the associated hypercatabolism increase ventilatory requirements that may not be well tolerated if respiratory reserve is decreased [43]. Thus, there are numerous potential indications for endotracheal intubation and mechanical ventilation in patients with TEN.

TEN is associated with a hypercatabolic state. Calorie and protein requirements are increased, although not as much as in burns of comparable BSA involved. Thus *nutritional support* must provide adequate nutrients to support the immune function, prevent infection, speed the epithelialization process, and support intestinal mucosal cell turnover [39]. There are no studies of the nutritional requirements of patients with TEN. In a series of 19 patients with TEN (mean BSA involved 75% ± [SD] 20%), weight stability and positive nitrogen balance were achieved by providing 2500 kcal per day [33].

Skin care is extremely painful, particularly on admission, when large areas of necrotic skin have to be debrided. Under these circumstances, *analgesia* with ketamine (iv boluses of 1 mg/kg until the desired effect is achieved), preceded by a small dose of midazolam (to decrease the risk of hallucinations), is adequate. This analgesic regimen induces the desired level of analgesia, and does not depress respiratory function, being very useful in nonintubated patients. In intubated patients, opiates, benzodiazepines, and muscle relaxants if necessary, are administered during wound care [44].

Nursing and general care includes a particular attention towards mucosal damage prevention and treatment. In general, mucosal damage has to be more aggressively treated during the first week, the period of time over which epithelial detachment and exudate formation with the subsequent risk of superinfection and formation of sequelae are most important. Oral mucosal care includes washings with clorhexidine 4–6 times a day as well as debridement of necrotic tissue in the oropharynx with swabs. These maneuvers avoid synechiae formation and obstruction of salivary gland ducts. External auditory duct also requires daily hygienic measures and debridement of necrotic tissue. Synechiae formation has to be prevented also in the genital mucosa, to prevent future dysfunction [45].

Conjunctival mucosa needs close monitoring, to treat the frequent and severely disabling sequelae that may appear (vide supra) [45]. An *ophthalmologist consultation* is required on the same day of admission and daily thereafter. Treatment includes administration of artificial tears, topical antibiotics, and conjunctival debridement. A few cases will still require surgical treatment [46–48]. We have recently included the administration of topical cyclosporin A (CSA) 2% every 6 hr as part of the eye treatment.

Adequate Immunosuppressive Treatment

Corticosteroid treatment is generally recommended in an attempt to inhibit antibody-mediated cytotoxicity [9, 19]. However, the practice of administering high-dose corticosteroids throughout the course of the disease has clearly fallen out of favor [10].

In early reports of TEN patients treated with corticosteroids, nearly 75% of patients treated with large doses of corticosteroids succumbed to sepsis, and patients with more than 50% BSA involved rarely survived [9, 10]. Compared with historical experience, treatment of TEN patients without corticosteroids was associated with a much lower mortality rate (33% versus 66%) [9].

The use of corticosteroids for more than 48 h was associated in a descriptive analysis of 37 patients with a two-fold increase in the incidence of infection (30% vs 64%), longer hospital stay (16 vs 40 days) and increased mortality rate (4% vs 50%) [8].

Although available evidence indicates that treatment with corticosteroids is of little benefit and may in fact be harmful [8, 32] the lack of a prospective randomized trial has made the assessment of the effectiveness of this therapy difficult [8–10, 32, 33, 49, 50].

Most centers stop systemic corticosteroids upon admission. The proponents of steroid therapy yet defend that the benefit is mostly seen in preexfoliative cases, and cases with slow progression [51–53].

Cyclophosphamide (CPM) has also been used as an immunosuppressive agent in TEN. Treatment with CPM is frequently associated with leukopenia, lymphopenia and a high infection risk [54–57].

Based on the clinical and histological similarities between TEN and GVHD, it was proposed that CSA could be effective in patients with TEN [18, 58]. CSA acts on CD4 lymphocytes, inhibiting IL-2 synthesis and release as well as the proliferation of activated T cells. CSA has no effect on CD8 lymphocytes or B cells [59, 60]. Only a total of nine cases of TEN treated with CSA (in conjunction with or after corticosteroids) have been reported in the literature [61–67].

We have treated with CSA at the moment of this writing 11 consecutive patients with TEN

TABLE 3. Comparison between some demographic and outcome measurements in patients with TEN treated with cyclophosphamide and corticosteroids or cyclosporin A

	Cyclophosphamide n = 6	Cyclosporin A n = 11	p (a)
Age (b)	56 ± 9	42 ± 20	0.12
% surface area (c)	77 ± 18	83 ± 17	0.52
Survived (d)	3/6	11/11	0.029
Delay to admission (e)	6.3 ± 3.2	7.4 ± 3.9	0.56
Time to arrest (f)	3.6 ± 1.5	1.4 ± 0.3	0.0002
Time to re-epithelialization (g)	17.6 ± 3.1	12.0 ± 3.6	0.0058
LOS (h)	15 ± 8	27 ± 25	0.31
Sepsis (i)	5/6	8/11	0.99
Organ failure (j)	2.3 ± 1.8	1.1 ± 1.2	0.11
Organ failure (≥4) (k)	3/6	2/11	0.029
Leukopenia (l)	4/6	0/11	0.006

(a) p value. Two-tailed unpaired Student's t test for quantitative variables or Fisher's exact test for qualitative variables
(b) Age in years
(c) Body surface area involved (%)
(d) Patients surviving to hospital discharge
(e) Time from initiation of signs of the skin disorder to hospital admission (days)
(f) Time from onset of treatment to arrest of disease progression (days)
(g) Time from onset of treatment to complete re-epithelialization (days)
(h) Intensive Care Burn Unit length of stay (days)
(i) Number of cases with sepsis, as defined in [29]
(j & k) Number of organs failing, as defined in [30], for the following organs or systems: lungs, cardiovascular, kidneys, liver, gastrointestinal, hematological, metabolic
(l) Patients with leukopenia (<1000 cells/μl), requiring administration of granulocyte colony stimulating factor. Data are mean ± SD.
Reproduced from J Trauma, with permission.

(Table 3) [68]. All patients had received corticosteroids, which were discontinued upon ICBU admission. Our experience with this immunosuppressive regimen, as compared with the historical control group treated with corticosteroids and cyclophosphamide, indicates that CSA treatment is associated with a more rapid arrest of the disease progression and reepithelialization rate, as well as with a lesser mortality. Although we recognize the limitations of the comparison with a historical control group, our study suggests that treatment with CSA is safe and probably more effective than with CPM.

Prevention and Early Treatment of Infection

The intimate relationship between the underlying disease (characterized by epidermal loss and immunocompromise) and the development of infectious complications help understand why treatment of infection is not just one more issue in the management of patients with TEN. All interventions aimed at achieving successful resuscitation (fluid therapy and maintenance of tissue perfusion), early wound healing (wound debridement and coverage with skin substitutes and immunosuppressive therapy), and supporting the immune system (enteral nutrition) are part of the infection prevention and treatment program.

Microbiological surveillance is an important aspect of infection control. We routinely obtain surveillance samples from the oropharynx, rectum and skin, on admission and twice a week from every patient admitted to our ICBU. Microbiological surveillance may help define the particular microbiological profile in our unit, and detect the state of carrier of resistant microorganisms. This information can then be used to (i) better define empirical antibiotic regimens for septic patients until culture results are received, (ii) eradicate resistant microorganisms.

In our series of 24 cases, 12 had bacteremia during the first week after ICBU admission (one case was due to two different microorganism). Causative bacteria included both Gram-negative bacilli in five cases (K. pneumonia, E. coli, P. mirabilis and E. cloacae in two cases) and Gram-positive cocci in another eight cases. Thus empirical antibiotic therapy must cover both Gram-positive and Gram-negative bacteria, including resistant strains (i.e., MRSA) in patients coming from other institutions, where they may have acquired these resistant pathogens. We also detected five more episodes of bacteremia after the first week of ICBU admission. The clinical utility of surveillance cultures is suggested by the finding that 11 of the 18 isolated microorganisms, the bacteria were cultured in a surveillance sample (wound or rectal exudate). In two more cases the bacteria growing in the blood were also detected in the tracheal aspirate culture, and in four cases in the catheter tip culture (some bacteria grew in more than one sample, i.e., in the wound exudate and in the catheter tip culture). In only four cases no source of the bacteremia could be detected. Thus performing the appropriate cultures helps anticipate which bacteria are causing infection and bacteremia in a septic patient.

We also diagnosed five cases of pneumonia, caused by Gram-positive cocci in all cases (S. Aureus in two, MRSA in two, and E. faecalis in one). Diagnosis was made between day 1 and day 14 of ICBU admission. Therefore, empirical treatment of pneumonia must cover Gram-positive cocci.

Given (i) the high incidence of infectious complications in TEN, (ii) the state of immunodeficiency of these patients, and (iii) the relationship between sepsis and mortality, we recommend the initiation of antibiotic treatment as soon as sepsis is suspected, until the diagnosis of infection is ruled out (i.e., when appropriate cultures turned out to be negative). A delay in this therapy may make the patient's clinical condition irreversible. In our series the diagnosis of severe infections very early after ICBU admission is not uncommon. Thus, the appearance of signs such as fever or hypothermia, or leukocytosis or leukopenia, should prompt an aggressive search for an infection source and the initiation of empirical antimicrobial therapy [27, 50].

Surgical Treatment: Dermal Coverage with Skin Substitutes

Surgical treatment of patients with TEN is based on the same principles as for burn patients. On admission, the BSA affected, the stage of the different lesions and the extent of mucosal damage have to be determined. This assessment can be performed in the ICBU under adequate analgesia [44]. Exhaustive debridement by mechanical abrasion of all affected areas is performed, leaving the affected dermis exposed. We generally use for this debridement liquid clorhexidine 0.1% [69, 70]. This procedure is repeated until all loose skin and blisters, as well a areas with positive Nikolski's sign (easy removal of apparently normal skin) are removed (Figures 1 and 2).

Thereafter, the exposed dermis have to be covered with a skin substitute, such as porcine xenografts or criopreserved allografts [9, 33, 71]. Skin coverage provides the dermis with an environment mimicking the normal skin. We prefer the use of Biobrane (Down Hickman Pharmaceuticals Inc.; Sugar Land, Texas), since availability limitations, risk of infection transmission, and requirement of special storage conditions make other biological coverings less desirable [72, 73]. Biobrane is a semisynthetic skin substitute composed of a net of nylon and purified porcine collagen, and an external layer of nylon, which allows the passage of fluids [74–76]. Sheets of Biobrane are fixed to the dermis by metallic of reabsorbible staples (Figure 2). After this procedure, the patient should remain in bed for two days to facilitate the adherence of the biomaterial to the underlying dermis. Elastic wrappings or the application of topical antiseptics are not required. The patient is free to move after adherence is observed, and staples can be retired. As the epithelialization process progresses, sheets of biobrane become brittle and spontaneously come off. These areas are trimmed as the underlying dermis heals, and the skin is covered with vaseline [45, 77, 78].

If a biological skin substitute such as Biobrane is used, it is of utmost importance to continue inspection of covered areas for the detection of purulent material that may accumulate between the dermis and the biomaterial. Failure to identify these focus of infection may promote bacterial overgrowth and severe sepsis. If purulent material is detected under the biomaterial, immediate drainage and removal of the sheets of the biomaterial have to be performed [78, 79].

Biobrane has the advantage of easy inspection of the epithelialization process and of the appearance of potential complications. It helps control pain, decreases fluid losses, prevents hypothermia, controls bacterial colonization, and possibly accelerates the epithelialization process. On the other hand, unlike other biological coverings, it does not require frequent changes [33, 34, 72, 75–80].

Conclusions

TEN is a systemic disease that is best treated in an ICBU, were expertise in the treatment of syndromes of extensive skin loss can be provided to attain the best clinical outcomes. Management is similar to that of superficial burns, including fluid resuscitation, nutritional support, and skin debridement and coverage with skin substitutes. In addition, immunosuppressive therapy, as well as treatment and prevention of mucosal damage (corneal involvement may lead to blindness) are important aspects in the therapy of patients with TEN.

Infections, particularly episodes of bacteremia, are very frequent complications in patients with TEN, sometimes appearing very shortly after their ICBU admission. Death is most frequently related to septic complications.

The risk of infection is increased due to epidermal loss, immunocompromise, aggressive wound care and mucositis. The risk of sepsis remains high as long as the skin has not healed. Thus, all those measures aimed at achieving early epithelialization, such as skin debridement, immunosuppressive therapy and skin coverage with skin substitutes, are part of the infection control program.

Since signs of sepsis may be indistinguishable from those of the underlying inflammatory disease, a high index of clinical suspicion is required for the diagnosis of infection. The high incidence of infections, the sepsis-related mortality and the immunocompromise of patients with TEN make it of the utmost importance the aggressive search of a focus of infections and the early initiation of antimicrobial therapy when infection is suspected.

References

1. Lyell A Toxic epidermal necrolysis an eruption resembling scalding of the skin. Br J Dermatol 68:355, 1956.
2. Bastuji-Garin S, Rzany B, Stern RS, Shear NH, Naldi L, Roujeau JC. Clinical classification of cases of toxic epidermal necrolysis, Stevens-Johnson syndrome and erythema multiforme. Arch Dermatol 129:92, 1993.
3. Patterson R, Dykewicz MS, Gonzales A. Erythema multiforme and Stevens-Johnson syndrome: descriptive and therapeutic controversy. Chest 98:331, 1990.
4. Wilkins J, Morrison L, White CR. Occulo-cutaneous manifestations of the erythema multiforme/Stevens-Johnson syndrome/toxic epidermal necrolysis spectrum. Dermatol Cline 10:571, 1992.
5. Roujeau JC, Kelly JP, Nalco L. Medication use and the risk of Steven's-Johnson syndrome or toxic epidermal necrolysis. N Engl J Med 333:1600, 1995.

6. Chan HL, Stern RS, Ardnt KA. The incidence of erythema multiforme, Steven's-Johnson syndrome and toxic epidermal necrolysis: a population-based study with particular reference to reactions caused by drugs among outpatients. Arch Dermatol 126:43, 1990.
7. Zoltie N, Verlende P, O'Neill S, McKenzie AW. Lyell's syndrome on a burn unit. Burns 204:368, 1994.
8. Kelemen III JJ, Cioffi WC, McManus WF, Mason AD, Pruitt BA. Burn center care for patients with toxic epidermal necrolysis. J Am Coll Surg 180:273, 1995.
9. Halebian PH, Madden MR, Finkelstein JL. Improved burn center survival of patients with toxic epidermal necrolysis managed without corticosteroids. Ann Surg 204:503, 1986.
10. Herndon DN. Toxic epidermal necrolysis: a systemic and dermatologic disorder best treated with standard treatment protocols in burn intensive care units without the prolonged use of corticosteroids. J Am Coll Surg 180:340, 1995.
11. Revuz J, Penson D, Roujeau JC. Toxic epidermal necrolysis: clinical findings and prognostic factors in 87 patients. Arch Dermatol 123:1160, 1987.
12. Roujeau JC, Stern RS. Severe cutaneous adverse reactions to drugs. N Engl J Med 331:1272, 1994.
13. Correia O, Chosidow O, Saiag P, Bastuji-Garin S, Revuz J, Roujeau JC. Evolving pattern of drug induced toxic epidermal necrolysis. Dermatology 186:32, 1993.
14. Prendiville JS, Hebert AA, Greewald MJ, Esterly NB. Management of Stevens-Johnson syndrome and toxic epidermal necrolysis in children. J Pediatr 115:881, 1987.
15. Saiag P, Caumes E, Chosidow O. Drug induced toxic epidermal necrolysis (Lyell's syndrome) in patients infected with the human immunodeficiency virus. J Am Acad Dermatol 26:567, 1992.
16. Roujeau JC, Revuz J. Toxic epidermal necrolysis: An expanding field of knowledge. J Am Acad Dermatol 31:301, 1994.
17. Parsons JM. Toxic epidermal necrolysis. Int J Dermatol 31:749, 1992.
18. Peck GL, Herzig GP, Elias PM. Toxic epidermal necrolysis in a patient with graft vs host reaction. Arch Dermatol 105:561, 1972.
19. Avakian R, Flowers FP, Araujo OE, Ramos Careo FA. Toxic epidermal necrolysis: A review. J Am Acad Dermatol 25:69, 1991.
20. Arévalo JM, Lorente JA. Necrolisis epidérmica tóxica. Tendencias terapeúticas. Anales de Medicina Interna (Madrid, Spain) (*in Spanish*) 15:67, 1998.
21. Chosidow O, Delcjier JG, Chaumette MT. Intestinal involvement in drug-induced toxic epidermal necrolysis. Lancet 337:923, 1991.
22. Whale D, Beste D, Conley SF. Laryngeal involvement in toxic epidermal necrolysis. Otolaryngol Head Neck Surg 6:796, 1992.
23. Lebargy F, Wolkenstein P, Gisselbrecht M, Lange F, Fleury-Feith J. Pulmonary complications in toxic epidermal necrolysis: A prospective clinical study. Intensive Care Med 23:1237, 1997.
24. Villada G, Roujeau JC, Clérici T, Bourgault Y, Revuz J. Immunopathology of toxic epidermal necrolysis. Arch Dermatol 128:50, 1992.
25. Paquet P, Pierard GE. Erythema multiforme and toxic epidemal necrolysis: A comparative study. Am J Dermatol 19:127, 1997.
26. Roujeau JC, Chosidow O, Saiag P, Guillaume JC. Toxic epidermal necrolysis (Lyell's syndrome). J Am Acad Dermatol 23:1039, 1990.
27. Arévalo JM, Lorente JA. Fiebre y leucopenia en un paciente con rash maculopapular progresivo tras un proceso gripal. In Rello J, Vallés J (eds). Casos clínicos en infecciones graves. Trucos y trampas. Barcelona: EdikaMed, 1998: 23.
28. Green D, Law E, Still M. An approach to the management of toxic epidermal necrolysis in a burn center. Burns 195:411, 1993.
29. Bone RC, Balk RA, Cerra FB. The ACCP/SCCM consensus conference committe. Definitions for sepsis and organ failure and guidelines for the use of innovative therapies. Chest 101:1644, 1992.
30. Marshall JC. Criteria for the description of organ dysfunction in sepsis and SIRS. In Fein AM, Abraham EM, Balk RA, Bernard GR, Bone RC, Dantzer DR, Fink MP (eds). Sepsis and multiorgan failure. Baltimore: Williams and Wilkins, 1997: 286.
31. Halebian P, Corder V, Herndon DN. A burn center experience with toxic epidermal necrolysis. J Burn Care Rehabil 4:176, 1983.
32. Khoo AKM, Foo CL. Toxic epidermal necrolysis in a burn center: A 6 year review. Burns 22:275, 1996.
33. Heimbach DM, Engrav LV, Marvin JA. Toxic epidermal necrolysis: A step forward in treatment. JAMA 257:2171, 1987.
34. Kucan JO. Use of Biobrane in the treatment of toxic epidermal necrolysis. J Burn Care Rehabil 16:324, 1995.
35. Arévalo JM, Lorente JA, Gordo F, Tejedor C, Pascual T, Esteban A. Cambios en la perfusión de la mucosa intestinal inducidos por dobutamina

en pacientes quemados críticos. Medicina Intensiva (Barcelona) 21:147, 1997.

36. Lorente JA, Ezpeleta A, Esteban A, Arévalo JM. Hemodynamic and gastric pCO2 changes in critically ill burned patients. Crit Care Med, 28:1728–1735, 2000.
37. Timsit JF, Mion G, Gulluche YL. Severe hypothermia occurring during the course of toxic epidermal necrolysis in patients treated with air fluidized beds. Arch Dermatol 127:147, 1991.
38. Arévalo JM, Lorente JA. Tratamiento de la necrolisis epidérmica tóxica. Med Clin (Barc) 111:27, 1998.
39. Finlay AY, Richards J, Holt PJA. Intensive therapy unit management of toxic epidermal necrolysis: Practical aspects. Clin Exp Dermatol 7:55, 1982.
40. Management of toxic epidermal necrolysis (editorial). Lancet 2:1250, 1984.
41. Marvin JA, Heimbach DM, Engrav LH, Harner TJ. Improved treatment of Stevens-Johnson syndrome. Arch Surg 119:601, 1984.
42. Canoso JJ, Barza M. Soft tissue infections. Rheum Dis Clin North Am 15:235, 1993.
43. Lorente JA, Gordo F, Arévalo JM. Cambios hemodinámicos en pacientes con quemaduras. In Lorente JA, Esteban A (eds). Cuidados intensivos del paciente quemado. Barcelona: Springer Verlag Ibérica, 1998: 353.
44. González-Arévalo A, Caro MM, Ortigosa E. Analgesia del paciente quemado. In Lorgnette JA, Esteban A (eds). Cuidados intensivos del paciente quemado. Barcelona: Springer Verlag Ibérica, 1998: 489.
45. Velasco P, Garcia E, Abad E, Lorente JA, Arévalo JM, Casado S. Cuidados de enfermería en el paciente con necrolisis epidérmica tóxica. Enferm Intensiva 10:174, 1999.
46. Bjornberg A, Bjornberg K, Gisslen H. Toxic epidermal necrolysis with ophthalmic complications. Acta Opthalmol 42:1084, 1964.
47. Howard GM. The Stevens-Johnson syndrome, ocular prognosis and treatment. Am J Ophthalmol 55:893, 1963.
48. Roujeau JC, Koso M, Andre C. Sjögren-like syndrome after drug induced toxic epidermal necrolysis. Lancet 2:609, 1985.
49. Lyell A. Toxic epidermal necrolysis, the scalded syndrome: a reappraisal. Br J Dermatol 100:69, 1979.
50. Revuz J, Roujeau JC, Guillaume JC. Treatment of toxic epidermal necrolysis. Creteil's experience. Arch Dermatol 123:1156, 1987.
51. Serfling S. Sudden onset of blisters and ulcerations in a healthy man. Arch Dermatol 129:776, 1993.
52. Tegelberg-Stassen MJAM, van Vloten WA, de la Faille HB. Management of non-staphilococcal toxic epidermal necrolysis: follow up study of 16 case histories. Dermatologica 180:124, 1990.
53. Parsons JM. Management of toxic epidermal necrolysis. Cutis 36:305, 1985.
54. Madalene C, Sunni G. Efficacy of cyclophosphamide in toxic epidermal necrolysis. J Am Acad Dermatol 25:778, 1991.
55. Razzaque AA, Hombal GM. Cyclophosphamide (Cytosan). J Am Acad Dermatol 11:111, 1984.
56. Hertl M, Bohlen H, Merk HF. Efficacy of cyclophosphamide in toxic epidermal necrolysis. J Am Acad Dermatol 129:92, 1993.
57. González-Herrada CM, Jiménez-Reyes J. Necrolisis epidérmica tóxica (síndrome de Lyell). In Lorente JA, Esteban A (eds). Cuidados intensivos del paciente quemado. Barcelona: Springer Verlag Ibérica, 1998: 63.
58. Biren CA, Barr RJ. Dermatologic applications of cyclosporin A. Arch Dermatol 122:1028, 1986.
59. Wagner H. Cyclosporin A: Mechanism of action. Transplant Proc 25:523, 1983.
60. Fredane LM, McCabe RE. The effect of cyclosporin A on lymphocyte subset in experimental allergic encephalomyelitis: functional loss of disease-supressing cells in vivo. Transplant Proc 15:2909, 1983.
61. Renfro L, Grant-Kels JM, Daman LA. Drug induced toxic epidermal necrolysis treated with cyclosporin A. Intern J Derm 28:441, 1989.
62. Hewitt J, Ormerod AD. Toxic epidermal necrolysis treated with cyclosporin A. Clin Exp Derm 17:264, 1992.
63. Szepietwski J, Wasik F, Szybejko-Machaj G, Maj M. Toxic epidermal necrolysis successfully treated with cyclosporin A. Report of three cases. J Eur Acad Dermatol Veneorol 9:169, 1997.
64. Zaki Y, Patel S, Reed R, Dalziel KL. Toxic epidermal necrolysis associated with severe hypocalcemia and treated with cyclosporin A. British J Derm 133:329, 1995.
65. Jarret P, Rademaker M, Havill J, Pullon H. Toxic epidermal necrolysis treated with cyclosporin A and granulocyte colony stimulating factor. Clin Exp Dermatol 22:146, 1997.
66. Jarret P, Ha T, Snow J. Toxic epidermal necrolysis and cyclosporin A. Clin Exp Dermatol 22: 254, 1997.
67. Sullivan JR, Watson A. Lamotrigine induced toxic epidermal necrolysis treated with intra-

venous cyclosporin A: A discussion of pathogenesis and immunosupressive management. Austr J Dermatol 37:208, 1996.
68. Arévalo JM, Lorente JA, González-Herrada CM, Jiménez-Reyes J. Treatment of toxic epidermal necrolysis with cyclosporin A. J Trauma, 48: 473–478, 2000.
69. Taylor JA, Grube B, Heimbach DM. Toxic epidermal necrolysis, a comprehensive approach multidisciplinary management in a burn center. Clin Pediatr 28:404, 1989.
70. Roher TE, Ahmed R. Toxic epidermal necrolysis. Int J Dermatol 30:457, 1991.
71. Yarbrough DR. Experience with toxic epidermal necrolysis treated in a burn center. J Burn Care Rehabil 17:30, 1996.
72. Prasad JK, Feller I, Thompson PD. Use of amnion for the treatment of Stevens-Johnson syndrome. J Trauma 26:945, 1986.
73. Bishop JF, Demling RH, Hansbrough JF, Hansbrough W, Kucan JO, Rodeheaver GT, *et al.* Indications for use of Biobrane in wound management. J Burn Care Rehabil 16:341, 1995.
74. Rodeheaver GT, Harstell MS, Brent C. Influence of Biobrane construction on adherence. J Burn Care Rehabil 16:321, 1995.
75. Smith DJ. Use of Biobrane in wound management. J Burn Care Rehabil 16:317, 1995.
76. Arévalo JM, Gaos L, Lorente JA. Cobertura de la quemadura. In Lorente JA, Esteban A (eds). Cuidados intensivos del paciente quemado. Barcelona: Springer Verlag Ibérica, 1998: 156.
77. Sowder LL. Biobrane wound dressing used in the treatment of toxic epidermal necrolysis: a case report. J Burn Care Rehabil 11:237, 1990.
78. Arévalo JM, Lorente JA. Skin coverage with Biobrane biomaterial for the treatment of patients with toxic epidermal necrolysis. J Burn Care Rehabil 20:406, 1999.
79. Al-Qattan MM. Toxic epidermal necrolysis: a review and report of the successfull use of Biobrane for early wound coverage. Ann Plast Surg 36:224, 1996.
80. Pruitt BA, Levine NS. Characteristics and uses of biologic dressings and skin substitutes. Arch Surg 119:312, 1984.

54. VASCULAR GRAFT INFECTIONS

Gary R. Seabrook and Charles E. Edmiston, Jr

Introduction

Infection of a vascular reconstruction is an infrequent, but ominous, complication. The patient is at risk not only from the infection but also from the potential for ischemia if the conduit must be interrupted, replaced or removed. Because vascular grafts function as substitute conduits in the arterial circulation, vascular graft infections are approached with a greater sense of gravity than other surgical wound or prosthetic implant infections. A vascular graft infection may be associated with sepsis, erosion of the graft into the gastrointestinal tract, dehiscence of the graft-artery suture line, and result in hemorrhage or false aneurysm formation or rupture of the graft itself. The incidence of infection is less when autologous tissue is used for artery replacement or bypass compared with prosthetic bypass grafting, and this observation remains a compelling reason to use autologous conduits in the management of arterial trauma where contamination is frequent. However, routine replacement of aortic segments for aneurysmal or occlusive disease cannot use autologous tissue, as there is no large enough segment of conduit that can be sacrificed. The inflammatory response associated with implantation of a foreign body appears to potentate the risk of infection, even when minimal bacterial contamination of a vascular bioprosthesis occurs.

The biology and epidemiology of vascular graft infections correlate with their clinical presentation, and provide direction for diagnostic and treatment strategies. It is important to understand how vascular grafts become contaminated, how bacteria resist host defense mechanisms, and the spectrum of symptoms and signs associated with a vascular prosthesis infection. A classification of vascular graft infections based on pathogenesis and timing after operation also helps guide the management of this complication.

Pathogenesis

Bacterial contamination of prosthetic vascular grafts is frequent, if not routine, occurrence. Contamination may occur when the graft is placed or at a time remote from surgical implantation. Contamination before implantation, due to improper sterilization or packaging of the graft, is a rare cause of graft infection. Prostheses may become infected after implantation by inoculation of the external graft surface or by hematogenous seeding. Moore *et al.* showed that bacteremia could induce a graft infection up to six months after implantation if the lumen of the graft did not become lined with a well-developed pseudointima [1]. The evidence in humans for vascular graft infection caused by bacteremia is anecdotal. Szilagyi and colleagues at Henry Ford Hospital pioneered work in aortic replacement, and in 1972 observed an infection of an aortic graft in a patient with an abscess of the hand, and postulated that it was hematogenous seeding of the prosthesis [2]. Goldstone and Moore postulated that prosthetic graft infections could be linked to a prior Gram-negative urinary tract infection [3]. It has been well documented that bacteria follows diagnostic instrumentation of the oral, gastrointestinal, and genitourinary tracts, but there have been few clinical reports of vascular graft infections as a consequence of dental or endoscopic procedures.

The greatest risk of vascular graft contamination occurs at the time of graft implantation. There are several routes by which microorganisms may come into contact with a vascular graft. A gross break in operative technique, permitting the graft to touch unprepared skin, would result in obvious contamination. Bacteria are also present within the dermal layer of skin, and are thereby protected from the bactericidal effects of the surgical scrub. Incisional margins, therefore, are theoretically contaminated sites, although the number of organisms is low. Colonization of prosthetic vascular grafts by bacteria residing in diseased arterial walls, to which the graft is anastomosed, has been implicated as an etiology of late graft infections. Ernst *et al.* reported that the incidence of graft infection in patients undergoing aortic surgery increased from 2% to 10% when aortic wall cultures were positive [4]. Macbeth *et al.* studied the arterial wall microbiology in patients undergoing elective aortic and extremity vascular reconstructions [5]. Cultures of the native artery, arterial thrombus, atheroma, and peri-arterial tissues were positive in 43% of the specimens studied. In a group of patients with clinical graft infections, there was a 57% incidence of anastomotic dehiscence in 14 of 20 patients with positive arterial wall cultures, compared with no occurrence of graft-artery disruption in patients with negative cultures. These data suggest that occult infection of diseased native arteries contributes to infection of vascular prostheses and may complicate the excision of infected grafts. Performance of a concomitant surgical procedure (e.g., incidental appendectomy, cholecystectomy, or colon resection) at the time a vascular graft is implanted may dramatically increase the risk of infecting the bioprosthesis with the patient's enteric flora. Newer evidence indicates that microbial aerosols can routinely be recovered from the operating room environment, and that the spectrum of organisms recovered closely matches the profile commonly responsible for vascular graft infections [6]. However, no direct link has been established with airborne bacteria and wound or prosthetic device infections.

The lymphatic system may also provide a route of contamination leading to the infection or a vascular graft. In the immediate postoperative period, prosthetic grafts implanted in the groin are bathed by lymphatic drainage from the distal extremity. These lymphatics may be draining the tissue of chronically infected ulcers or ischemic tissue where the normal protective barriers have been compromised. The potential for graft contamination by lymphatics is compounded by the transection of multiple lymphatic channels during routine arterial dissection, particularly in the femoral region where lymphatic drainage follows the course of venous tributaries. The graft may thus be contaminated by bacteria traveling through lymphatic and venous channels to the systemic circulation or by directly bathing the graft in contaminated fluid from disrupted lymphatic channels. Rubin *et al.* showed experimentally in a canine model that lymphatics could collect *Escherichia coli* and *Staphylococcus aureus*, and transport them to the site of a vascular graft [7].

Biomaterial implantation, bacterial contamination, and operative dissection will each incite an inflammatory response by the host. Inflammation is characterized by a local reaction of injured tissue and more importantly the blood vessels endothelium. The inflammatory response has two missions: neutralization of the offending agent, and repair of the injury. The inflammatory response usually eradicates any bacterial inocula and provides the framework for wound healing, which eventually results in vascular graft incorporation by surrounding structures. That the process is effective is evidenced by the low rate (<2%) of vascular graft infections in "clean" cases. In response to a bacterial challenge, an inflammatory reaction develops and stimulates the recruitment of leukocytes (primarily neutrophils and monocytes), plasma cells, and macrophages. Vasodilatation occurs at the site of the infection, with the opening of new arteriolar and venular beds, followed by an increase in vascular permeability. The activated neutrophils enclose the bacteria in a phagocytic vacuole, into which cytoplasmic granules containing collagenase, elates, and plasminogen activator are discharged. Derived from blood monocytes, tissue macrophages act against foreign matter, including bacteria, by phagocytosis and degradation with hydrolytic enzymes released from lysosomes. Mobile phagocytes are attracted to bacteria and to all sites of inflammation even in the absence of microbes.

Through the excretion of chemotaxins, bacteria and injured tissue stimulate the migration of leukocytes by means of a process that is chemically modulated through intracellular cyclic nucleotides. Phagocytosis is facilitated by coating the microorganisms or foreign material with serum factors called opsonins. These immunoglobulins exhibit a specificity for the surface receptors on macrophages and neutrophils. Antigenic binding also causes the foreign particle or bacterium to become situated in close proximity to the phagocyte, permitting it to be engulfed. Antibodies that attach to the surfaces of bacteria may alter ionic charges on the cell surfaces, so they are more easily ingested by the phagocyte. Biologically active components of the complement system participate in the inflammatory response by increasing vascular permeability and acting as chemotactic agents.

A bacterial infection occurring in the environment of a prosthetic vascular graft results in a pathological condition, in which the host is attempting to eradicate the infection as well as direct an inflammatory response against the foreign body. Both the bacteria and foreign body stimulate similar responses of the immune system. However, the presence of a foreign body also serves as a "decoy" by creating a reactive environment, and expending cellular energy of the inflammatory response while diminishing available reserves of phagocytic activity against bacterial invasion. The cellular and enzymatic activity at the site of the vascular prosthesis results in increased oxidative metabolism with the generation of oxygen free radicals that may be injurious to adjacent cells. The cytotoxic enzymes are more likely to damage or destroy host tissue than the vascular prosthesis.

Bacteriology

Initial reports of prosthetic graft infections identified *S. aureus* as the predominant pathogen [8, 9]. Szilagyi *et al.*, in an early comprehensive study of vascular graft infections, identified coagulase-positive staphylococci as the infecting organism in 13 of 40 graft infections [2]. Gram-negative organisms, including *E. coli*, *Proteus*, *Bacteroides*, and *Pseudomonas* accounted for another 14 graft infections. Liekweg and Greenfield also identified *S aureus* as the most common organism cultured, but observed an increased recovery of enteric pathogens through the course of the series [10]. The mean time interval to presentation was 27 weeks. All investigators have emphasized that the majority (two thirds) of graft infections involves the femoral component of the vascular prosthesis.

The organisms involved in early graft infections tend to exhibit virulent characteristics. Coagulase produced by staphylococcal species, such as *S aureus*, coats the microorganisms with a film of fibrin that allows them to clump together, organize within a wound or abscess cavity, and thus inhibit phagocytosis. Coagulase-positive staphylococci also produce lysins, which are hemolytic and responsible for cell necrosis and the killing of mobilized leukocytes. Coagulase production may contribute to antibiotic resistance.

Pseudomonas species have been notoriously associated with virulent infections involving vascular grafts. Geary *et al.* reported a significant increased incidence of anastomotic disruption and vein graft wall necrosis in a canine model when *Pseudomonas aeruginosa* was used to infect prosthetic and autologous vascular grafts [11]. The virulence of *Pseudomonas* species is associated with their ability to produce destructive endotoxins [12]. Elastase and alkaline protease, produced by the bacteria, act against the elastin and collagen in artery or vein graft walls, compromising structural integrity.

The presence of the prosthetic implant potentiates the infection when bacterial contamination is present. The vascular graft is not an innocent bystander to the infection; it amplifies the inflammatory response and enhances the pathological process. The environment created by the inflammatory reaction in response to a foreign body is conducive to bacteria survival and proliferation. Cellular debris surrounding the vascular prosthesis provides an acidic, relatively ischemic environment that provides appropriate nutritional sources for the bacteria, and protects them from the action of other phagocytes and from lysosomal enzymes that would normally be bactericidal.

Bacteria may also become sequestered in the interstices of a vascular graft and be further protected from polymorphonuclear leukocytes and macrophages by being incorporated in a mesh of fibroblasts, collagen, platelets, and fibrin. Proteolytic enzymes released during this inflammatory process may have little effect on sequestered microcolonies, and rather, may injure normal surrounding tissue, including the artery wall to which the graft material is anastomosed.

Surface characteristics of a vascular prosthesis, including porosity, hydrophobicity, and texture, influence the magnitude of the inflammatory response that occurs following implantation. More porous structures allow contiguous tissue in-growth over the surface of the prosthetic, rather than the formation of a fibrous capsular plane at the interface of the graft and host tissue. A prosthetic with a high degree of porosity permits tissue invasion with a decreased inflammatory response. Expanded polytetrafluoroethylene (PTFE) vascular grafts are formed by an extrusion process and have a structure that permits tissue incorporation but a porosity low enough to obviate the need for preclotting before insertion in the arterial stream. These characteristics also result in the formation of a pseudointima that is less thrombogenic than the lining of the more porous woven or knitted Dacron vascular grafts.

Colonization of a vascular graft with bacteria ensures that an ongoing inflammatory interaction within the host will occur. The resultant cellular and tissue response is manifest by clinical signs of inflammation including pain, fever, swelling, leukocytosis, and autolysis of surrounding tissue. The inflammatory response is successful if the foreign body and bacteria are digested and eliminated, as might occur after placement of an absorbable surgical suture, but such a benign outcome would not be expected following infection of a vascular prosthesis. For the latter, the inflammatory response results in the progressive involvement of surrounding tissue with graft erosion, sinus tract formation, or suture line dehiscence due to loss of tensile strength of the adjacent artery wall.

Over the past three decades, the opportunity to study a large population of patients with prosthetic grafts has become available. The incidence of early graft infection has decreased, and with long-term follow-up, a significant incidence of late graft infection has been chronicled. Late-appearing infections are more subtle in their presentation, and progress in a more indolent fashion than classic surgical wound infections. A decade after Szilagyi's review of graft infections. Bandyk *et al.* reported a series of aortofemoral graft infections that identified a mean time interval from operation to treatment of 41 months (range 14 to 80 months) [13]. The contrasting feature of this series, compared with prior reports, was that *Staphylococcus epidermidis* prevailed as the organism responsible for the infection in 60% of the cases. The clinical presentation of these infections differed from the familiar combination of pain, swelling, erythema, and incision break-down characteristic of a surgical wound infection and observed in most graft infections caused by *S aureus* or Gram-negative organisms. Clinical features associated with *S epidermidis* graft infections included anastomotic false aneurysm, a sinus tract communicating between the graft and the skin, and failure of the graft to become incorporated in the adjacent tissue with formation of a perigraft cavity containing an exudate. Typically, the perigraft fluid was composed of many polymorphonuclear leukocytes, but no bacteria. A more recent review of 45 anastomotic femoral pseudoaneurysms, which presented with no clinical signs of graft infection, also documented that many of the patients have characteristics associated with *S epidermidis* graft infections, as described previously [14]. The recovery of *S epidermidis* organisms from abnormal arterial tissue is not unusual. Macbeth *et al.*, in their survey of arterial wall microbiology, reported *S epidermidis* was the most common (71% of isolates) organism cultured from arteries, arterial thrombus, and atheroma of patients undergoing elective aortic and extremity arterial reconstruction [5].

The involvement of coagulase-negative staphylococci (CNS) with vascular graft infections involving the inguinal site is not unexpected. The highest staphylococcal concentrations on body skin surfaces are found in the axilla and the groin where the temperature and humidity provide an optimum environment for growth. Although CNS had previously been dismissed as nonpathogenic skin contaminants when recovered from prosthetic material, their role in infections involving implanted devices in humans has been confirmed. In addition to infecting vascular grafts, CNS have been implicated as the pathogenic organisms in infections of cardiac valves cerebrospinal fluid shunts and intravascular catheters [15–17].

We have shown that many vascular patients entering the hospital are colonized with multiple strains of slime-producing CNS. Twenty-one patients admitted to our institution for lower extremity arterial revascularization had body surface cultures of planned incision sites performed on admission, immediately preoperatively and 5 days postoperatively. A large number (n = 327) of CNS isolates were recovered, and *S epidermidis* was the predominant species isolated at all three sample times [18]. On admission to the hospital, the incidence of methicillin resistance was 15% for *S epidermidis* and 10.1% for the other CNS isolates. However, 5 days after operation, the incidence of *S epidermidis* methicillin resistance increased to 50% and the overall, and methicillin resistance of CNS strains incresed to 57%. The hospital environment, including perioperative antibiotic administration, results in an increased frequency of antibiotic-resistant CNS strains. This selection process can contribute to the pathogenicity of these organisms, especially in patients with prolonged hospitalization before surgery or those requiring re-operation, since routine antibiotic prophylaxis may not be as effective.

As vascular surgeons have become suspicious of occult infection, more sophisticated culture techniques have been used. Enhanced recovery of CNS is achieved when graft material is submitted for culture in trypticase soy broth and further improved by disrupting adherent bacteria from the graft fabric by using ultrasonic oscillation's. Glucose supplementation of the cryptic soy broth used for staphylococcal incubation may be required to recover colonies when only a few organisms are present in the initial sample of graft material submitted for culture. A prolonged (up to 14 days) incubation period for slow growing, fastidious organisms may be required.

There is no evidence that vegetative lesions occur, within arterial conduits infected by CNS similar to those that may be located on infected cardiac valves. Fever is seldom a presenting symptom with late graft infections, nor are other stigmata of cardiac valve infections typically present, such as Osler's lesions, Janeway's lesions, Roth's spots, petechiae, or splinter hemorrhages. The lack of these signs in graft infection caused by CNS points against a seeding and showering process as an etiologic factor in most late graft infections.

Natural History of Graft Infections

Szilagyi *et al.* classified graft infections in a three-tiered system based on the anatomic level of invasion. Grade I infections involved only the dermis; Grade II infections extended into the subcutaneous region but did not involve the prosthetic material; Grade III infections involved the arterial implant [2]. Because the Grade II infections and I were not involved with significant sequelae, they have not been studied in detail. Most Grade III infections result as a consequence of a surgical wound infection and probably evolve through the two previous phases during their clinical presentation. Szilagyi's classification scheme centered on the concept that contamination of the vascular graft occurs primarily through the surgical wound or via an enteric erosion. Indeed, these are the important mechanisms of early graft infections. More recent reports on graft infection have focused on pathogenesis and treatment of late-appearing infections, particularly graft-enteric erosions or fistulas. Investigators have emphasized the concept of bacterial adherence to the vascular graft material as a critical initial step in the infectious process. The time of onset following the primary operation for a graft infection to appear frequently predicts which pathogens are involved. The classification of graft infections as early (less than six months following implantation) or late is useful clinically, since different diagnostic and treatment strategies are required.

Early graft infections follow a clinical course of a surgical wound infection which, in fact is the likely etiology. During the perioperative period, the surgical wound is inoculated with bacteria and the graft becomes colonized. A local inflammatory response occurs, and an abscess involving the vascular conduit forms. The surgical wound, itself, is the focus of the infection, and any portion of the graft may be involved. The infection may extend along the external surface of the graft, to involve the suture line between the graft and the native arterial tissue, with a significant risk of anastomotic dehiscence.

Infections of autologous grafts occurring in the early perioperative period are frequently related to technical error, adjacent ischemic tissue, or a concomitant infectious process. Infected autologous tissue (e.g., vein grafts or patches, endarterectomized arterial segments) may necrose and rupture either at, or away from, suture lines. Most infections involving autologous conduits occur early and present as wound infections. They are treated with classic surgical techniques for wound management: drainage of abscess cavities; debridement of devitalized tissue; coverage of an uninfected conduit with viable tissue; or excision of an infected conduit. Late graft infections involving autologous vascular grafts are rare, and the incidence is not great enough to define etiologies and to formulate management within a classification scheme.

Early prosthetic vascular graft infections are usually the result of local wound contamination. These infections may be associated with a wound-healing complication such as dehiscence, hematoma, seroma, lymphatic leak, or skin edge necrosis. The graft becomes inoculated through the disrupted surgical incision or via an adjacent abscess cavity. The anastomotic suture lines of prosthetic grafts are dependent on the integrity of the native artery, because a union between the prosthetic and the implanted material via a proliferative process does not occur. In the early postoperative period, dehiscence of the suture line is associated with hemorrhage because, the prosthetic material will not have become incorporated by surrounding tissue to contain the force of arterial pressure.

As surgical technique and perioperative antibiotic therapy become increasingly rigorous, the relative incidence of early graft infection has decreased. Infections involving prosthetic grafts are more likely to occur late in the postoperative course. One group of these infections involves a previously incorporated, uninfected graft becoming contaminated by direct exposure

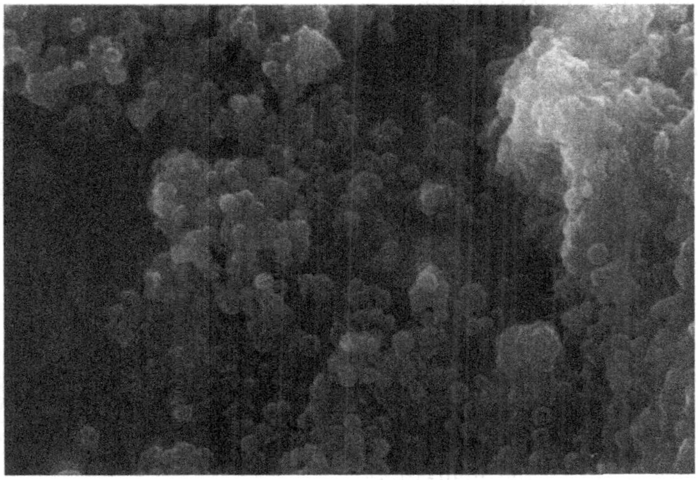

FIGURE 1. Scanning electron micrograph of *Staphylococci epidermidis* on Dacron graft fabric. Numerous adherent bacterial microcolonies are enclosed within an extracellular surface biofilm. These mucin-producing organisms become sequestered within the interstices of the prosthetic graft fabric leading to occult infection.

(graft enteric erosion) or hematogenous seeding from another systemic septic focus (e.g., pneumonia, urinary tract infection, dental abscess). These infections are likely to present with the patient exhibiting clinical signs of sepsis (e.g., fever, chills, lethargy, leukocytosis, vasodilatation, hyperdynamic cardiac activity, septic shock). Signs of wound infection may be absent and timely diagnosis delayed, because the infection is focused at the site of the graft that is located deep to the overlying healed surgical incision. The contaminated graft is targeted by host defenses as a septic focus, and an acute inflammatory response ensues. An exudative process will encircle the vascular prosthesis. As the infection extends along the external surface of the prosthetic material, the vascular anastomosis may become involved in the infection. The infecting organisms are virulent Gram-positive cocci or Gram-negative enteric pathogens. Successful treatment involves aggressive intervention with resection of the prosthetic material, extra-anatomic bypass, systemic antimicrobial therapy, and multisystem support of a critically ill patient.

The second group of late onset vascular graft infections follows a more cryptic process. Bacterial microcolonies contaminate the graft, are sequestered within the interstices of the prosthetic fabric, and become adherent to the graft surface at the time of implantation. These infections are most frequently caused by CNS. As the body incorporates the prosthetic graft, the contaminating bacteria are entrapped, and may be surrounded by an exopolysaccharide biofilm (mucin or slime), which protects the organisms from the host's immune defense system and systemic antibiotics (Figure 1).

There may be a latent period extending from months to years following prosthetic implantation when no clinical signs of infection are exhibited, and the integrity of the prosthetic anastomosis remains unaltered. Eventually, the microbial population grows beyond the surface of the graft, is recognized by host defenses, and a chronic inflammatory process develops. Cytolysins released from macrophages break down the matrix of collagen and fibroblasts that have coalesced around the prosthetic material, resulting in the graft becoming unincorporated from the host tissue. In this environment, the artery wall may become inflamed with a decreased anastomotic tensile strength at the graft-artery interface [20]. Persistence of the chronic inflammatory state may lead to the development of a pseudoaneurysm at the anastomotic site. This low-grade inflammatory process does not present as systemic sepsis, but is more commonly manifest by subtle changes at graft implantation. The incorporated graft becomes surrounded with a perigraft exudate or fluid collection and, with a continuous stimulus for inflammation, a sinus tract may form between the perigraft cavity and the skin surface, or a pseudoaneurysm may form at the graft-artery interface due to disruption of the anastomosis. If a pseudoaneurysm is explored during the evolution of this inflammatory reaction signs of infection (perigraft fluid, leukocytes, or bacteria on gram stain) may be evident. Treatment strategy depends on the recognition that these anatomic changes are due to an infectious process, rather than host vessel degeneration or an immune-mediated reaction directed at the vascular prosthesis. Identification of the pathogen in these circumstances requires the culture of the biomaterial itself, rather than culture of perigraft tissue or fluid. Failure to recognize a graft infection invariably leads to a future graft-healing complication, typically manifesting at an anastomotic site as either rupture or thrombosis of a false aneurysm.

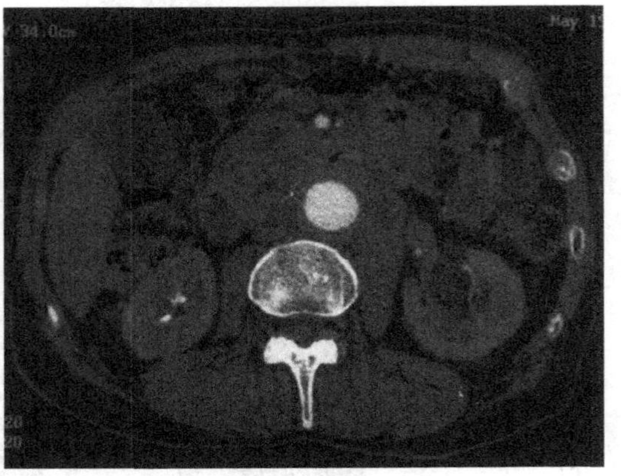

FIGURE 2. CT scan of a patient eight months following aortic grafting for aneurysmal disease. A gas pocket is present anterior to the aortic graft. The duodenum is involved with extensive inflammation surrounding the prosthesis extending into the left psoas muscle. At operation an aorto-enteric fistula was identified.

Diagnostic Imaging

Computerized tomography (CT) is the most useful and accurate modality to diagnose a vascular graft infection. Findings that will lead to the diagnosis of graft infection are perigraft air, perigraft fluid collections, and inflammatory changes in the retroperitoneal structures (Figure 2). Although residual intra-abdominal air may be present in the early post-operative period, particularly following aneurysm repair, after two months any air in the region of the graft should be considered pathologic. When perigraft air is found late (greater that six months) following implantation, the diagnosis of graft infection is almost certain. When vascular contrast is administered in association with axial imaging, the CT provides information to define the arterial anatomy that should obviate the need for angiography. Although CT scanning will seldom demonstrate an aorto-enteric fistula, it may provide information to argue against that diagnosis if it can be demonstrated that the duodenum is separated from the vascular structures by normal tissue planes with no inflammatory tissue changes.

Arteriography has more potential in formulating operative strategy than in establishing a diagnosis of prosthetic graft infection. An arteriogram may locate a graft infection by demonstrating a nonpalpable proximal pseudoaneurysm, but this modality never identified a fistulous tract independently diagnosed as primary graft infection. Arteriographic imaging of the native vascular anatomy allows the surgeon to plan the extra-anatomic arterial reconstruction.

Attempts to firmly establish the diagnosis of aorto-enteric fistula can be an arduous task. Patients with aorto-enteric fistula usually present with some form of gastrointestinal bleeding. It may be acute and severe making the diagnosis obvious, however, patients may initially present with only anemia or guaiac positive stools. Upper GI endoscopy is the most frequently performed diagnostic intervention, but it actually establishes the diagnosis in only a few patients. Endoscopy is more commonly employed to identify other pathology responsible for a source of significant blood loss in the esophagus, stomach, or duodenum. Most patients with vascular grafts and GI bleeding have GI sources of bleeding and not aorto-enteric fisitulae. However, the clinician must be wary not to implicate "esophagitis, gastritis, gastric erosions or duodenitis" when there is actually major blood loss. In such a setting avoiding the diagnosis of aorto-enteric fistula will only lead to a delay in establishing the correct diagnosis. Only an actively bleeding lesion or other demonstrable GI pathology that can account for the patient's symptoms should be considered a true source of hemorrhage as an alternative to an aorto-enteric fistula during this evaluation.

Treatment of Aortic Graft Sepsis

The principles of operative management consist of total excision of the infected aortic graft, debridement of the aorta to reach normal artery wall, debridement of retroperitoneal structures associated with the infectious process, longitudinal closure of the duodenum, oversewing the aorta followed by an onlay omental patch, placement of retroperitoneal drains if there had been an abscess cavity, and revascularization through an extra-anatomic route. Such an operation is one of the most taxing surgical procedures performed for both the patient and surgeon. If the patient is stable, it is preferable to perform the extra-anatomic revascularization as a staged procedure, followed in 24 hours with excision of the infected graft. This allows for two shorter operations with better ability to manage the patient's fluid status and the associated risk to the cardiac and pulmonary systems. In our reported series of 20 patients, 14 underwent aortic graft excision followed by extra-anatomic revascularization, while five patients had extra-anatomic revascularization performed prior to excision of the aortic prosthesis. Whether revascularization was performed before or after aortic graft excision did not alter the eventual outcome of the patients in our series. Although performing the revascularization prior to graft excision avoids the obligatory ischemic time to the lower extremities, there is the theoretical risk of bacteremic seeding of the new graft material if it is placed prior to removal of the infected prosthesis. However, the one patient in our series who developed an infection of his axillofemoral graft had it placed after excision of the aortic graft [19].

The most common technique for lower extremity revascularization is axillofemoral, femoral-femoral bypass constructed with PTFE graft material which has the lowest incidence of bacterial adherence [20]. If the aortic procedure has been confined to the abdomen, then the common femoral arteries can be used for the extra-anatomic reconstruction with little risk of contamination. However, when the aortic graft has been extended to the femoral segments, the revascularization must be taken more distally through uninfected tissue. If the patient's superficial femoral artery is open, the lower extremities are usually not at risk for ischemia, however when there is arterial occlusion of the superficial femoral segment, the reconstruction must target the profunda femoris or even the popliteal artery for runoff.

In our series, cultures from two patients who presented with clinical signs of sepsis recovered a polymicrobial mixture of aerobic and anaerobic organisms. Five of the nine patients with late-onset primary graft infection had only *Staphylococcus epidermidis* recovered. Despite having clinical evidence of graft infection (draining wound sinus, perigraft exudate, poor graft incorporation, anastomotic pseudoaneurysm) the four remaining patients had no isolates recovered [19].

Despite broad advances in medical technology, operative mortality (14–50%) and morbidity (25–70%, primarily from lower limb amputations) have remained considerable, when the standard treatment of excision of the infected graft and revascularization via an extra-anatomic approach, is followed [21, 22]. This has lead some authors to suggest alternative approaches such as simple repair of the fistula without regrafting, or *in situ* replacement of the prosthesis in the infected field [23, 24]. Although it may be necessary for vascular surgeons to have these options available in their treatment armamentarium, prosthetic material should not be permanently placed in an infected field.

Aortic stump dehiscence remains a significant late cause of death in patients surviving surgical treatment of aortic vascular graft infections. *In situ* replacement of grafts from patients with aorto-enteric fistulae resulted in a 16% incidence of recurrent fistula or dehiscence, and exsanguination at the proximal anastomosis [19]. Reilly *et al.* reported a 25% dehiscence and mortality in 25 patients following perioperative treatment for aorto-enteric fistulas, but no cases of aortic stump problems in patients treated for primary graft infection [22].

There are two factors that play a role in the pathogenesis of late aortic stump problems: persistent peri-aortic infection and bacterial virulence. The aorta must be debrided back to normal arterial wall to enable a secure closure. Attempts to close friable, edematous aorta predispose the patient to future complications. In addition, an attempt must be made to debride the surrounding retroperitoneal structures involved in the infectious process to remove sources of contamination. The second factor related to subsequent infectious problems with the aortic stump is related to the virulence of the organisms involved in the infectious process. Late stump dehiscence is more common following aorto-enteric fistulas than primary graft infections. Isolates from aorta-enteric fistulae are polymicrobial and involve more virulent organisms such as *Escherichia coli*, *S. aureus*, and *Pseudomonas*. In contrast, *Staphylococcus epidermidis* is the most common isolate recovered from late onset primary graft infections. The inherent low virulence of *S. epidermidis*, when combined with complete excision of the prosthesis, has resulted in the failure of this organism to be implicated in aortic stump dehiscence.

Following excision of an aotic graft the patient should be maintained on a course of antibiotic therapy to protect the patient from infection from residual microscopic contamination and to irradiate organisms still in the lymphatic system. If pre-operative blood cultures were positive, the susceptibility data from these cultures will guide therapy. However, the nature of biofilm infections may result in negative cultures from specimens collected at the procedure. Empiric therapy must then be instituted. We use a semi-synthetic penicillin with a Beta-lactam inhibitor or a quinolone, with additional coverage to both of these regimens if there is an indication that an anaerobic process is involved. Vancomycin is not routinely used. Intravenous therapy is routinely continued for two weeks and then the patient is converted to an oral agent, which is continued until there is evidence on follow-up CT scan that all of the intra-abdominal inflammatory process has resolved (Figure 3).

When long-term antibiotic therapy is prescribed, the consequences of this therapy must be considered, including the development of drug allergies, specific organ dysfunction such as nephrotoxicity, the development of supra-infections including pseudomembranous colitis, and the emergence of bacterial resistant organisms.

The most common risk factor factors that predisposes to infectious complications is multiple previous vascular procedures. Repetitive exposure of the graft increases the risk of contamination and a subsequent infection. Archer and Tenenbaum have demonstrated the emergence of

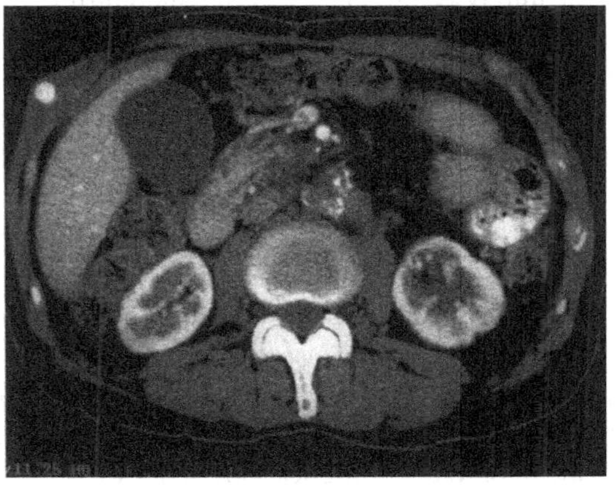

FIGURE 3. CT scan of the patient (Figure 2) six weeks after excision of the infected aortic graft and oversewing of the infrarenal aorta. An axillofemoral bypass was constructed to perfuse the lower extremities (right antero-lateral abdominal wall). The extensive inflammatory changes observed on the pre-operative CT have resolved.

antibiotic resistance in Staphylococcal strains recovered from cardiac surgery patients in the postoperative period [25]. The necessity for graft revision in the early postoperative period may greatly increase the risk of graft colonization by more virulent or resistant strains of the commensal skin flora.

In situ Replacement of Infected Grafts

The low virulence of coagulase-negative staphylococci and their unique characteristics of colonization via a surface biofilm permit treatment of some infected grafts by excision of the grossly involved graft segments, debridement of perigraft tissue and adjacent artery, and *in situ* replacement of another prosthesis. Several caveats must be emphasized in selecting this treatment option. First, it is essential that the patient has the correct microbiologic diagnosis. This technique is not appropriate or recommended for patients who have Gram-negative bacteria infections. The role of coagulase-positive staphylococci in these infections is not yet defined. In latent, indolent infections where coagulase-positive staphylococci are cultured, *in situ* replacement may be successful. Why some patients with coagulase-positive staphylococcal infections fail to mount the systemic reaction that is more classically associated with this infection is not understood. There may be a spectrum of virulence in these species in which some isolates act like the more benign coagulase-negative staphylococci.

Graft biofilm infections involving the femoral anastomosis are the cases where an *in situ* replacement technique will be most appropriately used. When an *in situ* technique is employed, the operative treatment must include total excision of the biofilm cavity and the involved graft. Because this often results in an extensive groin dissection, there is an increased incidence of lymphatic wound complications, particularly the occurrence of lymphocytes in the post-operative period. The use of muscle coverage is important because it provides vascularized tissue to surround the graft and be interposed between the skin and the conduit if wound complications occur. The treatment of lymphoccles should be aggressive, with operative ligation and drainage if they do not promptly resolve or begin to leak through the wound creating a potential tract for secondary infections.

Expanded PTFE is usually selected as a replacement interposition graft because our laboratory data has demonstrated that the bacterial adherence of slime-producing bacteria is significantly less to ePTFE than to knitted or woven Dacron [26]. Slime-producing coagulase-negative staphylococci adhered to the knitted Dacron 100 times greater than to PTFE. Because bacterial adhesion is the important first step in biofilm graft infection, the relative resistance to bacterial adhesion possessed by PTFE has significant potential advantages as an *in situ* replacement conduit.

A special note of caution needs to be raised for patients who have femoral limbs of their aorto-bifemoral grafts resected. Even after the replacement grafts have healed well and have demonstrated no evidence of recurrent infection, the residual aortic graft segment in the patient may subsequently develop changes suggestive of coagulase-negative staphylococcus infection manifested by the development of a perigraft cavity and fluid. Should this clinical presentation occur, it probably represents a latent infection that existed even at the time of the initial resection. Since replacement of the intra-abdominal portion of an aortobifemoral graft is fraught with the greatest potential for complications, it is reasonable to be cautious in making a decision to remove the aortic segment.

Because biofilm infections occur months and years after an initial vascular reconstructive procedure, the mortality rate from associated cardiovascular disease is high in this cohort of patients. The mortality rate for most series of patients with graft infections is at or above 50%, most of it caused by cardiovascular causes. Because of this high mortality rate, clinicians are curtailed in studying extended durability of this repair technique.

Conclusions

The most important factor in selecting treatment regimens for vascular graft infections is the proper analysis of the patient. The role of the infecting organism is primary in selecting less radical treatment of *in situ* repair as opposed to the traditional treatment of graft excision and extra-anatomic bypass to restore distal flow.

The pathobiology of vascular graft infections is affected by the microorganisms colonizing the graft, the site of implantation, and the character of the prosthetic material used in the reconstruction. Sensitive culture techniques are necessary to recover bacteria from graft infections when overt signs of sepsis are absent.

It is critical for the surgeon to identify patients with biofilm infections during follow-up surveillance. Because of the indolent nature of the infection and the low virulence of the organisms, the diagnosis can rarely be made definitely before graft removal and culture. The clinical presentation is typical enough so, that a tentative diagnosis can be reliably made. The principle components of this diagnosis include an infection occurring at a time remote from the previous vascular procedure (at least six months) and the absence of systemic evidence of toxicity. The use of CT scanning and duplex scanning is valuable to detect perigraft fluid and the presence of intra-abdominal false aneurysms.

Late prosthetic graft infections differ from classical surgical wound infections, and management of these complications requires the vascular surgeon to understand the etiology and natural history of the process. We do not recommend *in situ* replacement for Gram-negative infection and for coagulase-positive staphylococcus infections where the patient has systemic effects of infection and bacteria can be seen on gram stains of the perigraft fluid. In these situations traditional techniques of graft removal and autogenous or extra-anatomic revascularization are still the treatments of choice.

References

1. Moore WS, Rosson CT, Hall AD, *et al.* Transient bacteremia: a cause of infection in prosthetic vascular grafts. Am J Surg 7:342, 1969.
2. Szilagyi DE, Smith RF, Elliott JP, *et al.* Infection in arterial reconstruction with synthetic grafts. Ann Surg 176: 321, 1972.
3. Goldstone J, Moore WS. Infection in vascular prostheses. Arch Surg 97:872, 1968.
4. Ernst CB, Campbell HC, Daugherty ME, *et al.* Incidence and significance of intraoperative bacterial cultures during abdominal aortic aneurysmectomy. Ann Surg 185:626, 1977.
5. Macbeth GA, Rubin JR, McIntyre KE, *et al.* The relevance of arterial wall microbiology to the treatment of prosthetic graft infections: graft infection vs. arterial infection. J Vasc Surg 1:750, 1984.
6. Edmiston CE, Sinski S, Seabrook GR, Simons D, Goheen M. Airborne particulates in the OR environment. AORN 69:1169, 1999.
7. Rubin JR, Malone JM, Goldstone J. The role of the lymphatic system in acute arterial prosthetic graft infections. J Vasc Surg 2:92, 1985.

8. Javid H, Julian OC, Dye WS, *et al.* Complications of abdominal aortic grafts. Arch Surg 85:142, 1962.
9. Fry WJ, Lindenauer SM. Infection complicating the use of plastic arterial implants. Arch Surg 94:600, 1967.
10. Liekweg WG, Greenfield LJ. Vascular prosthetic infections: collected experience and results of treatment. Surgery 81:335, 1977.
11. Geary KJ, Tomkiewicz ZM, Harrison HH, *et al.* Differential effects of a gram-negative and a gram-positive infection on autogenous and prosthetic grafts. J Vasc Surg 11:339, 1990.
12. Rotschafer JC, Shikuma LR. *Pseudomonas aeruginosa* susceptibility in a university hospital: recognition and treatment. Drug Intell Clin Pharm 20:575, 1986.
13. Bandyk DF, Berni GA, Thiele BL, *et al.* Aortofemoral graft infection due to *Staphylococcus epidermidis*. Arch Surg 119:102, 1984.
14. Seabrook GR, Schmitt DD, Bandyk DF, Edmiston CE, Towne JB. Anastomotic femoral pseudoaneurysm: A prospective investigation of occult infection as an etiologic factor. J Vasc Surg 11:629, 1990.
15. Slaughter L, Morris JE, Starr A. Prosthetic valvular endocarditis: a 12 year review. Circulation 47:1319, 1973.
16. Bayston R, Pennym SR. Excessive production of mucoid substance in staphylococcus SIIA: a possible factor in colonization of Holter shunts. Dev Med Child Neurol 14:25, 1972.
17. Peters G, Locci R, Pulverer G. Adherence and growth of coagulase-negative staphylococci on surfaces of intravenous catheters. J Infect Dis 146:479, 1982.
18. Levy MF, Schmitt DD, Edmiston CE, Bandyk DD, Krepel CJ, Seabrook GR, Towne JB. Sequential analysis of staphylococcal colonization by body surface cultures on patients undergoing vascular surgery. J Clin Microbiol 28:664, 1989.
19. Schmitt DD, Seabrook GR, Bandyk DF, Towne JB. Graft excision and extra-anatomic revascularization: the treatment of choice for the septic aortic prosthesis. J Cardiovasc Surg 31:327, 1990.
20. Schmitt DD, Bandyk DF, Pequet AJ, Malangoni MA, Towne JB. Mucin production by *staphylococcus epidermidis*. Arch Surg 121:89, 1986.
21. O'Hara PJ, Hertzer NR, Beven EG, Krajewski LP. Surgical management of infected abdominal aortic grafts: review of a 25 years experience. J Vasc Surg 3:725, 1986.
22. Reilly LM, Altman H, Lusby RJ, Kersh RA, Eherenfeld WK, Stoney RJ. Late results following surgical management of vascular graft infection. J Vasc Surg 1:36, 1984.
23. Walker WE, Cooley DA, Duncan JM, Hallman GL, Ott DA, Reul GJ. The management of aortoduodenal distula by *in situ* replacement of the infected abdominal aortic graft. Ann Surg 205:727, 1987.
24. Thomas WEG, Baird RN. Secondary aortoenteric fistulae: towards a more conservative approach. Br J Surg 73:875, 1986.
25. Archer GL, Tenenbaum MJ. Antibiotic-resistant *staphylococcus epiderminidis* in patients undergoing cardiac surgery. Antimicrob Agents Chemother 17:269, 1980.
26. Schmitt DD, Bandyk DF, Pequet AJ, Towne JB. Bacterial adherence to vascular prostheses. J Vasc Surg 3:732, 1986.

55. ACUTE MEDIASTINITIS

David K. Warren, Thoralf M. Sundt, III and Louis B. Polish

Mediastinitis is an infection of the structures in the thorax excluding the lungs and pleural space. Most cases of mediastinitis are secondary to spread of infection from a distant site or direct inoculation of organisms secondary to trauma or esophageal perforation due to malignancy. The last 30 years have seen a dramatic increase in the annual number of cardiac surgical procedures performed. Consequently, post-sternotomy surgical site infections have accounted for an increasing number of cases of mediastinitis. Despite significant advances in antibiotic therapy, surgical technique, and intensive care management, mediastinitis continues to have a high morbidity and mortality. This chapter will focus on three major categories of mediastinitis, including descending necrotizing infections, mediastinitis secondary to esophageal perforations, and post-sternotomy surgical site infections, and will discuss the pathogenesis, presentation, diagnosis, and management associated with each. The anatomy of the neck and mediastinum, with is crucial to understanding the pathogenesis and complications of mediastinitis, as well as unusual causes of mediastinitis will also be reviewed.

HISTORICAL OVERVIEW

The first major review of suppurative mediastinitis was by Pearse [1] who reported 110 cases in 1938. In this series, 58% of cases were due to esophageal perforation and the remainder were secondary to descending infections of the head and neck, along with post-surgical complications. Mortality in the pre-antibiotic era without surgical drainage was 85%; with surgical intervention mortality decreased to 35%. The need for surgical drainage was particularly stressed in these early reports.

With the increasing use of the median sternotomy incision demonstrated by Julian in 1957 [2], a new cause of mediastinitis rapidly became apparent. Overall, the surgical site infection rate for median stermotomy is low, but given the volume of patients who undergo this procedure for cardiac surgery each year, even a low rate translates into a potentially large number of patients with mediastinal infections as a post-surgical complication. In a 1976 review by Culliford *et al.* [3] mortality ranged from 7% in the group that was recognized early to 20% among patients diagnosed late post operatively. The surgical management of these infections has evolved from initial debridement with closure by secondary intention, to primary closure with closed irrigation, to the use of omental and muscle flaps.

The advent of antibiotics did little alone to change the outcome of mediastinitis. In 1983, Estera *et al.* [4] reviewed 21 cases of descending necrotizing mediastinitis from 1960–1980 and reported a mortality of 42.8%, with the majority of these cases being diagnosed at autopsy. This high mortality rate was attributed to the frequent lack of both physical and radiographic findings early in the course of the disease. The development of computerized tomography (CT) has increased the capacity for earlier diagnosis of disease and improved pre-operative planning of surgical management. An analysis of 48 cases of mediastinitis from 1990–1998 revealed that the mortality for descending infections had

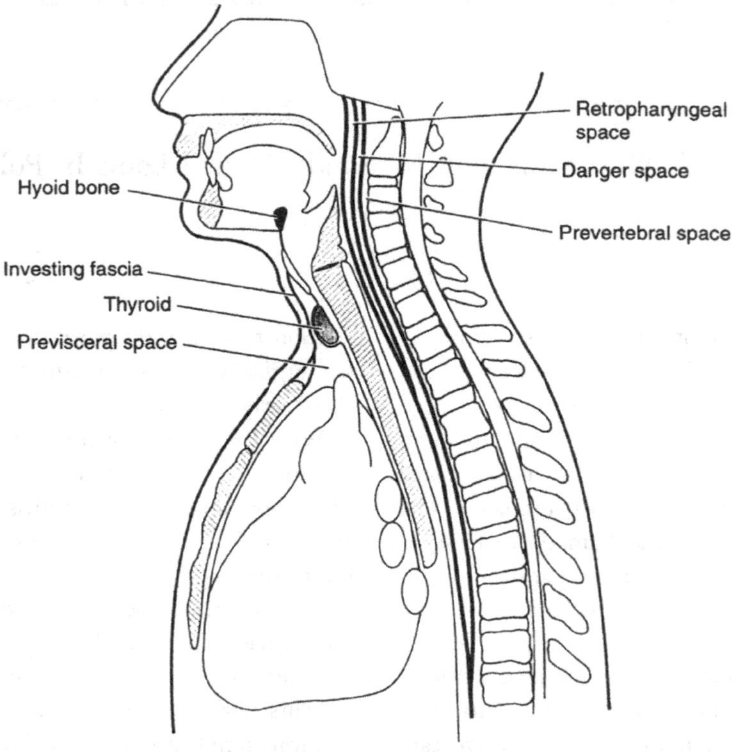

FIGURE 1. The deep fascial layers of the neck and their relationship to the mediastinum.

improved to 23% [5], which the authors attributed to the availability of CT.

ANATOMY OF THE NECK AND MEDIASTINUM

Understanding the pathogenesis, complications, and successful management of mediastinal infections requires knowledge of the anatomical relationships between the organs and vascular structures of the neck and mediastinum. The mediastinum contains the heart, great vessels, trachea, esophagus, paratracheal lymph nodes, and the thymus. This is bordered anatomically by the thoracic inlet superiorly, the diaphragm inferiorly, the sternum anteriorly, the vertebral bodies posteriorly, and the pleural cavities laterally. It is further divided into superior, anterior, middle, and posterior mediastinum, however in understanding the spread of infection in the chest, the utility of this division is unclear [6]. Of greater importance are the fascial planes of the head and neck. The most important of these include the retropharyngeal, visceral, prevertebral, lateral pharyngeal, and previsceral spaces which communicate directly with the mediastinum, and determine the mechanism by which perforations in the cervical esophagus and infections of the oropharynx can spread to the thorax.

The clinically important areas in the neck are divided into three sections determined by their relationship to the hyoid bone (Figure 1). The retropharyngeal and the visceral spaces extend both above and below the hyoid bone. The retropharyngeal space, or retrovisceral space, is limited anteriorly by the middle layer of the deep cervical fascia and the deepest layer of the deep cervical fascia, or the alar fascia posteriorly. This space exists behind the hypopharynx and esophagus from the base of the skull to the superior mediastinum. Retropharyngeal infections in this space can descend easily into the superior mediastinum. This was recognized early to be the space most likely involved cervical esophageal perforations [1, 6, 7]. This space is often involved in extension of infections of the cervical vertebra. Just posterior to the retropharyngeal space, between the alar fascia and the prevertebral fascia is an area called by some authors the "danger space" [7] which extends from the base of the skull to the crus of the diaphragm and is a source of potential dissemination of retropharyngeal or lateropharyngeal infection to the base of the posterior mediastinum and the retroperitoneal space [4, 7].

The visceral space is located within the carotid sheath and includes all three layers of the deep cervical fascia. Infections in this space less commonly extend down to the mediastinum, but given their location in relationship to the great vessels, can cause internal jugular vein septic thrombophlebitis and carotid artery rupture. Classically, suppurative lymphadenitis, peritonsillar abscess, and Ludwig's angina were causes of infections in this space; however, any of the structures of the pharynx and neck can serve as a source.

Above the hyoid bone are the submandibular space, the lateral pharyngeal space, the masticator space, and the parotid space. The submandibular and masticator spaces are most involved with dental infections, with Ludwig's angina being a result of submandibular space infection. The lateral pharyngeal space communicates with many of the spaces in the neck and is associated with infections of the pharynx, teeth, tonsils, or parotids. The parotid space communicates directly with the "danger space" and the lateral pharyngeal space. Therefore, infections in the parotids can rapidly extend throughout the mediastinum.

Below the hyoid bone is the anterior visceral or previsceral space. This extends from the hyoid bone superiorly to the anterior mediastinum inferiorly. It is bordered by the strap muscles anteriorly, and surrounds the trachea, with the esophagus forming its posterior border. The pretracheal investing fascia is attached to the pericardium and the parietal pleura, which can result in pericarditis and empyema from infection in this space. The most common causes of infection in this space include tracheal or esophageal disruption. Finally, the course of the esophagus is important to review, as esophageal perforation is a significant cause of mediastinitis and the complications of this can be predicted partially from the site of the perforation. The upper two-thirds of the thoracic esophagus lies in close proximity to the right pleural space, while the distal third deviates to the left to enter the diaphragmatic hiatus. Perforations of the lower thoracic esophagus are more likely to cause left-sided empyemas and possible retroperitoneal extension [6].

PATHOGENESIS

The causes of mediastinitis are multiple (Table 1). However, most cases can be divided by source, which explains the microbiology of the infection and also in part determines treatment strategies. A division, which is helpful, is to discuss head and neck sources of mediastinitis, esophageal perforations, and post-sternotomy mediastinitis. Other more unusual causes of mediastinal infection will also be addressed.

Descending Necrotizing Mediastinitis

Descending necrotizing mediastinitis is an unusual infection arising from the structures of the mouth, neck and pharynx. This begins as a localized infection, which then descends inferiorly via the fascial planes of the neck into the thorax. Several factors facilitate the spread of these infections to the mediastinal structures,

TABLE 1. Selected causes of mediastinitis

Descending necrotizing mediastinitis	**Iatrogenic**
Odotogenic[2,7–11]	Esophagogastroduodenoscopy[45,53]
Ludwig's angina[15,44]	Esophageal dilation[51]
Peritonsillar abscesses[2,6,7,15–17]	Nasogastric tube[53]
Parotitis[19]	Esophageal sclerotherapy[53]
Facial cellulitis[24,26]	Esophageal surgery[50,53]
Epiglottitis[23]	Dislodged cervical fixation device[54]
Pharyngitis[2,15–18]	**Cardiothoracic surgery**
Infectious mononucleosis[18]	Coronary artery bypass grafting[67–126]
Cervical lymphadenitis[1]	Cardiac valve replacement[71–73,76,104–107]
Iatrogenic	Cardiac transplantation[88–90,100–102]
Tooth extraction[8,13,14]	**Dissembinated spread**
Air-turbine dental equipment[8,13,14]	Bacteremia[78,137–140]
Oral[9,21] or nasal[22] intubation	Pneumonia or empyema[1,134–139,142]
Post-tracheotomy[23]	
Thyroidectomy[1]	
Central venous catheterization[145,146]	
Esophageal perforation	
Emesis[46,64]	
Carcinoma[47,48,53]	
Foreign body[56,57]	
Penetrating trauma[52,59,60]	
Blunt trauma[55,56,59]	
Trauma hyperextension[51]	

including gravitational drainage, negative intrathoracic pressure with inspiration, and the lack of significant barriers in the retropharyngeal space, the most common path of descent. The fascial planes of the neck can be penetrated by these kinds of infections, and subsequently involve all compartments of the neck and mediastinum. Often, patients can rapidly progress with overwhelming infection, including septic shock, multi-system organ failure, and death unless adequate surgical therapy is initiated.

Odontogenic infections account for 30–70% of all cases of descending mediastinitis [4, 7–10]. While infections in the 1st molar have been reported as causing mediastinitis [11], infections involving in the 2nd and 3rd mandibular molars are particularly dangerous. The reason for this association is felt to be due to the fact that the 2nd and 3rd molars roots extend below the hyoid ridge while the 1st molar roots do not. This anatomic observation is believed to be crucial because apical abscesses in the 2nd and 3rd molar roots can often rupture through the mandibular bone into the submandibular space, causing Ludwig's angina or gaining access to the deeper spaces of the neck. Occasionally, these infections will be occult or minor [12, 13]. Dental procedures which result in increased oral pressure and subcutaneous emphysema, such as tooth extraction, root canal therapy, high speed air-turbine dental equipment, and laceration of oral soft tissue have been also associated with mediastinitis [8, 13, 14].

Peritonsillar and retropharyngeal infections account for most of the remaining cases of descending necrotizing mediastinitis. Peritonsillar abscesses complicating bacterial tonsillitis [4, 6, 7, 15–17] or infectious mononucleosis [18] are frequently reported. Retropharyngeal abscesses may develop from extension of a peritonsillar disease, penetrating trauma to the pharynx [4], parotitis [19], epiglottitis [20], either oral or nasotracheal intubation [9, 21, 22], or post-tracheotomy [23]. In one study 50% of patients with parapharyngeal neck infections had some evidence of mediastinal involvement by CT [24].

Other rare causes of descending necrotizing mediastinitis include facial cellulitis [25, 26] and transnasal sinus drainage [10]. Though common in the pre-antibiotic era, suppurative cervical lymphadenitis, cervical discitis, and post-thyroidectomy surgical site infections rarely cause mediastinitis currently.

MICROBIOLOGY

Descending necrotizing mediastinitis is generally a mixed or polymicrobial infection. Combinations of aerobic and anaerobic organisms, reflective of the flora of the oropharynx, are usually recovered. Mediastinal tissue, pericardial fluid, and pleural fluid have multiple organisms seen on Gram stain. Anaerobic bacteria which have been recovered in the past include *Bacteroides* sp., *Fusobacterium* sp., anaerobic *Streptococcus* sp. *Peptostreptococcus* sp., and *Prevotella denticola* [14, 21, 27–29]. Studies in the 1970s showed that on average three to four anaerobic organisms were isolated per culture specimen [16]. Aerobic organisms most frequently recovered include aerobic *Streptococci*, *Staphylococcus aureus*, and *Enterobacteriaceae*, of which *E. coli*, *Klebsiella* sp., and *Pseudomonas* sp. have been reported. Several authors [4, 30, 31] have theorized that the altered redox potential due to aerobic bacterial metabolism and the closed spaces of the fascial planes of the neck leads to an area in which organisms can thrive, particularly anaerobes. This results in a high organism count and rapid tissue destruction.

SIGNS AND SYMPTOMS

Many patients with mediastinitis present with fever, neck and chest pain or non-specific symptoms. Often, individuals are on antibiotics for dental infections or presumed bacterial pharyngitis [4]. Mediastinitis can be missed initially unless clinical suspicion is high. Individuals with infections of the head and neck who suddenly develop chest pain should arouse suspicion of mediastinal spread [7]. As mediastinal infection progresses, brawny induration of the upper chest and neck can occur, along with pitting edema and subcutaneous crepitus. This process can then extend to the upper extremities in some cases [10]. However, even these signs are felt to lack sensitivity [10]. Loss of the sternal notch and the clavicular landmarks can also be seen. If these signs are noted they are highly suggestive of the diagnosis. Though dysphagia has been more commonly associated with esophageal perforation, this can be seen in cases of posterior mediastinitis in which the esophagus is compressed by abscess formation [32]. Airway compromise due to compression of the central airway and pharynx from inflammation is common and can lead to dyspnea and ultimately respiratory collapse. Epigastric and abdominal pain mimicking an acute abdomen has been reported with descent of the necrotizing process into the retroperitoneum [4].

Given the tendency for descending necrotizing mediastinitis to progress rapidly and frequent delays in diagnosis, patients often present with complications. As discussed earlier, complications are dependent on the anatomy of the mediastinum. The most frequent complication is rupture of a mediastinal abscess through the parietal pleura, resulting in an empyema. Transudative effusions have been reported, however, direct extension of the infection resulting in purulent fluid in the pleural space is more common. Bacterial pericarditis with friction rub or tamponade has been described, which is also believed to be secondary to direct extension. This is especially true of infections in the pretracheal space. Involvement of the cranial nerves in the neck can lead to focal neurological deficits. As the disease progresses, tracheal and esophageal fistulas can develop [33]. Vascular structures in both the neck and thorax are also susceptible to involvement. The internal jugular vein can be thrombosed or the carotid artery can rupture when the carotid sheath is infected [11]. The great vessels in the thorax can erode from direct infection [4, 10, 34] resulting in rapid exsanguination. The innominate vein and artery frequently have been involved in case reports. Anterior mediastinitis can rarely result in superior vena cava obstruction with head and neck cyanosis, edema, and neck vein distention [32].

DIAGNOSIS

Rapid diagnosis is crucial to improving long-term survival in this disease. Early reports noted that 60% of patients presenting to medical attention with necrotizing mediastinitis due to an odontogenic infection did so within 48 hours from the onset of symptoms. Later reviews however, noted that the delay could be as long as 15 days [7]. Because of this, many cases of mediastinitis are diagnosed late in the process. Several reviews have noted a delay from admission to diagnosis on average of 2.5 days [4, 7, 10]. As clinical signs are often non-specific or do not become apparent until wide-spread tissue destruction has already occurred, radiological diagnosis has long been recognized as paramount [4, 7, 9, 10, 35].

Radiographic findings in descending necrotizing mediastinitis can be identified in both lateral simple neck x-rays and the PA and lateral chest x-rays. Lateral neck radiographs may reveal subcutaneous air in the soft tissue of the neck, swelling of the prevertebral soft tissue (suggestive of retropharyngeal abscess), loss of cervical spine lordosis, or air in the retropharyngeal space. Chest radiographs can show mediastinal widening, pneumomediastinum, anterior displacement of the thoracic trachea due to abscess formation, mediastinal air-fluid levels, enlarged cardiac silhouette, and pleural effusion. Plain radiography, however, is usually negative early in the disease, with findings only becoming present after sepsis has developed [35].

Most authors agree that the most rapid and effective way to diagnose descending mediastinitis is by (CT) [4, 7, 9, 10, 35]. Magnetic nuclear resonance (MRI) can similarly show fascial planes and chest involvement, however patients generally are too unstable to undergo MRI in a timely manner. CT is particularly helpful in assessing extent of disease and guiding surgical therapy. The benefit of CT became apparent in the review by Estrera *et al.* in 1983 [4] when mediastinal involvement was noted in these patients by CT when plain films had been unrevealing. Fluid collections, loss of distinct tissue planes, mediastinal inflammation, and air in the mediastinum are easily seen by CT (Figure 2). Pericarditis and empyemas can also be assessed by this method.

TREATMENT

The effective management of this life-threatening illness requires rapid recognition of the extent of disease. Aggressive fluid resuscitation, stabilization of the compromised airway, early empiric antibiotic therapy, and surgical drainage of infection are the mainstays of therapy.

The dramatic inflammatory reaction often seen in mediastinal infections results in a significant amount of third space sequestration. This requires intravascular volume resuscitation with intravenous fluids. The extensive amount of pharyngeal edema and inflammation seen in descending necrotizing mediastinitis, particularly in cases which arise from a submandibular space infection can rapidly compromise the airway. Many authors recommend tracheotomy for all patients with descending necrotizing mediastinitis to assure airway patency, and to avoid the risk of accidental dislodgment of an endotracheal tube, which may be impossible to replace in the face of tissue edema [4, 10, 35–37]. Endotracheal intubation causing the traumatic rupture of a parapharyngeal abscess into the pharynx, with subsequent aspiration of purulent material has been reported [10]. More recent authors, however, have taken the approach of perfoming a tracheotomy only when there is evidence of impending airway compromise by

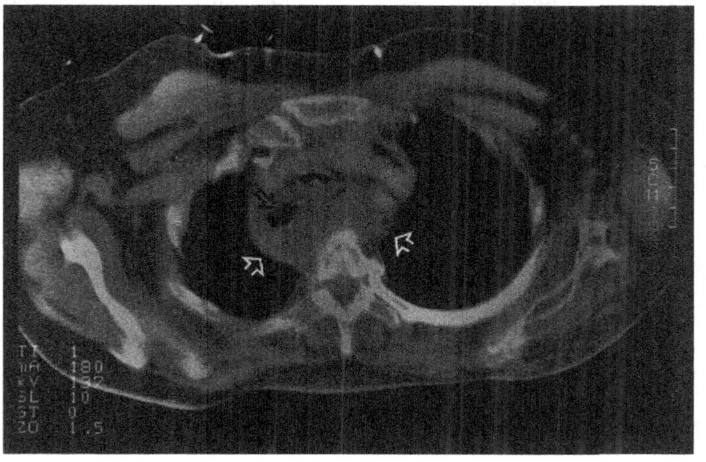

FIGURE 2. Descending necrotizing mediastinitis diagnosed by computer tomography. A large mediastinal abscess (white arrows) with gas present in the abscess (black arrow) is seen displacing the trachea and great vessels anteriorly.

clinical criteria or by CT [9, 38]. This is in part due to the risk of introducing infection into the lower airway perioperatively during the procedure [9, 39–41]. Regardless, a low threshold for performing tracheotomy would be prudent in any patient who presents with serious deep neck infections.

Descending necrotizing mediastinitis is a surgical emergency. As noted previously, despite the onset of improved imaging, the mortality of this disease has not changed dramatically in the last 20 years. This is felt in part by many to be a result of inadequate initial surgical drainage and debridement. Though there are some reports of successful antibiotic mangagement alone [24] and CT-guided drainage of focal mediastinal abscesses [42], most agree that aggressive surgical drainage is the cornerstone of therapy [4, 7, 10, 33–35, 38, 43]. Transcervical drainage was the traditional approach to descending necrotizing mediastinitis, however this was felt by many to be inadequate, particularly when there was extension of necrosis below the level of the fourth thoracic vertebrae [4, 44]. In cases that involve the anterior mediastinum a subxiphoid incision combined with submandibular incisions has been used [34, 35]. However, most surgeons advocate drainage by thoracotomy when mediastinitis involves the pleural or pericardial cavity, or where there is involvement of the inferior mediastinum [10, 16, 38, 43]. Post-operative fever that persists, or lack of clinical improvement, should prompt a repeat CT to search for undrained sources of infection [10].

Antibiotic therapy is a necessary component in the management of descending necrotizing mediastinitis. Empiric coverage should be initiated as soon as possible. Antibiotic coverage should be broad and directed toward those organisms most likely to be implicated in this infection. Regimens with activity against Gram-positive organisms, including *Streptococcus* and *Staphylococcus* spp., parapharyngeal facultative anaerobes, and Gram-negative aerobic organisms, are most appropriate. Penicillin G has coverage against the oral flora both aerobic and the facultative anaerobic bacteria and can be used as part of an initial regimen. However, many of the *Prevotella* sp. have acquired β-lactam resistance, so clindamycin or metronidazole would be necessary, along with another antibiotic with Gram-negative activity. Alternatively, single-agent empiric therapy with a β-lactamase resistant penicillin, such as imipenem, piperacillin/tazobactam, ticarcillin/tazobactam, or ampicillin/sulbactam, which would cover

Gram-positive cocci, anaerobes, and Gram-negative bacilli can be used. Antibiotic therapy can be further refined once surgical culture results become available. Anaerobic coverage should be continued regardless of culture results, however, given that they are frequently difficult to recover. The duration of antibiotic therapy must be tailored to the clinical response of the patient but frequently is on the order of weeks to months.

Mediastinitis Resulting from Esophageal Perforation

Disruption of the esophageal wall for various reasons results in the spillage of salivary secretions and food particles directly into the mediastinum. Prior to the onset of modern cardiothoracic surgery this was the most common inciting mechanism for mediastinitis during the first half of the twentieth century [1]. Because of the role oropharyngeal flora plays in its pathogenesis, mediastinitis due to esophageal perforation shares many similarities to mediastinitis arising from head and neck infections, however, there are significant differences in presentation, diagnosis, and surgical management between the two entities.

The most common causes of esophageal perforation are iatrogenic [45–48] and are generally secondary to endoscopy, esophageal dilation procedures, complications of variceal banding or electrocautery, breakdown of surgical anastomoses after esophageal resection, or inadvertent perforation during head and neck surgery [49–52]. The patients who develop perforation after instrumentation generally have some underlying esophageal disease [45, 53]. Case reports of migration of dislodged cervical fixation devices or cervical bone fragments eroding into the esophagus have been noted [54]. Hyperextension injuries of the cervical spine and other trauma to the neck and chest are also causes of esophageal rupture. Glatterer *et al.* [52] reviewed 26 cases of traumatic esophageal perforation and found that 21 of these cases were due to cervical injury, with the four of those due to blunt trauma. The thoracic cases in that study were all due to penetrating trauma, however deceleration injury resulting in thoracic esophageal perforation has been reported [55]. Another cause of esophageal injury is erosion due to foreign bodies lodged in the lumen of the esophagus, particularly in children or adults with underlying esophageal pathology [56, 57]. Finally, malignancy, ingestion of caustic substances, and emesis are well-recognized sources of perforation. Perforation due to malignancy, in particular, has been noted have a worse outcome, though this may be related to a tendency towards a more conservative approach [47, 48, 53].

Because esophageal injury results in the spillage of oropharyngeal secretions into the mediastinum, the microbiology is very similar to that found in mediastinitis secondary to odontogenic disease. These infections are generally polymicrobial in nature. Gram-positive organisms such as *Streptococcus* and *Staphylococcus* sp. along with facultative and obligate anaerobes form the oropharyngeal flora are frequent causative pathogens. Gram-negative enteric bacteria are also identified from culture regularly. In a review of 16 patients with esophageal perforation due to various causes, Burnett *et al.* found *Streptococcus*, *Pseudomonas*, and *Candida* spp. to be the most commonly isolated organisms [49]. *Candida* spp. often colonize the human esophagus and have been isolated in over 25% of normal hosts [46].

SIGNS AND SYMPTOMS

Mediastinitis frequently arises as a complication of esophageal perforation because the perforation it often missed. Immediately after an injury occurs, the classic symptoms of chest pain and subcutaneous emphysema are often absent. Particularly in individuals with multiple trauma to the head and neck, the diagnosis may be obscured by more apparent injuries. Patients may present with chest pain, shortness of breath, nausea, and malaise. Dysphagia and odynophagia have been reported, especially when a foreign body is lodged in the esophagus. Pediatric cases of foreign body ingestion can have excessive salivation or what appears to be new onset asthma [57]. Cervical esophageal injury can present with pain and tenderness in the neck, resistance in the neck to passive motion, cough, stridor, hoarseness, or bleeding in the mouth. Lower thoracic injuries can present as a rigid or tender abdomen, along with a mediastinal crunch on auscultation due to pneumomediastinum. In individuals with blunt or penetrating trauma to the neck or chest, subcutaneous emphysema, hematoma of the neck, and blood return from nasogastric tube have also been associated with perforation [52]. As the process advances, neck erythema, swelling, and fever become apparent, finally progressing to septic shock and multisystem organ failure.

As with infections arising from the head and neck, mediastinitis from esophageal perforation will often present with complications of infection by the time the patient comes to medical attention. Extension of pathology into the pleural space can lead to pneumothorax, hemothorax and empyema. Purulent pericarditis can be seen. Esophageal fistula formation is a late complication of infection, with can result in communication with the skin, respiratory tract, or vascular structures in the mediastinum and neck [49, 52, 58]. Exsanguination from aorto-esophageal fistulas has been reported [49, 57].

DIAGNOSIS

There is no single best test to diagnose esophageal perforation. Oral contrast studies performed with a water-soluble material, such as Gastrografin, will often reveal a disruption. This is generally the safest method for rapid diagnosis an should be the first step in evaluation of a suspected esophageal perforation. However, in several reviews water-soluble contrast studies have been associated with a false-negative rate of between 20–50% [52, 59, 60]. Most recently, Buecker, *et al.* [61] showed that in 18 patients with an initially negative water-soluble contrast study 22% had evidence of perforation on immediate follow-up barium fluoroscopy. This has led some authors to recommend performing barium swallow studies or endoscopy if the initial water-soluble study is unrevealing [52, 57]. Other imaging modalities, such as CT and MRI are useful in defining the extent of mediastinal involvement, however they still lack the detailed visualization of esophageal anatomy that contrast imaging affords. Plain radiography can give some clues to the underlying diagnosis of an esophageal perforation and mediastinitis, but lacks adequate sensitivity [52]. Cervical or mediastinal air, mediastinal widening, pleural effusion, pneumothorax, or mediastinal air-fluid levels can all be seen. Occasionally, a foreign body can be identified on plain film. The migration of a foreign body from the neck to the stomach on serial films confirms the presence of an esophageal perforation [52].

TREATMENT

Success in treating mediastinitis secondary to esophageal perforation rests partially on the rapid diagnosis of the underlying perforation. A detailed history is important to identify risk factors for disruption such as violent emesis, recent endoscopic procedures, and ingestions. Often in trauma cases a history is unavailable and instead a high index of suspicion must be present, particularly in injuries to the neck and penetrating chest wounds. Contamination of the paraesophageal space with saliva and bacteria occurs early in the course of injury, and delay in diagnosis leads to extension of infection. Several authors have shown increased mortality if the delay in diagnosis is greater than 12–24 hours [49, 58]. However, more recent studies have shown less of an association with outcome and time to diagnosis [47, 53]. When esophageal perforation is suspected, the patient should be made NPO to minimize further contamination and empiric antimicrobial therapy should be instituted.

As with descending head and neck infections rapid institution of broad-spectrum antimicrobials to cover Gram-positive bacteria, anaerobic organisms, and Gram-negative enteric bacteria is essential. *Candida* sp., as noted above, is frequently isolated from culture and empiric antifungal therapy, particularly in patients at high risk for invasive fungal disease (e.g., prolonged ICU stay, prior broad-spectrum antibiotic use, and neutropenia) should be considered [46].

Surgical management of esophageal perforation remains somewhat controversial. Some have advocated conservative management with antibiotic therapy, nothing by mouth, and interventional radiology-placed drainage, nasogastric drainage, and supplemental enteral or parenteral nutrition for contained perforations without sepsis [53, 62, 63]. The use of esophageal stents [64] to contain perforations and thorascopic drainage of the mediastinum [65] have also been reported. Most do agree, however, that in patients with circumfrential or multiple disruptions of the esophagus, intra-abdominal perforations, uncontained perforations, and evidence of mediastinitis or sepsis surgical intervention is warranted [46, 48, 62, 63]. Surgical techniques of repair perforations vary by surgeon and center, and are influenced by the underlying co-morbidities and overall risk of operation in a particular patient. Some of these procedures include primary repair with or without pleural or muscular buttress, esophagectomy, T-tube drainage, and cervical esophagostomy.

Studies in recent years have shown some improvement in overall mortality from infections due to esophageal leaks, with rates of 4–25% [45, 47, 48, 53, 62, 63], compared to rates of 15–44% [49, 52, 62] in the mid-to-late 1980s. There has not been a significant change in the time to diagnosis [53], however. Whether advances in intensive care management or refinement in selection of surgical approach account for the decreased death rate is unclear. Despite this, infections due to esophageal perforation remain a significant source of morbidity and mortality.

Mediastinitis as a Complication of Cardiac Surgery

Though the idea of the median sternotomy approach was discussed as early as the late 1800s [66], it was not until the advent of cardiopulmonary bypass that the modern era of cardiothoracic surgery became a reality. It was recognized early that infections of the sternum could easily spread into the mediastinum from direct extension and carry serious consequences. Though the incidence of post-operative deep wound infection has been between 0.23–2.7% in most large scale studies [67–76], the mortality has been between 14–41% [68, 69, 71–73, 77]. There is also significant morbidity associated with these infections, with a median hospital length-of-stay that is double that of non-infected patients [77]. Additionally, many patients need to undergo repeat surgical procedures for treatment or reconstruction. Both the prolonged hospital stay and repeated surgical procedures contribute to an excess cost approximately three times that of uncomplicated post-operative stays. Often, patients are left with chronic pain and significant chest wall deformity if they do survive the infection. Despite the relatively low incidence of mediastinitis from cardiac surgery, the shear number of procedures performed each year have made it the most common cause of acute mediastinitis encountered in modern practice.

Host factors predisposing to mediastinitis after cardiac surgery include diabetes mellitus [73, 74, 78–82], obesity [67, 73, 75, 78, 79, 83], and extended preoperative length of stay [68, 76, 81]. Perioperative risk factors include those which reflect a more debilitated patient population, such as use of intra-aortic balloon pump or other inotropic support [68, 75, 78], excessive aortic cross-clamp and by-pass time [67, 84], re-exploration or emergent surgery [68, 73, 75, 84] prolonged post-operative mechanical ventilation [85, 86], and concurrent saphenous vein graft harvest site infection [73].

Several procedures associated with the particulars of cardiac surgery, such as, pre-operative chest hair removal by shaving [74], the reliance on electrocautery for dissection [84], and the use of bilateral internal mammary arterial grafting in diabetics [75] have all been sited as contributing to the pathogenesis of deep sternal wound infections. Francel *et al.* showed in cadaveric studies that the inferior sternal/xiphoid area has an intrinsic paucity of vascular supply, which is further compromised by the classic internal mammary artery harvest and may then serve as a nidus for infection [87].

Cardiac transplantation procedures warrant special discussion. Several studies have documented sternal wound infection rates following cardiac transplant of approximately 2.5% [88, 89]. Risk factors specifically associated with mediastinitis after cardiac transplant include prior mediastinotomy, ischemic cardiomyopathy, and early acute rejection requiring the use of steroids and murine-monoclonal CD–3 antibody (OKT3) [88, 89]. Donor to recipient transmission of bacteria as a cause of mediastinitis has also been reported [90].

MICROBIOLOGY

The microbiology of mediastinitis following cardiac surgical procedures is different in nature from those infections arising from head and neck or esophageal sources. This is due to the skin being the supposed primary site of entry in the majority of cases. Several studies have noted an approximately 60% positive culture rate when sternal wounds were explored. Gram-positive organisms are the predominate organism isolated in sternal wound cultures [67, 69, 71, 73, 75–77, 81, 82, 91], with *Staphylococcus aureus* as the most common organism isolated, followed by coagulase-negative *Staphylococcus*, and *Enterococcus* sp. Some more unusual organisms, such as *S. pnuemoniae*, have been reported as causative agents [92]. Gram-negative bacteria represent approximately 20–40% of clinical isolates in several studies [67, 68, 72, 73, 77, 81, 82, 91]. The most common of these include *E. coli*, *Enterobacter* sp., *Serratia* sp., *Klebsiella* sp., and *Pseudomonas* species. Yeast, specifically *Candida* sp. [93–95], has been seen as pathogen and has been associated with prolonged pre-operative antibiotic use. The rate of fungemia in these patients appeared to be as high as 75% in one study [93]. Anaerobes, such as *Proprionobacterium acne*, *Bacteroides* sp. [96, 97] have been indentified as causative agents in a number of cases. Other more unusual pathogens, such as *Corynebacterium xerosis* [98], and *Mycoplasma hominis* [99] have been rarely reported. *M. hominis* can be missed due to slow growth in anaerobic media. Post-operative mediastinitis can be polymicrobial in nature [76, 82, 91], but is much less common than in the other causes of mediastinitis, generally 10% in case reviews. Mediastinitis after cardiac transplantation also is most frequently due to *Staphylococcus* sp., followed by Gram-negative bacilli, however, some opportunistic organisms, such as *Nocardia* sp. [88, 89, 100, 101] and *Aspergillus* sp. [102], have been reported. Bacteremia occurs in 25–57% of patients with mediastinitis and has been associated with increased mortality [68]. Conversely, in individuals who are bacteremic after coronary artery by-pass, deep sternal wound infections were the cause in 67% of the cases in one study [94]. There have been cases of hematogenous seeding of the wound site from catheter-associated bacteremia [103]. A heightened index of suspicion for deep sternal wound infections in the bacteremic patient would seem to be prudent.

An unusual group of pathogens seen as a particular cause of post-sternotomy mediastinitis are the rapid-growing mycobacterium. *M. fortuitum, M. chelonei*, and *M. smegmatis* have all been isolated from deep sternal wound infections. Porcine heterograft valves contaminated with *M. chelonei* [104–106], and ice for cooling cardioplegic solution contaminated with *M. fortuitum* [107] have been responsible for epidemic outbreaks of mediastinitis in cardiothoracic units.

Several other cases have been presented in which case clusters have been identified and an environmental source suspected, but never clearly determined [108–110]. Clinically, infections with the rapid-growing mycobacterium tend to be more indolent, with the formation of cold abscesses and fistulas [111] or minimal inflammatory signs [112]. However, case reports have noted the tendency for these organisms to cause breakdown of vein graft anastamotic sites and aortic psuedoanuerysms due to vasculitis [107, 110, 113]. Rapid-growing mycobacterium should be considered in those patients with clinical evidence of deep sternal wound infection post-sternotomy, but in whom routine cultures have remained negative [114].

SIGNS AND SYMPTOMS

The symptoms of mediastinitis after cardiac surgery can occur as early as a few days post-procedure, to as late as 3–6 months afterwards, however, the average time to presentation has been reported as 7–15 days from the time of surgery [68, 71, 77, 95]. Wound drainage, which occurs in 70% to 100% of cases, erythema, increased pain at the operative site, and fever have been observed in case reviews of post-surgical mediastinitis [68, 71, 95, 115]. Though wound drainage is frequently present, it is non-specific. Sternal instability and sternal dehiscence either partial or complete, are indicators of underlying deep infection, however they are reportedly present in only 25–60% of mediastinitis patients [67, 95]. In one study dehiscence was observed to occur 24–48 hours after onset of wound drainage [73]. Drainage through the sternotomy wound that bubbles with respiratory chest wall motion is indicative of deep infection in the mediastinum. In an early pediatric study by Jimenez-Martinez *et al.* all patients with this clinical finding had anterior mediastinal involvement at the time of surgical exploration [115]. Laboratory data is generally limited in usefulness. Leukocystosis [71, 73, 115] is the most common laboratory finding in mediastinitis. In a small percentage of patients, leukocytosis and persistent fever may be the only presenting signs of mediastinal infection.

As with others forms of mediastinitis, post-sternotomy infections can be associated with complications. Empyemas and pericarditis from direct extension of infection can be seen, along with sepsis, and multisystem organ failure. Endocarditis has been seen in valve replacement surgery and cardiac transplantation [101]. Coronary artery graft anastomotic breakdown and aortic graft dehiscence with fatal exsanguination have also been reported [77, 95].

DIAGNOSIS

The diagnosis of post-operative mediastinitis is based on a high clinical index of suspicion, as no single test is definitive. Several studies have looked at the utility of wound and epicardial lead cultures in the diagnosis of mediastinitis. Surface wound cultures in one review were not sensitive, yielding the causative pathogen in only 6 of 15 cases [77]. Cultures of epicardial pacemaker leads, given their position in the anterior mediastinum and ease at which they can be removed under sterile conditions for culture, have been looked at as a diagnostic tool. The studies are mixed. One early report showed a high sensitivity at diagnosing deep infections and good correlation with follow-up intra-operative cultures [116]. However, a larger, more recent study showed that the positive predictive value of epicardial cultures was only 11.6%, and only slightly better with *S. aureus* positive cultures at 32.3% [69]. The role of chest radiography is limited in the diagnosis of deep sternal wound infections. Indium scanning has been evaluated in a small study, which showed an 83% sensitivity rate [116]. Computerized tomography can be used for diagnostic purposes [88, 116], but again there are conflicting reports of the sensitivity and specificity of the technique. CT can identify fluid collections, which can then be sampled for evidence of infection. It is also useful in following patients after debridement and drainage. Sternal aspiration can be done at the bedside and can be useful in making a diagnosis and obtaining early culture results to guide antibiotic therapy [117].

TREATMENT

The management of post-sternotomy mediastinitis focuses on both antimicrobial and surgical therapy. Antibiotic therapy alone for mediastinitis is inadequate, and should be viewed as an adjuvant to surgical treatment. Antimicrobial therapy should be empirically started when post-operative infection is suspected. Coverage should include anti-Staphylococcal coverage and, given the significant proportion of cases in which Gram-negative organisms are isolated, a broad-spectrum antibiotic with activity against cephalosporinase-producing organisms, such as *Enterobacter* sp., should be given. Therapy should then be tailored to cover organisms found in intra-operative specimens and, while no evidence-based guidelines are available, is generally on the order of 4–6 weeks of intravenous therapy, with longer courses in cases with significant amounts of sternal osteomyelitis. Initial surgical management of mediastinitis in the past consisted of debridement of necrotic or infected tissue, especially sternal bone, with the mediastinum left packed open to close by secondary intention. This approach resulted in a high morbidity, often complicated by pneumonia [115], prolonged hospital stay, abnormal thoracic wall mechanics, and cosmetic deformity.

Surgical treatment at present varies, and is partially dependent on the viability of the sternum at the time of surgery Approaches in which the sternum is relatively intact include debridement with rewiring of the sternum, and percutaneous drainage, either as single staged procedure, or after several days of open irrigation. Some have also advocated the use of continuous sternal irrigation with antibiotic or providone-iodine solutions either in a closed procedure [118], or as follow-up of open debridement and re-wiring. Closed continuous sternal irrigation is able to maintain normal chest wall mechanics compared to open procedures, however, has been reported to have a high failure rate and an association with iodine toxicity when providone-iodine was used as an irrigant [119, 120]. Several studies have looked at rigid fixed closure or modified re-wiring of the sternum after open debridement [82, 121]. When there has been significant evidence of sternal destruction or recurrence of infection, frequently a large dead space is present after debridement. This often requires the use of muscle or omental flaps to both obliterate the dead space and achieve closure of the wound. Generally, this has been done as a staged procedure, particularly if a significant amount of infected, devitalized tissue is present, but in some series patients with relatively clean wound margins have had closure with myocutaneous flaps at the time of initial debridement and irrigation [122]. While major plastic surgery allows for chest wall closures, long-term it can result in chronic pain, paresthesia, sternal instability, or shoulder weakness [123]. There are also rare reports of myocardial hemorrhage post-debridement, with puncture of the myocardium by the sternal edge or tearing at the myocardial-sternal interface [124–126]. The ideal surgical management for patients with post-sternotomy mediastinitis remains to be defined.

Chronic Fibrosing Mediastinitis and Other Uncommon Causes of Mediastinitis

There are several infectious causes of mediastinitis, which can present with a more insidious course consisting of adenopathy and progressive fibrosis of mediastinal structures. This can result in pulmonary artery fibrosis with pulmonary hypertension, tracheobronchial stenosis, esophageal obstruction or esophago-respiratory fistulas, and superior vena caval obstruction. *Histoplasmosis capsulatum* is the organism most frequently associated with mediastinal fibrosis [127, 128], though *Mycobacterium tuberculosis* [129–132], *Blastomyces dermatitidis* [133, 134], and *Wuchereria bancrofti* [135] have been reported to result in similar syndromes. In the case of

H. capsulatum, it is theorized that after primary infection, the ongoing seepage of fungal antigens from granulomas in the mediastinal tissue causes a host hypersensitivity response with fibroblast activation and resulting fibrosis [136].

Hematogenous seeding of the mediastinum is unusual but has been reported. *Salmonella* sp. has been associated with hematogenous dissemination from a subcutaneous abscess complicating a raccoon bite [137] and superinfection of a benign mediastinal mass after an episode of enteritis [138]. Group A *Streptococcus* [139] and *S. aureus* [140] have also resulted in mediastinitis after bacteremia.

Inhalational exposure to the spores of *B. anthracis* may result in a mediastinitis. This has received attention in recent years due to concerns of the use of anthrax in biological warfare [141–143]. The infection results in a primary focal hemorrhagic, necrotizing pneumonia in some patients, but more striking is the development of rapidly progressive hemorrhagic thoracic lymphadenitis and mediastinitis [142]. The significant amount of third-space fluid shift into the mediastinum can result in stridor, chest pain, and cyanosis from compression of the tracheobronchial tree [144]. Patients can rapidly progress to intravascular collapse and death. As with other causes of mediastinitis, a widened mediastinum can be seen on chest radiographs.

Finally, mediastinitis has been observed as a complication of central venous catheterization. Migration of the catheter out of the vessel into the mediastinum has resulted in the infusion of total parenteral nutrition solution [145] and chemotherapeutic agents [146]. Infiltration of the infusate can result in a significant chemical mediastinitis.

Mediastinitis continues to be a challenge for the clinician. For descending necrotizing mediastinitis an understanding of the anatomy of the head and neck is important in recognizing mediastinal infections which originate in these structures. Likewise, in patients with either esophageal disease or procedures performed on the esophagus, signs or symptoms of infection should warn the clinician of possible perforation. Understanding risk factors for mediastinitis after cardiac surgery and that deep sternal wound infections can often lack clear clinical indicators is important. CT still remains the diagnostic test of choice for mediastinitis secondary to descending infection. For cases in which esophageal perforation is suspected, an oral contrast radiographic study can aid in diagnosis. While no single diagnostic test has proven superior for post-cardiac surgery mediastinitis, CT is helpful in guiding the surgical approach. The treatment of mediastinitis requires a high index of suspicion and prompt initiation of both broad antimicrobial therapy and surgical evaluation. This currently offers the best chance of survival in these critically ill patients.

References

1. Pearse HE Jr. Mediastinitis following cervical suppuration. Surg Gynecol Obstet 157:588, 1938.
2. Julian OC. The median sternal incision in intracardiac surgery with extracorporeal circulation. Surgery 42:753, 1957.
3. Culliford AT, Cunningham JN Jr, Zeff RH, Isom OW, Teiko P, Spencer FC. Sternal and costochondral infections following open-heart surgery. A review of 2594 cases. J Thorac Cardiovasc Surg 72:714, 1976.
4. Estrera AS, Landay MJ, Grisham JM, Sinn DP, Platt MR. Descending necrotizing mediastinitis. Surg Gynecol Obstet 157:545, 1983.
5. Kiernan PD, Hernandez A, Byrne WD, Bloom R, Dicicco B, Hetrick V, Graling P, Vaughan B. Descending cervical mediastinitis. Ann Thorac Surg 65:1483, 1998.
6. Payne WS, Larson RH. Acute mediastinitis. Surg Clin North Am 49:999, 1969.
7. Marty-Ane CH, Alauzen M, Alric P, Serres-Cousine O, Mary H. Descending necrotizing mediastinitis. Advantage of mediastinal drainage with thoracotomy. J Thorac Cardiovasc Surg 107:55, 1994.
8. Steiner M, Grau MJ, Wilson DL, Snow NJ. Odontogenic infection leading to cervical emphysema and fatal mediastinitis. J Oral Maxillo Surg 40:600, 1982.

9. Temes RT, Crowell RE, Mapel DW, Ketai L, Pett SB Jr, Wernly JA. Mediastinitis without antecedent surgery. Thorac Cardiovasc Surg 46:84, 1998.
10. Colmenero RC, Labajo AD, Yanez VI, Paniagua J. Thoracic complications of deeply situated serous neck infections. J Craniomaxillofac Surg 21:76, 1993.
11. Zachariades N, Mezitis M, Stavrinidis P, Konsolaki-Agouridaki E. Mediastinitis, thoracic empyema, and pericarditis as complications of a dental abscess: report of a case. J Oral Maxillofac Surg 46:493, 1988.
12. Haraden BM, Zwemer FL Jr. Descending necrotizing mediastinitis: complication of a simple dental infection. Annals Emerg Med 29:683, 1997.
13. Phelps R, Jacobs RA. Purulent pericarditis and mediastinitis due to Peptococcus magnus. JAMA 254:947, 1985.
14. Rubin MM, Cozzi GM. Fatal necrotizing mediastinitis as a complication of an odontogenic infection. J Oral Maxillo Surg 45:529, 1987.
15. Gilchrist BF, Valerie EP, Nguyen M, Coren C, Klotz D, Ramenofsky ML. Pearls and perils in the management of prolonged, peculiar, penetrating esophageal foreign bodies in children. J Pediatric Surg 32:1429, 1997.
16. Wills PI, Vernon RP Jr. Complications of space infections of the head and neck. Laryngoscope 91:1129, 1981.
17. Albertsen J, Thomsen EM. Nonclostridial deep gas-producing infection in the neck. Arch Otolaryngol 92:383, 1970.
18. Kopec SE, Irwin RS, Mello CJ, Umali CB. Bilateral anaerobic empyemas complicating infectious mononucleosis. Chest 112:833, 1997.
19. Guardia SN, Cameron R, Phillips A. Fatal necrotizing mediastinitis secondary to acute suppurative parotitis. J Otolaryngology 20:54, 1991.
20. Chong WH, Woodhead MA, Millard FJ. Mediastinitis and bilateral thoracic empyemas complicating adult epiglottitis. Thorax 45:491, 1990.
21. Lu DC, Chang SC, Chen HC. Polymicrobial bacterial pericarditis with mediastinitis after endotracheal intubation. Diagnos Microbiol Infect Dis 23:115, 1995.
22. Seaman M, Ballinger P, Sturgill TD, Maertins M. Mediastinitis following nasal intubation in the emergency department. Am J Emerg Med 9:37, 1991.
23. Bishop MJ. Epiglottitis in the adult. Anesthesiology 55:701, 1981.
24. de Marie S, Tjon ATR, van der Mey AG, Meerdink G, van Furth R, van der Meer JW. Clinical infections and nonsurgical treatment of parapharyngeal space infections complicating throat infection. Rev Infect Dis 11:975, 1989.
25. Perfect JR. Mediastinitis complicating cellulitis of the head and neck. South Med J 73:1378, 1980.
26. Calandra GB, Mackowiak PA. Retropharyngeal abscess, mediastinitis, and pleural effusion complicating streptococcal facial erysipelas. South Med J 74:1031, 1981.
27. Murray PM, Finegold SM. Anaerobic mediastinitis. Rev Infect Dis 6(Suppl 1):S123, 1984.
28. Mukau L. Dissecting retropharyngeal abscess due to Fusobacterium necrophorum in an adult. South Med J 78:476, 1985.
29. Brondbo K, Rubin A, Chapnik JS, Mucklow MG, Steinhardt MI. Ludwig's angina following dental extraction as a cause of necrotizing mediastinitis. J Otolaryngology, 12:50, 1983.
30. Economopoulos GC, Scherzer HH, Gryboski WA. Successful management of mediastinitis, pleural empyema, and aortopulmonary fistula from odontogenic infection. Ann Thorac Surg 35:184, 1983.
31. Stone HH, Martin JD Jr. Synergistic necrotizing cellulitis. Ann Surg 175:702, 1972.
32. Pane GA, Hamilton GC, Call E. Nontraumatic suppurative mediastinitis presenting as acute mediastinal widening. Ann Emerg Med 12:777, 1983.
33. Kruyt PM, Boonstra A, Fockens P, Reeders JW, van Lanschot JJ. Descending necrotizing mediastinitis causing pleuroesophageal fistula. Successful treatment by combined transcervical and pleural drainage. Chest 109:1404, 1996.
34. al Ebrahim KE. Descending necrotising mediastinitis: a case report and review of the literature. Eur J Cardio-Thorac Surg 9:161, 1995.
35. Wheatley MJ, Stirling MC, Kirsh MM, Gago O, Orringer MB. Descending necrotizing mediastinitis: transcervical drainage is not enough. Annals Thorac Surg 49:780, 1990.
36. Lalwani AK, Kaplan MJ. Mediastinal and thoracic complications of necrotizing fasciitis of the head and neck. Head & Neck 13:531, 1991.
37. Maisel RH, Karlen R. Cervical necrotizing fasciitis. Laryngoscope 104:795, 1994.
38. Sugata T, Fujita Y, Myoken Y, Fujioka Y. Cervical cellulitis with mediastinitis from an

odontogenic infection complicated by diabetes mellitus: report of a case. J Oral Maxillofac Surg 55:864, 1997.
39. Zeitoun IM, Dhanarajani PJ. Cervical cellulitis and mediastinitis caused by odontogenic infections: report of two cases and review of literature. J Oral Maxillofac Surg 53:203, 1995.
40. Ogiso A, Tamura M, Minemura T, Kurashina K, Kotani A. Mediastinitis caused by odontogenic infection associated with adult respiratory distress syndrome. Oral Surg Oral Med Oral Pathol 74:15, 1992.
41. Harrison GA, Schultz TA, Schaberg SJ. Deep neck infection complicated by diabetes mellitus. Report of a case. Oral Surg Oral Med Oral Pathol 55:133, 1983.
42. Marsh MD, Amorosa JK, Abassi M, Nosher JL, Gross SC, Alcid DV. Salmonella mediastinitis – a rare disease. Computerized Radiology 8:375, 1984.
43. Bonapart IE, Stevens HP, Kerver AJ, Rietveld AP. Rare complications of an odontogenic abscess: mediastinitis, thoracic empyema and cardiac tamponade. J Oral Maxillofac Surg 53:610, 1995.
44. Snow N, Lucas AE, Grau M, Steiner M. Purulent mediastinal abscess secondary to Ludwig's angina. Arch Otolaryngol 109:53, 1983.
45. Altorjay A, Kiss J, Voros A, Sziranyi E. The role of esophagectomy in the management of esophageal perforations. Ann Thorac Surg 65:1433, 1998.
46. Bauer TM, Dupont V, Zimmerli W. Invasive candidiasis complicating spontaneous esophageal perforation (Boerhaave syndrome). Am J Gastroenterol 91:1248, 1996.
47. Bufkin BL, Miller JI Jr, Mansour KA. Esophageal perforation: emphasis on management. Ann Thorac Surg 61:1447, 1996.
48. Reeder LB, DeFilippi VJ, Ferguson MK. Current results of therapy for esophageal perforation. Am J Surg 169:615, 1995.
49. Burnett CM, Rosemurgy AS, Pfeiffer EA. Life-threatening acute posterior mediastinitis due to esophageal perforation. Annals Thorac Surg 49:979, 1990.
50. Holinger PH, Schild JA. The Zenker's (hypopharyngeal) diverticulum. Annals Otol Rhinol Laryngol 78:679, 1969.
51. Gertler JP, Brophy C, Elefteriades J. Esophageal rupture after routine Maloney dilatation. A proposed mechanism. J Clin Gastroenterol 8:175, 1986.
52. Glatterer MS Jr, Toon RS, Ellestad C, McFee AS, Rogers W, Mack JW, Trinkle JK, Grover FL. Management of blunt and penetrating external esophageal trauma. J Trauma 25:784, 1985.
53. Lawrence DR, Moxon RE, Fountain SW, Ohri SK, Townsend ER. Iatrogenic oesophageal perforations: a clinical review. Ann R Coll Surg Engl 80:115, 1998.
54. Lew TW, Darby J, Marion DW. Candida mediastinitis and septic shock following occult esophageal perforation in a patient with posttraumatic quadriplegia. J Trauma 39:805, 1995.
55. Micon L, Geis L, Siderys H, Stevens L, Rodman GH Jr. Rupture of the distal thoracic esophagus following blunt trauma: case report. J Trauma 30:214, 1990.
56. Kamath MP, Shanmugam Shetty AB, Prasad KC. A rare complication of an impacted foreign body in the cricopharynx. Am J Otolaryngology 19:61, 1998.
57. Komatsu ES, Costa F, Marchese LT, Villari FS. Abscess of the mediastinum: a case report. J Pediatr Surg 24:1125, 1989.
58. Salo JA, Isolauri JO, Heikkila LJ, Markkula HT, Heikkinen LO, Kivilaakso EO, Mattila SP. Management of delayed esophageal perforation with mediastinal sepsis. Esophagectomy or primary repair? J Thorac Cardiovasc Surg 106:1088, 1993.
59. Splener CW, Benfield JR. Esophageal disruption from blunt and penetrating external trauma. Arch Surg 111:663, 1976.
60. Weaver AW, Sankaran S, Fromm SH, Lucas CE, Walt AJ. The management of penetrating wounds of the neck. Surg Gynecol Obstet 133:49, 1971.
61. Buecker A, Wein BB, Neuerburg JM, Guenther RW. Esophageal perforation: comparison of use of aqueous and barium-containing contrast media. Radiology 202:683, 1997.
62. Santos GH, Frater RW. Transesophageal irrigation for the treatment of mediastinitis produced by esophageal rupture. J Thorac Cardiovas Surg 91:57, 1986.
63. Altorjay A, Kiss J, Voros A, Bohak A. Nonoperative management of esophageal perforations. Is it justified? Ann Surg 225:415, 1997.
64. Eubanks PJ, Hu E, Nguyen D, Procaccino F, Eysselein VE, Klein SR. Case of Boerhaave's syndrome successfully treated with a self-expandable metallic stent. Gastrointest Endosc 49:780, 1999.
65. Roberts JR, Smythe WR, Weber RW, Lanutti

M, Rosengard BR, Kaiser LR. Thoracoscopic management of descending necrotizing mediastinitis. Chest 112:850, 1997.

66. Milton H. Mediastinal surgery. Lancet 1:872, 1897.
67. Bitkover CY, Gardlund B. Mediastinitis after cardiovascular operations: a case-control study of risk factors. Annals Thorac Surg 65:36, 1998.
68. Munoz P, Menasalvas A, Bernaldo de Quiros JC, Desco M, Vallejo JL, Bouza E. Postsurgical mediastinitis: a case-control study. Clin Infect Dis 25:1060, 1997.
69. Maroto LC, Aguado JM, Carrascal Y, Perez A, Perez-de-la-Sota E, Cortina JM, Delgado R, Rodriguez E, Molina L, Rufilanchas JJ. Role of epicardial pacing wire cultures in the diagnosis of poststernotomy mediastinitis. Clin Infect Dis 24:419, 1997.
70. El Oakley RM, Wright JE. Postoperative mediastinitis: classification and management. Ann Thorac Surg 61:1030, 1996.
71. Kutsal A, Ibrisim E, Catav Z. Tasdemir O, Bayazit K. Mediastinitis after open heart surgery. Analysis of risk factors and management. J Cardiovasc Surg (Torino) 32:38, 1991.
72. Engelman RM, Williams CD, Gouge TH, Chase RM Jr, Falk EA, Boyd AD, Reed GE. Mediastinitis following open-heart surgery. Review of two years' experience. Arch Surg 107:772, 1973.
73. El Oakley R. Mediastinitis in patients undergoing cardiopulmonary bypass: risk analysis and midterm results. J Cardiovasc Surg (Torino) 38:595, 1997.
74. Ko W, Lazenby WD, Zelano JA, Isom OW, Krieger KH. Effects of shaving methods and intraoperative irrigation on suppurative mediastinitis after bypass operations. Ann Thorac Surg 53:301, 1992.
75. Hazelrigg SR, Wellons HA Jr, Schneider JA, Kolm P. Wound complications after median sternotomy. Relationship to internal mammary grafting. J Thorac Cardiovasc Surg 98:1096, 1989.
76. Risk factors for deep sternal wound infection after sternotomy: a prospective, multicenter study. J Thorac Cardiovasc Surg 111:1200, 1996.
77. Bor DH, Rose RM, Modlin JF, Weintraub R, Friedland GH. Mediastinitis after cardiovascular surgery. Rev Infect Dis 5:885, 1983.
78. Ryan T, McCarthy JF, Rady MY, Serkey J, Gordon S, Starr NJ, Cosgrove DM. Early bloodstream infection after cardiopulmonary bypass: frequency rate, risk factors, and implications. Crit Care Med 25:2009, 1997.
79. Sethi GK, Copeland JG, Moritz T, Henderson W, Zadina K, Goldman S. Comparison of postoperative complications between saphenous vein and IMA grafts to left anterior descending coronary artery. Ann Thorac Surg 51:733, 1991.
80. Vuorisalo S, Haukipuro K, Pokela R, Syrjala H. Risk features for surgical-site infections in coronary artery bypass surgery. Infect Control Hosp Epidemiol 19:240, 1998.
81. Nagachinta T, Stephens M, Reitz B, Polk BF. Risk factors for surgical-wound infection following cardiac surgery. J Infect Dis 156:967, 1987.
82. El Gamel A, Yonan NA, Hassan R, Jones MT, Campbell CS, Deiraniya AK, Lawson RA. Treatment of mediastinitis: early modified Robicsek closure and pectoralis major advancement flaps. Ann Thorac Surg 65:41, 1998.
83. Roy MC. Surgical-site infections after coronary artery bypass graft surgery: discriminating site-specific risk factors to improve prevention efforts. Infect Control Hosp Epidemiol 19:229, 1998.
84. Nishida H, Grooters RK, Merkley DF, Thieman KC, Soltanzadeh H. Postoperative mediastinitis: a comparison of two electrocautery techniques on presternal soft tissues. J Thorac Cardiovasc Surg 99:969, 1990.
85. Kouchoukos NT, Wareing TH, Murphy SF, Pelate C, Marshall WG Jr. Risks of bilateral internal mammary artery bypass grafting. Ann Thorac Surg 49:210, 1990.
86. Farinas MC, Gald PF, Bernal JM, Rabasa JM, Revuelta JM, Gonzalez-Macias J. Suppurative mediastinitis after open-heart surgery: a case-control study covering a seven-year period in Santander, Spain. Clin Infect Dis 20:272, 1995.
87. Francel TJ, Dufresne CR, Baumgartner WA, O'Kelley J. Anatomic and clinical considerations of an internal mammary artery harvest. Arch Surg 127:1107, 1992.
88. Karwande SV, Renlund DG, Olsen SL, Gay WA Jr, Richenbacher WE, Hawkins JA, Millar RC, Marks JD. Mediastinitis in heart transplantation. Annals Thorac Surg 54:1039, 1992.
89. Baldwin RT, Radovancevic B, Sweeney MS, Duncan JM, Frazier OH. Bacterial medias-

tinitis after heart transplantation. J Heart Lung Transplant 11:545, 1992.

90. Burket JS, Chenoweth CE, Meyer TL, Barg NL. Donor-to-recipient transmission of bacteria as an unusual cause of mediastinitis in a heart transplant recipient. Infect Cont Hosp Epidemiol 20:132, 1999.
91. Gottlieb LJ, Beahm EK, Krizek TJ, Karp RB. Approaches to sternal wound infections. Adv Card Surg 7:147, 1996.
92. Maroto LC, Aguado JM, Carrascal Y, Rodriguez JE, Cortina JM, Rufilanchas JJ. Fulminant mediastinitis due to Streptococcus pneumoniae following cardiac surgery; report of a case. Clin Infect Dis 22:594, 1996.
93. Clancy CJ, Nguyen MH, Morris AJ. Candidal mediastinitis: an emerging clinical entity. Clin Infect Dis 25:608, 1997.
94. Kohman LJ, Coleman MJ, Parker FB Jr. Bacteremia and sternal infection after coronary artery bypass grafting. Ann Thorac Surg 49:454, 1990.
95. L'Ecuyer PB, Murphy D, Little JR, Fraser VJ. The epdidemiology of chest and leg wound infections following cardiothoracic surgery. Clin Infect Dis 22:424, 1996.
96. Czachor JS, Hawley HB. Anaerobic wound infection: Bacteroides mediastinitis after cardiovascular surgery. Heart Lung 17:335, 1988.
97. Cerat GA, McHenry MC, Loop FD. Median sternotomy wound infection and anterior mediastinitis caused by bacteroides fragilis. Chest 69:231, 1976.
98. King CT. Sternal wound infection due to Corynebacterium xerosis. Clin Infect Dis 19:1171, 1994.
99. Sielaff TD, Everett JE, Shumway SJ, Wahoff DC, Bolman RM III, Dunn DL. Mycoplasma hominis infections occurring in cardiovascular surgical patients. Annals Thorac Surg 61:99, 1996.
100. Thaler F, Gotainer B, Teodori G, Dubois C, Loirat P. Mediastinitis due to Nocardia asteroides after cardiac transplantation. Intensive Care Med 18:127, 1992.
101. Toporoff B, Rosado LJ, Appleton CP, Sethi GK, Copeland JG. Successful treatment of early infective endocarditis and mediastinitis in a heart transplant recipient. Heart Lung Transplant 13:546, 1994.
102. Byl B, Jacobs F, Antoine M, Depierreux M, Serruys E, Primo G, Thys JP. Mediastinitis caused by Aspergillus fumigatus with ruptured aortic pseudoaneurysm in a heart transplant recipient: case study. Heart Lung 22:145, 1993.
103. Weinstein RA, Jones EL, Schwarzmann SW, Hatcher CR Jr. Sternal osteomyelitis and mediastinitis after open-heart operation: pathogenesis and prevention. Ann Thorac Surg, 21:442, 1976.
104. Tyras DH, Kaiser GC, Barner HB, Laskowski LF, Marr JJ. Atypical mycobacteria and the xenograft valve. J Thorac Cardiovasc Surg 75:331, 1978.
105. Levy C, Curtin JA, Watkins A, Marsh B, Garcia J, Mispireta L. Mycobacterium chelonei infection of porcine heart valves. N Engl J Med 297:667, 1977.
106. Laskowski LF, Marr JJ, Spernoga JF, Frank NJ, Barner HB, Kaiser G, Tyras DH. Fastidious mycobacteria grown from porcine prosthetic-heart-valve cultures. N Engl J Med 297:101, 1977.
107. Kuritsky JN, Bullen MG, Broome CV, Silcox VA, Good RC, Wallace RJ Jr. Sternal wound infections and endocarditis due to organisms of the Mycobacterium fortuitum complex. Ann Intern Med 98:938, 1983.
108. Yew WW, Wong PC, Woo HS, Yip CW, Chan CY, Cheng FB. Characterization of Mycobacterium fortuitum isolates from sternotomy wounds by antimicrobial susceptibilities, plasmid profiles, and ribosomal ribonucleic acid gene restriction patterns. Diagnos Microbiol Infect Dis 17:111, 1993.
109. Wallace RJ Jr, Musser JM, Hull SI, Silcox VA, Steele LC, Forrester GD, Labidi A, Selander RK. Diversity and sources of rapidly growing mycobacteria associated with infections following cardiac surgery. J Infect Dis 159:708, 1989.
110. Robicsek F, Daugherty HK, Cook JW, Selle JG, Masters TN, O'Bar PR, Fernandez CR, Mauney CU, Calhoun DM. Mycobacterium fortuitum epidemics after open-heart surgery. J Thorac Cardiovasc Surg 75:91, 1978.
111. Sethi GK, Simons WJ, Scott SM. Mycobacterium fortuitum infections of the mediastinum. J Cardiovasc Surg (Torino) 26:307, 1985.
112. Robicsek F, Hoffman PC, Masters TN, Daugherty HK, Cook JW, Selle JG, Mauney CU, Hinson P. Rapidly growing nontuberculous mycobacteria: a new enemy of the cardiac surgeon. Ann Thorac Surg 46:703, 1988.
113. Jauregui L, Arbulu A, Wilson F. Osteomyelitis, pericarditis, mediastinitis, and vasculitis due to

mycobacterium chelonei. Am Rev Respir Dis 115:699, 1977.

114. Hoffman PC, Fraser DW, Robicsek F, O'Bar PR, Mauney CU. Two outbreaks of sternal wound infection due to organisms of the Mycobacterium fortuitum complex. J Infect Dis 143:533, 1981.

115. Jimenez-Martinez M, Arguero-Sanchez R, Perez-Alvarez JJ, Mina-Castaneda P. Anterior mediastinitis as a complication of median sternotomy incisions: diagnostic and surgical considerations. Surgery 67:929, 1970.

116. Browdie DA, Bernstein RV, Agnew R, Damle A, Fischer M, Balz J, Bernstein RV. Diagnosis of poststernotomy infection: comparison of three means of assessment [published erratum appears in Ann Thorac Surg 52:900, 1991.]. Annals Thorac Surg 51:290, 1991.

117. Rosenbaum GS, Klein NC, Cunha BA. Poststernotomy mediastinitis. Heart Lung 19:371, 1990.

118. Albat B, Trinh-Duc P, Boulfroy D, Picard E, Wintrebert P, Thevenet A. Mediastinitis in heart transplant recipients: successful treatment by closed local irrigation. Cardiovasc Surg 1:657, 1993.

119. Campistol JM, Abad C, Nogue S, Bertran A. Acute renal failure in a patient treated by continuous povidone-iodine mediastinal irrigation. J Cardiovasc Surg (Torino) 29:410, 1988.

120. Glick PL, Guglielmo BJ, Tranbaugh RF, Turley K. Iodine toxicity in a patient treated by continuous povidone-iodine mediastinal irrigation. Ann Thorac Surg 39:478, 1985.

121. Gottlieb LJ, Pielet RW, Karp RB, Krieger LM, Smith DJ Jr, Deeb GM. Rigid internal fixation of the sternum in postoperative mediastinitis. Arch Surg 129:489, 1994.

122. Nahai F, Rand RP, Hester TR, Bostwick J III, Jurkiewicz MJ. Primary treatment of the infected sternotomy wound with muscle flaps: a review of 211 consecutive cases. Plast Reconstr Surg 84:434, 1989.

123. Ringelman PR, Vander Kolk CA, Cameron D, Baumgartner WA, Manson PN. Long-term results of flap reconstruction in median sternotomy wound infections. Plast Reconstr Surg 93:1208, 1994.

124. Piwnica A, Abdelmeguid I, Mesnildrey P, Laborde F, Menasche P, Romano M, Guedon C. Rupture of the right ventricular free wall. An unusual complication of mediastinitis after cardiac surgery. Euro J Cardio-Thorac Surg 2:172, 1988.

125. Georgiade G, Levan TA, Anthony J, Oldham N, Julio H, Milano C, Ritter E. Management and prevention of cardiovascular hemorrhage associated with mediastinitis. Ann Surg 227:145, 1998.

126. Cartier R, Diaz OS, Carrier M, Leclerc Y, Castonguay Y, Leung TK. Right ventricular rupture. A complication of postoperative mediastintis. J Thorac Cardiovasc Surg 106:1036, 1993.

127. Camacho MT, Edelman M, Rozenblit A, McKitrick JC, Pinsker K, Fell SC. Mediastinal histoplasmosis causing massive hematemesis. J Thorac Cardiovasc Surg 111:1283, 1996.

128. Mathisen DJ, Grillo HC. Clinical manifestation of mediastinal fibrosis and histoplasmosis. Ann Thorac Surg 54:1053, 1992.

129. Suzuki T, Suzuki S, Kamio Y, Hori G, Endo S, Suzuki H. Mediastinal tuberculous lymphadenitis diagnosed and treated by thoracoscopy. Thorac Cardiovasc Surg 45:140, 1997.

130. Lee JY, Kim Y, Lee KS, Chung MP. Tuberculous fibrosing mediastinitis: radiologic findings. Am J Roentgenol 167:1598, 1996.

131. Shah P, Ramakantan R. Hoarseness of the voice due to left recurrent laryngeal nerve palsy in tuberculous mediastinitis. Arch Otolaryngol Head Neck Surg 116:108, 1990.

132. Ramakantan R, Shah P. Dysphagia due to mediastinal fibrosis in advanced pulmonary tuberculosis. Am J Roentgenol 154 61, 1990.

133. Lagerstrom CF, Mitchell HG, Graham BS, Hammon JW Jr. Chronic fibrosing mediastinitis and superior vena caval obstruction from blastomycosis. Ann Thorac Surg 54:764, 1992.

134. Neuzil KM, Mitchell HC, Loyd JE, Lagerstrom CF, Hammon JW Jr, Graham BS. Extrapulmonary thoracic disease caused by Blastomyces dermatitidis. Chest 106:1885, 1994.

135. Gilbert HM, Hartman BJ. Short report: a case of fibrosing mediastinitis caused by Wuchereria bancrofti. Am J Trop Med Hyg 54 596, 1996.

136. Goodwin RA Jr, Nickell JA, Des Perez RM. Mediastinal fibrosis complicating healed primary histoplasmosis and tuberculosis. Medicine 51:227, 1972.

137. Nordmann P, Commare MC, Ronco E, Barois A, Nauciel C. Mediastinitis due to non-typhi Salmonella. Clin Infect Dis 18:255, 1994.

138. Snider JM, Hannah H, McNabney WK, Pemberton LB. Salmonella mediastinal abscess. Ann Thorac Surg 56:556, 1993.

139. Henkel JS, Armstrong D, Blevins A, Moody

MD. Group A beta-hemolytic Streptococcus bacteremia in a cancer hospital. JAMA 211:983, 1970.

140. Dreyfuss D, Djedaini K, Bidault-Lapomme C, Coste F. Nontraumatic acute anterior mediastinitis in two HIV-positive heroin addicts. Chest 101:583, 1992.

141. Bioterrorism alleging use of anthrax and interim guidelines for management – United States. MMWR 48:69, 1999.

142. Abramova FA, Grinberg LM, Yampolskaya OV, Walker DH. Pathology of inhalational anthrax in 42 cases from the Sverdlovsk outbreak of 1979. Proc Natl Acad Sci USA 90:2291, 1993.

143. Atlas RM. The medical threat of biological weapons. Crit Rev Microbiol 24:157, 1998.

144. Sekhar PC, Singh RS, Sridhar MS, Bhaskar CJ, Rao YS. Outbreak of human anthrax in Ramabhadrapuram village of Chittoor district in Andhra Pradesh. Indian J Med Res 91:448, 1990.

145. Keung YK, Gendreau J, Barber A, Cobos E. Acute mediastinitis secondary to leakage of parenteral nutrition from a migrated central venous catheter in a patient undergoing autologous bone marrow transplant. Bone Marrow Transplant 17:871, 1996.

146. Anderson CM, Walters RS, Hortobagyi GN. Mediastinitis related to probable central vinblastine extravasation in a woman undergoing adjuvant chemotherapy for early breast cancer. Am J Clin Oncology 19:566, 1996.

INDEX

Note: Page numbers followed by *f* refer to figures; page numbers followed by *t* refer to tables.

9781461356745V02